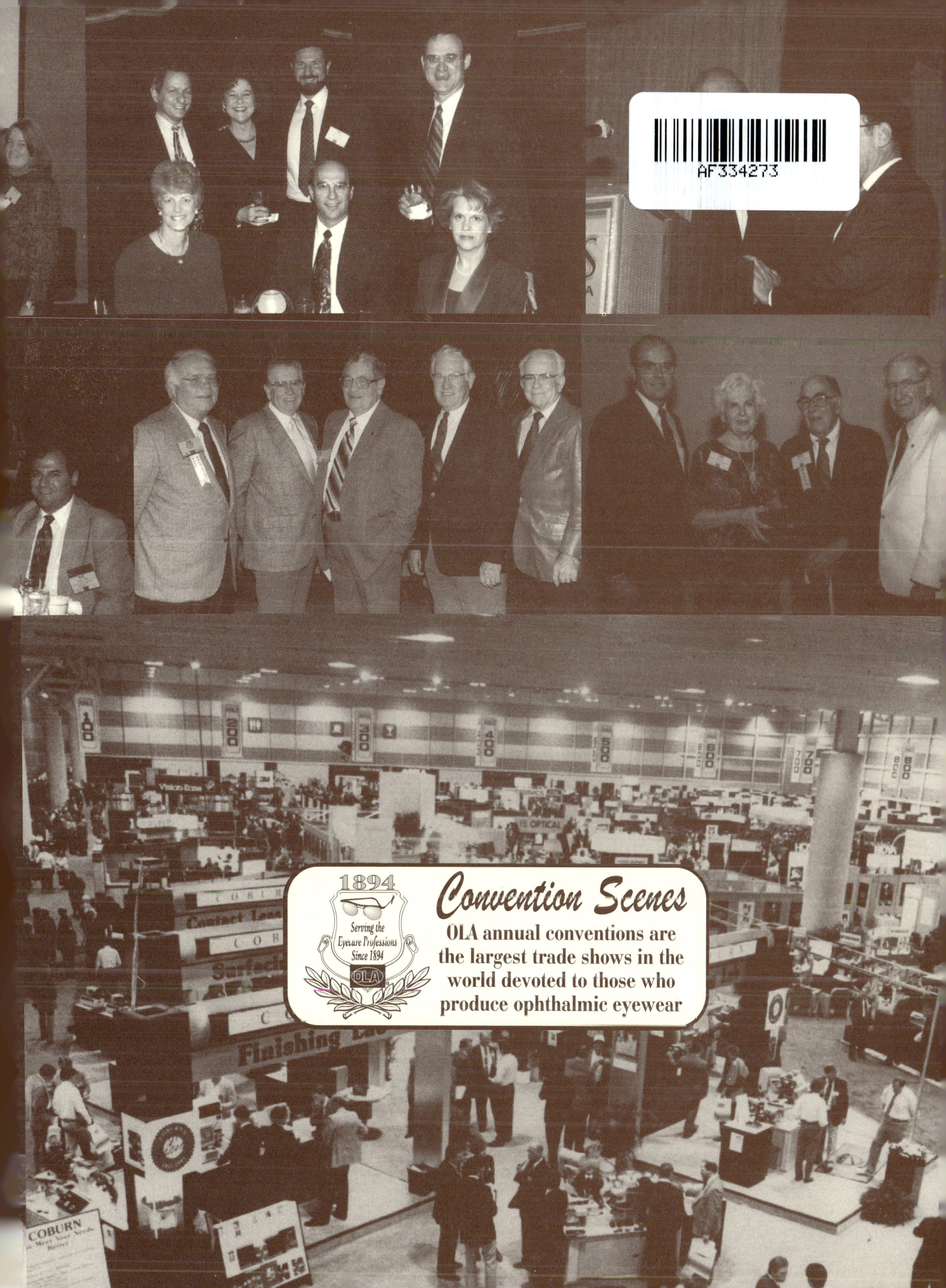
1894
Serving the
Eyecare Professions
Since 1894
OLA
Convention Scenes
OLA annual conventions are
the largest trade shows in the
world devoted to those who
produce ophthalmic eyewear

LOOKING BACK

An Illustrated History
of the American Ophthalmic Industry

Joseph L. Bruneni

Optical Laboratories Association
Publishing Division
2908 Oregon Court, Suite I-2
Torrance, CA 90503-2637

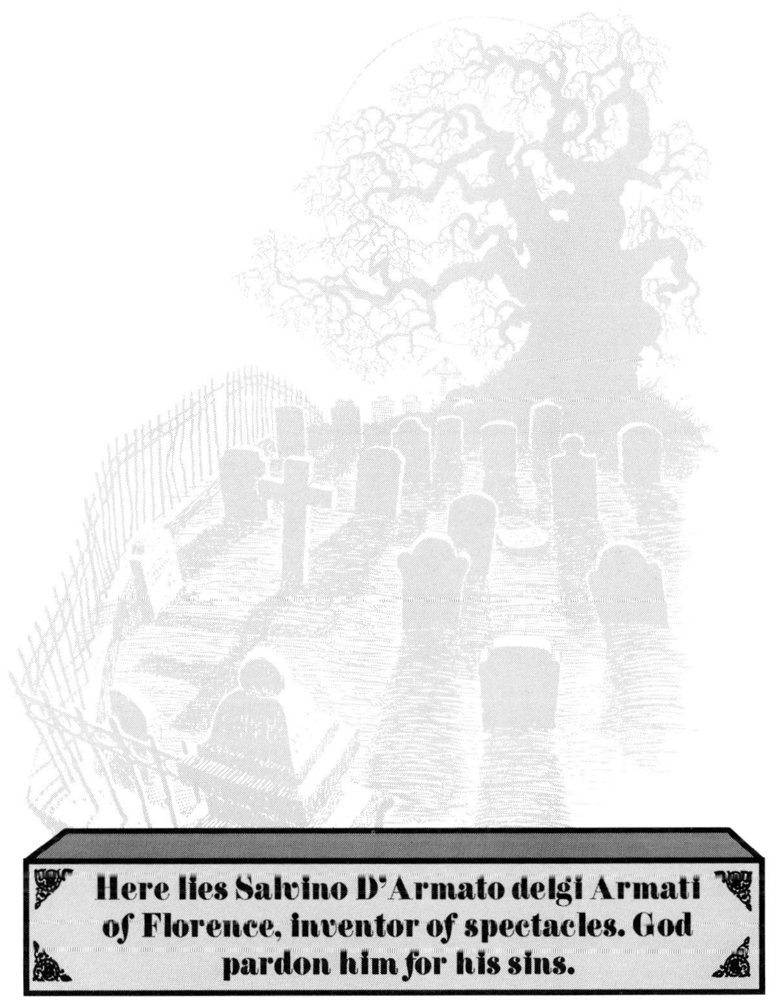

A tomb in the church of Santa Maria Maggiore in
Florence, Italy bears this inscription. Armati died in 1317.

LOOKING BACK

An Illustrated History of the American Ophthalmic Industry

© 1994 by Joseph L. Bruneni

Published by:
Optical Laboratories Association
Publishing Division
2908 Oregon Court, Suite I-2
Torrance, CA 90503-2637

Library of Congress Card No. 94-68862
ISBN 1-886308-00-4
First Edition - November, 1994

Printed in the USA by:
Hawthorne Printing Company
Gardena, CA 90249

Book Design and Layout:
Cindra Shields

Cover Photography:
Bill Milne

"That men do not learn very much from the lessons of history is the most important of all the lessons that history has to teach."

Collected Essays (1959), Aldous Huxley

"There is properly no history; only biography."

History, Ralph Waldo Emerson

Introduction

In an effort to make this illustrated history more meaningful to anyone familiar with today's optical business we chose to make this a history of individual companies and the interesting personalities who built them, creating in the process the optical industry we know today. These personal stories have been included because so many companies making up the industry are products of and resulted from the endeavors of some remarkable people. We have tried to include the stories of representative companies from each segment of the industry. To the many worthy companies not included in this history, we can only confess to the restrictions imposed by limited time and limited space. It is by no means a reflection on their contributions to the history of this industry.

Knowing the past can lead to a better understanding of how the industry grew into its present form. Readers will discover many names appearing in more than one story. Sometimes it's because these individuals' influence carried into multiple aspects of the industry. Other times it's because of the close, often personal, relationship that so often existed between the people who created and operated those pioneer companies.

Readers will notice multi-generations of the same family appearing as the years go by and this is no accident. It has often been said that, once an individual is involved in the optical industry, others in their family become involved - sometimes in the same company and sometimes in completely unrelated organizations. Nowhere is this more true than with optical laboratories. Some OLA laboratories profiled in this book represent two, three and even four generations of the same family - something that has come to be a hallmark of the optical business.

This, then, is the story of those families and those individuals and, as readers discover how the industry evolved, they can take even greater pride in being a part of it. You'll discover colorful characters, inventive geniuses, brilliant organizers and some spectacular failures among the individuals who created the industry that has become such an important part of our lives.

Joseph L. Bruneni
Optical Laboratories Association
September, 1994

Acknowledgments

Lionel Topaz, born in Russia in 1875, sailed to England in 1897 and eventually landed in the United States in 1903. Seven years later, he established THE OPTOMETRIC WEEKLY in Chicago. In 1919, he founded The Professional Press, Inc. which would be run by three generations of the Topaz family, publishing six magazines in the medical, paramedical and trade fields and a full line of textbooks and directories.

Lionel took to the optical industry and it took to him. By 1940, he had developed personal relationships with virtually every person of significance in the industry. It was in that year that he announced his intention of writing and publishing a history of the optical industry. Lionel began his research by writing people all over the country. He also met with many of them on his extensive travels. In 1940, it was still possible to find active people who could tell personal stories dating back to turn-of-the-century days in the optical business. He collected personal letters from hundreds of individuals who played important and not-so-important roles in the development of the industry.

Unfortunately, Lionel Topaz passed away on July 23, 1942. By then he had collected a lot of material for his book but hadn't completed what was intended to be his crowning achievement. His son, Marty Topaz, stored this research material with the intention of some day completing his father's work but the project was never completed.

The Optical Laboratories Association and the author are indebted to Marty Topaz and his family for their contribution of Lionel's research material to this OLA industry history.

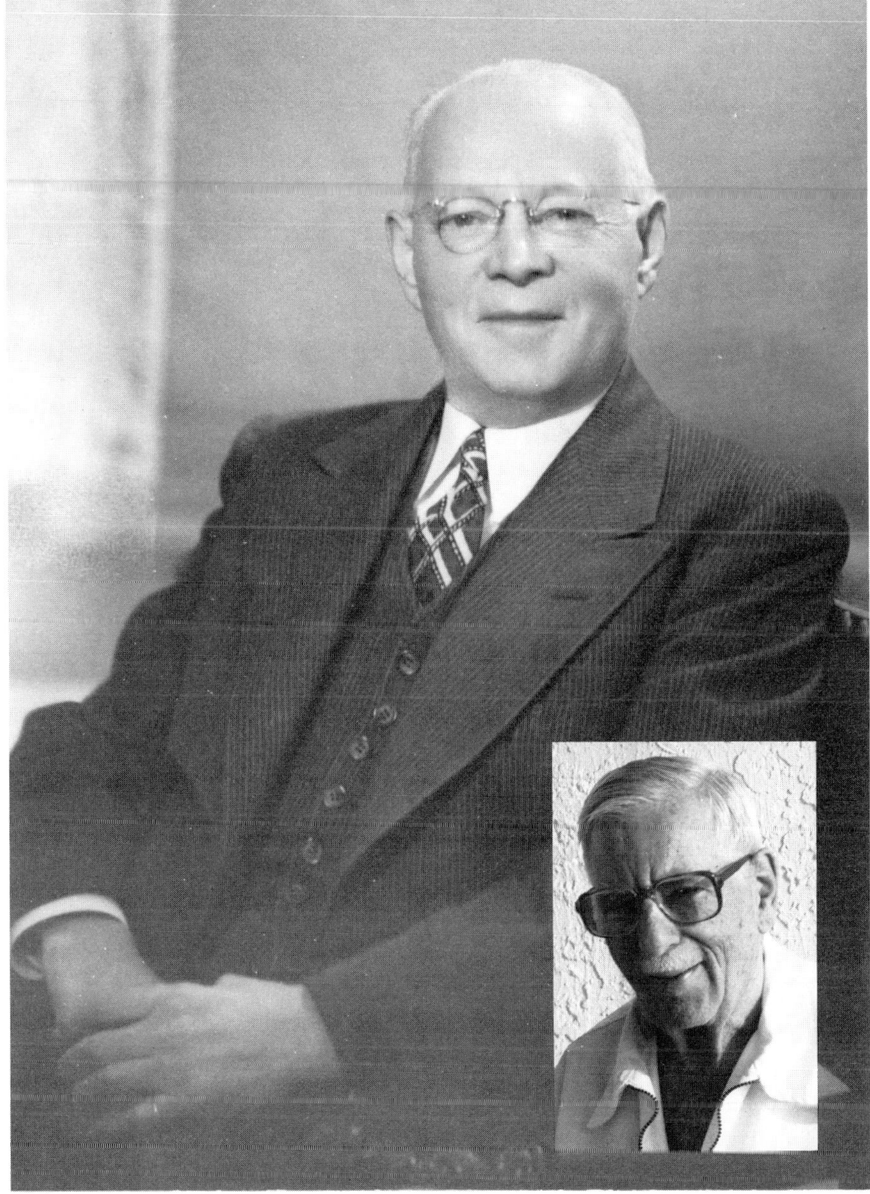

Inset – Martin Topaz

This was a valuable repository of personal memories from many people who helped shape the industry. In letters to his correspondents, Lionel Topaz often made the comment that "the job [*writing a history of the industry*] is bigger than I ever thought it would be, and I only hope I live long enough to see it completed". He did not, of course, but we believe he would be pleased that the personal material he researched during the years 1940-42 added so significantly to this history written more than 50 years after his death.

Valuable input was received from too many individuals to list here. They know who they are and as they read this history, they will find their contributions enriching these stories. To all those who searched their files, their basements and their attics for the many illustrations we used, we tried to acknowledge each contributor with an illustration credit. A special "thank you" is owed to President Richard Hopping, O.D. and Librarian Patricia Carlson of the Southern California College of Optometry. Their help in making SCCO's extensive files available was invaluable. John M. Young *(Essilor of America)* provided helpful material from his unpublished "Some History of Eyewear" manuscript.

Table of Contents

The Cover Photo

The photo montage on the dust jacket was created by photographer Bill Milne. Bill is from Toronto but has operated a studio in New York since 1985. His food photography has appeared regularly in major publications in the United States and Canada. LADIES HOME JOURNAL, GOURMET, WEIGHT WATCHERS and NEW CHOICES are some of his more recent editorial assignments.

Eight books have been published solely with his work plus several other books where he served as contributing photographer. The main core of his studio work is for advertising clients, including American Express, General Foods, AT&T, US Postal Service, Apple Computer and many others. In addition to his photography, he is creative director of EYEQUEST MAGAZINE, a trade journal distributed to 40,000 eyecare professionals across the United States.

Antique artifacts used for the cover montage are from the collection of J. Wm. Rosenthal, M.D., New Orleans, La. Dr. Rosenthal has been collecting antique optical artifacts since 1956, starting with items collected by his father.

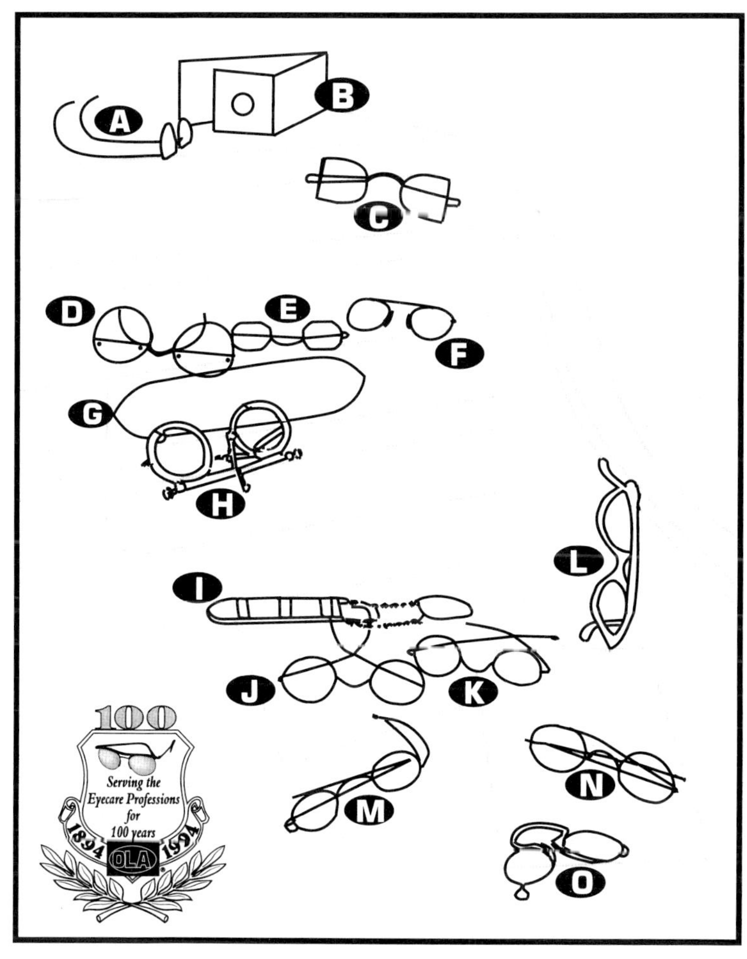

He established the Jonas W. Rosenthal Memorial Ophthalmic Museum at Tulane University in memory of his father. His antique collection ranges from 1300 A.D. to the 1990's and includes European, Chinese and American items. Dr. Rosenthal was Chief Curator of the American Academy of Ophthalmology Museum for its first eight years and still serves as Curator for Vision Aids. He has been a consultant to the Smithsonian Museum since 1963.

A   Rimless pulpit glasses, known as half eyes today. 1912

B   Self testing device for use by persons ordering mail order eyeglasses. 1912.

C   Horseshoe or Railway double glasses with side shields. 1820

D   Shuron Rimway rimless mounting. 1937

E   McAllister 14K gold. 1820

F   Bar spring 10K gold. 1885

G   Frog mouth case from retail office started by John Jacob Bausch. 1880

H   Early trial lens frame. 1894

I   Chatelain Case. 1900

J   Perfection Bifocal in a Standard Optical frame. 1890

K   Landscape shooting glass. 1880

L   Shell frame. 1923

M   Early 14 K gold McAllister frame with -13.50D lenses. 1798

N   Franklin bifocals in blue steel frame. 1880

O   Hard rubber frame. 1870

Close-up photos of each of these items are included in this history.

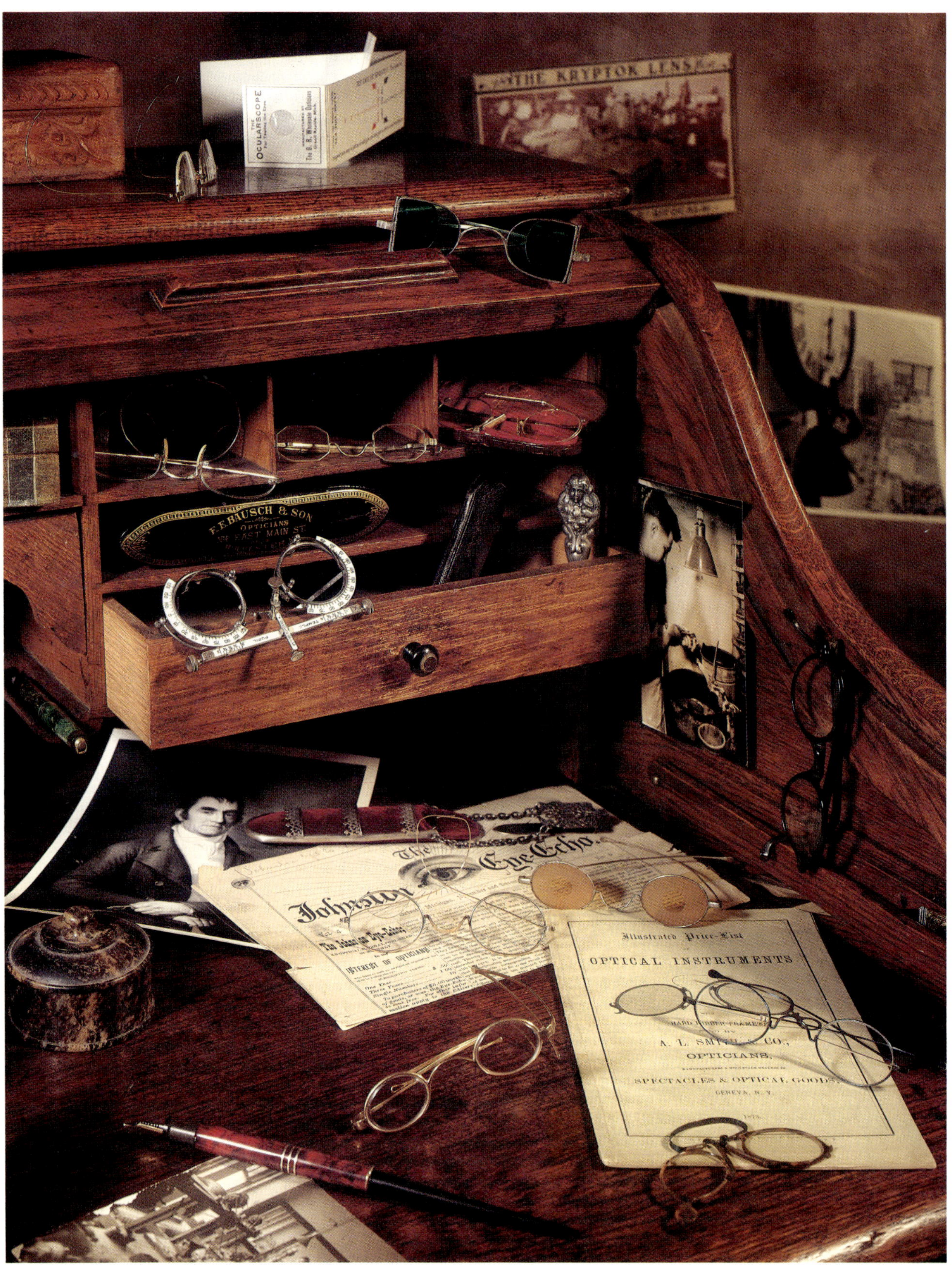

Chapter 1
Synopsis

The first optical lenses that can be traced were most likely used as magnifying lenses. These were first mentioned by an Arab physicist al-Hazen *(996-1038)* in a famous treatise on optics. He made the observation that a segment of spherical glass, i.e. a plano-convex lens, would magnify images. Italians called magnifiers *Lapides ad legendum (stones for reading)*. The earliest origin of eyeglasses, however, is a matter of some dispute. During the 13th century, the English Monk/Philosopher Roger Bacon wrote that their origin was Tuscany or perhaps Pisa or Florence. In his famous "Opus majus", Bacon described how a convex lens would magnify and suggested that such a lens might help anyone with vision problems. *"With this instrument anyone whose eyes are sick will be able to see much better even the smallest of letters"* was how he described such lenses. Bacon is not considered the actual inventor of glasses, but there is little doubt that their first use started during Bacon's time.

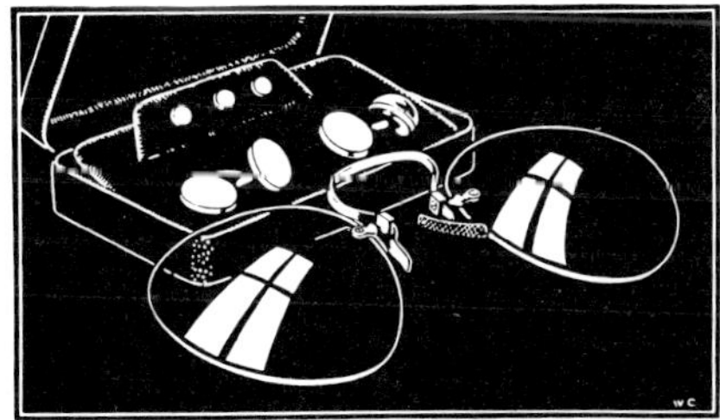

Nero's emerald "eyeglass" started a fad.

The Origin

The exact origin of spectacles has been debated over the centuries but most scholars attribute the earliest eyewear to the City of Venice where records indicate they were being produced during the middle of the 13th century. No trace or mention of them can be found prior to that period. It's believed the early Romans utilized some form of magnification but no one during the Roman period seemed to have connected the concept of using magnifying lenses as an aid for close work or reading. That may be simply because few of the world's population at that time knew how to read. Printing wouldn't be invented for another 300 years and little reading was done outside the Church.

The Emperor Nero was said to view his games through an emerald lens. The cool green color was probably the reason for choosing an emerald. There's good reason to believe that artisans cutting the stone to its final shape probably gave the lens a slight concave shape. This may have helped a near-sighted Nero see better. The true facts are lost in the mists of history, but we do know that Nero's "eyeglass" started a fad that was widely copied by nobles of that day.

A manuscript written in Florence in 1299 included a statement that will sound familiar to anyone over 45 years of age: *"I find myself so oppressed by age that I can neither read nor write without those glasses they call spectacles, lately invented for the great advantage of old men when their sight grows weak"*.

Crystal Lenses

The first spectacles are believed to have been produced by Venetian glaziers *(called Cristallieri)*. They utilized lenses made from quartz or rock crystal which were fashioned by gold craftsmen trained to work with those materials. All crafts in that part of the world were governed by individual statutes that applied to everyone engaged in the craft. The Cristallieri received their own code in November, 1284. This is significant because it reveals that making spectacles was by then common enough to require their own regulations. It's interesting that their code specifically banned any temptation members might have to substitute rock crystal with clear glass.

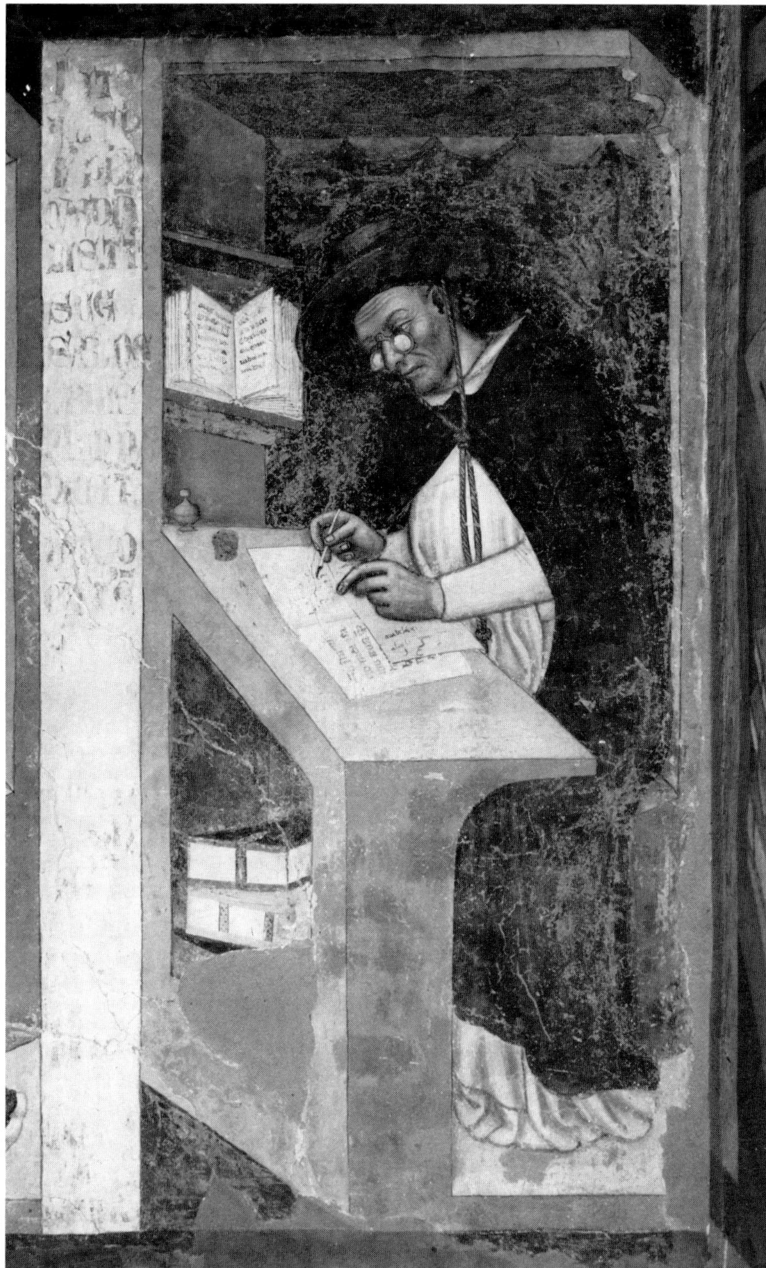

Bishop Ugone da Provenza, the first painting to show eyeglasses.

A Balancing Act

The biggest problem for wearers of early spectacles was keeping them balanced on their nose. It would be many years before the idea of holding them in place with temples was conceived. During that period spectacles were usually held in place by hand, resting precariously on the wearer's nose. In the late 1500s, someone came up with the bright idea of fastening glasses in place with ribbons or cords tied behind the ears. This was an important development because it made it possible for spectacle wearers to see clearly as they moved about. This must have been an exciting and practical improvement for eyeglass wearers. This idea of tying eyewear in place gradually migrated to the Far East, where it was introduced by early missionaries.

Strangely enough, the Chinese had not yet invented eyeglasses. An amusing tale is told of the Mandarin who was so impressed by the first pair of glasses he saw that he traded his horse for them on the spot and returned home on foot. Dignitaries in China who had no need for glasses took to wearing them, usually with tinted lenses - to protect them from the glare of the sun and spare them from looking at evil spirits. Eyewear held in place with string or ribbons was still being used in the Far East in the late 1700s.

Earliest Visual Record

The first historical figure known to wear glasses was a Dominican, Bishop Ugone da Provenza. He was portrayed in a painting by Tomaso da Modena in the year 1252. This earliest record of a person wearing spectacles can still be seen in the church of St. Nicolo in Treviso near Venice. Those first glasses were simple magnifiers with short handles, riveted together so they could perch on the nose.

None of those earliest riveted frames were known to have survived. We had only the paintings to show how they looked. Then a chance discovery occurred in 1953 while workmen in a monastery in Wienhausen were removing the oak floor beneath a choir section. Underneath, they found two perfect specimens of riveted eyeglasses along with fragments of nine others. The frame rims were made of wood and the lenses had a light green or yellow tint. They were plano-convex form and measured between +3.00 and +3.50.

Printing Marks the Beginning

Widespread use of spectacles didn't really begin until the mid 1500s when Gutenberg invented the printing press. That momentous development marks the real beginning of the need for correcting sight with eyeglasses. The first lenses produced were biconvex and used primarily to correct presbyopia. A short while later,

Crystal was very expensive and the authorities wanted to make sure customers got exactly what they paid for. Those early artisans were permitted to use glass but only so long as they made no claims that the lenses were quartz. The fact that counterfeiting of eyeglasses was so tightly controlled at that time *(1301)* seems to indicate that eyeglass making was already widespread. On June 15, 1301, the rules in Venice were liberalized so that any person could make reading spectacles from glass, providing they took an oath in front of judges that they would never misrepresent the lenses as anything other than glass.

biconcave lenses appeared as an aid for nearsighted persons. By the year 1500, a man named Johannes Kepler had conceived a way of grading lenses by their focal values. Prior to that, lens powers were categorized solely by the age of the person wearing them.

Meniscus Lenses

Kepler was very aware of the distortion that was created as wearers looked away from the center of those early flat lenses. He suggested front curves be curved more steeply so the eye would have a wider, more sweeping view. He coined the term "meniscus" for these lenses. Unfortunately, scientists at that time were more interested in lenses for telescopes and microscopes so there was little improvement made in ophthalmic lenses for centuries. Flat lenses were still widely used well into the 20th century.

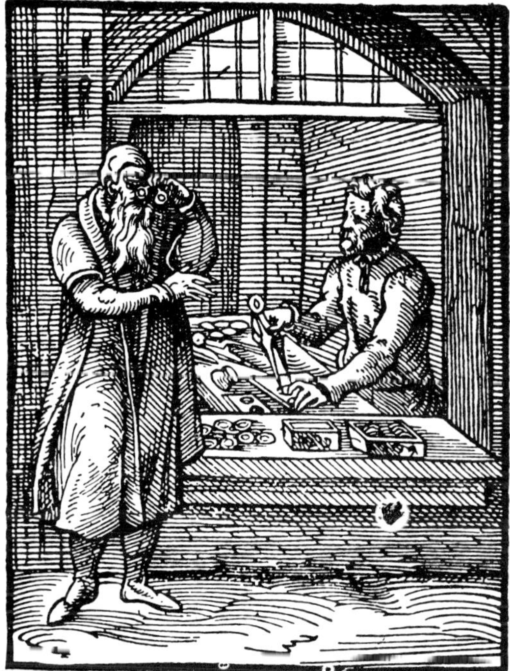

19th Century

By the time American Optical Company started operations in 1833, the population of the United States was still less than twenty-five million. Communications and transportation were difficult and time-consuming. Most of the country's population, in any case, was located along the eastern seaboard. Distribution of optical goods was accomplished in limited quantities through wholesalers or large retailers. As the 19th century progressed, it gradually became easier to travel as the road network and railroads brought the nation closer together. Mass production began to replace goods previously produced by hand-crafted methods.

At the start of the 19th century, glasses were often sold in hardware stores but as gold and silver came into use as frame materials, jewelers became logical successors to hardware merchants, although the latter continued to handle spectacles for some years. These retailers carried ready-made glasses, purchased one dozen to the box and sold under an "inch-number" system. Away from the large cities *(which were mostly on the East coast)*, peddlers became a vital part of eyeglass distribution. Most goods sold by peddlers came from European sources or, in some cases, American jewelry factories. Traveling was difficult in those days and there were few opticians to service the vast, nearly empty stretches of the growing nation. Spectacle peddlers filled this gap, primarily serving presbyopes and often carrying other items along with their optical goods.

Prospective buyers would try on different glasses with varying strength lenses until they found a pair that gave them adequate vision *(lens powers were always the same in both eyes)*. This self-refraction was the custom for many years. During the second half of the 19th century, a few dedicated peddlers took to carrying trial lens kits and began to help their customers select their eyewear. Some of the more aggressive peddlers would make outlandish promises. These traveling eyeglass peddlers were looked down on by local opticians who often had no more qualifications than the peddler but, because they remained in one place, considered themselves more reliable and more professional. In fact, many local opticians were simply peddlers who had tired of traveling and drifted off the road to establish a local optical business.

Bifocals

Every student learns that Ben Franklin invented bifocals in the late 1700s. This myth is actually rooted in fact.

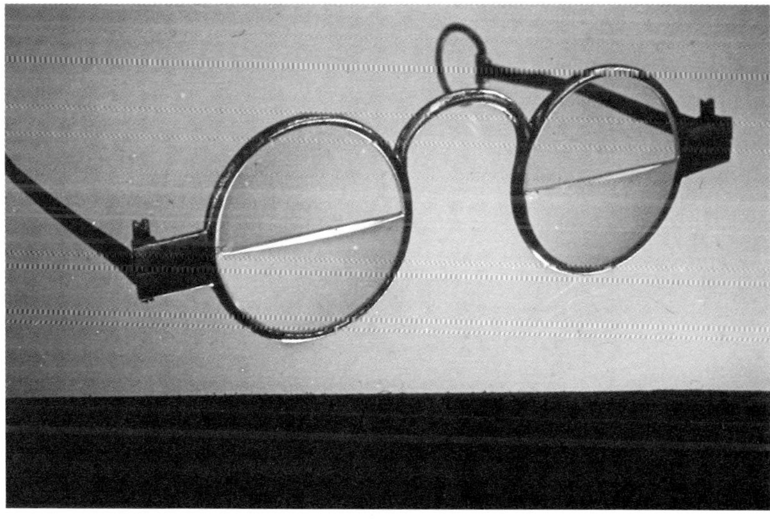

Early Franklin bifocal

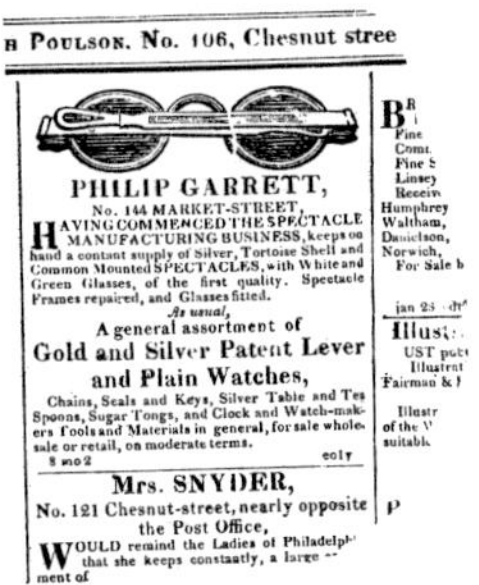

Early optician's ad.
OLA OPTICAL INDUSTRY MUSEUM

Franklin was certainly an early wearer of bifocals and did design the ones he wore. Biographies describe him as carrying a crab-tree stick and wearing glasses. By August, 1784 he found he could not do without them *(". . . not distinguish a letter even of large print")*. Before that year he had always kept two pair of glasses with him. *". . . two pair of spectacles which I shifted occasionally, as in traveling I sometimes read and often wanted to regard the prospects. Finding this change troublesome and not always sufficiently ready, I had the glasses cut and half of each kind associated in the same circle."* In this way, he "discovered" bifocals. *"This I find more particularly convenient since my being in France, the glasses that serve me best at table to see what I eat not being the best to see the faces of those on the other side of the table who speak to me; and when one's ears are not well accustomed to the sounds of a language, a sight of the movements in the face of him that speaks helps to explain; so that I understand French better by the help of my spectacles."*

It's hard to believe that no one else had thought of combining distance and near lenses before Franklin. Two other individuals, S. Pierce in 1760 and A. Smith in 1783 are credited for having independently conceived and produced bifocals prior to Benjamin Franklin.

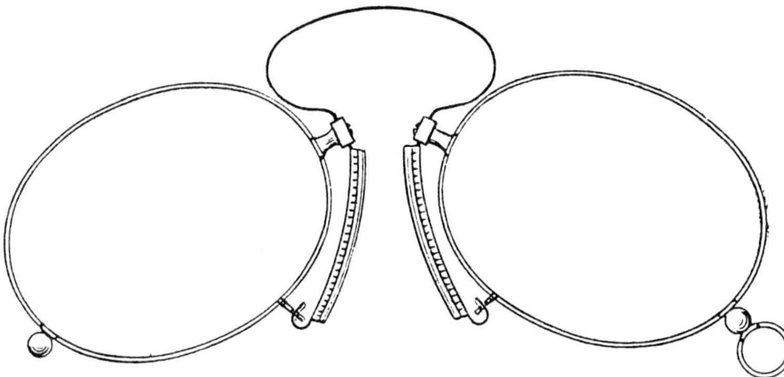

OLA OPTICAL INDUSTRY MUSEUM

Early Forms of Spectacles

Lorgnette: This French term refers to eyeglasses that neither perch on the nose nor touch the face but are held by hand in front of the eyes at appropriate times. Some lorgnettes were produced in the form of pendants that hung around the neck. One form came to be called "scissors lorgnette" because their shape resembled that of scissors.

Pince-nez: These were widely used during the early 1900s. The first patent for folding glasses without a nosepiece was issued to a French optician named Berthiot. They maintained their position by gripping the nose through a spring action of the flexible bridge. They often featured a chain or ribbon to catch them when they fell off the nose *(a rather common occurrence)*. These were called *Zwicker* or *Kneifer* by Germans but

English-speaking people learned to call them by the French term *Pincenez*. A great variety of patents and designs were devoted to producing Pince-nez frames that would minimize the agony of those pincher-like nose pads. Pince-nez wearers could always be identified, even without their glasses because of tell-tale indentations in their nose. Nevertheless, they were considered the ultimate in eyeglass elegance.

Monocles: This innovative eyewear corrected vision in only one eye. Never widely used in the United States, they were seen primarily on the stage and in the movies since their appearance quickly established characters as very European, somewhat "foppish" or arrogantly military (usually German).

An Optical Milestone

Early opticians were continually looking for a way to hold lenses in front of the eyes. Early on, there were vain attempts to fasten eyeglass frames to hat brims and Henry the Eighth had a pair of lenses fastened into his armor helmet. It took 350 years from the time when spectacles first appeared to the time someone thought of holding glasses in position with cords tied around the ears. Later, a Parisian optician named Marc Thomin devised the brilliant idea of adding arms to eyeglasses. His side pieces, however, only extended to the temples because of the wigs customarily worn by men of property *(the only people who could afford glasses)*. The short arms had large rings at the end to provide a comfortable grip on the head. In German these were called *Schlafenbrillen* or "temple glasses". In the early 1700s,

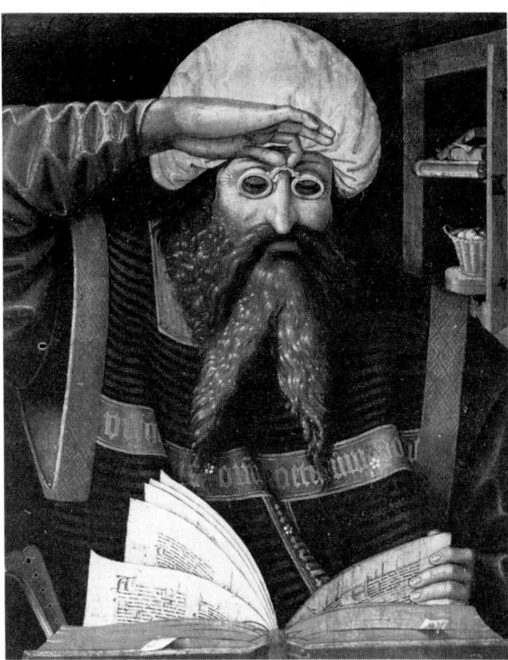

Early eyeglasses were simply held in place by hand.
PAINTING COPY – OPTISCHE WERKE G. RODENSTOCK, MÜNCHEN

GEORGE WASHINGTON'S GLASSES

One of George Washington's most cherished gifts was a lorgnette presented to him by his good friend and comrade-in-arms Marquis De Lafayette. It is assumed that they were of French origin since almost all eyeglasses at that time were manufactured in Europe. The lenses were mounted in iron rims, joined at the top of a flat handle of mother-of-pearl. The rims folded into the handle. It was reported in a 1936 issue of the Optical Journal-Review that the lorgnette was in the National Museum in Washington at that time.

OLA OPTICAL
INDUSTRY MUSEUM

Edward Scarlett, a long-forgotten English optician, proposed using rigid arms extending over the ears as a way to hold glasses firmly in place. His invention was called temples and endures to this day.

As printing spread and more of the world's population learned to read, the acceptance and use of spectacles continued to grow. Laboratories producing custom ordered eyeglasses began appearing in Great Britain, France, Austria and eventually the United States. An optical industry has only existed in an organized manner in the United States for the past 150 years. Probably the first mention of spectacles in America was an announcement found in the Pennsylvania Gazette on October 27, 1737. It stated that the post office of the United States would be found in Benjamin Franklin's printing shop on Market Street. They listed over 50 articles which Franklin had for sale, in and out of his shop. These ranged from stationery, books and soap to a four-wheeled chaise and horse that could be used for riding or driving. Among the articles mentioned in the announcement were spectacles, undoubtedly imported from England.

An Early Astronomer/Optician

David Rittenhouse, the first American astronomer, was born in 1732 and by 1770 was living in Philadelphia. He had been highly recommended to the Colonial Assembly for appointment to trustee of the Loan Office. Local city fathers wanted to give Rittenhouse some income so he would be encouraged to devote time to the manufacture of optical and mathematical instruments which had never before been produced in America. Those needing such instruments had to order them from England and many of those received in the Colonies were shoddy and ill-finished.

By the time the Revolutionary War was over, Rittenhouse had become an accomplished spectacle maker. A good idea of how skilled he was can be determined by the following story. At the time of the Provisional Articles of Peace between Great Britain and the Colonies, Mr. Rittenhouse, enthused with the splendor of the American victory, decided to make and send a pair of spectacles

and a pair of reading glasses to General George Washington at Army Headquarters. They were intended to be a small testimonial of Rittenhouse's respect for the character and service of that great man. A copy of General Washington's letter of acknowledgment has survived the years.

Newburgh, New York

16 February, 1785

I have been honored with your letter of the 7th and beg you to accept my sincere thanks, for the favor conferred on me, in the glasses which are very fine; but more particularly, for the flattering expression which accompanied the present. The spectacles suit my eyes extremely well as I am persuaded the reading glasses also will, when I get more accustomed to the use of them. At present I find some difficulty in coming to a proper focus but when I do obtain it, they magnify perfectly, and show those letters very distinctly which at first appear as a mist blended together and confused.

With greatest esteem and respect, I am, sir, your most obedient and humble servant,

(signed) George Washington

Grinding and polishing the lenses given to Washington appear to be David Rittenhouse's own workmanship. It is evident from Washington's letter that David Rittenhouse taught himself to grind and polish spectacle lenses as well as telescope lenses.

Washington was no stranger to eyeglasses. Another episode occurred in March, 1783 when Washington was faced with a group of officers who had grown dissatisfied with a foreign policy he had outlined in a paper. Meeting with these discontented officers, he drew a pair of glasses out of his coat and said, *"Gentlemen, allow me to put on my eyeglasses, because I have grown not only gray, but nearly blind in the service of my country."* There's no record of what followed, but it is assumed the General was able to soothe his unhappy officers.

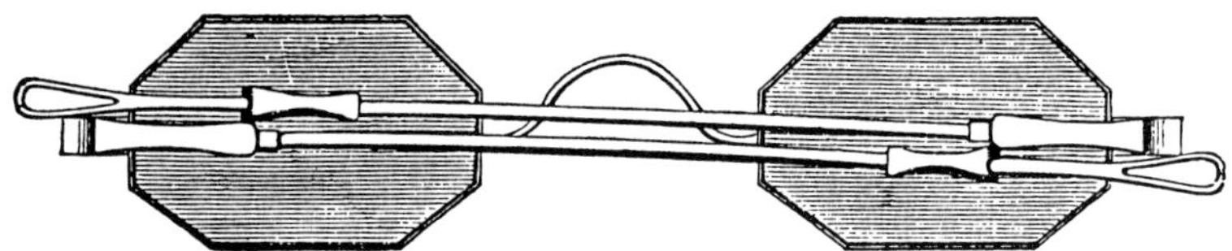

McAllister spectacle from their 1867 catalog. OLA Optical Industry Museum

An Industry Develops

In the 1830s, a few hardy entrepreneurs in the United States began to produce frames and lenses, using primitive mass-production methods. This was during a time when the optical professions were just beginning to develop. Oculists utilized crude refracting techniques to determine visual requirements; opticians were learning how to help their customers determine their visual needs and improved optical equipment slowly began to appear. Oculists were few in number so opticians began to help customers determine their visual requirements by means of self-administered tests. In many cases, these tests would be mailed to the patient with instructions on how to use them. Since only spherical corrections were available for most of the 19th century, this system worked reasonably well.

Vision requirements had been relatively modest before the 19th century. Gutenberg's invention of movable type in about 1450 gave early impetus to the world's developing need for visual aids. Few people could read or write until the 19th century so near vision needs weren't considered essential. With no television, movies or automobiles until the 20th century, there was little need for sharp, clear distance vision. Another often overlooked contributing factor is that, prior to the 20th century, life expectancy was less than 50 years. This reduced presbyopia needs to a minimum. Only as modern inventions of the last 100 years began to appear did a real need for better vision arise. This growth of technology, accompanied by increased visual demands all combined to provide a major impetus to the fledgling optical industry.

Birth of an Industry

Early lens efforts in this country were primarily concentrated on the design and manufacture of optical instruments, mostly telescopes and microscopes. Development of these scientific products often aided development of eyeglass materials. In Germany, Carl Zeiss expanded a retail optical business he established in 1846 for selling instruments as he started manufacturing the items he sold. He was aided by Professor Ernst Abbe, who held a full time job as a professor at the University of Jena while directing the early growth and operations of the Zeiss Company.

In the United States, the earliest efforts showed up in New England in 1833 when some Massachusetts farm boys developed special equipment to produce optical frames. Their early efforts resulted in the formation of what ultimately became the American Optical Company, an organization that eventually led and controlled the entire industry for more than 50 years. John J. Bausch, who shifted from carpentry to opticianry in 1853, eventually sold his retail optical business to his brother and began producing frames and lenses in Rochester, N.Y. His company, Bausch & Lomb, went on to become a second industry-controlling giant, in company with American Optical.

Well into the 19th century, many optical retailers were jewelers or watchmakers with their optical business serving merely as a sideline. Supplying these retailers was the function of jewelry wholesalers who sold mostly glazed goods for the correction of presbyopia. During the 19th century, all lenses and most frames were imported from Europe. Retailers simply fashioned spectacles or eyeglasses to each individual's needs *(At that time the term "spectacles" was the term used for frames having temples. Those with no temples and clinging to the nose by spring action were called "eyeglasses". Today, the industry makes no distinction between the two terms).*

Retailers bought ready-made prescription lenses from manufacturers or, sometimes, laboratories. Some of these early optical retailers taught themselves to perform subjective eye examinations, *(i.e. "Which is better, this or this?")* and began to fill their own prescriptions. Ordering eyeglasses by mail was common during the latter half of the 1800s with the patient determining his or her needs from a catalogue/price list supplied by the optician. The catalog came complete with an eye testing apparatus for which the patient paid in advance, receiving credit against his new spectacles upon return of the testing set and receipt of his self-determined prescription.

Trial Frames

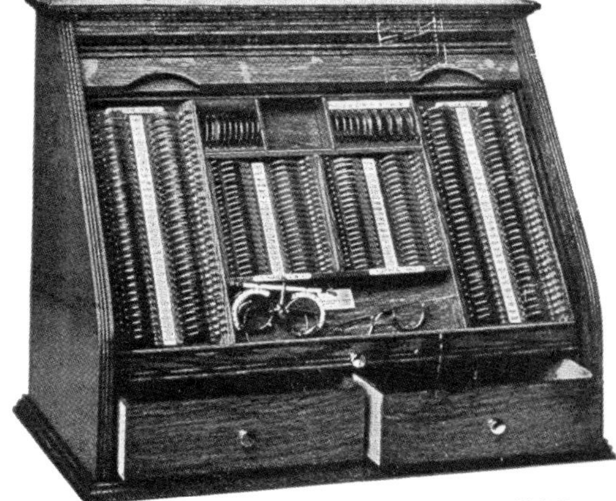

OLA OPTICAL
INDUSTRY MUSEUM

As opticians began to "refract", they needed some way to determine the Rx in advance. Trial lenses made this possible.

Trial frames and cases were unknown until 1860 when Donders devised a case of trial lenses containing cylinders. Dr. Ezra Dyer, a surgeon connected with the Wills Eye Hospital in Philadelphia had worked with Donders and Snellen in 1861 in Europe. He overheard Dr. Donders suggest to Snellen that test letters devised on a scientific principle would be helpful. When he returned from Europe in 1862, Dyer had a test card printed, based on Snellen's principles. He actually proceded Snellen by several months in creating a test card. Dr. McClure, also of the Wills Eye Hospital, designed a trial frame to be used in solving the intricate problems of astigmatic refraction. It was made by J.L. Borsch, a Philadelphia optician of whom much is recorded elsewhere in this history. Before the McClure trial frame was accepted as practical, Philadelphia optician Ivan Fox produced a trial case with wide cells that had convenient notations on the handles.

Several developments were notable in 1886. Natchet of Paris devised a metric system of lens notation *(lenses had been categorized by the age of the patient and in later years by expressing the focal length in inches)*. Dr. George T. Stevens of New York City created a terminology for functional and organic disturbances of extra-ocular muscles and Charles Prentice, an optician who later became an optometrist, announced his prism dioptry measurement system.

In 1893, American Optical introduced a standardized case of trial lenses. In connection with the history of the trial case, the American Ophthalmological Society passed a resolution in 1879 adopting Javal's notation for prescribing cylindrical and prismatic glasses. This suggested that the zero point be taken at the left of the horizontal meridian and the inclination of the cylinder axis or position of the base of the prism be expressed in degrees counting upward around the circle from that point. This is the system still in use today.

The 1905 Sears Roebuck and Company's catalogue included a complete self-testing kit for $27.50. The kit enabled the customer to perform a primitive "do-it-yourself" refraction. Many times these Sears kits were also used by local opticians to order glasses for their retail customers.

The Eyecare Professions

Anyone selling eyeglasses during the 19th century knew there had to be a better way to determine eyeglass needs. Eventually, it became apparent that it ought to be possible to test *(refract)* the eye and determine what kind of lens would best aid the patient. Physicians who had special training in diseases of the eye and eye surgery were called "Oculists". They performed medical eye exams, along with surgery, sometimes learning refraction techniques from local opticians, sometimes

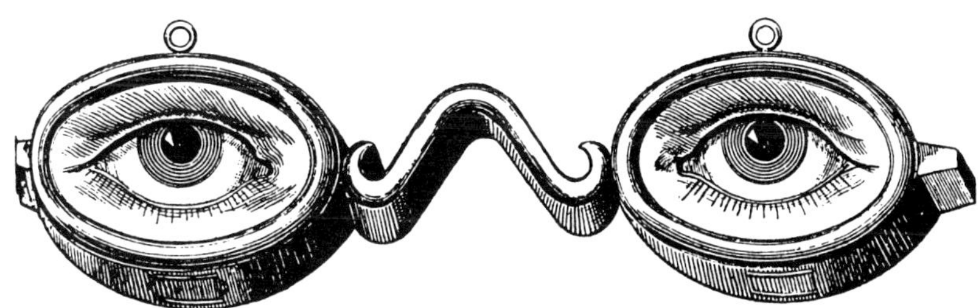

Optician's sign dating from the turn of the century.

OLA OPTICAL INDUSTRY MUSEUM

teaching the opticians. In this way, mid-19th century oculists and opticians often learned and worked together.

As more was learned about refracting the eye, refractions were often performed by opticians who had been taught subjective methods of refraction by understanding physicians. These doctors understood that the demand for eye refractions required more refractionists than the relatively few MD's who refracted. Early opticians also worked in conjunction with the many oculists who did not refract, but instead, relied on opticians to perform this service for their patients.

As the science of refracting was refined and refractions became the accepted way to provide eyecare, opticians gradually divided into two camps. The first group considered themselves "prescription opticians". They were usually closely allied to the physicians and limited themselves to providing spectacles on the prescription of the physician. The second group called themselves "refracting opticians" because they both refracted and supplied spectacles.

The separation between the two classes of opticians broadened as the use of diagnostic drugs was adapted by physicians. The Retinoscope had been introduced in 1873 and its use was made easier through use of a drug that would dilate the patient's eyes making it easier for the physician to view the retina. Using drops also enabled the doctor to conduct the examination without requiring subjective accommodative responses from the patient.

OLA OPTICAL INDUSTRY MUSEUM

Refracting Opticians

As a result of these changes, "refracting opticians" wanted a legal definition of their function and eventually chose the name "Optometry" to define their profession. In the early 1900s, refracting opticians banded together to establish legal recognition of their new profession. By the 1930s, optometry had been fully established as a separate and legal profession. Opticians who did not refract considered themselves "prescription opticians". Eventually they adapted the term "dispensing opticians" as a more descriptive way of defining their role in providing eyecare.

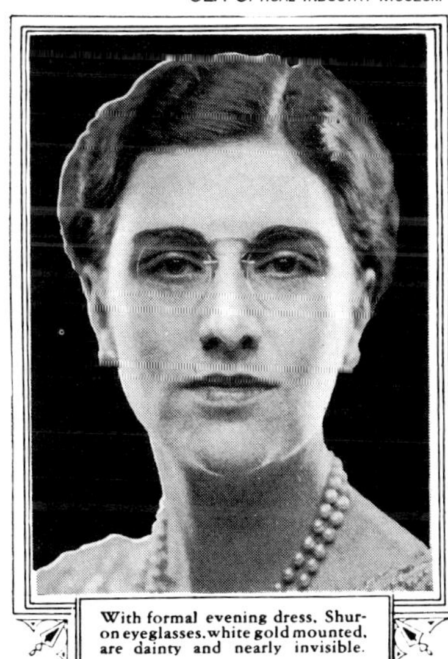

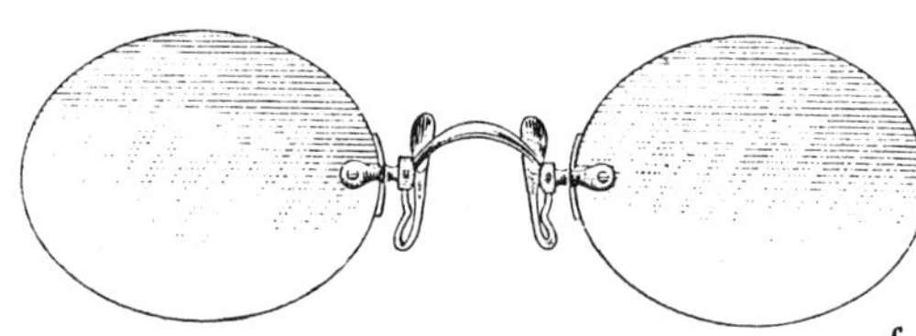

Original Shur-on mounting, from which Shuron took their name.

The oculist's eyeglass prescriptions were usually filled by local area opticians except for "country doctors" who were far removed from metropolitan areas and had only a few prescriptions to fill. These remote doctors would sell their own glasses, buying them from city laboratories or opticians. Because most corrections were spherical, this worked reasonably well until late in the 19th century. Complicated cases in those days were referred to larger, better equipped city opticians.

Growing Domination by the Big Two

As the century drew to a close, the two leading manufacturers, American Optical and Bausch & Lomb, began to formalize their sales efforts by establishing greater sales representation over a wider area. The Wells brothers *(the three sons of George Washington Wells),* as part of their training, traveled the country extensively, carrying the American Optical label nationwide and internationally as well. Henry Lomb set up a sales office for Bausch & Lomb in New York City with distribution facilities aimed at better serving the company's customers. In the first part of the 20th century, both companies set up stock offices throughout the country including the major population centers of Chicago, Philadelphia, Boston, Atlanta, Dallas, Denver, and San Francisco.

Meanwhile, in Rochester, N.Y., Kirstein Optical Company, founded in 1864, established a laboratory and extended their lens service to include frames and, later, machinery, instruments and cases. Over a period of several decades, the company began mass production of single vision and bifocal lenses, often by acquiring other manufacturers to expand their line. Kirstein worked closely with A.L. Smith and Company, Geneva, N.Y., a frame manufacturer that would later become Standard Optical *(STOCO).* In 1925, Kirstein and Standard merged under the name "Shur-On". This name came from one of their most popular products, a finger-piece mounting that sat so firmly on the nose it was called Shur-On. Shur-on broadened their distribution by setting up independent laboratories to distribute their expanding product line.

By the early 1920s, most distribution of these major manufacturers was accomplished through large wholesale chains that also sold to the public. Wholesalers selling at retail came about because most oculists did not sell optical goods such as eyeglasses. Many of the opticians previously used by oculists were now examining eyes and eventually would become Optometrists. Oculists did not care to chance losing patients by sending them to these refractionists. Large wholesale opticians, often with their own surfacing facilities, were more than willing to see the oculists' patients and fill their prescriptions for eyeglasses.

Selling Optical Goods

Sales to optical retailers were conducted by sales representatives who were often owners of the company they represented. These hardy travelers covered great distances over extended periods of time to show goods to hungry retailers. Indeed, as late as the 1950s, the Fehrs, who owned Western Optical Company in Salt Lake City, Utah, had a company policy that guaranteed an order to any optical salesman dedicated enough to make the effort to visit them in Salt Lake City. Utah was off the beaten path and Western Optical wanted to be sure they stayed current on developments in the industry.

Rebating

During these years, a number of schemes were established, all accomplishing the same goal — providing substantial rebates to doctors who referred eyeglass patients to a wholesale/retail optician. One such scheme involved "charge and send" in which the doctor sent patients to the optician who would take appropriate measurements, offer a frame selection, produce and assemble the lenses, adjust them to the patient, and return the patient to the doctor. The doctor was charged wholesale pricing for the glasses, plus a fitting fee. The doctor, in turn, would collect the full retail price, which had already been quoted by the optician. Refracting fees at the time were often no more than $5 *(taxable)* and the 40 percent difference between the "charged" price and the resale price was generally at least $10 *(nontaxable),* so the arrangement was satisfactory to the doctor. Wholesale opticians were satisfied to collect their full wholesale Rx price for the glasses, plus a fitting fee. Other schemes involved direct rebates of up to 40 percent, expensive "presents", or participation arrangements. With few exceptions, this was how medically prescribed glasses were handled, particularly in the mid-west, south, southwest, and the west. These rebate schemes lasted up to the 1940s when a Federal law suit put an end to all of them.

AO and B&L Build Lab Network

In the early 1920s, American Optical and Bausch & Lomb started buying up their wholesale customers to insure distribution of products made at the factory. AO absorbed their acquisitions and established a national chain of laboratories, all under the name "American Optical Company". Companies acquired included Potter & Schnackenburg *(New York),* R. Mohr and Sons *(San Francisco),* F. A. Hardy *(Kansas City),* Merry Optical *(Chicago),* and many others. B&L acquired Colonial Optical Company *(Boston and New York),* McIntire

McGee & Brown *(Philadelphia)*, S. Galeski *(Richmond, Va.)*, Riggs Optical Co. *(started in Omaha, Neb., but set up as two companies: one in Chicago, the other in San Francisco)*, and White Haines Optical Co. *(Columbus, Ohio)*. B&L preferred that their acquisitions retain their own names, usually with substantially the same management. Their laboratories became known as "the affiliates" *(B&L owned 75 to 90 percent of each company)* and operated relatively independently as company-owned wholesalers dedicated to promoting Bausch & Lomb products. Soon two-thirds of the production of both factories were being sold through their wholesale divisions.

Since most of these acquired companies had retail businesses as well, this put AO and B&L solidly in the retail business. At their peak shortly after World War II, AO had 375 branches and B&L more than 300. Most branches sold at both retail and wholesale. In addition, AO controlled many large retailers through generous financing of their purchases and substantial entertainment which exerted a considerable influence over their purchasing.

In this way the two largest manufacturers also became the largest wholesalers and retailers in the country. Further, AO controlled major patents in the frame business *(Ful Vue, Numount, and Rimway)* and, together with B&L and Shuron, were the only major manufacturers supplying machinery and instruments. The fascinating aspect to this period of history is that all this power rested in the hands of one man, George W. Wells, President and major owner *(together with the Wells family)* of American Optical Company. He was able to dictate price, policy, and product at all levels of the industry. Fortunately, he was reasonably benevolent. The industry was basically a small, family business in which everyone knew all the players, but there was never a doubt in anyone's mind that American Optical's needs came first.

Frame Distribution

Frame manufacturers, because of AO's tight patent control, were told what to produce, who they were permitted to sell to and at what price. Lens manufacturers were provided price parameters each year. Wholesale prices in the industry were completely guided by what AO and B&L labs charged - even to the extent that these two companies could, and sometimes did, reduce their prices below cost in certain cities when they wanted to eliminate bothersome competition. Those were monopolistic days in which the Fair Trade Act *(i.e. controlled retail price of a branded retail product)* was enforced by the federal government to assure that no Fair Traded goods were sold at discount prices. No one in the industry was big enough to quarrel with AO. B&L's policy

was to listen carefully and then follow what AO said. The rest of the industry accounted for only one-third of the total industry volume and had little choice other than to follow AO's lead regarding price and sales policies.

Large retailers were often favored with "big dealer" discounts which bypassed wholesale laboratories and kept these retailers as faithful accounts of the two major factories. They also enjoyed prolonged credit to the extent that ultimately AO exercised control over any retailer who found himself unable to bring his account up to current status.

The Consent Decrees

In this way American Optical ruled supreme from the early 1920s until 1948. At that time, an extensive investigation of the industry, which had been in process for some years, ended in three major consent decrees affecting AO, B&L, most lens and frame manufacturers, and all dispensing opticians. In the first of these, the government enjoined AO *(and anyone else in the industry)* from restrictive product licensing: the rule became "license one, license all". Further, the licensee could not be told what prices to charge and, for two years, resale prices from wholesale to retail could not be published. This last restriction was not very effective since AO and B&L both published resale prices for their own wholesale branches and expected their distributors to follow these prices.

The second decree mandated that AO and B&L withdraw from the retail business within a reasonable time *(B&L was out by 1950, AO continued in retail until 1951)*. Further, the practice of rebates was firmly eliminated with stringent penalties to be imposed for any violations. As an example, Fred Hushea *(Canton, Ohio)* and Tom Lilly *(Wilmington, NC)* were actually jailed for a year for refusing to divulge how much they had rebated and to whom. It was rumored that Hushea, on returning from incarceration, dropped a key on the desk of each of his referring doctors explaining that this was a key to his safe deposit box where his records were kept and suggested they continue to refer patients to him. They did and he prospered until he sold to Kindy Optical in 1965, when the business ultimately slowed to almost a stop.

The divestiture of AO and B&L retail businesses created a new generation of optical dispensers. AO sold each branch to its branch manager, a local employee, or an outsider; B&L preferred to select buyers more carefully, choosing those who were better liked, yet, paradoxically, often refusing to continue selling to those who bought their branches. Many

William Waldert (founder of Rochester's Waldert Opticians) was a sales rep for E. Kirstein Company.

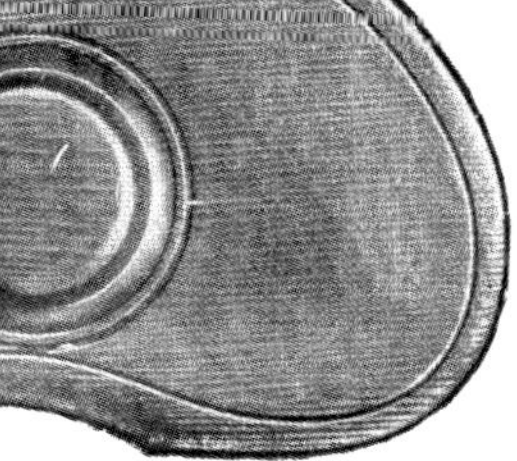

Case for non-folding oxford. Metal cup in center prevented the nose guards from becoming bent.

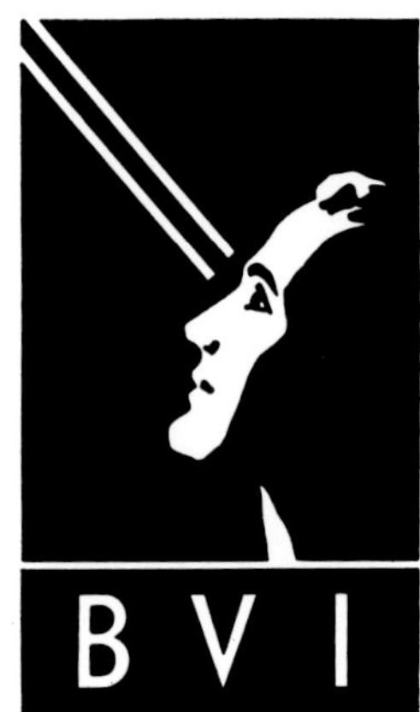

The Better Vision Institute was (and still is) a major public relations vehicle for promoting eyecare.

former B&L and AO employees did very well in their new retail businesses and some, entering the wholesale business, created new competition for their former employers. In general, former AO employees tended to remain loyal to AO whereas former B&L personnel did not retain this bond.

Almost all wholesale dispensers were required to sign this federal decree as well and rebating in this country generally ceased. Many ophthalmologists *(oculists by now had renamed themselves)* began dispensing eyeglasses to make up for the painful loss of income from rebates. Today, many Ophthalmologists are dispensing eyewear in their office.

AO's Diminishing Influence

AO's control was further weakened by a number of factors:

1) There was further litigation including a suit in Dallas in which Dal-Tex, one of the earliest "Texas large labs" set up to sell at lower prices than those prevailing at the time, sued AO and B&L for restraint of trade since they could not buy product from either company. The defendants *(considered "foreign corporations" by the Texas courts)* lost and were enjoined from not selling for any illegal reason *(such as failure to uphold mandated prices)*. Further, they were told to give appropriate quantity discounts for lens and frame product "when this was earned". This was an industry first.

2) Madison Optical was a small wholesale dispenser in Milwaukee. In 1964, they were delisted by B&L and AO for price cutting, a normal custom in those days. A complaint to Wisconsin's Senator Alexander Wiley resulted in a federal investigation. The federal government *(represented by the same attorney who had handled the 1948 consent decrees)* sued AO and B&L for restraint of trade under the Sherman Anti-Trust Law, as an extension to the consent decrees of 1948. The federal government brought in many witnesses who had previously held high positions at AO and B&L *(both companies were undergoing substantial corporate restructuring and replacing of older hands)* and was able to obtain significant evidence of violation of these laws.

In the settlement, AO and B&L were enjoined from removing anyone from their wholesale lists for illegal reasons. Further, they were enjoined, for 20 years, from opening new wholesale branches or from operating any branch at a loss for more than two consecutive years, in which case they must close or sell that branch. Even further, the government defined what their profit should be.

The first commercially successful bevel edger, manufactured and sold by Arthur Lemay.

Profit meant the net amount received after determining cost of product *(including that supplied by their own factory)* on the same basis as anyone else buying similar quantities. This included machinery supplied to the branch by the factory.

The factory was also required to allocate an appropriate amount of factory overhead to each branch. These were severe restrictions which effectively eliminated AO's control of the wholesale industry. AO and B&L were also enjoined from engaging in dispensing for five years *(this restriction was subsequently extended)*. Penalties included loss of the complete wholesale setup.

One of the more significant results of these mandates was an almost complete disruption of relations between AO and B&L personnel. From that point on, company personnel did not dare meet so as to avoid any appearance of "conspiring". These decrees were undoubtedly a major factor in the decline of AO and B&L during the following 10 years.

A Changing Industry

The industry began to acquire a different complexion as a result of these factors. Added to this was the fact that the founding families of AO and B&L were aging and the heirs had little interest in continuing the family business. They had become comfortably wealthy and many had developed other interests.

The Wells family sold their stock gradually, starting in 1947 and in 1954, Warner-Lambert, a large pharmaceutical concern, acquired the company. American Optical had tried for several years to attract executives from other industries but these executives had difficulty with optical marketing techniques, as well as the low pay scale of the optical industry. The low volume did not

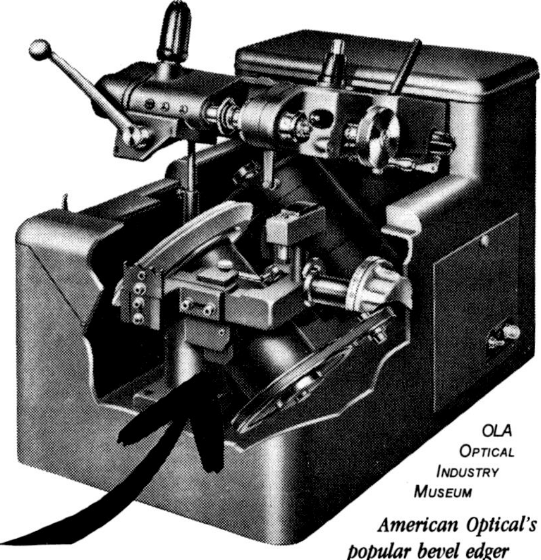

American Optical's popular bevel edger used a distinctive ceramic wheel set at a 45 degree angle. A diamond wheel version was also produced, with very limited success.

provide enough money, at their accustomed percentages, to operate as they would in other industries. Warner-Lambert had a similar experience, particularly since the attitudes of the professions regarding consumer advertising virtually prohibited the company from advertising as they did in other industries. The loss of AO's former leverage meant their direction had to change. The Bausch family also sold its stock and the new, publicly held company was taken over by non-optical executives with similar results in the optical arena.

The laboratory setup at both companies had become antiquated. AO's machinery division produced surfacing machinery only for their branches *(which were dwindling in numbers)* and for international accounts. B&L had no budget for refurbishing their labs. AO and B&L branches gradually became less competitive and independent labs took over the field. Further, non-optical executives were driving the better optical people out of both companies because of unreasonable demands, poor marketing policies, inadequate products, inability to produce quality work at the branch level, and inadequate wages. Finally, when frames started becoming more and more important to the retail industry, AO and B&L remained noncompetitive in that area as well. By the time B&L divested their laboratories in 1981, along with their frame and lens operations, AO and B&L had been out of power for at least 15 years, even though both companies retained large businesses in all areas of the ophthalmic industry.

Retail Chains

The power vacuum left by AO's relinquishing of control was never filled. Leadership shifted gradually to the retail chains who increased in size and power during the 1980s. Chains were able to demand special treatment, special prices and special products. The lens industry no longer had a leader although SOLA and Silor exercised growing influence. The frame business had no single leader and importers gradually took over the market place. Wholesale laboratories found their frame sales gradually eroding as direct sellers proliferated. This loss of sales, however, was largely offset by the growing importance of lens add-ons such as high index, polycarbonate, aspherics and progressives.

Recent years have seen a resurgence of frames ordered from laboratories and the concept of ordering frames and lenses from a single source is growing. Retail power shifted to the major chains: Pearle Vision *(with both company owned and franchised operations),* Cole National *(controlling most Sears stores and other departments as well),* Lenscrafters *(who started the super-store trend)* and many other small to medium retail chains. Mass warehouse operations have discovered

the optical business and are a growing influence at both retail and wholesale levels.

The industry has prospered, however. In 1970, total industry sales at the retail level were $1 billion; in 1991, sales increased to $15 billion plus $3 billion in refractions, a total of $18 billion. This astonishing growth was accomplished without the aid of the two major industry leaders who, without question, had been responsible for creating the industry. AO and B&L had led the industry from a scattered group of artisans producing hand-crafted eyewear for only the wealthy to mass-produced eyeglasses, affordable to everyone.

Each of the subjects reviewed in this Synopsis is explored in greater depth in succeeding chapters of this history. For specific subjects, consult the Index at the back of the book.

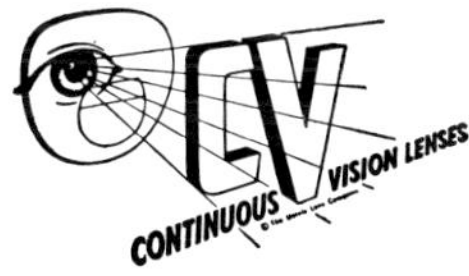

Feeling the name "trifocals" intimidated patients, Univis coined a new name for these multifocals.

OLA OPTICAL INDUSTRY MUSEUM

EARLY SEATTLE MEMORIES

John H. Burke, then manager of Riggs Optical's Los Angeles branch wrote in 1941 of his early memories of working in Seattle.

"What glorious opportunities there were in those days (1906). Seattle had a number of optical stores and a few upstairs men. The prices averaging about $10 a pair, but most upstairs men had pretty tough picking. They were the professional pioneers and their offices had a decidedly pioneer aspect. Trial case, Snellen's Chart and a couple of kitchen chairs. How things have changed."

"One character who stands out in my memory was Dr. Todd Morcum, long since dead. An old fair worker, came up through the gutters, a fine looking, handsome chap, always immaculately dressed. This fellow made $50,000 out his little store on First Avenue. He was absolutely illiterate, couldn't sign his own name, yet he was one of the brightest, shrewdest men I ever met."

"I remember another old friend who operated in a long narrow dirty store. He was dirty too, especially his hands. I sat and watched him many times wondering what attracted patients to him, I guess it was low prices. He used to spit on his patient's glasses and wipe them off with the end of his necktie. He had a pot bellied stove in his store on which he usually had some kind of a stew simmering and from time to time while waiting on a patient, he would leave his seat, go over to the stove and stir up the concoction he was cooking."

"Of course, there were honest and sincere men as well as humbugs. The humerous [sic] stands out because most of them were honest rascals and didn't kid those who knew them and about their remarkable ability. The country was too new for the sanctimonious type. This fact stands out. In 1906, there were 14 or 15 people engaged in the wholesale business in Seattle and they were able to take care of the business of that enormous territory. By 1919 when we sold out to Riggs, there were laboratories in British Columbia, Tacoma and Spokane, cutting down on business but there were still at least 50 people engaged in the wholesale business in Seattle."

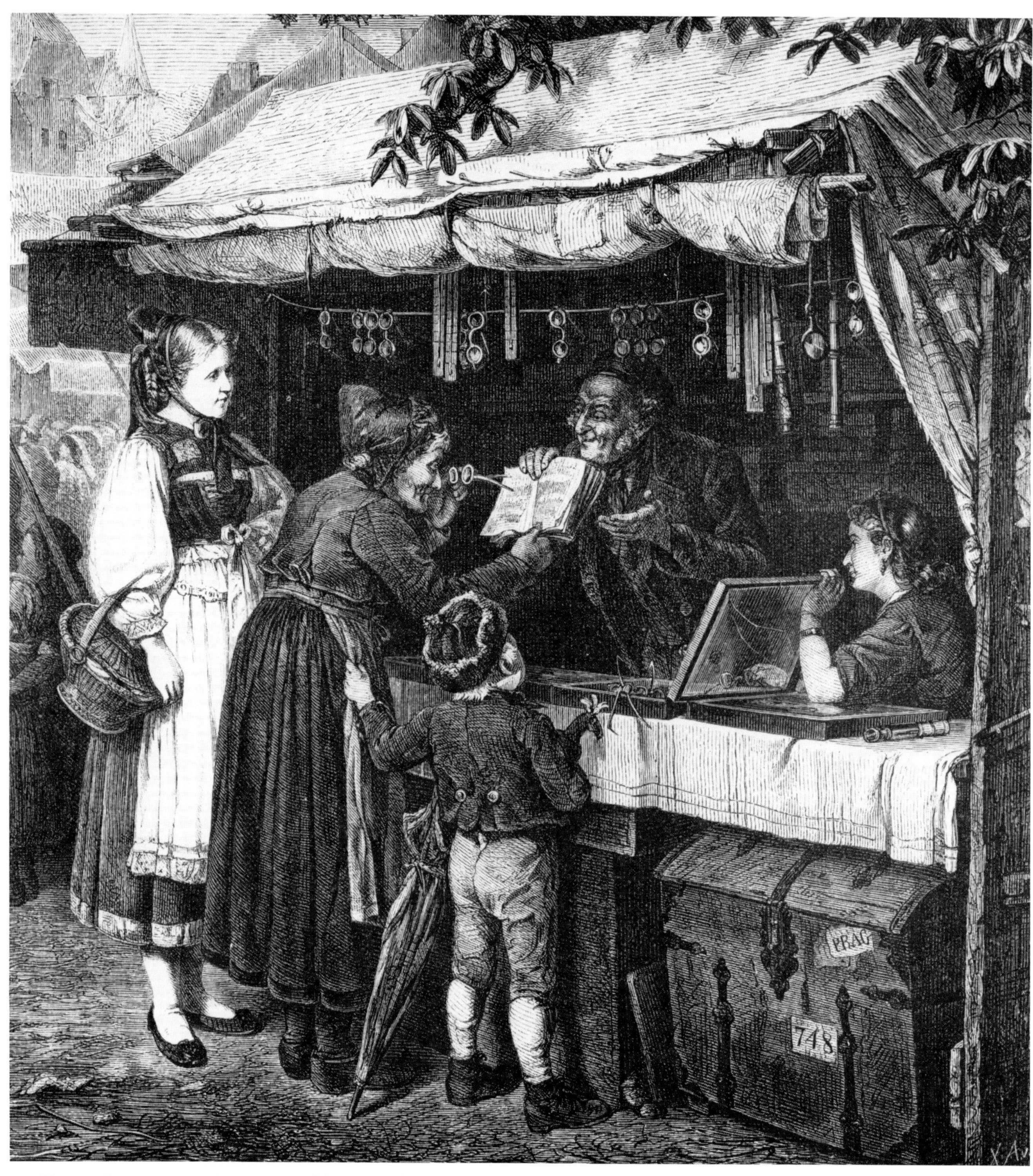

Until late in the 1 800's, eyeglasses were sold as a complete unit, frame and lenses together. To determine their prescription, wearers would simply try on one pair after another until a pair that worked was found. Eyeglasses were often found in general stores, hardware stores, later drug stores or jewelry stores and frequently were sold by traveling peddlers or at fairs and other open-air gatherings as shown in this German woodcut.

Chapter 2
The Optical Professions

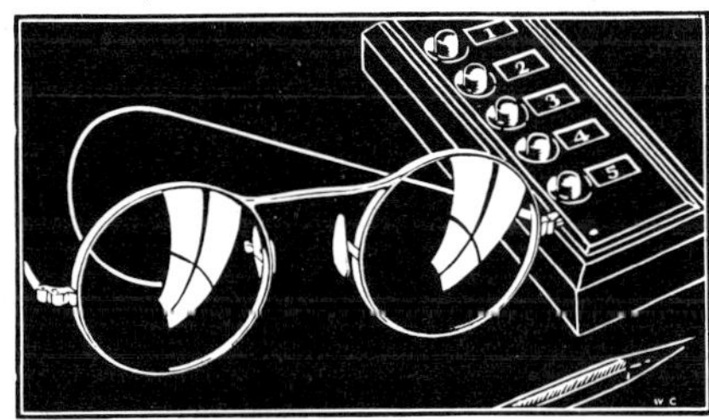

It is difficult to relate the optical retailer of today with those in the industry's early days. There have been so many changes and modifications in the way retailers have operated through the years, it's like comparing apples with oranges. Optometrists and opticians sprang from common roots until a significant fork in the road was reached. At that point, refracting opticians went one way to become what we know as Optometrists. Non-refracting opticians remained basically technicians and merchants, usually supporting Ophthalmologists, at least until recent years.

Today there has been a great blurring of the lines of distinction. Optometrists sometimes work for opticians and vice versa and ophthalmologists often employ either or both Optometrists and Opticians. Ophthalmologists are sometimes employed by opticians or optometrists. This is further confused by laboratories that may own retail outlets or, more likely, are owned by retail outlets. So the definition and chronology of the three O's *(opticianry, optometry, and ophthalmology)* is interrelated and difficult to define - historically and currently.

Colonial Days

During Colonial days, there were few opticians in the United States, mostly in New York, Philadelphia, and Boston. Southern, mid-western, and western areas were served primarily by "peddlers" or by mail order from eastern opticians. Peddlers acquired their goods from wholesale companies *(most of whom were in the jewelry trade)*. At first, these wholesalers purchased finished goods from Europe. Then gradually they started making their frames, usually inserting imported finished lenses. Prescriptions were entirely spherical until the end of the 19th century with the variety of frame styles and sizes severely limited.

Peddlers

Peddlers offered eyeglasses, sometimes as an exclusive line of eyewear, but more often as a side line to other wares. Some peddlers were conscientious, learning their trade through experience, and some were unscrupulous, gouging customers and using high pressure sales methods, often with promises impossible to fulfill. Over time, many of the more conscientious peddlers settled down, opened optical stores, and acquired optical knowledge as best they could. Even in their new, settled locations, they often continued traveling to rural areas on a regular basis to serve their widespread customers.

Training

Training was available from several sources. A few ambitious medical doctors had set up training and correspondence courses. One such school, the Klein School of Optics, was founded in 1894 by Dr. August Klein, a prominent Boston oculist. Initially Klein provided clinical instruction to physicians only, but soon began teaching the use of the ophthalmascope to opticians so they could recognize and refer eye abnormalities. This school eventually became the Massachusetts College of Optometry. The refracting school initiated in 1872 by George and J.B. McFatrich in Chicago under the name Northern Illinois College of Ophthalmology and Otology merged in 1926 with the Needles Institute of Optometry and became the Northern Illinois College of Optometry. In 1955, after a bitter fight with the Chicago College of Optometry, the two merged to form the present Illinois College of Optometry.

Other training, of a less formal nature, was provided by wholesale or manufacturing firms, such as the Spencer Optical Company of New York and Julius King *(founded by Dr. Julius King)* of New York and Cleveland, Ohio. Both companies gave brief "familiarization" correspondence courses and awarded diplomas upon successful completion of the course. It's doubtful that much was learned, or taught, but this was better than nothing and provided the prospective *(or working)* optician a smattering of technical knowledge to help in refracting and dispensing.

Licensing

In the late 19th century, there were no restrictions or qualifications required to operate a retail optical store. Anyone could sell eyeglasses, examine eyes and make eyewear. It didn't take long before this chaotic situation created major conflicts between the oculist *(who was*

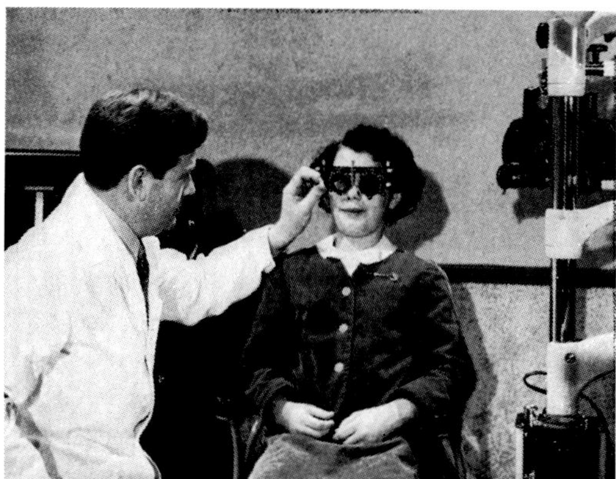

Typical refracting scene from the late 1930's.

emerging as an ophthalmologist) and sight-testing opticians. Medical doctors argued that no one could examine eyes unless they were qualified in medicine. Opticians stated that many medical doctors were not qualified to perform optometric functions and those trained in the science of optometry *(which, they claimed was based on physics and mathematics, not medicine)* could do a better job of refracting while referring any pathology to competent medical doctors.

Optometrists argued that optometry was based on the science of refraction of light and an eye examination was not a medical function and had nothing to do with the physiology of the eye. They probably had a point because few early medical men were trained in what was required for determining corrective lenses for the patient and only a few knew anything regarding lenses.

Optometry

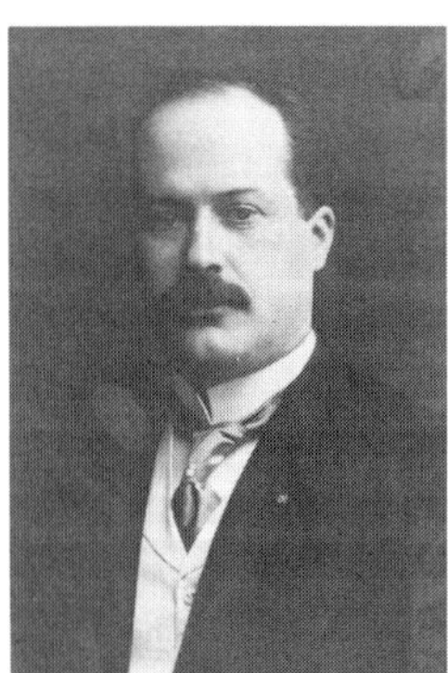

Dr. J.B. McFatrich — he and his brother George founded No. Illinois College of Ophthalmology and Otology (the present Illinois College of Optometry)

Frederic Boger was the first to suggest an organization be established to represent opticianry and optometry *(in 1897)*. He was founder and publisher of THE JOURNAL, started in 1885, containing material of interest to jewelers and opticians. It was renamed THE OPTICAL JOURNAL in 1891. Subscriptions were $1 per year, payable in advance.

Following up on Boger's suggestion, opticians Andrew J. Cross and Charles F. Prentice sent out a call to action. On October 10, 1898, the would-be association held a meeting at the famous Broadway Central Hotel in New York City with 183 members representing 31 states and three Canadian provinces. It was a rather hodgepodge group who sold "optical, philosophical, and photographic goods". They chose to name their new association "The American Optical Association". Some members refracted and some did not.

Initially, "dispensing opticians" controlled this association, primarily because the first president was a

New York optician named Charles Lembke. However, he was succeeded in 1900 by Andrew Jay Cross, a New York optometrist who would be remembered as "the father of optometry". The group eventually became exclusively optometric.

Opticians Who Refracted

Refracting opticians had a great deal of difficulty in deciding what to call themselves. By 1904, many were calling themselves "optometrist" *(meaning "one skilled in the practice of physiological optics")*, a term proposed by John Eberhardt. Other suggested names included "optician", "sight-testing optician" and "opticist". The last name was the name coined and preferred by Charles Prentice, backed by the prestige of the internationally recognized prism dioptry system he had formulated. All these names were used interchangeably until 1919 when "optometry" and "optometrist" became the officially adopted names for the new profession. The fact that many ophthalmological publications and texts on refraction used the term "optometry" when referring to refraction, added credence to that name. In 1904, at the organization's meeting in Milwaukee, the members adopted the name "optometrists". It's interesting to note that, three years before, in 1901, Minnesota passed the first optometry law, using the word "optometrist".

Their association was founded under the name "American Association of Opticians" and operated under that name until the 13th convention in 1910 when the name was changed to "American Optical Association". However, it wasn't until 1918 that the association changed its name to "American Optometric Association". In some states it was necessary to amend the laws to ensure the word "optometrist" was used on business cards, stationery, etc. The honorific title of "Doctor" was seldom used before 1922.

The Association was not necessarily the arbiter of optical matters since only a small percentage of retailers were members and some of these were disaffected with the early results attained by the association. During a convention of the new association in Atlantic City, N.J., in 1904, a to-the-point question was addressed to the chair, "What do I get for my $1 annual dues? We think we are being gypped."

Education

Meanwhile, as fighting over a name continued, advances were being made in the field of education. Optical correspondence courses had become popular, springing up all over the country. Once tuition was paid and the few lessons completed, students received a diploma giving them the right to practice and, in many cases, the use of the title "Doctor". Dr. Brown established his Philadelphia Optical College in 1892, and a Mr. Thomson started the South Bend College of Optics in Indiana. In 1894, the largest of these schools was started in Chicago by brothers J. B. and George McFatrich. They called their school the Northern Illinois College of Ophthalmology and Otology, which was shortened to Northern Illinois College of Optometry in 1925. During the school's first 20 years, more than 7,000 graduated. In addition to a successful correspondence course, the school gave lectures. Courses lasted one to six weeks, at a cost of $25 a course.

Around 1898 or 1900, the McCormick Neurological School, later the McCormick Medical School, was giving courses. In 1900, C.L. Merry started a school in his building in Kansas City to provide his growing laboratory with new customers. Named the Southwestern Optical College, it was later turned over to Dr. E.A. Lane to operate. A jeweler could take a few lessons, buy a trial case, receive a prescription order book and be ready to practice. This school became so profitable that competition sprang up. Merry withdrew his support of Dr. Lane and encouraged Dr. William B. Needles, a young man who had just finished a course at the McCormack Medical College, to start a new school in Kansas City. The year was 1909 and the Needles Institute of Optometry flourished in the years to come.

Educational standards gradually improved as the practice of optometry was legalized in every state. Practitioners had to fulfill certain requirements in order to be licensed. It took 23 years to get an optometric law in every state. By 1924 when Calvin Coolidge put his signature to the last law *(District of Columbia)*, 20,000 optometrists were registered throughout the country.

One of the more gratifying developments in the field of optometric education was the initiation of optometry courses by several large universities. In 1910, Colombia University added optometry to its curriculum; Ohio State University followed in 1914 and California in 1923 when optometrists of that state underwrote the course. A yearly registration fee of $10 for optometrists was established, $8 of which went to the university as an income for the optometry course. The University of Rochester also conducted an optometry course for a while.

State Licensing

The American Optometric Association promoted the concept of professionalism for their members and urged state laws demanding high qualifications for optometry.

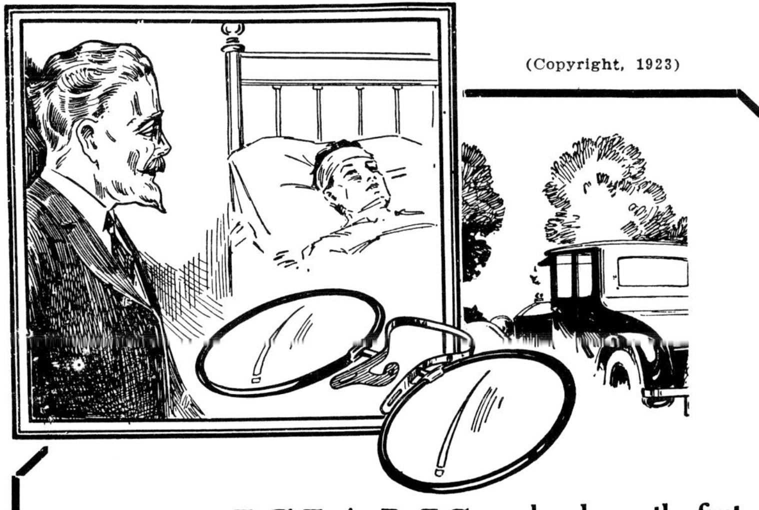

As optometrists refined their skills, they were sometimes prone to overstating the efficacy of the eyewear they prescribed. This 1920s ad mat made glasses sound better than vitamins.

OLA OPTICAL INDUSTRY MUSEUM

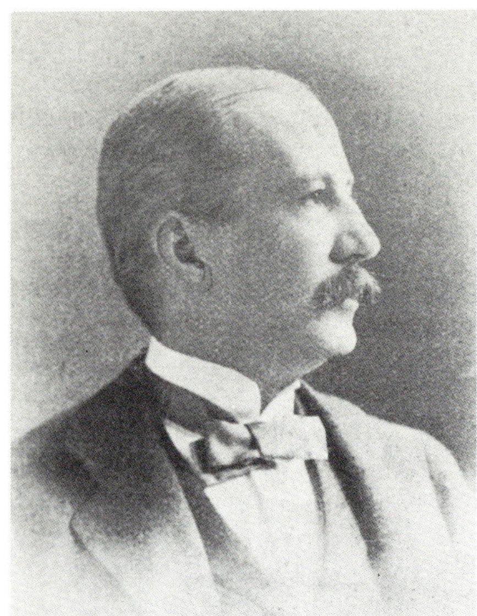

Andrew Jay Cross

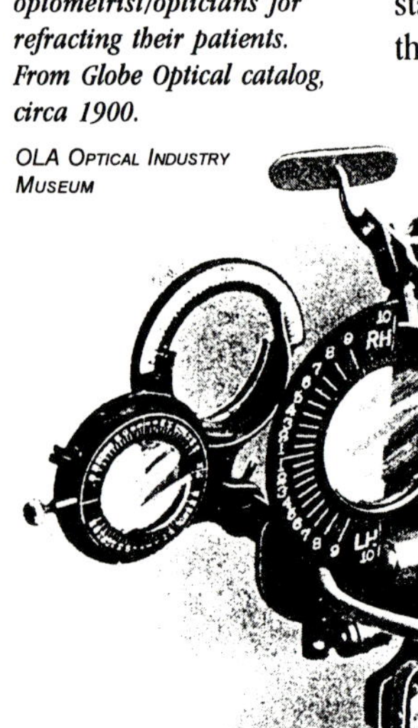

Oliver's Model Phoro-Optometer. This 3-cell trial frame included a rotary prism, a Maddox Multiple Rod and a Stephens Phorometer. Prior to the development of the refractor, this was the type of instrument used by modern optometrist/opticians for refracting their patients. From Globe Optical catalog, circa 1900.

Prospective optometrists, under the new rules, had to be approved by local boards. Those who were already refracting were exempt from taking board examinations under a "grandfather clause". It would take a while for optometry to come out of the "dark ages". Current thinking was, "how could an optometrist charge for a refraction when the oculist received only $5 for a medical refraction?" As it turned out, for many years optometrists who charged for eye examinations defied the medical field which was strongly opposed to nonmedical men charging for what they perceived to be professional medical services.

Yearly conventions held by the AOA helped firm up their concepts. An idea of the interest in group actions by American optometrists can be deduced by the attendance figures of their national conventions. In 1898, the first convention in New York City attracted 32; in 1899, 175 attended the second convention in Rochester; in Detroit, in 1900, there were 300; in 1906, in Rochester, N.Y., 1,000 were in attendance with this figure climbing to 1,071 in Providence, R.I. in 1916.

Interprofessional Competition

Optometry chose many ways to fight the fierce attempts by medical refractionists to eliminate their profession, including use of a rather obvious slogan no one could deny, *"A lens is not a pill"*. In 1914, the medical profession in Pennsylvania was able to pass a law which stated that optometry was a "minor branch" of medicine that should be supervised by the Medical Examining Board. Optometry successfully fought this law through the courts who, on appeal, reversed the law. The court agreed that optometry and medicine overlapped but decided optometry required a proper academic, educational background as well as competence in refracting - that their experience in refractive techniques often predated medical participation in this area. The conclusion was that optometry belonged to the world of science rather than the profession of medicine, and was a function of physics.

New York state had problems as well. The title of "Doctor" was not officially authorized until the late 1950s *(although it was in common usage)*. The New York State Optometric Association had its origins years before when a group of New York City and upstate opticians formed the Optical Society of the State of New York. Founding members included Prentice *(the first President)*, Cross *(Treasurer)*, Boger *(Secretary)*, and George B. Bausch, J. J. Bausch's brother *(vice-president)*. Friction arose between Prentice and Cross. Charles Prentice, a partner with his famous optician father, James, used knowledge gained in studies in Europe and with various, leading American optical and scientific firms in 1874 to develop impressive new instruments and theories. He wrote a book "Ophthalmic Lenses" in 1886 which became the definitive work on this subject and built the Astigmatic Eye Model. The model illustrated Prentice's discovery of the 16 laws he found that applied to combinations of cylindrical lenses in the correction of astigmatism. He is also credited with developing and promoting use of the dioptric measuring system, replacing various inch and metric measuring systems.

Andrew Jay Cross trained as a watchmaker while living in Visalia, Calif. and Walla Walla in the soon to be state of Washington. After traveling as a watch repairer, he became interested in optics, training with a Philadelphia optical firm. He opened an upstairs practice in New York City in 1894, later moving downstairs but still maintaining a professional atmosphere. Cross developed many instruments but was mainly known for discovering the principles of dynamic skiametry.

Both Prentice and Cross believed that present day refractions required a higher standard of practice but disagreed on how to achieve this. Prentice wanted immediate legislation to regulate the profession; Cross believed that the general educational level of the nonmedical refractionist should first be improved. Further, Prentice advocated the "Ideal Ophthalmologist" should be well-trained in medicine and all ophthalmic matters, and have a sound knowledge of many topics that opticians considered their field. Simultaneously, Prentice wanted the medical man to stay out of the province of the optometrist. Many optometrists felt that the "Ideal Ophthalmologist" was an infringement on their prerogatives and sided with Cross against Prentice.

In 1892, a battle began between Prentice and Dr. Henry D. Noyes, Chairman of the Section of Ophthalmology of the New York Academy of Medicine. Noyes objected to Prentice charging for refractions as he felt the public would assume that Prentice had qualifications that entitled him to charge a fee for advice. Prentice responded that he had charged for services for five years, the same as any competent designer charged for plans and specifications and, furthermore, he referred any pathology to competent oculists.

Defending Opticianry

The ensuing conflict involved medical opinion on both sides and continued in the New York state legislature. It was fiercely debated until, finally, the New York Optometric Law was enacted in 1908. In the course of this legislative fight, Prentice introduced his famous "Defense of the Optician". In this treatise, Prentice stated that medical doctors had little interest in eye refractions until the publication in 1864 of Donders' "Accommodation and Refraction of the Eye" and that oculists did not have full sets of trial lenses until the 1880s. Opticians had carried out most eye refractions and Chamblant of Paris had prescribed for astigmatism in 1849 with McAllister of Philadelphia doing so in 1854.

Prentice emphasized the work of opticians through the years, enumerating their developments and inventions, and accused medical men of becoming fascinated with "physico-mechanical jobs" because of the fees that could be charged. Prentice, however, abstained from most of the legislative fight, except for continually circularizing legislators with his treatise. He had been replaced by Cross as president of the New York State Society in 1897. Prentice had a goal to also establish regulation of New York state dispensing opticians but legislation accomplishing this would not pass until 1946.

In 1929, there were legal skirmishes in Pennsylvania on the basis that optometry was part of medicine just as dentistry had been until its break-away. Optometry stressed that it was an "optical science" and had never been part of medicine. Optometrists stated that they "refracted better without drugs than oculists could with drugs". Oculists argued that proper refractions could only be done with dilating drugs, such as atropine, which only medical doctors were permitted to use.

New York was the 13th state, in 1908, to pass an optometric law. The last area in the United States to pass an optometric law was the District of Columbia. President Calvin Coolidge signed the law in 1924 making optometric regulations prevalent in all states *(the first had been Minnesota in 1901)*.

The American Plan

Many have forgotten the impact the American Plan had on early optometry. This program had been developed by American Optical during its heyday. This was not entirely an unselfish plan as AO had problems in many branches maintaining sales to optometrists since AO's prices were higher than those of many independent labs. Optometrists, many struggling to make a living *(the median*

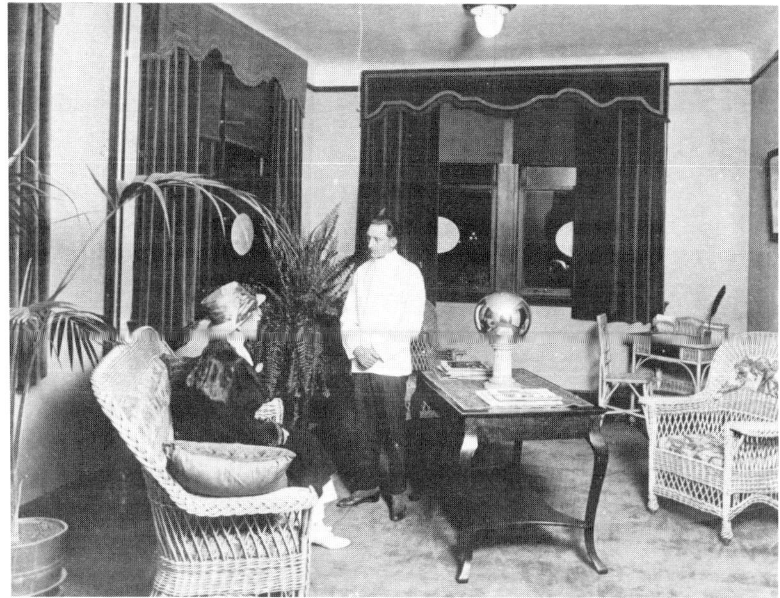

income for optometry in 1945 was $2,500/year - in 1990 it was over $50,000), were eager to take advantage of lower priced independent labs, many of whom used lenses made by companies other than AO or B&L.

So, AO put on a "dog & pony show" to promote professional optometry and the "American Plan". Optometrists were told to remember they were professional men. They were urged to move to upstairs professional offices, severely restrict their advertising and charge a "fee for service". AO pointed out that if oculists could charge $5 for an examination, the OD could charge at least $2 *(the value of these fees in the days when opticians earned $5 per week, were substantially higher than they are today)*.

They further suggested that "materials" and "therapeutic devices" *(i.e. lenses and frames - possibly the first reference to these products as "materials")* be included in their total fee based on double their cost. Obviously, an AO lab's high price would command a higher fee when doubled - few took the time to figure out they could charge that higher price even if they bought lower cost "materials" from independents.

The plan worked - to a degree. Many optometrists who moved upstairs proceeded to starve to death economically, cut off from both street traffic and advertising.

Dr. Amand DeKeyser was a founder of the optometry program at Pacific University. This is his reception room in downtown Portland, circa 1920.

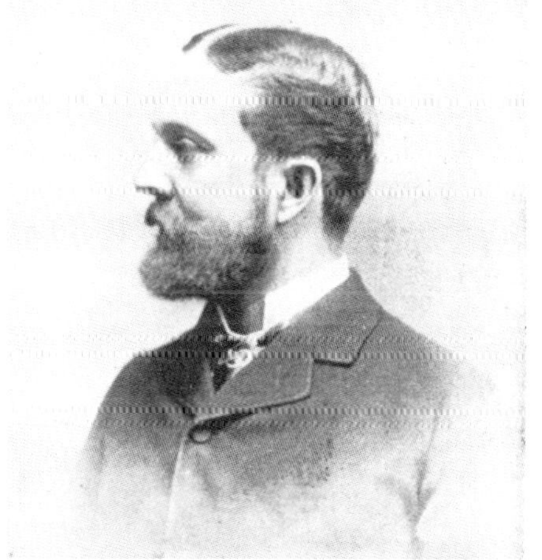

Charles Prentice developed and promoted the dioptric measuring system which replaced earlier inch categories for prescription lenses.

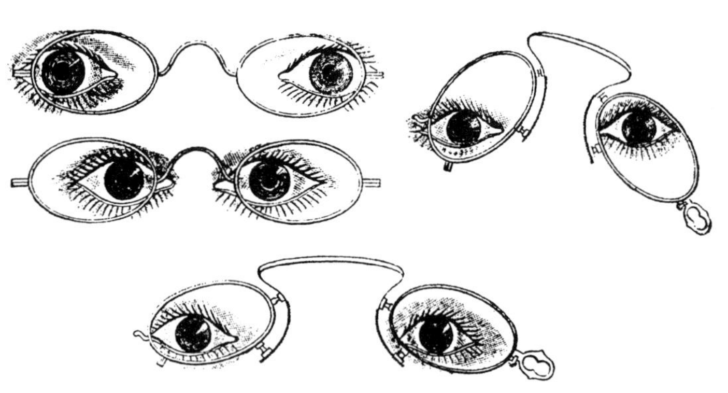

From an early catalog of Dr. S. Galeski, Consulting Optician in Richmond, VA, circa 1880. Prior to the turn-of-the-century, it was common practice to mount all lenses "on center". Therefore, it was very important to fit the frame PD to the patient's PD, either by varying the bridge or the lens size. Many of the opticians ordering glasses from Dr. Galeski's catalog had no formal training and he was attempting to demonstrate the importance of centering lenses in front of the pupil.

They donned white coats and started charging fees for all services and materials. They were aided, however, by the advent of World War II when everything was in short supply and the public had more money to spend than ever before. Those "upstairs" professional optometrists pioneered today's professional optometry.

Glasses By Mail

This interesting development originated with Montgomery Ward, who had started business in 1872. The first optical mail order house was the Dr. Haux Mail Order Spectacle Company started in St. Louis in 1900. It was later owned by brothers Maurice and Harry Goldman who changed the name to St. Louis Spectacle Company. From 1901 until the Federal Government shut them down, the brothers made a fortune. Unfortunately, they spent most of it fighting government actions.

Another prominent mail order operation was set up in Chicago by Juda Ritholz. He left the business to his sons, one of whom, Ben, brought some ingenious and profitable methods to the business. He accumulated a list of over a million names, most of them farmers. He approached other firms that might be interested in selling to this huge market. Clothing firms, shoe dealers, jewelers, razor manufacturers and dozens of others agreed to pay him to print and mail their pieces along with the Ritholz' optical materials. In this way, he not only made enormous profits on eyeglass sales, but did it with no selling expense while making a profit from other advertisers.

During the 20 golden years that mail order glasses flourished, large fortunes were made. In 1934, it all came to an end when the Federal Government began an investigation of mail order glasses. On May 2 of the following year, Karl Crowley, Solicitor of the Post Office Department recommended issuing a fraud order which read, *"The evidence shows, and I so find, that this is a scheme for obtaining money through the mails by means of false and fraudulent pretenses"*. The firms cited were: the U.S. Spectacle Company, International Spectacle Company, International Spectacle House, Self-Test Optical Company, World Optical Corporation, Shur-Fit Optical Company, Clear Sight Spectacle, Ritholz Spectacle and a number of others. Some selling of eyeglasses by mail continued but the fraud order marked the end of the big mail order concerns. Reading this history of mail order glasses makes one wonder what will come out of the present trend of mail order contact lenses.

Optical Departments

A.T. Stewart opened the first department store in New York City in the 1870s. He later sold out to John Wanamaker who is generally credited with originating most of the features of a first class department store. One of Wanamaker's innovations was opening an optical department in his Philadelphia store in 1886 with James Wilson in charge. The Brandeis store in Omaha also takes credit for the first optical department. In 1905, the man in charge of the Brandeis optical department, then known as the Boston Store, claimed he had been running it for 25 years. Whoever started it, the concept spread and by 1940 almost every city of any size had at least one department store with an optical department.

It wasn't uncommon for one man to own a chain of such departments, among them Benjamin Gainsburg and Samuel A. Hollender who each operated 18 to 20 stores. Credit jewelers who sold glasses on credit were quick to copy this idea. By the 1940s, there were thousands of jewelry optical departments, many set up as retail chain operations.

World War II

The war helped optometry because ODs were accepted by the Navy as medical officers. The army continued to utilize their services as enlisted men until after the war. Naval optometrists, however, worked side by side with medical colleagues in performing optometric services. This added prestige and the mutual respect gained by optometrists working closely with ophthalmologists helped when the war ended.

By the 1950s, optometry had grown more professional with four-year optometric schools, staffed with optometrically-trained professors *(following an obligatory two or more years of college level study)* and stiff state boards. Continuing education was required to maintain licenses. Professional fees soared, aided by third party payments *(now averaging a third of the income of many practices)* and greater affluence among their patients. Major optical chains developed in the 1970s and optometry was once more threatened by giants.

Retail Chains

Just as AO and B&L commanded a third of the retail business in 1950, the chains captured close to that share by 1990. The difference was that chains required optometrists to work for them - at high salaries but still as employees. Independent optometry was once more under siege, losing patients to the chain's advertised enticements and losing colleagues to the security of working for chains.

In their favor, optometry is benefiting from present day high fees and price levels, third party support, and an increasing need for eye care. They are able to take advantage of modern instrumentation, such as auto-refractors and electronic keratometers, which makes the work more comprehensive, often easier and justifies higher fees.

Optometrists also have contact lenses which, for some years, offered substantial profits but have become less profitable because of intensive competition *(including, once again, mail order operations)*. They can take advantage of computer point-of-sales systems that enable them to perform regular patient recalls, target marketing, and obtain statistics to pinpoint weaknesses and opportunities in their practices.

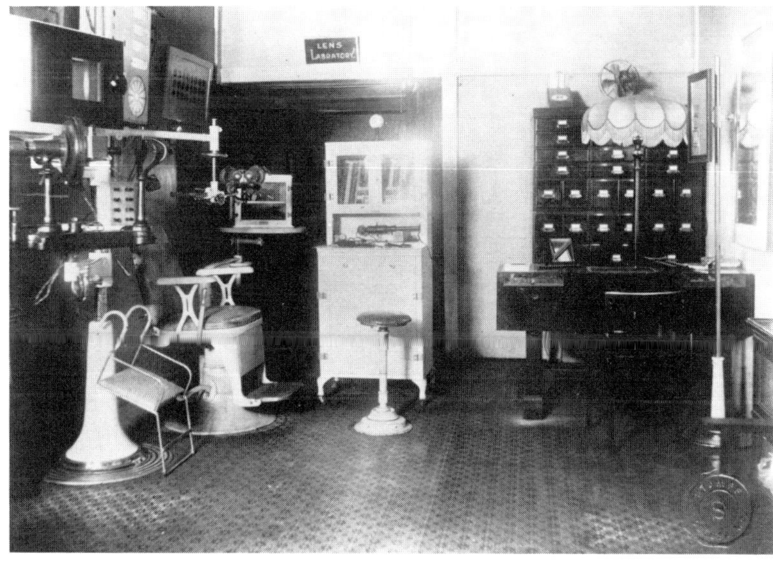

The trend today is to incorporate medical prerogatives into optometry, such as the application of therapeutic and diagnostic medication and even the use of lasers. Optometry is attempting to achieve a prominent position as a primary health provider which once more puts them in direct conflict with ophthalmology.

Dr. Robert L. Searfoss, Sr. practiced in Odessa, Missouri. His refracting room is typical of a properly equipped optometric office of that day (1910), even to the booster chair for his young patients.

Ophthalmology

Unlike optometrists, oculists did not evolve from a lower level. Early oculists often drifted into eye care from general medicine, primarily to do eye surgery and treat ocular diseases. For centuries, the medical profession considered eyewear to be harmful to the health. Religious leaders were also against eyewear, seeing it as a "tool of the devil". During the mid-1700s, a number of itinerant charlatans and quacks were treating eye diseases with such careless abandon that Dr. Adam Spencer chose to speak out on the subject. Addressing an audience in what would become Independence Hall, his lecture on the eye was "to account for the Faculty, the Nature and Diseases of that Instrument of Sight." This was the first known lecture on ophthalmology in the United States. Typically, early American physicians were foreign-trained and practiced a very broad spectrum of medical care. Dr. Spencer was an unusual physician. His scope was so broad and authoritative that no less a person than Benjamin Franklin acknowledged a personal indebtedness to Spencer for the knowledge of electricity that he acquired from Spencer's lectures.

During most of the first half of the 19th century, eye diseases were cared for by what is best described as "part-time" ophthalmologists. The first acknowledged American eye specialist was Elisha North, who actually never had a medical title until he received an honorary degree in 1813. He attended the University of Pennsylvania Medical School from 1793 to 1795 but did not graduate. He seemed to enjoy telling the world about his talents in medicine, midwifery and surgery. He advertised in an 1812 issue of the Connecticut Gazette that he would *"with promptness and pleasure attend to all such calls in the line of his [sic] profession as I may receive."* Two years later he advertised that *"Information is hereby given that the operation for cataract is performed."*

Dr. North founded the first eye infirmary in New London, Conn. in 1817. No refracting was done there but eye problems were treated. He wrote at the time, *"We had attended to eye patients before that time, but it occurred to us that we might multiply the number of cases and thereby increase our knowledge, advising the public in regard to an eye institution. Our success or exertions probably hastened in this country the establishment of larger and better eye infirmaries."* His clinic was shut down 12 years later but stands as a milestone, being the first American hospital to specialize in treatment of the eye. The New York Eye and Ear Infirmary opened in 1820 and is still in operation.

The first American work on ophthalmology was written by

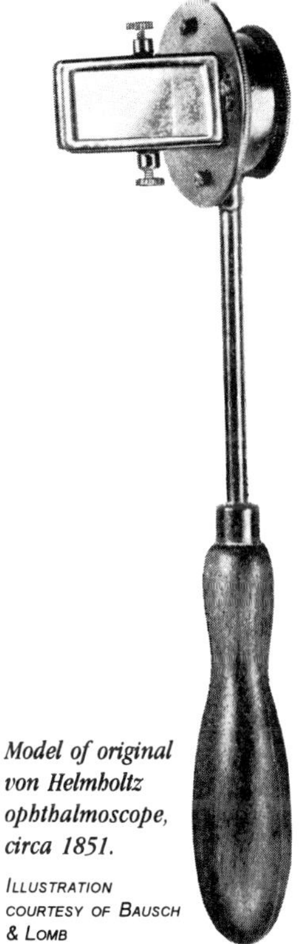

Model of original von Helmholtz ophthalmoscope, circa 1851.

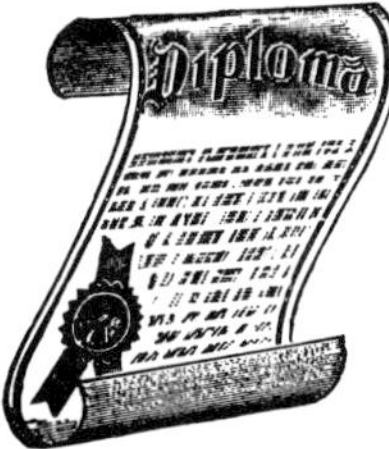

DON'T YOU WANT A DIPLOMA?

We would certainly recommend all workers in the field of optics, to take a course of study and secure a graduates *Diploma*, if their means and time will permit of it. There can be little doubt that the time is coming, and not so far distant either, when all States will legislate and require all Opticians and Dealers in Glasses, to be a graduate and possess a Diploma from some reputable College, as is now done in the case of Druggists, Doctors and Dentists. The signs of the times all point in that direction, so you would probably only anticipate matters a little, if you take a course now. You would find it a paying investment at any rate, for you would be able to do better work, largely increase the volume of your business and get better pay for it.

We have two courses to offer you—attendance or correspondence—either one of which entitles you to a Diploma: One, to come to our city and attend College until you graduate— or remain at home and at work, and take a correspondence course. The latter offers many advantages, and as a rule, we would recommend this course in preference. Much time and expense can be saved, and after completing the Correspondence Course and receiving the Diploma, you are cordially invited, if you see fit, to spend a week at our College in Chicago, without extra charge—although this addition to the course is not necessary, as we thoroughly equip the graduate for his practical work before granting the Diploma or conferring the degree of "Doctor of Optics." If convenient, however, and you do come, we can promise you that one week spent with us in reviewing, will accomplish more than two months, if the rudiments of the subject were not understood before.

Our course is thorough, practical and simple, and the advancement of our students depends upon their application to the work and their own ability.

Our methods of instruction are absolutely effectual—they not only give the student a technical knowledge, but the practical work is perfectly comprehended. We avoid as much as possible all technicalities and endeavor to select the practical points that are applicable in every day business.

Six weeks is the usual time required by our correspondence students and four weeks by our attendant students; we have had exceptional cases where the work was mastered in a less time. But an attractive feature of our course is, that students are not limited to a specified time, but progress as leisurely or as rapidly as they are able to comprehend the work.

Full particulars to those interested, sent on application.

Many early opticians didn't want training as much as they wanted the status provided by a diploma. Responding to this need, many wholesalers offered training and the important diploma. This is from a Coulter Optical ad, circa 1897.

George Frick, a Baltimore physician who received his medical degree in 1815 from the University of Pennsylvania and later studied abroad. In 1823, he published his famous book "A Treatise on the Diseases of the Eye". North and Frick both practiced general medicine with particular attention to the eye. Elkanah Williams, a Cincinnati doctor, however, is considered the first physician in America to confine his practice to diseases of the eye, ear, nose and throat. After receiving his degree from the University of Louisville and studying ophthalmology abroad, Williams returned to Cincinnati in 1855 and practiced his specialty exclusively. Dr. Henry Willard Williams of Boston seems to have been the first to give a clinical course in ophthalmology to a class at Harvard Medical School in 1850. He was one of the founders, in 1864, of the American Ophthalmological Society and its president for many years.

Ophthalmology Centers

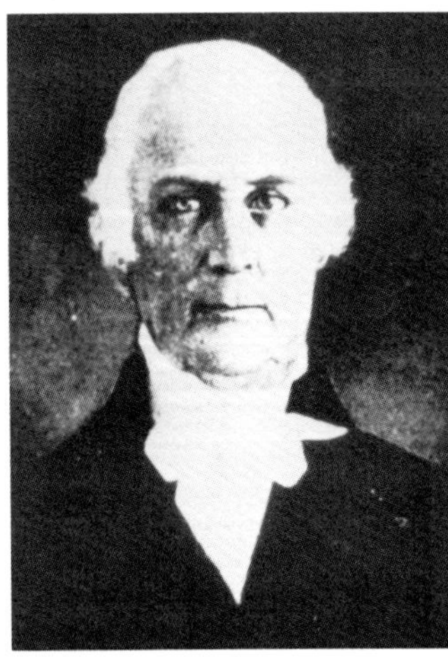

Elisha North is acknowledged as the first American eye specialist and founded the first American hospital specializing in treatment of the eye.

Ophthalmology centered in New York, Philadelphia, and Boston in the mid-19th century but doctors still depended on European training and innovations. Until mid-century, most medical doctors had no professional titles, little training and did few refractions. The discovery that was mainly responsible for ophthalmology's emergence as a specialty was the development of the Ophthalmoscope in 1850 by Hermann von Helmholtz, a German oculist. The information about the eye revealed by this new instrument was a major milestone in the advancement of ophthalmology. The Trial Case, introduced in 1881, made it easier for professional men to conduct refractions. This development; combined with the Ophthalmoscope, enabled the oculist *(as well as the sight-testing optician or optometrist)* to conduct better refractions.

Oculists and Opticians

By late 19th century, however, it was often the medical profession that determined how opticians would fit the glasses they prescribed as oculists began to realize that poorly fit glasses could invalidate their prescriptions. So, oculists would examine the eyes, determine the pupillary distance, the vertex distance required, the pantoscopic tilt of the frame desired and the eye and bridge sizes. In other words, just about everything that the "manufacturing optician" needed to make, or supply the glasses prescribed.

As the 19th century waned, the oculist progressed in both knowledge and ability and by the early part of the 20th century was becoming the ophthalmologist we know today. Ophthalmologists performed surgery in the 19th century and as their surgical techniques improved, the scope of their operations became broader. Their knowledge of the eye, optics and vision requirements increased rapidly. Meanwhile "manufacturing opticians" gradually became "dispensing opticians" and manufacturing came to be the province of lens or frame manufacturers and optical laboratories.

Academy of Ophthalmology

The American Academy of Ophthalmology and Otolaryngology was formed in 1896 and only ophthalmologists who satisfied the rigid requirements of the Academy were permitted to join. By the 1950s, their annual convention *(held at the Palmer House in Chicago)* was one of the largest conventions held in any profession or industry in the United States - attended by more than 10,000. In fact, the Academy became so large that, in 1979, the Otolaryngologists spun off to form their own association. In 1990, attendance at the Academy of Ophthalmology convention in Atlanta, Georgia was more than 20,000 *(including a large foreign contingent who have their own Pan American division)*. It seems almost a commentary on the times that, when the Academy held its convention in Las Vegas in 1988 with attendance over 15,000, this enormous convention was eclipsed a few weeks later when the computer industry met and attracted almost ten times as many participants.

Rebates

Ophthalmologists benefited directly from their association with opticians and with AO and B&L when these two manufacturers entered the retail business. Better patient care could be provided because of coordinated efforts of refractionist, dispenser and manufacturer. A less visible benefit, however, was the widespread practice of accepting direct or indirect rebates from dispensing houses. It's quite understandable how the practice started. Fees charged by Ophthalmologists were so low,

($5 was typical for an examination fee and less than $100 for cataract surgery) rebates became essential to maintain a comfortable living standard. When the practice of rebating ceased in 1948, many Ophthalmologists started dispensing, making up what they had lost from rebates by serving as their own opticians. At first the Academy *(under William Benedict, MD, who ran the Academy for many years as Executive Director, and A.D. Ruedeman, MD, his principal assistant, with a large practice in Detroit)* was against this practice. Younger men, however, took over, many of whom operated dispensing operations in their offices. The Academy's attitude changed to the point that today many ophthalmologists are now dispensing.

There was a time, in the 1980s, when many ophthalmologists soured on dispensing, not because of the headaches involved but because they were benefiting from other extraordinary income. In the 1960s, many benefited from contact lenses but competition gradually reduced the number of contacts dispensed by the medical profession *(optometrists and many opticians also fitted contact lenses)* as well as the fees that could be charged.

Intra-Ocular Lenses

Then came intra-ocular lenses *(IOLs)* which proved to be a bonanza for the profession. Each eye could mean gross income of $3,000 or more - most of it paid by third party *(Medi-Care, insurance, etc.)*. A physician doing only two or three implants a week could get by very well. There was panic in the late 1980s when the Social Security Administration, deciding that IOL costs were too high, started cutting back fees. Ophthalmological incomes plummeted, setting off a renewed interest in dispensing.

In today's market, there is a sharp division between ophthalmologists who serve private patients and those who concentrate on Health Maintenance Organizations *(HMOs in which the federal government pays a group of medical doctors so much per person signed up for that group to provide complete medical services without further cost to the government)*. Most eye doctors now practice in groups that tend to be either HMO-oriented or aimed at private patients

Ironically, the relationship between ophthalmology and optometry has never been better as ophthalmologists depend on optometrists for a large percentage of referrals for IOLs. The new concentration of optometric services in what has been considered traditional medical areas may change this.

Opticianry

It wasn't until the middle of the 19th century that opticians handling only optical merchandise began to spring up around the country. Some of the earliest ones were in Philadelphia, following the lead of McAllister, Zentmayer, *(he has the distinction of being the first to limit his business to fitting spectacles from ophthalmologists' prescriptions)* and followed 25 years later by Ivan Fox, John L. Borsch, George Mayer and Wall & Ochs a little later. In 1853, the year the railroad was completed between Rochester and Syracuse, N.Y., Edward E. Bausch, a brother of John Jacob Bausch *(B&L)* began selling eyeglasses. He would diagnose the problem, grind the lenses and fit them into frames. For a while, his firm was known as Bausch & Dransfield, but later used the name E. E. Bausch & Sons, Inc.

Early American opticians were located mostly in the east. A major center was Philadelphia which boasted a large community of German-trained opticians. They helped to expand businesses such as those started by William Richardson *(he owned a hardware business and sold optical goods to customers like Thomas Jefferson)* and John McAllister, a Scotsman who took over Richardson's business in 1799 as a supplement to his own factory manufacturing canes and whips. Besides selling eyeglasses, most early opticians also sold binoculars, telescopes and other optical-type goods.

McAllister and his son, John Jr., *(See Chapter 3)* who joined his father in 1811, would insert lenses imported from Germany into frames they manufactured. It was 1825 before they had ready access to minus power lenses to supplement their convex lens stocks. McAllister is credited for manufacturing the first cylindrical correction for astigmatism in the United States in 1828, 40 years before a cylindrical correction was written by an oculist. They also produced what they called "cylindrical lenses". These were actually

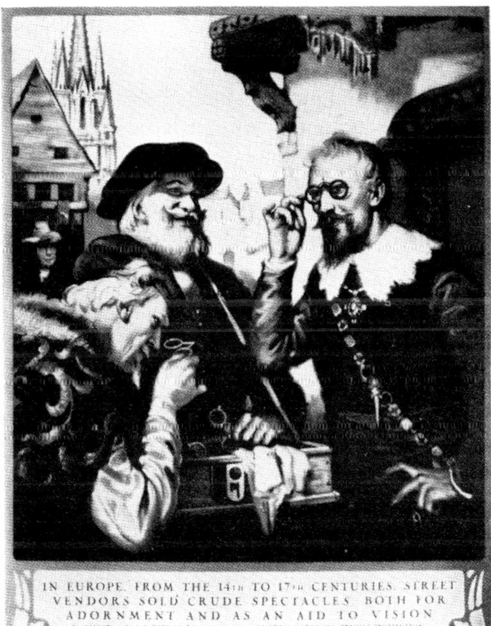

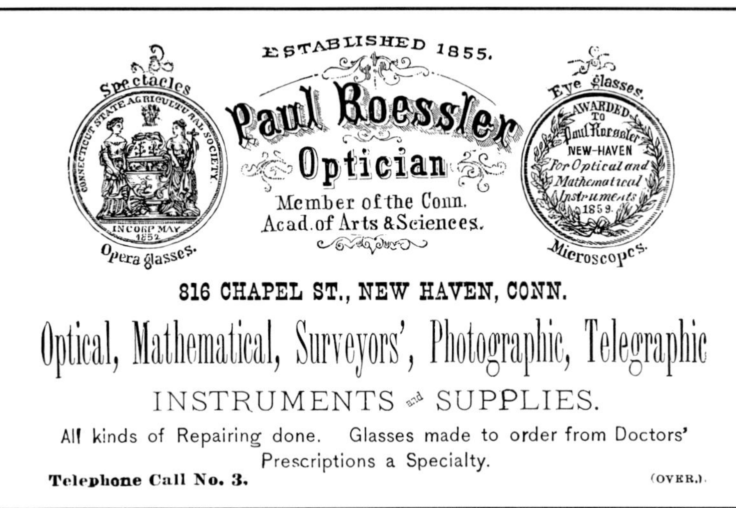

This interesting specimen of 19th century advertising was written by Paul Roessler, founder of the firm now called Fritz and Hawley. Notice the telephone number "Call No. 3", indicating Roessler was an early subscriber in the first commercial telephone exchange in the world.

COURTESY OF FRITZ AND HAWLEY

cross cylinders which acted like spherical lenses but corrected certain aberrations. True cylinder lenses, as we know them, would not be available until mid-19th century. McAllister also imported microscopes, prisms and other precision optics. When John McAllister, Jr. retired in 1853, he had accumulated $400,000, a huge fortune by mid 19th century standards.

Refracting

It was John McAllister, Jr. who first tested eyes at the Wills Eye Hospital. Testing was basically a trial-and-error method of trying different powers until one enabled the patient to see better - all corrections were spherical and both eyes were always given the same power. The major criteria considered were the patient's age, sex, and the distance at which the patient could read small print. After the death of John, Sr. in 1830, the McAllister business continued with James W. Queen, Walter B. Dick, and W. Y. McAllister *(son of John, Jr.)* until Queen, an apprentice to the McAllisters, left to form his own business in 1853. The McAllister family heirs continued operating McAllister's until 1928.

A Modern Dynasty

One of the oldest optician firms still going strong today is Fritz & Hawley of New Haven, Connecticut. The firm began in 1855 when Paul Roessler, an optician with a German science degree opened the first optical store between New York and Boston as well as the first one in Connecticut. Four years later the State Agricultural Society awarded Roessler a medal of excellence for optical and mathematical instruments. In 1910, the company was purchased by the Fritz & Hawley Company. Gustave G. Fritz was president and George Hawley, a former apprentice of Fritz, was vice president and partner.

Fritz & Hawley became charter members of the newly formed Guild of Prescription Opticians. In 1934, they installed air conditioning becoming the first retail store

in Connecticut to do so. The store was redecorated and a miniature theatre for demonstrations and private showings of motion picture films was installed. In 1954, the company set up an "Eye Style Center", the first of its kind in New England. B&L, AO, the Guild and the BVI all made special presentations at the company's 100th anniversary in 1955.

Craig Fritz and Russell Fritz, Jr. assumed ownership in 1985 and remain partners. Today the company operates three stores. G. Fritz, Ed Fritz and Russell Fritz are all past presidents of the Guild. Russell Fritz, Sr. was president of the OAA. Pam Fritz, wife of Craig Fritz, has been a well-known national lecturer and marketing consultant for over 20 years. In many ways, the firm of Fritz & Hawley typifies the best in professional retail dispensing.

Guild of Prescription Opticians

The Guild of Prescription Opticians was founded as a local association in Philadelphia in 1915 by the "Chestnut Street Opticians". These were a long row of Opticians that included Wall & Ochs, J. E. Limeburner, Bender & Off, Street, Propper and Lindert, Bonschur & Holmes, and Joseph Zentmayer.*(a highly respected and skillful optician in the late 19th century).* These companies represented the more ethical of the nation's non-refracting opticians, having received training at McAllister or Queen. About the same time another group was established in New York City with E. B. Meyrowitz as president.

Peter Meyer, however, dreamed of a national organization. In the early months of 1926, he approached Lionel Topaz, editor of the newly founded OPTICAL INDEX distributed to every dispensing optician in the country. Topaz was asked to help support a national Opticians Guild. The organizing went smoothly and a charter was granted in 1927. The previous fall, Peter Meyer had been elected president and Harry Shimwell of Philadelphia was secretary. Among the founding members were E. B. Meyrowitz of New York City, Carpenter & Hughes of Syracuse, N.Y., Waldert Opticians and Whelpley & Paul of Rochester, N.Y., Buffalo Optical and Prechtel Optical of Buffalo, N.Y. and Fritz & Hawley in Connecticut. The purpose was to promote ethical *(i.e. non-refracting)* opticianry and support medical doctors.

In March, 1927, the Guild took out a full-page ad in the OPTICAL INDEX soliciting members. This was so effective that when the Guild met formally in Buffalo a few months later, the membership had trebled. Reporting on this second annual meeting, the INDEX reported: *"It can be looked upon as one of the most important gatherings in the annals of dispensing opticians . . . It (the Guild) has gathered about itself the progressive element of the dispensing men, who were alert to recognize the profit to be derived through the influence of an organized body."*

Guild opticians did not refract and, for this reason, parted company with optometry. Highly conservative in their principles and quite restrictive in their membership, they paralleled the American Optometric Association, with considerable rivalry, however. In 1970, they changed their name to Opticians Association of America, extended their membership to include more opticians, and continued to promote Opticianry through a membership which today includes both individual and chain opticians. In 1991, several major chains dropped their membership because of conflicting views on proposed restrictive legislation which was considered to be contrary to the best interest of the continually expanding chains. Traditional opticians reached their peak in the 1960s and then began to shrink in numbers as smaller optician chains were acquired by bigger chains.

Optician Chains

Opticianry chains existed throughout the nation as early as the turn of the century. E. B. Meyrowitz, besides a number of branches in New York, had branches in St. Paul, Minn., and Seattle, as well as Paris and London. This company also had a substantial wholesale business and, through the Kryptok Company which Meyrowitz controlled, mandated who could handle bifocals and at what prices. They manufactured the bifocals in their lens factory which ultimately became General Optical, later acquired by Shuron.

M. H. Harris and John F. Hill also had substantial retail businesses in New York. Montgomery-Frost and Andrew J. Lloyd *(run by the Collinson family who were very influential with Shuron)* had multi-branch locations in Boston and other parts of New England. Edmonds Opticians and Franklin Opticians *(who fitted lenses to Abraham Lincoln)* were in Washington DC. S. Galeski in Richmond, Va. and the Shenandoah Valley, after selling their business to B&L, later repurchased the retail business in 1948 when B&L was forced out of retail. Other chains included Ballard's in Atlanta; Barnett Opticans in New Orleans, Shadford & Fletcher and Symonds-Atkinson in Denver, Superior Optical and Spratt Optical in Los Angeles and Western Optical in Seattle. Jenkel Davidson in San Francisco had 65 stores in the Bay area by 1956. All of these were large, multi-location retail operations and most operated their own laboratories. Many of them also serviced ophthalmologists with instruments, often on extended credit terms and with reciprocal referrals.

Benson Optical

Benson Optical, for example, acquired Shaler and Crawford in Pittsburgh, L. M. Prince in Cincinnati, J. H. Penny in New York, House of Vision in Chicago, Bayne in Detroit, Shadford-Fletcher and Symonds Atkinson in Denver. Jenkel-Davidson, Parsons, and Wooster in San Francisco, and others in the Northwest, Texas, New Mexico, and the East. Several of these optician chains had been acquired by House of Vision before Benson swallowed them up. Benson, in turn, was acquired by Frigitronics, a publicly listed small manufacturer of medical and surgical devices, who also owned Ostertag Opticians, a major dispensing chain headquartered in St. Louis, Mo., and Oklahoma City. Ostertag was then combined with Benson's stores.

Benson suffered severe financial reverses *(as did all those companies acquired by them)* because of changing conditions in the optical business. Ophthalmologists started to dispense in larger numbers, eliminating the optician's prime source for referrals. Competition from price advertisers became fierce, the super-store concept began, and Benson's non-optical managers were unable to cope with the peculiarities of the industry. The General Electric Credit Corporation sold controlling interest in Benson to a financial group headed by Martin Franklin, who hired new management. Tim McKissick, whose optical experience included Lenscrafters, resigned in 1992 and, after a short interim period, Martin Franklin took over as chairman with Jack Gunion *(whose experience includes other retail chains)* as president. The company has closed or sold a number of stores and embarked on an acquisition program which included the 38 store Superior Optical operation in Southern California and stores owned by Franklin Optical in Northern California.

As this book was written, Benson was completing efforts to purchase Optical Radiation Corporation, primarily to acquire The Omega Group, a major wholesale chain of laboratories and has announced publicly that they intend to divest themselves of their retail businesses.

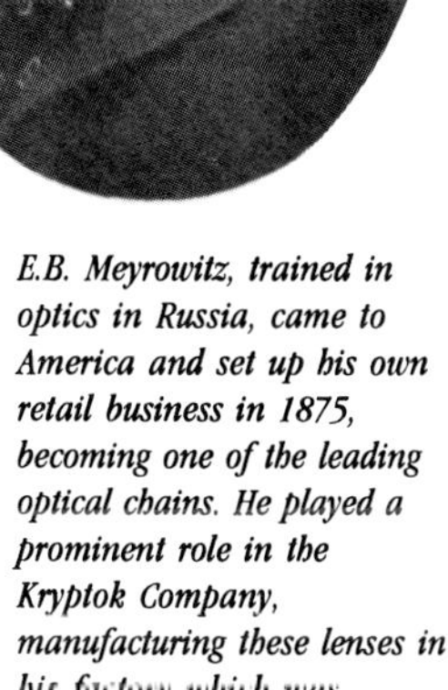

E.B. Meyrowitz, trained in optics in Russia, came to America and set up his own retail business in 1875, becoming one of the leading optical chains. He played a prominent role in the Kryptok Company, manufacturing these lenses in his factory which was ultimately acquired by Shuron.

Retailers who had a Kryptok license made sure everyone knew they could supply this new bifocal. This attractive window display won an award from the Kryptok Company for this office. Circa 1915.

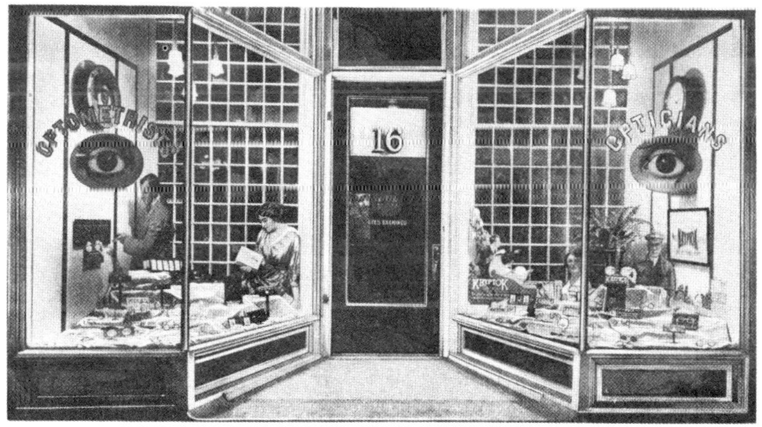

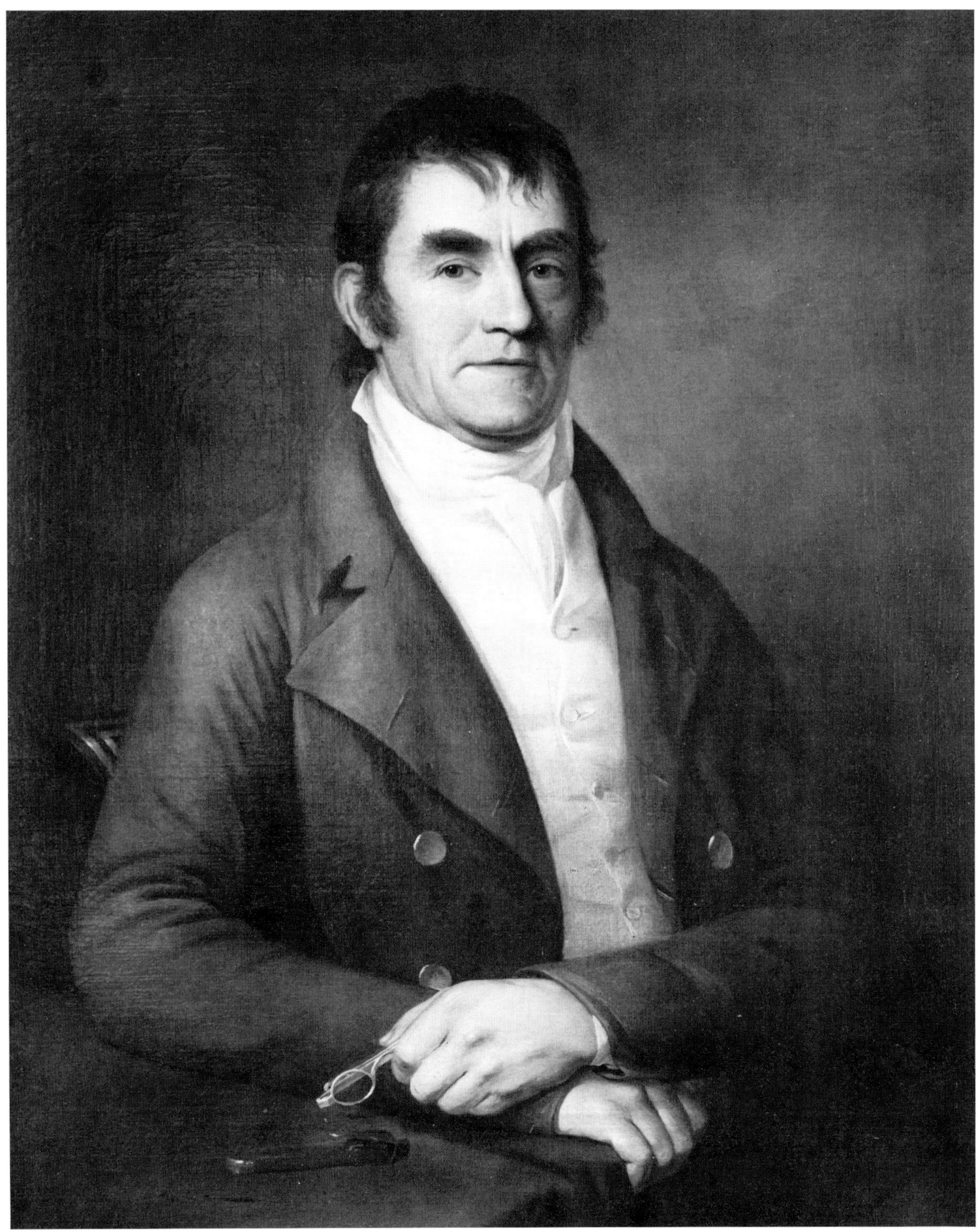

John McAllister - painted by James Peale in 1812.

John McAllister can truly be called the father of the American ophthalmic industry. He set up the firm of McAllister & Company in 1783 in Philadelphia and has the distinction of founding a profession and an industry. He was a man who started out as a shopkeeper and died a man of science and founder of a profession. He and his son were the first in the New World to grind cylinder lenses in 1828. Clients of his firm included Thomas Jefferson (whose glasses were made from drawings supplied by Jefferson) as well as Presidents Madison, Monroe and Jackson.

After the Wills Eye Hospital was established, their surgeons relied on the McAllister firm to test eyes as well as produce eyewear for their patients. The company survived well into the 20th century under a variety of McAllister names. John McAllister died on May 12th, 1830.

Chapter 3
Optical Pioneers

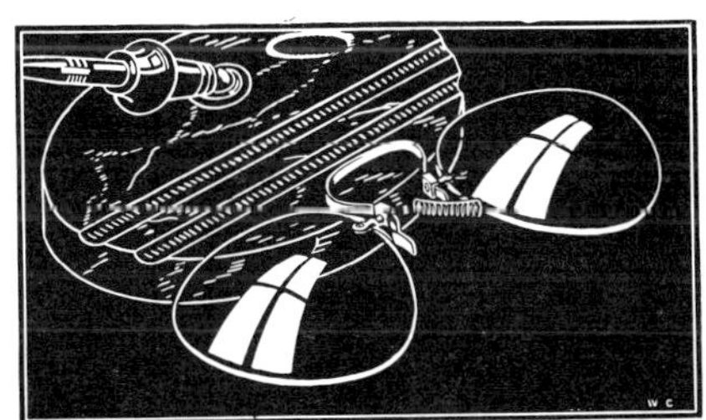

George Washington Wells

Emerson once wrote, "An institution is the lengthened shadow of a man". It would never be more true than in the story of American Optical Company and George Washington Wells. Here was a New England farm boy with little education but lots of vision who went on to become head of one of America's great industries. He was a man with a dream that probably contributed more to the optical industry than any other single event. It is the story of that Southbridge pioneer - George W. Wells, a man mostly forgotten today. It is impossible, however, to tell a true history of the industry without including the story of George Wells.

He was born at Woodstock, Conn., April 15, 1846. Descended from English stock, his ancestors on both sides came from England less than twenty years after the historic landing of the Mayflower. His boyhood was spent on the family farm. He was an engaging young man who enjoyed everything about farming but he had an unfortunate accident at age four. While playing some boyish game, he fell and broke an ankle. It might not seem serious today, but for 10 years after the accident, Wells was only able to walk with the aid of crutches. He was determined to keep this from becoming a handicap and, by the time he was 14, he walked, played, and worked like any of his friends. He never referred to this infirmity and in later years, friends never knew of it.

Only 15 when his father became totally disabled, young Wells had to run the farm for two seasons. Luckily, he loved farm work and did what was required with good will. This is undoubtedly where his reputation for enduring and enjoying hard work began. He had been the last of nine children born to John Ward Wells and Maria Cheney Wells and had barely a year of formal schooling at Woodstock Academy. The rest of his education came from his sister Elizabeth who taught him at home. She must have done a good job because at the age of 17 he was teaching school at Naversink Highlands

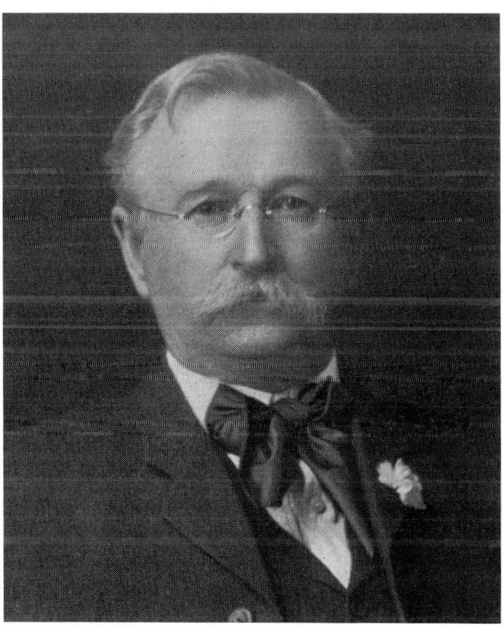

George Washington Wells

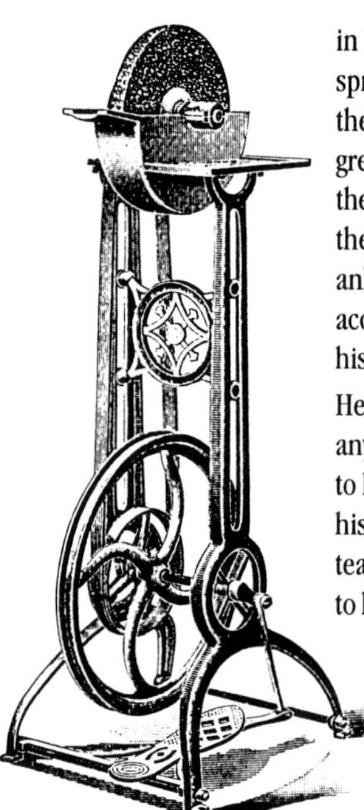

Opticians handstone (circa 1880). Notice foot treadle so operator could turn the stone as they edged the lenses.

in Red Bank, N.J. Once the school term was over in the spring of 1864, he returned to the farm. Perhaps from the influence of his grandfather Captain Henry Wells and great-grandfather Thomas Wells, both of whom fought in the Revolutionary War, the 17 year old volunteered for the Union Army. He was rejected because of his weak ankle and it was a big disappointment - his brother was accepted and remaining on the sidelines was a blow to his pride and ambition.

He tired of teaching. He had always been interested in anything of a mechanical nature and he was determined to learn a trade to gain experience and take advantage of his mechanical abilities. He had saved $50 while teaching. Taking this, along with an additional $50 left to him by his mother, the tall, handsome farm boy went to Southbridge, Massachusetts to live and work with his brother Hiram, who was already working in the optical business.

Optical Career

On April 2, 1864, still not 18 years old, he was hired as one of 11 employees at R. H. Cole & Co. The custom at the time was to serve a three year apprenticeship, but his natural aptitude for mechanical things made this unnecessary. His quick intelligence and unusual ability to concentrate on a task made him a fast learner at the art of making complete spectacles. William Freeman taught him how to make silver spectacles and how to set lenses in frames. His first month's pay was $15.

Three months later, incoming orders slowed and George was "laid off". Within nine months, however, he was back with Cole learning how to make spectacles from steel. Steel frames were an exciting innovation and it took him just a month to acquire skills that usually took years to master. During this period he began to tinker with materials. He wanted to improve the way things were made, to find shortcuts or to eliminate waste.

Once he gained the ability to make steel spectacles, he left Cole and went to work for E. Edmonds & Son, another small spectacle shop that had sprung up down the street. His previous boss missed Wells because of his ability to design and build all the new tools and dies his mind would devise. Cole was determined to get him back and offered him the unheard of pay of $3 a day. In later life he often wondered, "Why the firm could afford to pay a boy of 19 this phenomenal wage is yet an open

question." Cole evidently knew exactly what he was doing because later events proved that when he hired George W. Wells, he gained a mechanical genius.

Completely engrossed in his work, Wells now plunged into the job of changing the nature of optical manufacturing. Some machines he built during that period were still in use 75 years later. Basic principles he developed were used throughout the optical industry. Here are a few of his developments. While they may not seem revolutionary today, they were remarkable concepts at the time he initiated them.

> He discovered a new and better way of edging split bifocal lenses (these were state-of-the-art bifocals at the time but a monster to manufacture).

> He designed eccentric rolls used to taper spectacle stock material.

> He built the first lens cutting machine, only slightly modified for use some eighty years later.

> He created equipment for fitting in endpieces, for automatic milling and tapping of spectacle endpieces and for jumping and forming spectacle bridges.

> He discovered the wonderful cutting properties of the Cragleith stone, widely used from that point on for the edging of lenses.

At this point he decided to go into business for himself. It was 1869 and he looked at locations in New York and New Jersey but, in the end, came back to the area he knew best, familiar Southbridge. George and brother Hiram bought out H.C. Amnidown & Company and brought in C.S. Edmonds as a minority stock holder. At this same time, his previous boss Mr. Cole made one last offer for George to come back to R.H. Cole & Company, this time as a partner. George was most concerned about his brother Hiram so, after a great deal of negotiations, it was decided to merge the two firms and incorporate as a new company. No one knows who came up with the idea but the imposing name chosen for the merged company was "American Optical Company". This was just five years from the time George Wells left the family farm. He was 23 years old.

The New Company

By agreement, the partners decided George would serve as clerk of the new firm (an old English designation for "secretary") owning 40 out of the 400 shares of stock and R.H. Cole would be president. In describing the purpose of the new company, the original incorporation papers stated the company was "incorporated to manufacture and sell spectacles of gold, silver, steel and plated

Advertisement for steel spectacles. Frames made of steel were first produced by American Optical, starting a fad that lasted for more than sixty years. Steel frames usually had bluing applied to protect the finish from rusting (much like gun barrels).

metals, also rings, thimbles and such other articles as said company may from time to time desire to make."

Up to now, Wells had devoted his mechanical genius to manufacturing methods. In spite of the fact that all these new methods were fitting into a definite pattern, his real vision (and genius) was concern for the new company's future. Vague shapes were beginning to take form in his imagination.

By 1891, Wells had been elected president of American Optical and the United States was undergoing a rapid and remarkable economic and industrial expansion. By now railroads had joined the North with the South, the East with the West and the new American empire was welded together with thousands of miles of steel track. Up to now, distribution of manufactured goods had been restricted by primitive transportation. The railroads now opened up these far-flung markets.

Wells visualized a vast industry employing hundreds, maybe even thousands of workmen with highly specialized skills, turning out better spectacles faster and cheaper than ever before. In his mind's eye, he could see a day coming when spectacles would no longer be a luxury for the wealthy few. He believed that economies of large scale production could bring spectacles within everyone's reach. He even believed the day would come when European ships would no longer bring optical goods into American harbors. Instead, American ships would carry optical goods to all the ports of Europe.

Wells knew standardization of optical goods with interchangeable parts had to come about. As president of the American Optical Company, he had the power to make this vision come to pass. The plant expansion, mechanical operations, financing, patents, machinery, selling and trade relations were all designed to fit his master plan.

There was a time when Wells felt threatened by shoddy foreign goods coming into the country. He lobbied successfully for a protective tariff to eliminate this threat. The interests of the American Optical Company took him into almost every state in the Union and on frequent trips abroad. This provided Wells with an extensive personal network of influential optical people, both in America and abroad.

From a small factory on the Quinebaug River employing 11 employees making spectacles by the dozen, Wells built up an industry that ranked with the leading commercial enterprises of the nation, employing thousands of skilled workers turning out products known throughout the optical industry and traded in every country in the world. George Washington Wells died in 1912 at age 66 but his family continued to manage the affairs of American Optical Company until 1949.

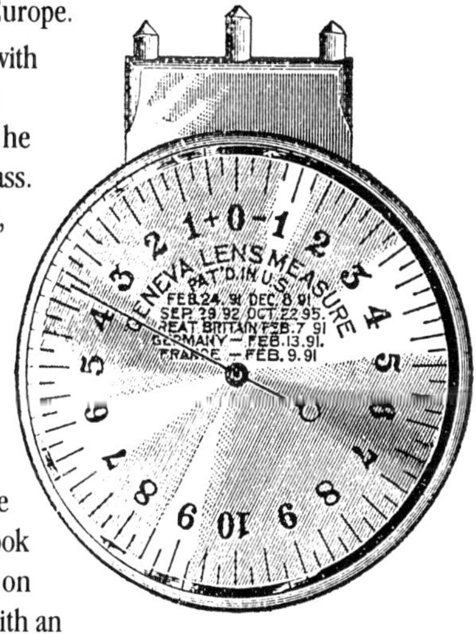

Lens clock. Patented in 1891, this was a necessary tool for every optician in the days before lensometers. The same basic instrument is still used today.

John Jacob Bausch

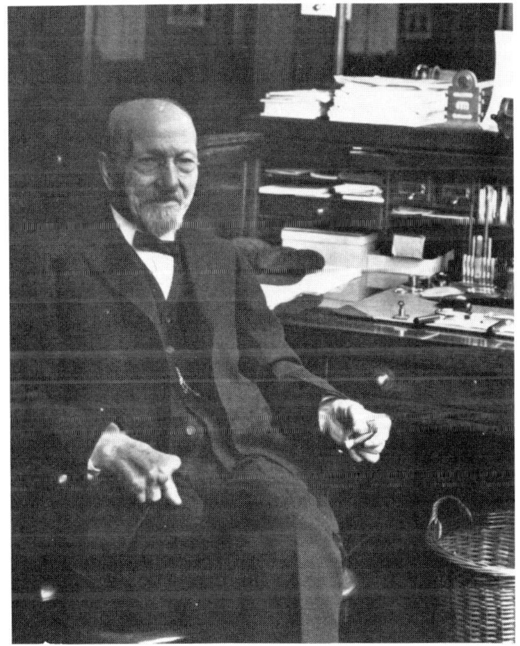

John Jacob Bausch - One of the last photographs taken before his death in 1926.

John Jacob Bausch was one of those tenacious men who hang on, determined to succeed in their goals in spite of whatever comes their way. Young Bausch was born in Gross Suessen, Germany on July 25, 1830. Early on, he became an apprentice in the optical field, learning to grind lenses and make spectacle frames out of horn. Looking to advance himself in his new field, he set out on foot to Berne, Switzerland to continue his optical education. There, he landed a job as the only worker in a small optical shop where he made spectacles and sold them for 6 cents a pair. He was able to make six pairs a day by working from morning to night.

Times were bad in Europe and, like so many others, Bausch heard wondrous tales of America, where fortunes could be made overnight. On the 26th of April, 1849, he set out for the New World. It took 49 days to cross the ocean to New York City. Landing in 1849, he was told New York was full and he should head west. After two days on the train, he arrived in Buffalo only to find a cholera epidemic raging with most of the population fleeing the city. The only work he could find was as a cook's helper, then a porter. There were no opticians in

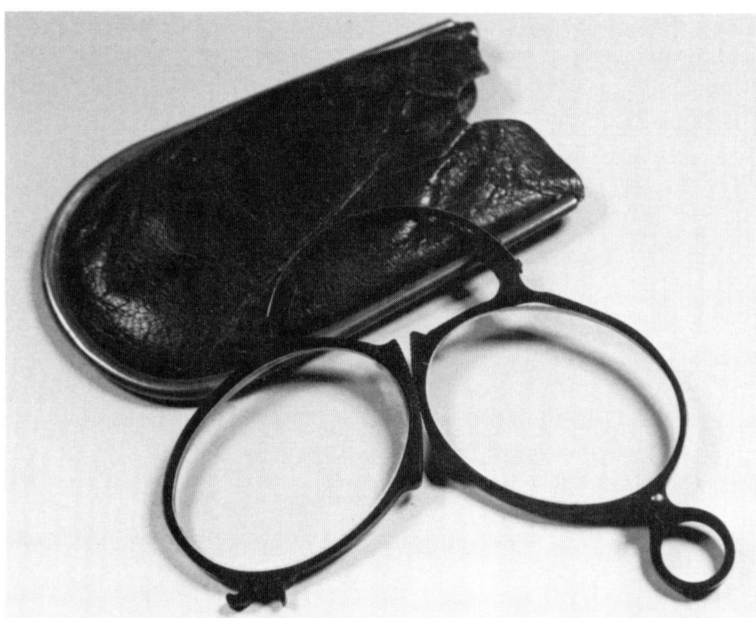

Hard rubber Pince-Nez frame manufactured by Bausch & Lomb with original case. Frame folds together to fit in case.

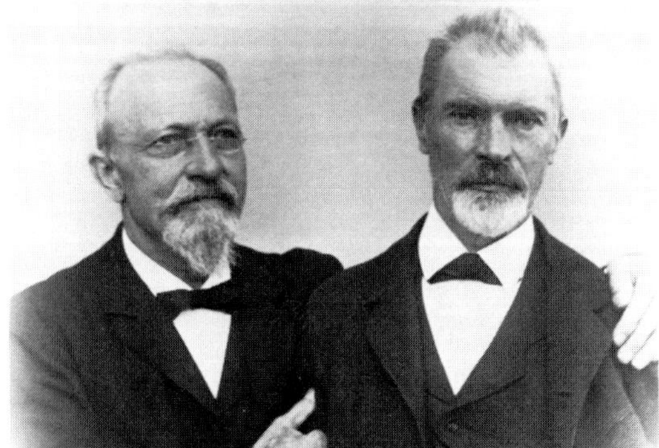

John Jacob Bausch and his partner Captain Henry Lomb.

Buffalo so he couldn't continue in his chosen field. Moving to Rochester, N.Y., he found a job in a wood turning establishment for $1 a day. In 1853, he married Barbara Zimmerman and, seven weeks into the marriage, suffered an accident in the wood shop, losing two fingers of one hand. The accident happened on Monday morning. All the young couple had to their name was $7.50, his wages from the previous week.

The following day, his friend Henry Lomb took up a collection from Bausch's friends and brought the couple $28. During his convalescence, Bausch and his wife spent their time discussing the future. He revealed his longtime ambition to set up his own optical business. In the meantime, however, they needed the income from his woodworking job. He wrote his brother in Germany, asking for two hundred gulden's worth of goods which he would pay back over a six month period. Selling the spectacles from his home by advertising in the local paper, he was able to pay off the first loan and send for a second order. Now, at last, he could give up his woodworking job.

The New Shop

He found a 4' by 6' space in the front half of a shoemaker's store in the gallery of Reynold's Arcade in Rochester and set up an optical shop. The furniture consisted of a table and two chairs with a wire strung across the window with frames hanging from it. The room was heated by an old-fashioned stove and fuel for the stove consisted of old shoe parts, creating an aroma not exactly propitious for a retail business. Years later, he would say, "Perhaps it was just as well that few people came to see me, for no one could have remained in the store very long."

Needing more goods for the optical shop, he approached his friend Lomb. Henry was unmarried and had been able to save a little money. Bausch, discovering his friend had saved up $62, borrowed the entire sum from his friend with an unusual promise of security. He promised that if the business ever grew to where it could support a partner, Henry would come in on the same terms as Bausch. No papers were signed. There was never anything but a gentlemen's agreement between them. A short while later, Bausch decided the business would prosper if he had a larger stock of goods. He decided to go to Germany to borrow money. Henry agreed to look after the business while he was gone. When Bausch returned, he took their new goods out to sell in cities and villages in the area while Lomb continued watching the store. Later, Lomb took over the traveling and Bausch ran the store. Borrowing from one friend or another and paying back each loan as it came due, the firm managed to struggle along. Lomb had moved in with the Bausch family and was able to put more money in the business than John Bausch. By the time the Civil War began, the business had produced a net loss. In addition, Bausch now owed Henry Lomb $1,000. He began to worry whether he would ever be successful.

The Civil War was the turning point in the fortunes of John Jacob Bausch. Henry Lomb went in the Army and managed to send most of his Army pay back to Bausch while he was gone. Their fortunes were further helped by the rapid appreciation of the gold dollar. It began to look like the firm might survive.

Frames

Bausch had been making a few frames for his customers out of horn and one day, while walking home to lunch, he spied a piece of hard rubber on the sidewalk. Idly picking it up as he walked, he began to think how well this material might work as a spectacle frame. He began making frames of rubber, preparing the stock of rubber by heating it on his kitchen stove. A watch manufacturer observed what he was doing and placed an order for some watch cases made of rubber. These worked and he came back for more. Meanwhile, the rubber frames were also selling. By the time Lomb came back from the war *(as a Captain),* the company had paid their debts and had $800 in the bank.

In the early days, all turning and polishing was accomplished by foot-power. A move from the Arcade to a small one room location in a two story building at the corner of Andrews and Water Streets was a momentous occasion. The new location included water power from the nearby Genesee River. No more pedaling! They began building what came to be the first power machinery in America for grinding of lenses.

Not that they didn't find problems along the way. Company savings were quickly exhausted as the company grew. There were even times when they were forced to send out invoices before any goods had been shipped. By now, the pressure of the growing business necessitated Bausch selling the retail store to his brother, E. E. Bausch. Christian Altpeter had shared space with the retail business for his watch repair business, but gave up that business to join the young optical company.

Some three years later, Bausch received a letter from the American Hard Rubber & Comb Company offering them exclusive rights to manufacture hard rubber eyeglass frames for the remainder of their patent life. Altpeter, who had already announced he was setting up his own frame business, traveled to New York with Bausch to see the American Comb Company. Bausch even permitted Altpeter to see the Comb Company people first. It didn't help because the company had already decided they preferred Bausch for the contract. Altpeter was shocked to find out he had no source for rubber and told Bausch that he was going to give him a run for his money with the horn eyeglasses he planned to make. It was a sordid ending to a trip that should have been an occasion for joy. The final arrangements with the rubber company were completed several weeks later (1866).

The rubber patent expired six years later. During that period, Bausch and Lomb realized a good profit and later bought the rubber company. They were now operating under the name Vulcanite Optical Instrument Company. Lomb had moved to New York to look after the company's sales, remaining there for 10 years until they decided sales could be handled out of the Rochester office. By now the company had begun manufacturing microscopes and the name "Vulcanite" didn't make much sense. The company name was changed to "Bausch & Lomb Optical Company".

In 1874, the first building on St. Paul Street was built. Bausch's eldest son Edward, who built his first microscope at age 14, won a scholarship to Cornell. At age 22, Edward was put in charge of the B&L booth at the Philadelphia Centennial Exposition where he saw his microscopes win awards. It had been a dream of the founders to make Bausch & Lomb the first in America to manufacture precision optical instruments. B&L microscopes, first manufactured in 1874, grew to rival those produced in Europe, accomplishing that dream.

John Jacob Bausch's son Edward went on to a lifetime of awards, including a medal from the American Society of Mechanical Engineers for "meritorious mechanical developments in the field of optics". Son William was responsible for finding a way for B&L to produce their own glass during the early days of the first World War. By May, 1915, William produced the first successful optical glass. Both sons spent their entire career with their father's company.

Henry Lomb died in 1908 but partner John J. Bausch remained active head of the company he founded for a full three quarters of a century, longer than the average span of life. He continued working until a few months before his death at age 96 in 1926. He was succeeded as company president by his son Edward.

John McAllister

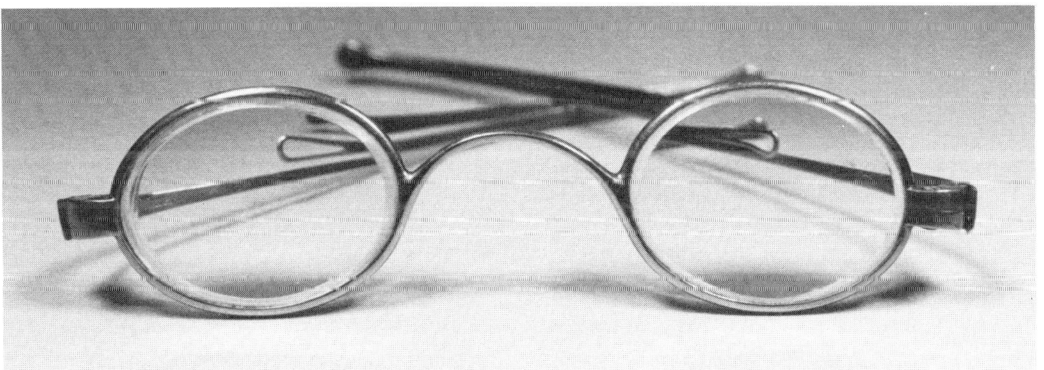

Made of 14 K solid gold, this frame has -13.50 lenses measuring 28 mm by 31 mm Glasses were manufactured by McAllister in 1815. Notice the hinged temples, permitting them to be worn with or without a wig. The beautiful artistry of the frame and the value of the frame material indicate these were undoubtedly made for a very important Philadelphian. This eyeglass is marked "M" in cover photo.

While John McAllister is third on this list of optical pioneers, in point of time, he is the first. Starting out as a seller of whips and canes, then adding glasses, his little store in Philadelphia was located just a few short blocks from where Thomas Jefferson penned the Declaration of Independence and close to the building where the founding fathers framed the Constitution.

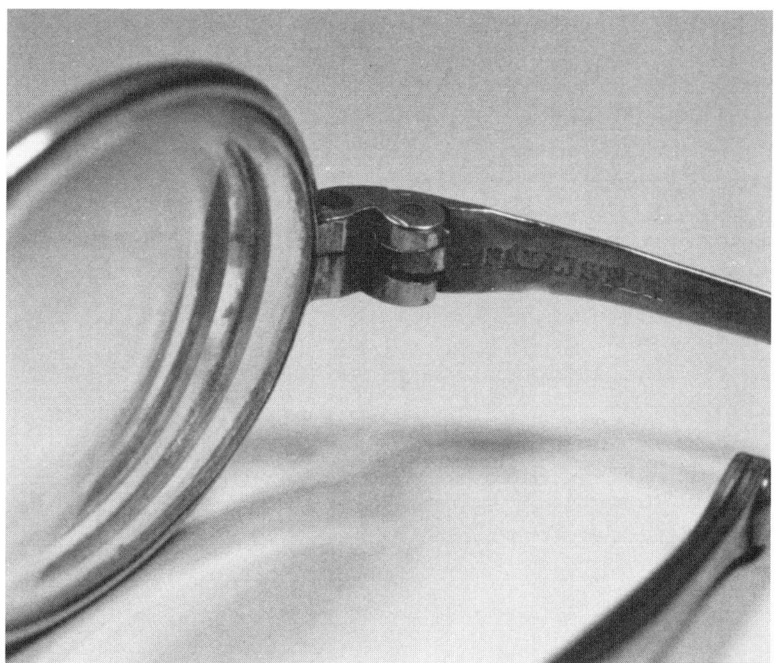

Close-up of the hinge construction of glasses shown on page 29. Notice the McAllister trademark stamped into the temple. This eyeglass is marked "M" in cover photo.

The Founder

McAllister was the first spectacle seller in America to recognize that glasses were not merchandise like the whips and canes he had been selling. He enjoys the unique distinction of founding both a profession and an industry. It was to John McAllister, his renowned son and his firm that the medical profession turned to for advice and guidance in the refracting of eyes. That phase of the activities of the Wills Eye Hospital in Philadelphia revolved around the house of McAllister for many years. Two years before he died, he, or more likely his son, produced the first cylindrical lens ever ground in America for the correction of astigmatism.

This extraordinary Scotchman started out as an ordinary shopkeeper, but died a man of science and the founder of a tradition still honored today. He was born in Scotland in 1753 and arrived in America in 1774. He worked as a journeyman wood turner for some years. McAllister had only been in the country for a year when the Revolutionary War began. He was present at the birth of the nation and as the country grew and prospered, so did McAllister. He holds undisputed claim to being the first important figure in the optical field of his adopted country and was a pioneer in every sense of the word. The optical industry and the McAllister firm owe equal regard to his son, John McAllister, Jr., who carried on the tradition begun by his father.

With the end of the Revolutionary War, McAllister, Sr. went to Philadelphia and started selling whips and canes. The year was 1783 and times were unsettled. His trade was humble but he made it an important one. He added hardware and plated goods and, in 1788, he led the journeymen working for him in a festive parade honoring the adoption of the Constitution. By this time McAllister had become a man of substance in Philadelphia.

Until 1799, his business was confined primarily to making and selling whips and canes. He had bundles of whips delivered from his factory to his store three times a week. The whips were often sold before they could get them in the store. That spring, a Mr. Richardson, well known as a vendor of spectacles, decided to move to the country. McAllister thought these spectacles might make a nice addition to his other goods. He purchased what remained of Richardson's spectacle stock, described by him as *"about as much as we would fill a half peck measure."* The company ran a newspaper ad in 1800 announcing "They mean also to keep a large assortment of spectacles, reading glasses, concave glasses, magnifiers, goggles, etcetera and to put new glasses in old spectacle frames." In 1806 telescopes and microscopes were added to their stock.

McAllister took a keen interest in his new line. He did not prescribe spectacles according to age as was the custom, because he decided age was an undependable way to determine lens power. When new glasses were needed, he advised patrons to send or bring a portion or all of the glasses that gave them good reading vision. He numbered George Washington among his customers *(Philadelphia was the nation's capital at that time)*.

Business was good and getting better. He started a factory near Mt. Airy to produce whips and canes, later manufacturing spectacles there as well. The spectacles were all low priced imported goods of iron, tortoise shell or plated metal. By the time his son entered the firm in 1811, the firm was prospering. Then, in quick succession, came the War of 1812 and another embargo. A diary of the McAllister family noted, *"The embargo of 1812 on imported goods put us to great trouble as neither frames nor glasses were made here."* About 1815, McAllister began producing silver and gold spectacles. *"The silver were heavy sliding sides weighing nearly a dollar"* he wrote a friend.

Whips, in the meantime, were becoming an unprofitable line. Families of the New Bedford whalers, looking for something to do while the family men were at sea, started producing whips as a home industry. Before long they were selling their products for far less than McAllister charged.

Notable Customers

John McAllister, Jr. was now a partner and the firm became known as John McAllister and Son, Dealers in Optical and Scientific Instruments. Many notables of the day came to McAllister's for spectacles. A special pattern was made for Thomas Jefferson while he was president from drawings furnished by Jefferson himself (1796). Grandson William McAllister was to later describe in his diary, *"The glasses were not larger than a ten cent piece and were much used by Jefferson's personal friends in Virginia . . . John Randolph of Roanoke and Presidents Madison and Monroe were often customers."* It was reported that Chief Justice Tilighman *(1815)*, Count Joseph Bonaparte *(1818)*, Henry Clay *(1828)* and President Andrew Jackson *(1841)* were all customers of McAllister.

From that time on, the history of the McAllister family was the story of their business. The father died in 1830 and by that time, the firm had achieved some memorable accomplishments. In 1801, Thomas Young, an English scientist had discovered the principle of astigmatism. In 1827, Sir George Airy, the famous astronomer, applied cylindrical lenses to correct this error of vision. In 1828 the McAllisters became the first opticians in the new country to grind a cylinder lens.

The story was told by the physician Isaac Hay. *"After Sir George Airy had discovered and corrected the myopic astigmatism of his own eyes, an American clergyman, Reverend Mr. Goodrich, who was also nearsighted, had noted in addition that when he looked at lines or branches of a tree or the rigging of a ship, that the parts of objects having a vertical direction were more distinct than those having a horizontal direction."* The good Reverend consulted with the McAllisters who, after studying his case and making tests, furnished him with glasses that had a glass ground plane *(flat)* on one side and a section of a cylinder on the other. The patient's vision was materially improved. Some forty-four years later, these same lenses were to come into the possession of Dr. Henry Noyes of New York. Reverend Mr. Goodrich had made a notation on a sheet of paper that were with

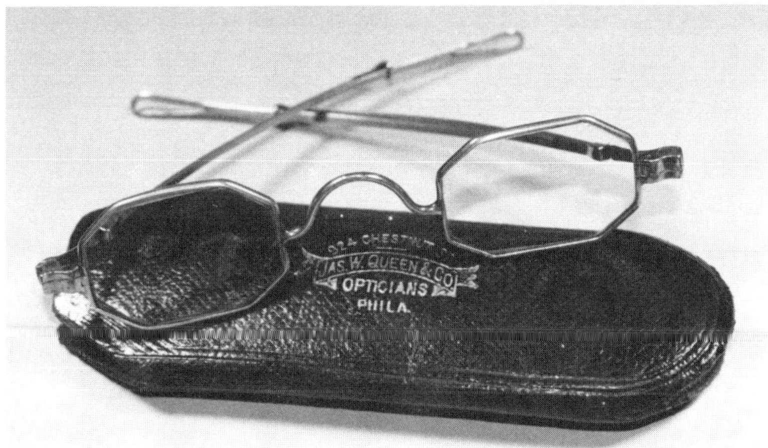

the glasses. The note said, *"Number 7 French number, cylinder concave, got of McAllister, May 1828."* There's little doubt that these were the first plano-cylindrical lenses ground in this country for the correction of astigmatism.

By the time the elder McAllister died in 1830, his name was one of the most famous and honored in Philadelphia. His son only added to its luster. John, Jr. remained with the firm until 1835 when he turned it over to his son William. After the Wills Hospital was established, patients needing glasses were sent to McAllister's. Wills' surgeons relied on them to test eyes as well as grind lenses. John, Jr. also gave Philadelphia the present system of numbering houses by blocks of 100, 200, etc., a system that was copied in Washington and eventually everywhere. He died in 1877 at age 91.

The company survived well into the 20th century under a variety of McAllister names, certainly a remarkable record for any company and a worthy testimonial to the original John McAllister, truly an optical pioneer.

Another example of a McAllister eyeglass (circa 1820). Case was supplied by Queen, a leading wholesaler during the late 1800s. Notice that this pair features sliding temple extensions rather than hinged extensions as on the earlier McAllister frame. This eyeglass is marked "E" in cover photo.

GLASSES FROM DR. WM. ROSENTHAL COLLECTION

A PIONEER OPTICAL JOURNALIST

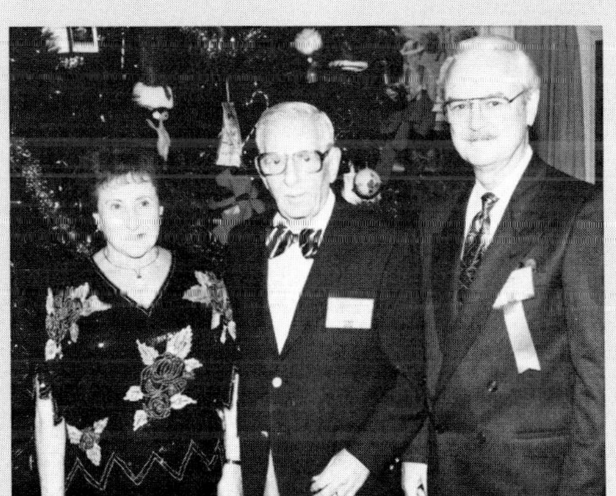

During the 1989 OLA Convention in Nashville, Tenn., the Directors' Choice Award of Excellence was presented to Martin Topaz, long-time publisher and President of the Professional Press. The Topaz family devoted close to 70 years to the growth and betterment of the ophthalmic industry. Marty and his wife Marge were familiar faces at hundreds of optical conventions and meetings. Elliott Shane tells of the time he and his wife met Marty and Marge *(who were on their honeymoon)* for dinner during the 1942 California Optometric Convention in Santa Barbara. A Japanese submarine chose that night to lob a few shells at Santa Barbara *(the only shelling of the U.S. mainland during the war)* and the resulting emergency blackout left them eating in the dark. Marty and his wife are shown with the OLA's Joe Bruneni on the evening of Marty's Award.

PHOTO - OLA OPTICAL INDUSTRY MUSEUM

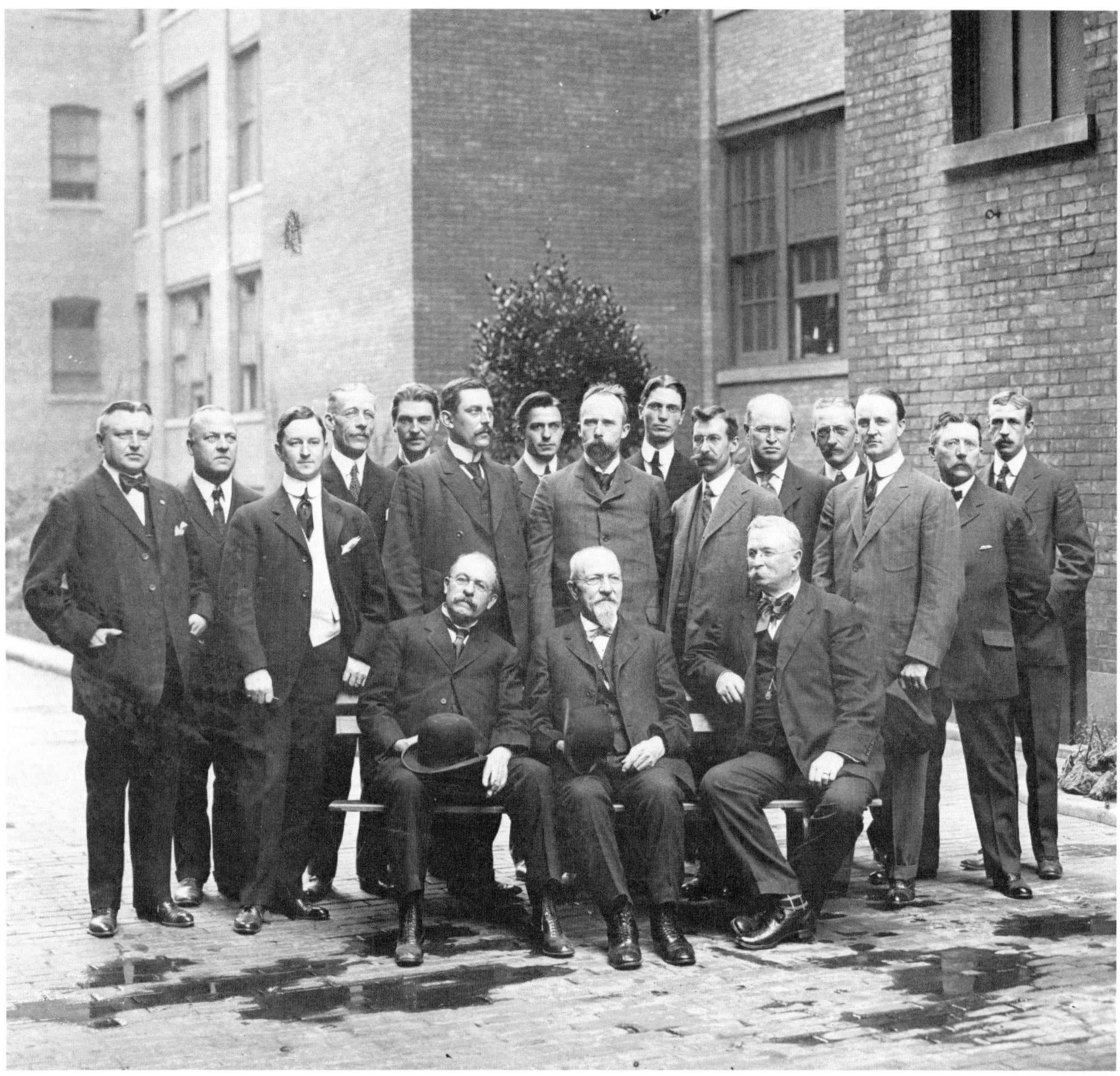

As mentioned elsewhere in this history, the Wells family (AO) and the Bausch family (Bausch & Lomb) were close friends and maintained a cordial working relationship. In this remarkable photo, taken in 1908, the two families had gathered in front of the factory (no one knows which factory) *for this informal portrait of a group of men who controlled more than half of the optical industry at that time.*

Back row: Wm. A.E. Drescher (Bausch's son-in-law), William Bausch, Henry Bausch, Adolph Lomb, George Saegmuller, Jr., Henry Lomb, Jr., Albert Wells, Edward Bausch, Carl F. Lomb (cousin), Lee Seagmuller. Center row: Cheney Wells, Dr. Rudolph Straubel, Dr. Paul Fischer, Fred Saegmuller, Channing Wells. Seated: Fred B. Saegmuller, John Jacob Bausch, George Washington Wells (Note: Bausch's partner Henry Lomb died June 13th of that year).

Regarding these people: William Drescher was married to Bausch's daughter, Anna Julia and rose to position of treasurer. William Baush was John's son. His most notable contribution was development of the company's glass making and he served as B&L's vice president. Henry Bausch, a son, died the following year at age 49. Adolf and Henry were the sons of company co-founder Henry. Edward Bausch was a son of John and served as president of B&L from 1926 when his father died until his death in 1944. He was a noted inventor with a particular interest in scientific instruments. Carl Lomb was Henry's cousin and husband of Caroline Bausch, John's daughter. He was a company vice president. Fred B. Saegmuller had owned a company making astronomical instruments and surveying equipment. He invented the Bore Sight Telescope used on U.S. Naval warships. Bausch & Lomb had been making lenses for their instruments for years and, in 1905, acquired the Saegmuller Company.

Chapter 4
The Major Manufacturers

For much of the 20th century, the major suppliers to independent laboratories were three in number and called "the majors". They were American Optical, Bausch & Lomb and Shuron Optical.

Shuron's strength was their alliance with the independents. From early in the 1920s and for the next 30 years, American Optical

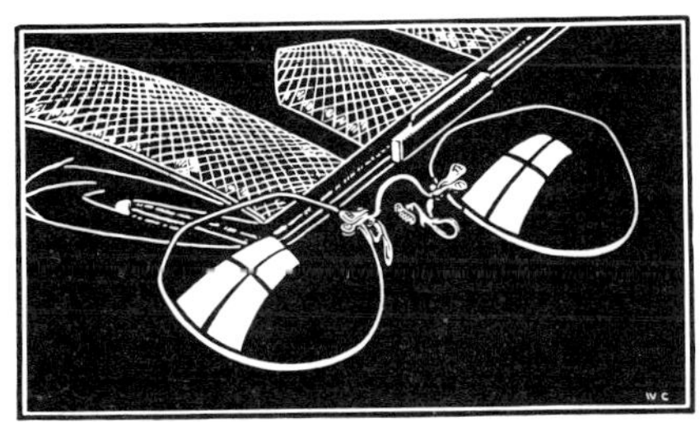

and Bausch & Lomb existed primarily to supply their own laboratories *(and retail dispensaries)*. While a few independent laboratories had AO or B&L listings, they were usually only companies too strong in the marketplace for AO or B&L to ignore. As a rule, independent labs *(not owned by AO or B&L)* turned to Shuron first for a listing, and when unsuccessful at Shuron, turned to Continental or Titmus *(usually in that order)*.

American Optical

It was 1826 when William Beecher founded the Beecher Jewelry Shop in Southbridge, Massachusetts but optical goods weren't added to the products they sold until 1833 *(American Optical always dated the birth of their company to the year 1833)*. The town of Southbridge had 1,600 inhabitants and Beecher's spectacles were the first to be made in that town. Between 1833 and 1840, Beecher employed seven craftsmen making spectacles *(from gold, silver, or steel)* at a rate of one frame per man per day.

By 1839, the business had grown enough to be moved from the jewelry shop to the company's first factory. The following year, Beecher created the first spectacles ever made of steel in the United States, starting a vogue for steel frames that lasted for 60 years. L. H. Ammidown, a competitor, purchased Beecher's interest and, in 1850, R. H. Cole, a Beecher apprentice, became a partner. By

1862, Cole and his son, E. Merritt Cole, owned the company and changed its name to R. H. Cole & Company.

George Washington Wells

George Washington Wells joined the firm as an apprentice in 1864, leaving a Connecticut farm at the age of 17, urged to do so by his brother who worked for Cole. Within three years, Wells was designing and improving the machinery used for manufacturing metal frames.

George Wells, wanting to get ahead in the world, left the firm to buy another frame manufacturer in Southbridge, started by H. C. Ammidown, Beecher's former partner. Cole realized he still needed Wells and after negotiating, the two firms merged so Cole could take advantage of Wells' technical expertise. Upon completion of the

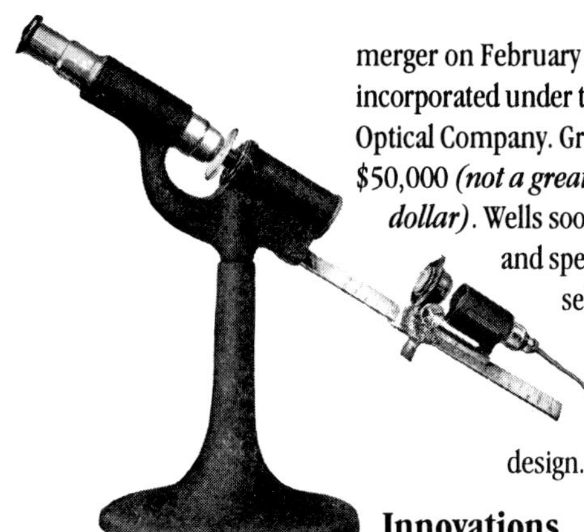

merger on February 26, 1869, the companies were incorporated under the impressive name of American Optical Company. Gross sales for the first year were $50,000 *(not a great deal even translated into today's dollar)*. Wells soon owned 26 percent of the stock and spent much of his time on the road selling. In 1879, he was elected treasurer and his responsibilities increased, but still included production and machinery design.

Innovations

George Wells had a flair for organization and administration and was considered a master builder in the young optical industry. By the time he died in 1912, the company under the administration of George Washington Wells had introduced a number of industry "firsts".

1874	Rimless spectacles
1883	The country's first lens plant
1884	Trial frames
1889	Oculist trial cases
1891	Automatic lens edgers
1891	Gold-filled spectacles
1894	First company catalog
1895	Eyeglass chains
1897	Eyeglass cases
1898	Standardized trial lens sets
1900	Toric lenses
1902	First traveling rep - W.R. Hurlbert

During this period, in addition to domestic expansion, the company opened branches in London (1905), in Chicago (1909), in New York (1910) and San Francisco (1911).

George Washington Wells and his three sons, Channing, Albert and Cheney were all administrators of the company from 1891 to 1912, giving the sons an opportunity to work directly with their father. During the period from 1900 to 1910, a new plant was constructed, much of which still exists today as American Optical headquarters. George Wells spent much of his time between 1879 and 1894 traveling as the company's only salesperson. The three sons were never pampered. They left school and, in 1891, went to work in the company plant, learning the business from the ground up. By the year 1910, the company was doing $9,000,000 a year in sales. Upon George Well's death in 1912, Channing was elected president. Training of the sons had been detailed and the three provided a perfectly balanced administration that enabled the company to continue to prosper.

Lenses

AO continued to grow and the inadequate supply of lenses from Europe began to choke the infant U.S. industry. Optical glass was made in Sheffield, England, ground in Birmingham and shipped to American Optical by Purdam and Boyd. Wells was totally disenchanted with the quality of lenses he was receiving. For one thing, the focus numbers were widely inaccurate *(lenses were categorized at that time by a number, not by foci)*. He felt he had to do something to improve lens quality. No one in the United States had the slightest knowledge about manufacturing lenses but Wells had heard of a family of lens grinders named Wilson who had come over from Sheffield and settled in Mt. Kisco, New York. Tracking them down, he found them grinding lenses on crude machinery in their farm house. Wells offered the senior Wilson a job in Southbridge. He turned the offer down but suggested his son Charlie for the job. Charlie Wilson, who came to be called "Pop", directed the installation of lens-making equipment and served as head of AO's lens production in Lensdale for the next 26 years.

Leaving AO in 1909, Wilson established his own lens plant. By 1912, his first buildings were completed, the start of the United States Lens Company. "Pop" retired after consolidating with Standard Optical and Kirstein Optical in 1925. His grandson, Bob Whiting, went to work for Shuron in 1934, working on a replica of a machine made by his grandfather.

It helps to keep in mind that lenses at this time were biconvex or biconcave *(basically flat)* and spherical in power. Starting with wooden machinery, American Optical produced their first lenses on January 18, 1884. By the fall, Wells was unhappy with the production and condemned all of the new equipment. He had "Pop" Wilson remake all of it in iron, the first iron lens-making machines anywhere in the world. By 1893, the company had added cylinder and compound lenses to their production. It wasn't until the year 1900 that they began producing periscopic or meniscus lenses. These modern, far superior lenses had both concave and convex surfaces and were designed to replace the flat lenses previously used.

B&L had started manufacturing lenses in 1878. By 1884, when America's dependence on European manufacturers lessened considerably, the two industry giants started producing spherical lenses of better quality than those previously imported from Europe. Both companies were able to offer reasonable delivery instead of European delivery that could take as long as a year.

The Wells Family

Wells became President of AO in 1891 when R. H. Cole retired. Gradually the Wells family became the major stockholders of American Optical. The Cole family maintained a minority interest which they constantly used to slow down any progress the Wells family tried to achieve. G. W. Wells turned over responsibility for operations to his sons in 1906 so they could "serve their apprenticeship in management" while he was still able to supervise them. This he managed to do until his death in 1912 at the age of 66. Channing Wells became president and handled sales, J. Cheney Wells left his medical career to run the technical side as well as research and development, and Albert Wells served as treasurer, ran the factory and supervised production. The brothers worked closely together and traveled selling the company's products.

During the many years the industry was controlled by AO and B&L, a close, personal friendship existed between the Wells and the Bausch families. Their two companies enjoyed a strange mixture of fierce competition. A follow-the-leader relationship eventually developed, with Bausch & Lomb usually acceding to policies decreed by AO.

Meanwhile, in 1917, after years of acrimonious relations, Albert Cole finally agreed to sell out to the Wells family who became sole stockholders of American Optical. The three brothers always presented a unified front to the industry although in private their relationship was not always quite so harmonious. All three were as dedicated as their father, George Washington Wells, to the building of the AO empire. Long days at the factory were relieved only by sales trips. The "work ethic" that G. W. Wells had instilled in his sons was passed down to the grandchildren as well. Under the aegis of the three brothers, the company continued to grow and by the 1920s, they controlled at least 40 percent of the entire optical industry.

Although the brothers had children, none of the next generation figured prominently in AO management. The rivalry for succession narrowed down to John, Cheney's son, and George B. Wells, Albert's son. These two vied against each other through prep school and Harvard and joined the company *(together with Greg and Turner, Channing's sons)* in the autumn of 1924. They worked their way up through management until John opted to pursue his interests in aviation in 1939. In 1936, George B. Wells replaced his uncle, Channing, as president of American Optical but was forced to contend with a management committee. A financial executive named Ira Mosher had the title of general manager. The committee, headed by Mosher, included Charles Cozzens as chief sales executive.

The three brothers were still around and subordinate executives soon discovered they could bypass the president and discuss policy directly with the senior brothers. This created problems for George who threatened on several occasions to resign and finally did so in 1946, giving way to Charley Cozzens. Cozzens was the first non-Wells family member to hold the title of president of AO. Cozzens died unexpectedly in 1947 and George returned to take over again. In 1949, he once again relinquished the title to Walter Stewart, a Canadian protégé of Cozzens, who assumed the presidency but established a "committee" type of management.

Instruments

AO had entered the instrument field early in the 20th century, acquiring such companies as Spencer Lens Company, a major instrument manufacturer in Buffalo, since 1892, having started as the Microscope and Telescope Department of Geneva Optical Company, Geneva, N.Y. AO also purchased De Zeng Instrument Company, another instrument manufacturer in New Jersey since 1896. De Zeng developed the phorometers *(an early phoropter which mechanized the eye exam by placing all the refractive lenses required in easy-to-use holders in front of the patient)* and the first phoropters which further streamlined this process. Other instrument makers were also added.

This heavy involvement in instruments enabled the company to gain a handle on oculists who often became dependent on AO for instrumentation, usually financed by AO. As a result the oculists usually referred patients to AO retail branches coming into the retail market in the 1920s. AO also manufactured cases and expanded their frame line to include plastic frames as this new material became available.

At the turn of the century, AO entered the scientific field, producing microscopes, diagnostic instruments, and scientific instrumentation. They helped establish the safety eyewear market, producing frames and special lenses as well as safety equipment and artificial eyes. They were able to offer the retailer - and the public who patronized their retail stores - a complete optical service, with the majority of it manufactured "in house".

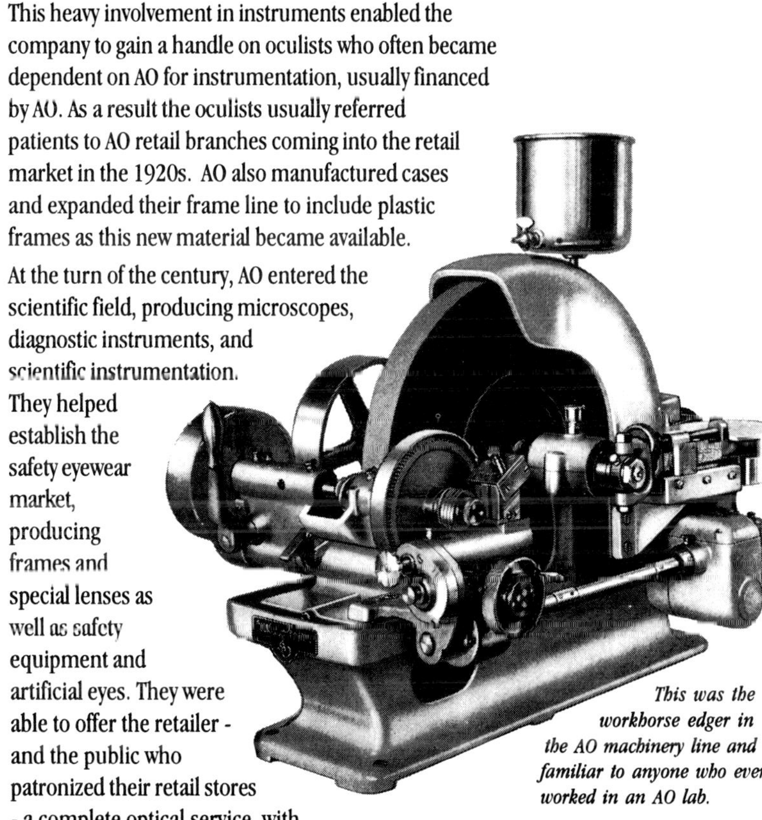

This was the workhorse edger in the AO machinery line and familiar to anyone who ever worked in an AO lab.

Tillyer

A major technical factor for AO was the work of Dr. Edgar Tillyer who joined the company in 1916. Tillyer invented the first lensometer, which enabled anyone to read the power of sphere and cylinder, determine the axis of the lens, and locate the optical center. This was a remarkable development when one considers the cumbersome and time-consuming process of hand neutralization that had been the only previous way to determine lens foci. Tillyer patented 73 inventions in the following years and developed AO's corrected curve lens series *(similar to Zeiss' Punktal and B&L's Orthogon)* that was to bear the Tillyer name.

AO's wholesale-retail business increased dramatically in the 1920s through acquisition of many large wholesale-retail chains. The company became the largest manufacturer, wholesaler and retailer in the optical business, controlling prices, distribution and product. This put the company in substantial control of much of the optical industry.

Wholesale Acquisitions

In 1923, AO made a decision that was to have a lasting effect on independent laboratories and the industry. American Optical, not content to compete with other manufacturers for distribution of their products, determined to take over distribution of their own products. The next few years saw a feverish round of buying or acquiring of a national network of independent stock houses and laboratories.

One of the first companies acquired was the Julius King Company *(Julius King had been the first president of the AAWO laboratory association)* a purchase that included an Industrial Eye Protection division. This was moved to Southbridge where it became one of the more important divisions of the company. During World War II, the Safety division was called on to produce millions of fliers' goggles, industrial goggles and sun glasses for government orders.

AO's acquisition of optical laboratories made a dramatic impact on the industry. Some of the companies that became part of this mushrooming industrial giant represented the largest and most dominant wholesalers in their regions. The following list shows only some of the companies acquired during this acquisition period.

1923

F.A. Hardy   40 branches

F.A. Hardy of Texas	6 branches
F.A. Hardy of California	5 branches
Merry Optical Company	32 branches
Merry Optical of Texas	2 branches
Merry Optical Agents	2 branches
Geo. S. Johnston Company	12 branches
Geo. S. Johnston Agents	2 branches
Geo. S. Johnston of California	3 branches
D.V. Brown	2 branches
Globe Optical Company	12 branches
Federal Optical Company	4 branches
Julius King Optical	2 branches
Rodney Pierce Optical	1 branch
Bohling, Gibbs & Lehmann	3 branches
New Orleans Optical	5 branches
Smith & Mercer	6 branches
Southerland Optical	2 branches
Cambria Optical Company	1 branch
Klein Optical Company	1 branch

1928

W.A. Jones Company	7 branches
W.P. Hitchcock	1 branch

Each of these companies continued to operate under their original name for several years in order to preserve and protect their contractual rights to distribute Kryptok and Ultex bifocals. These were the dominant bifocals of the '20s and could only be sold through laboratories authorized by the manufacturer. By 1941, American Optical was able to acquire or establish branches in 276 principal cities of the United States and Canada.

Machinery

By the turn of the century, AO's interests expanded to include optical machinery, needed for their factory and wholesale laboratories purchasing their lens products. By controlling machinery sales, they exercised further control of their customers by carrying notes issued for credit purchases of machinery and through contracts that required customers to buy lens product from the factory. These contracts included important agreements requiring customers to follow suggested resale prices. Notes could be called for infringements of any of these accords giving them the power to put that laboratory out of business or force them to become an AO branch.

During World War II, much of AO's manufacturing activities were involved in the war effort. During 1942 and 1943 alone, as the armed forces grew rapidly, AO was to supply 18 million pairs of lenses to the armed forces and, at the same time, try to maintain reasonable

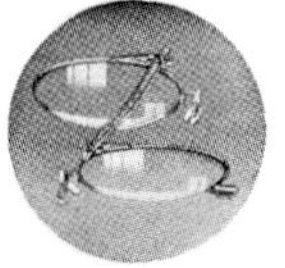
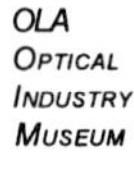

Ophthalmometer, circa 1924.

The "Z-Fold Oxford" was the newest developments in Oxford frames. Its unique design prevented lenses from rubbing against one another and scratching as the usual folding Oxford did. Lenses were always edged "on center" at this time and the fact that this frame could be ordered with different bridge widths to match the PD made it a real improvement.

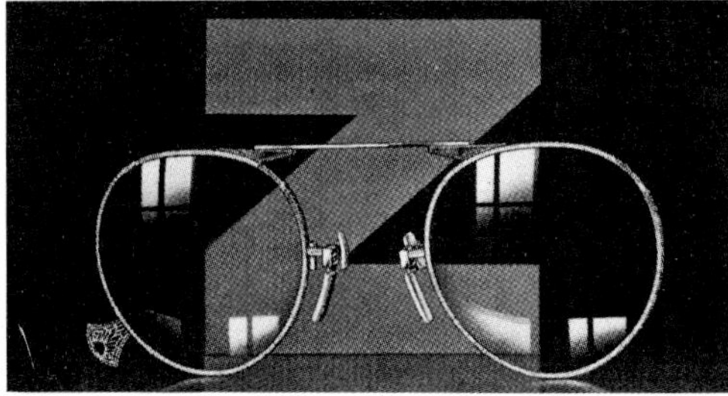

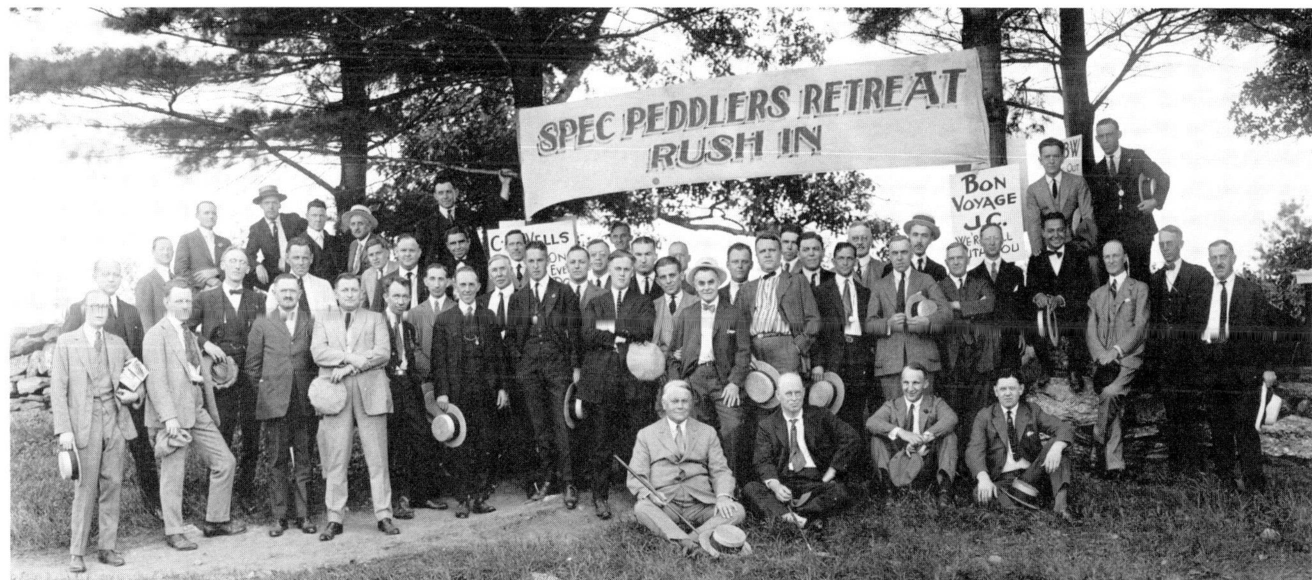

deliveries of civilian requirements. Immediately after the war, the company developed additional products including the famed Todd-AO process for wide-screen movie projection *(which received an Oscar)*.

The Wells Family Depart

As the Wells family sold out, starting in 1949, the traditional leaders disappeared. The two other vice-presidents who were at AO when Stewart assumed the presidency soon left: Al Marsters went to Bausch & Lomb to became Vice President of Sales, and Irv Wilson retired. Weldon Schumacher, a manufacturing executive *(whose father had been a prominent factor in the development of manufacturing processes)* assumed the presidency after Stewart. He guided the company through some difficult years until the company was sold. In spite of all the industry problems of that day, Schumacher's philosophy of building the best product at the best cost enabled the company to do well in all divisions including an expanded international division which opened *(or acquired)* laboratories in Canada, England, Germany, Switzerland, and Southeast Asia.

In 1957, the company decided that they had to have new blood and become more sales-oriented. A search was made outside the industry for a new vice president of marketing. Forest Frazier, who had been a consultant to the company, was vice president for a few weeks when he died suddenly on the train to Rochester. His replacement was Victor Kniss, a hard-hitting Westinghouse and Firestone executive who came to AO, along with many of his Westinghouse branch managers.

Kniss had expected to operate in the optical industry the same way he did at Firestone and Westinghouse, but he soon found the going very tough. The volume in the optical business was infinitesimal compared to what he was used to and the pay scale considerably less. AO branch managers failed to click their heels and respond as had his Westinghouse branch managers who were paid many times the salary then prevailing at AO. He did, however, depend on middle management to help further the programs he was implementing.

New Owners

The consent decrees of 1948 *(and subsequent litigation in Dallas and Milwaukee)* ultimately forced AO to alter direction drastically. New management, operating under the constraints of government decrees and faced with a rapidly changing industry, sold out in 1967 to Warner-Lambert, a major pharmaceutical company. The new owners saw in American Optical a great opportunity to apply their superior management and marketing skills to what they viewed as a backwards optical industry, even with its substantial gross profits. Victor Kniss opposed the sale of the company and soon after left.

Warner-Lambert's new management attempted to implement policies that had worked well in their own industry, but quickly discovered that these methods did not work in the optical industry, despite the addition of contact lenses and solutions *(AO arrived in this market late, becoming a me-too instead of a leader)*. Many of the better executives reached retirement age, or simply left the company for greener pastures, often because of politics. AO's laboratory division had became a real liability by this time. These labs were burdened with antiquated machinery and were only permitted to procure new machinery from their own factory. This was hampered though, because the factory's only market was the dwindling AO lab division along with a very uncertain international market and no new machinery was developed. Further, there was now strong competition

American Optical maintained a country retreat called *Wellsworth* where they would entertain visitors. *F.A. Hardy & Company* was AO's largest distributor (later acquired by AO) and the *Hardy* sales force spent 4 days at *Wellsworth* in August, 1921. Even though this was an informal, outdoors picnic, the *Hardy* men all turned up in coats, ties and snappy straw hats. The two men seated in the center are John Hardin, left, Hardy's president (later AO V.P.) and George W.'s son Albert B. Wells.

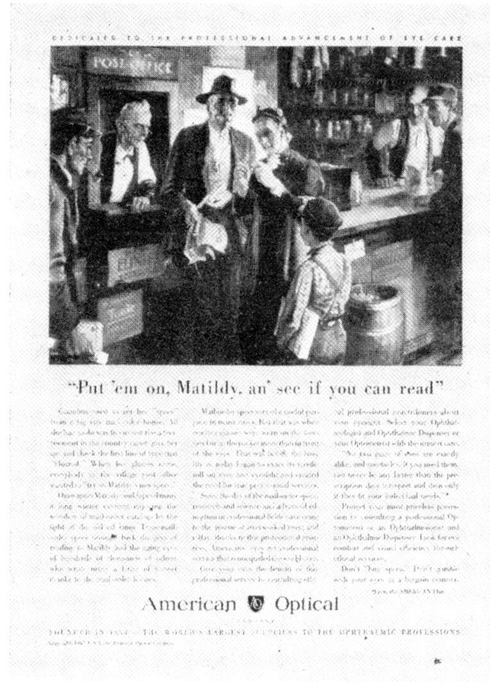

On June 22nd, 1942, AO launched a national P.R. campaign at the A.O.A. convention in Dallas. Aimed at increasing eyewear awareness, ads similar to this appeared in Life magazine and other publications. *OLA OPTICAL INDUSTRY MUSEUM*

For its day, this was a sophisticated lens cutter that permitted all sorts of adjustments. Unfortunately, Shuron soon developed a workborse of a lens cutter that didn't require all these refinements. These cutters were mostly found in AO labs.

from independents at the lab level and American Optical wasn't used to this strange phenomenon.

Schumacher continued to head the AO division until he was replaced by S. W. Pach, a Gillette executive, who was succeeded by a number of short-lived executives. None were able to maintain the high profits that the Cool-Ray *(sunglass)*, safety, ophthalmic, and instrument divisions had produced at the time AO was acquired by Warner Lambert.

As a result, in 1982, Warner-Lambert sold American Optical to private investors headed by Morris Cunniffe who is alleged to have bought the company for $35 million *($5 million down and the balance on a leveraged basis)*. The company was grossing almost half a billion dollars at the time but this volume accomplished little or no profit.

Dismantling

The new owners promptly closed the labs or sold them for low prices. The contact lens division, valued primarily for their contact lens solutions, was sold to Allergan for $85 million. When the government disapproved the sale because it would give Allergan too large a market share, AO turned around the following week and sold the division to Ciba-Geigy for $90 million. Frame production was shut down and the company later attempted to reenter the frame market as a "trader", but eventually pulled out of the frame market completely.

The year 1987 saw the beginning of a gradual dismantling of the company's lens production. Production of all glass bifocal products was shifted to IALO, a company AO acquired in Brazil. When this turned out to be difficult because of questionable product delivery and quality with minimal profits, they pulled out of the American lens market. IALO still sold products to the rest of the world but, in 1991, the company was sold. Single vision

glass lenses were procured for a year or so from factories in Thailand and Hong Kong but these were soon discontinued as well. By 1989, AO was totally out of the domestic glass lens market, a market they had dominated for 75 years.

Plastic lens production was shifted to Tijuana, Mexico, near the American border. The only production retained at the once-powerful factory in Southbridge were glass Executive bifocals *(demand for which had all but disappeared)*, molds for plastic lens production, and some specialized lens production such as the Omni and other progressive lenses, much of which has since been transferred to Mexico as well. In 1987, AO acquired United Kingdom Optical from a mini-conglomerate catering company. By this time, AO's worldwide volume was down to $200 million and the UK acquisition added $50 million to the company's sales.

For many years, it was rumored a secret cartel arrangement existed between the American giants, AO and B&L, and their German counterpart, Zeiss. Under this alleged arrangement, Zeiss stayed away from the American hemisphere and the American factories stayed out of Europe *(no one seemed to care about the rest of the world)*. Until the second World War, therefore, neither AO nor B&L had any major activities in international business - except for Latin America. AO established agencies in most Latin countries between the two World Wars. Several agents were self-consumers. Puerto Rico Optical in San Juan and Scadron Optical in Panama had by far the biggest businesses in their respective areas and sold only to the public, using AO as a brand name. In other countries, distributors or retailers bought directly from AO. Eventually, AO established companies in Mexico, Brazil, and established their Latin headquarters in Puerto Rico.

Postwar Growth

Following World War II, AO set up wholesale branches in Germany and Switzerland and established agents in other countries. In England, they set up their own company and attempted to manufacture lenses but the British operation was eventually acquired by UK Optical *(which had also absorbed B&L's London operation)* - ironically, this was the same UK Optical which would ultimately be acquired by AO.

In Southeast Asia, a network of branches was set up that did Rx work as well as distributing AO and other optical products. AO had branches in Singapore, Hong Kong, Bangkok, Manila, and Tokyo and other cities. In 1982 a decision was made to close or sell all Southeast Asia branches except Singapore and, subsequently, to build up the Singapore branch by putting in LOH machinery. The Singapore operation handles all AO business in Southeast Asia, even buying frames in Japan with the AO brand name to sell in the Singapore market. Singapore does retail advertising and sales there of the Omni progressive lens are substantial.

In 1989, AO sold their safety division, headquartered in Southbridge including four major labs located around the country, for a reputed $120 million to Cabot Industries, a safety-oriented company in Massachusetts. Today, AO's optical business in the United States consists solely of very profitable, higher priced progressive and specialty lenses while their international business *(except for UK)* thrives. Most of American Optical's current volume is in non-optical companies acquired since the original acquisition of AO by the Cunniffe group.

Today, American Optical's business is primarily outside the ophthalmic area with operations in abrasives, research, and other industries. Their optical operations are still significant but considering the way this company once completely dominated and influenced an entire industry, it's hard to believe it is the same company. Many who lived through the days when AO was "king of the hill" remember that as a time of distrust and fear of American Optical. Yet, in retrospect, the company, due in part to the Wells family, exerted their control in a way that was relatively benign and, in the long run, contributed a great deal to the growing industry.

Bausch & Lomb

Bausch & Lomb's development paralleled that of American Optical Company. John J. Bausch arrived in Buffalo, N.Y., in 1849. He was 18 years old and with no money, tried his hand as a woodturner *(there were no opticians at that time in Buffalo)*. Like the rest of the country, Buffalo was in a depression so, after a few months, he moved on to Rochester but still had little success in finding work.

He eventually found work but was involved in an industrial accident, catching his hand in a saw and losing two fingers. His recuperation was aided by the donation of $26 from friends, collected by his good friend Henry Lomb, a fellow carpenter. Unable to find further work in carpentry, Bausch resorted to the trade he learned from his older brother in Germany plus a short apprenticeship in Berne, Switzerland. He opened one of the first optical shops in Rochester in 1853 with goods imported from his brother in Germany *(on six months' credit terms)*. When timely payment was made for the first importation, other merchandise followed.

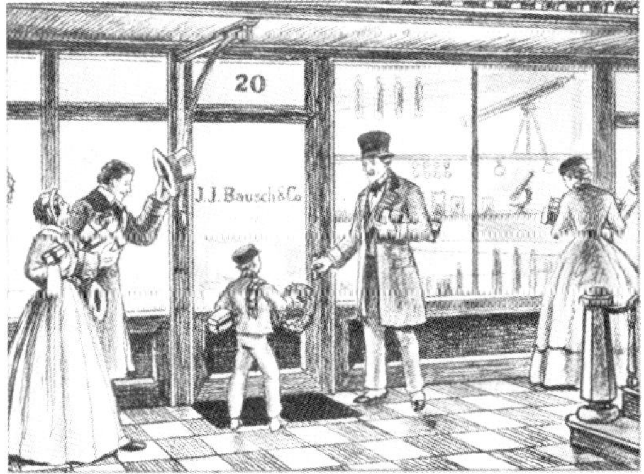

J. J. Bausch's second retail office was in room #20 on the ground floor of the Rochester's Reynolds Arcade.

The original store was in a shoemaker's establishment which smelled in wintertime of old shoes burned to heat the premises. With $62, again borrowed from his good friend, Henry Lomb, a new store was found. That rent was too high, so Bausch moved again to the Reynolds Arcade. Lomb's loan was repaid by giving him 50 percent interest in the business, which he retained until his death in 1908.

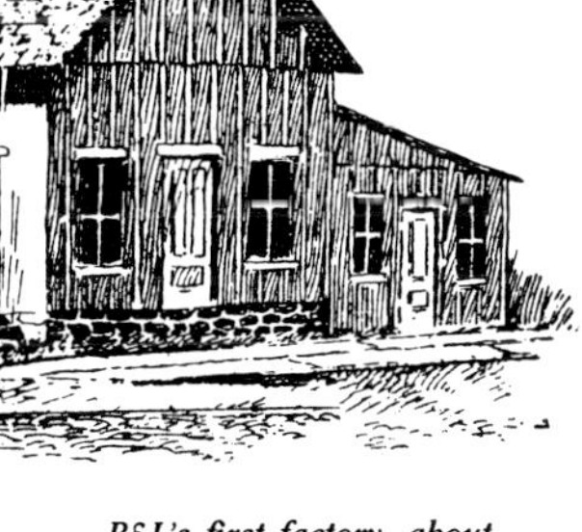

B&L's first factory, about 1866.

During the Civil War, Lomb enlisted in the New York State Volunteers for two years, the term of the regiment. He was elected first sergeant, promoted to first lieutenant and finally appointed captain. During his army service, he sent much of his meager salary to Bausch to help support the business. On returning from the war in 1870, Lomb set up a national sales office for the company in New York City, giving up the carpenter trade to head sales for the new business. For the rest of his life, Lomb would be called Captain Lomb.

Frames

Meanwhile, in 1861, Bausch had picked up a piece of vulcanized rubber on the street one day and, deciding this material would make a fine optical frame, began experimenting on his home kitchen range, heating rubber so it could be cut and shaped. He eventually was able to make decent frames from this material. He opened a factory near a good source of water power at the corner of Andrews and Water Streets and reorganized

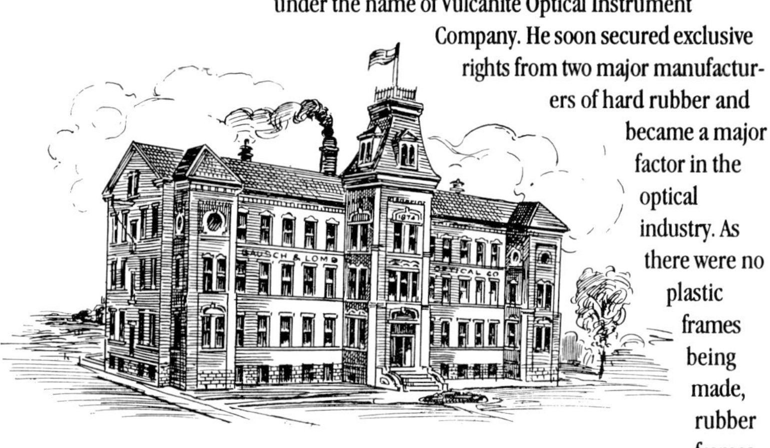

B&L's factory at St. Paul and Vincent streets, 1874.

under the name of Vulcanite Optical Instrument Company. He soon secured exclusive rights from two major manufacturers of hard rubber and became a major factor in the optical industry. As there were no plastic frames being made, rubber frames were one of the few alternatives to bone or metal frames. He also started taking orders for watch cases made of rubber and the business started to grow. Bausch's brother, E. E. Bausch, took over the retail business and John J. concentrated his efforts on manufacturing.

In 1874, the company moved to St. Paul Street and began developing a manufacturing complex which would house them for almost 100 years. In the 1870s, after changing the name to Bausch & Lomb Optical Company, they started manufacturing microscopes under the direction of Edward Bausch, J.J.'s oldest son. Spherical lenses were produced in 1878. B&L was the first American manufacturer to use mass production processing of lenses. By 1883, photographic lenses were being produced and they made Kodak's lenses until 1912. By the end of the century, the company was producing cylindrical lenses and had entered the optical instrument business as well.

During this period, Bausch & Lomb helped put an important revolutionary idea into effect. Glasses had always been sold as a complete unit, including both frame and lenses. B&L led the movement to standardize spectacle lenses so frames and lenses could be sold separately, providing practitioners greater variety from their inventories. The change met with immediate approval in this country and, before long, lenses made on the interchangeable method were being shipped to Europe. In 1896, the company produced the first meniscus lenses in America.

Instruments

In the early '90s, the company made arrangements with the Carl Zeiss Optical Works to manufacture an anastigmat camera lens developed by Zeiss. This relationship worked well for both companies and, in 1908, an allianace was consumated between B&L and Zeiss providing free exchange of technologies and product development. Edward Bausch, working with George Eastman, produced lenses for the first Kodak camera. By this time, George N. Saegmuller of Washington, D.C. had joined the company and was overseeing the manufacture of engineering and astronomical instruments for B&L. Their biggest customer was the U.S. Government who was delighted to have a domestic source for range finders and other optical instruments previously only available from offshore sources. In addition to scientific instruments which included binoculars, motion picture projection equipment, and fire control instruments for the armed forces, B&L entered the optical instrument field. Starting in the 1890s, they helped develop and manufacture instruments such as the Vertex Dioptometer *(an early phoropter utilizing a refracting system developed by B&L called Vertex Refraction)*, an ophthalmoscope *(in conjunction with Professor Allvar Gullstrand of Uppsala, Sweden)* and the Keratometer *(a version of which is still in use today)*. B&L also made the Green's refractor *(or phoropter)*, still used in many refracting offices. A significant development was the Model 90 and Model 70 Vertometers, competing with AO's Lensometer. These had been developed by Michael Friedman who ran B&L's machinery division and later their laboratories

B&L also began manufacturing laboratory machinery for their own wholesale chain as well as for other laboratories *(with the same conditions attached as AO required for their machinery)*. They produced several generations of sphere and cylinder polishers until, as a result of the Milwaukee case in 1966, their machinery manufacturing was closed. From that time on, they contracted with Coburn Optical for all machinery needs.

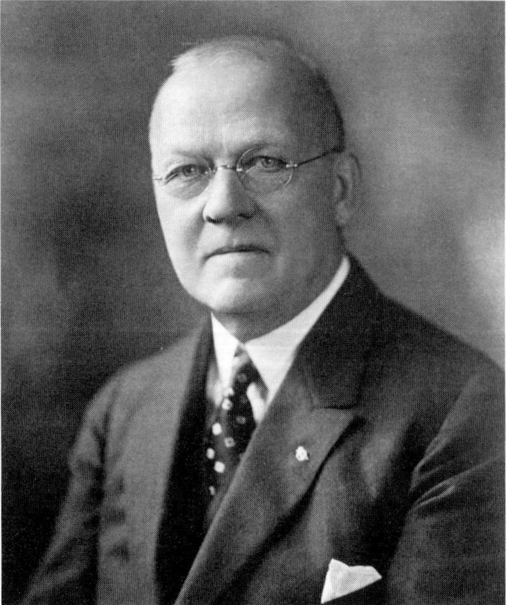

William Bausch, the man responsible for getting B&L into glass manufacturing. Notice his Ultex trifocals, B&L's premier lens of that day.

Optical Glass

One of the most significant contributions made by B&L was the opening of their ophthalmic glass plant, producing the first optical glass in volume in the United States. Under the direction of William Bausch, John J. Bausch's second son, B&L started producing glass in 1915, in time to provide America with excellent quality optical glass for World War I. This wasn't an easy task. Previously, their glass had come from Germany, France and England but none of these producers was willing to reveal their formulas. Furthermore, there was virtually no literature on the subject of making optical glass. With a world war raging in Europe, this was a serious problem for the United States armed forces.

William Bausch *("Uncle Billy"),* assisted by Jack Kurtz, mixed hundreds of batches of glass in small porcelain crucibles, firing them cautiously and then checking the results. Months of trial-and-error experiments eventually produced suitable barium crown, light crown, flint and dense flint glass in May of 1915. By March, 1917, one month before the United States declared war on Germany, imported stocks of optical glass were virtually depleted. The Carnegie Institution in Washington reported the only optical glass suitable for military instruments was being produced by B&L.

B&L worked closely with the Navy, producing superior periscopes and fire-control instruments, as well as range-finders, binoculars, gun sights, telescopes, and many other optical needs. Two-thirds of the armed services' glass requirements of 600,000 pounds in World War I was produced by B&L, with the balance drawn from existing glass inventories. By the end of 1917, the

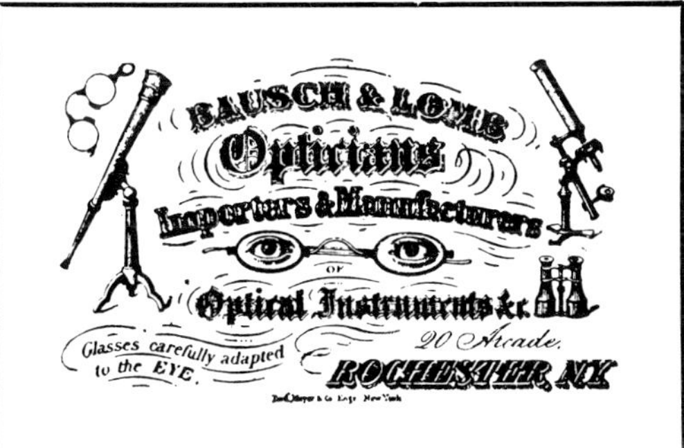

An early Bausch & Lomb business card, about 1864.

ILLUSTRATION – BAUSCH & LOMB

company was producing upwards of 40,000 pounds of glass per month. They also supplied most of the Navy's eyeglass requirements while still satisfying the home market.

B&L's new plant was the first to produce ophthalmic glass in the USA and the only plant owned by a lens factory *(this plant continued producing glass until the summer of 1986 when the company discontinued glass manufacturing).* Other lens manufacturers continued to buy from Europe and then from Pittsburgh Plate Glass, later acquired by Schott, or from Corning Glass when their factories opened. B&L's plant developed a better crown glass for ophthalmic use and a new barium crown glass which, when adapted to Kryptok bifocal production, eliminated most of the objectionable color fringes produced in the fusing process. Known as "Nokrome", the lens had no noticeable color or dividing line.

Edward Bausch was elected president in 1926, following John J. Bausch's death in February at age 95. In 1930, using the Hammon patent, B&L began producing the Panoptik bifocal. Originally the bifocal was to be marketed by Soft-Lite Lens Company, but was turned over to B&L because that company needed a bifocal to compete with the newly introduced flat top. The Panoptik was a fused flat top bifocal featuring a reading segment with rounded top edges. It could be produced with or without prism in the seg and commanded a premium price.

This product was added to B&L's bifocal line which included Kryptoks, Nokrome, and Ultex in various sizes and shapes. All B&L lenses, single vision or bifocal, were available as Orthogon *(corrected curve series)* or Certified *(non-corrected).* The policy of all lens manufacturers *(strictly enforced by AO)* was to sell only first quality products in the American market, selling all sub-quality lenses internationally where optical standards accepted inferior products without question.

Frames

In 1922, B&L purchased Stevens & Company in Providence, R. I., an old-line manufacturer of metal frames and cases and moved their production to Rochester. Stevens produced an excellent quality gold-

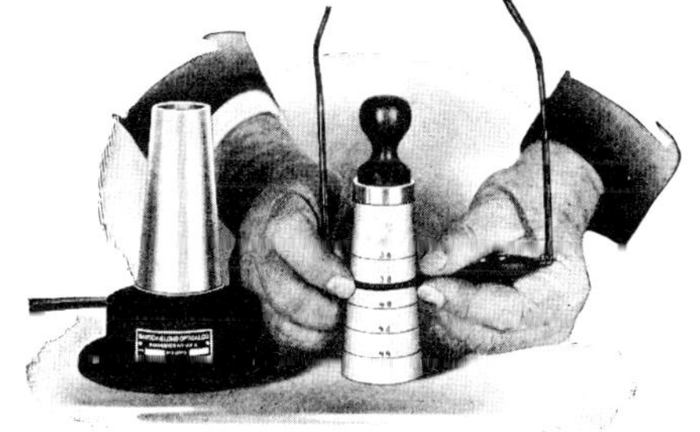

S-T-R-E-T-C-H
Zylonite Frames
the easy way

Anyone working with zyl frames 30 or more years ago will remember that every salt pan had a cone beside it for stretching zyl frames. Most offices only carried one or two cone shapes (usually P-3) and stretching some of the newer upswept shapes as they were introduced in the late forties required a great deal of hand skill.

OLA OPTICAL INDUSTRY MUSEUM

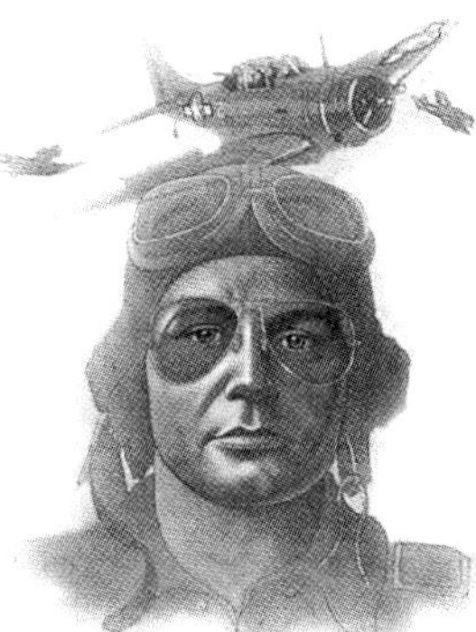

The famous Ray Ban aviator's goggle, still a top-selling sunglass fifty years later.

filled frame as well as a broad line of eyeglass cases enabling B&L to expand their line. They soon added plastic frames to their production and became a major factor in the frame business.

There had always been a close, personal relationship between the Bausch and Wells families, beginning with George Washington Wells and John Jacob Bausch. During the 1920s, B&L worked diligently to keep up with AO in product manufacture, wholesale laboratories, and the retail business. B&L began buying up independent laboratories to distribute their products during the '20s, the same period American Optical was setting up their laboratory division. B&L's philosophy was to follow AO's lead: whatever AO said, B&L did. By 1953, B&L had three sales and service divisions — Pacific, Northeastern and Central. San Francisco's Riggs Optical, acquired in 1926, became the Pacific Division in 1948. The following year the Northeastern Division was formed by a merger of two B&L affiliates, Colonial Optical of New York and McIntire, Magee & Brown of Philadelphia. In April of 1950, Riggs Optical of Chicago with 57 branches in 19 states became the Central Division. Including 33 branches of Southeastern Optical, an affiliate of B&L since 1929, the company now had 156 laboratories.

Sunglasses

Six years before Lindbergh's flight, an Army Air Corps lieutenant flew non-stop across the Atlantic. MacCready's flight, however, was in a blimp and has pretty much been ignored by history. He did, however, accomplish one other feat that should be remembered. In the late 1920s, Lt. MacCready asked Bausch & Lomb to develop an absorptive glass for use in flier's goggles. Pilots flying above the clouds were experiencing brutal headaches from glare reflected by the clouds. The results of B&L's research was the first Ray-Ban green glass, far exceeding the Air Corp's requested specifications.

In 1936, B&L took a bold step. Sunglasses were commonly sold for twenty-five cents. B&L introduced a plastic frame with prescription-quality lenses made from their new green glass. They coined a name "Anti-Glare Goggles" and put a $3.75 price tag on them. By 1937, knowing they had a winner, they took two important steps. First, knowing they could never protect the trademark "Anti-Glare", they changed the name to "Ray-Ban" and registered the name in March, 1937. The name has since become one of the most recognized trade names in the world and is one of Bausch & Lomb's prime assets. From 1942 to 1945, Ray-Ban production was devoted to the war effort and these goggles were standard government issue. For many years after World War II, Ray Bans were a major item of barter in Southeast Asia and still are one of the best selling sunglass lines in the world, with many styles featuring designs originally introduced in 1937.

The War Effort

In 1941, as the United States was gearing up to aid Great Britain in their war with the Nazi's, B&L played an important part by turning over to the British Purchasing Commission blueprints and specifications on two types of prism binoculars. Busy with their own U.S. war preparations, Bausch & Lomb provided these so Great Britain could secure bids from other binocular manufacturers. They also offered to supply glass pressings to those manufacturers, if needed. They provided technical assistance in setting up Research Enterprises, Ltd. to help the Canadian government produce optical glass and precision instruments. The company also agreed to train Canadian workers in their Rochester plant.

In 1944, control of Bausch & Lomb passed on to the third generation with the death of both Edward and William. Sons-in-law M. Herbert Eisenhart, Carl Hallauer, Joseph Taylor, and Theodore Drescher served as vice-presidents, president and chairman of the board in succession. Carl Bausch, the only male of the third generation to work in the company, made significant contributions in the research area. The fourth generation figured as well with Joseph W. Taylor serving as secretary and Richard Eisenhart handling various

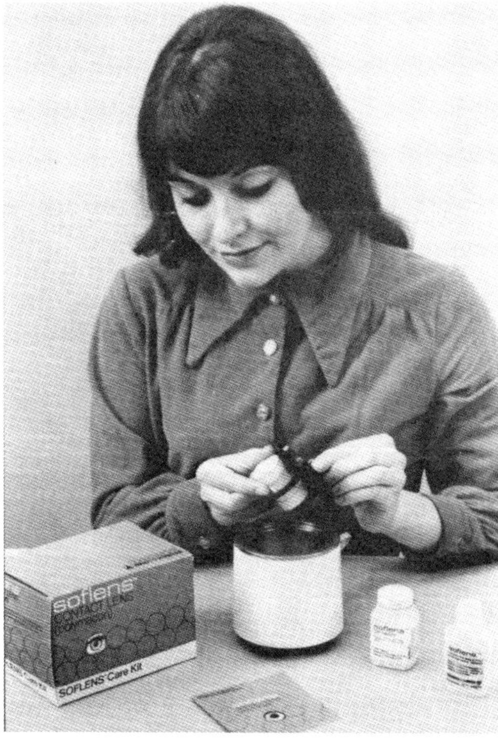

When B&L introduced the first soft contact lens (Soflens), every patient was given a lens care kit that included a heating unit for disinfecting lenses, a bottle of salt tablets and a mixing bottle.

sales responsibilities. The only outsiders were William McQuilkin, first as counsel to the company, then treasurer, and finally the first non-Bausch to become president and Ben Ramaker who served as vice-president of sales for many years.

Public Ownership

Henry Lomb's stock had reverted to the Bausch family on his death. The Bausch family continued as the only stockholders of the company until 1958 when the company's stock *(as usual, following AO's lead)* was first listed on the New York Stock Exchange. The name changed in 1960 to Bausch & Lomb, Inc. to enable the company to logically expand their operations into non-optical fields. Sales exceeded $100 million in 1966 and $1 billion dollars in 1989 - a far cry from the small shop started by J. J. Bausch in 1853. Bausch's constant efforts and meaningful contributions to the optical industry produced no significant profits until he was 60 years old and had been operating the company for 37 years *(1890)*.

Contact Lenses

A major change of direction occurred in 1971 with the approval by the Food and Drug Administration of B&L's soft contact lens. A license from the Czechoslovakian inventors permitted B&L to become the sole producer of this popular new product. Production costs were low since the lens was cast *(a patent prevented any competition from other cast lenses until 1989 - all competitors had to lathe-cut their lenses, a much more expensive process)*. Without competition, the Soflens commanded a high price and contributed substantially to B&L's profit and growth. Extremely profitable contact lens solutions, often costing less than the bottle, were added to the line, significantly increasing volume and profits.

By this time, the Bausch family was gone - retired, dead, or pushed out. William Schumann, with a financial background, guided the company into the contact lens era. Daniel Gill, with expertise in marketing in the pharmaceutical area was brought in. This new executive generation took a more sophisticated view of the business and made major changes. Schumann's decisions, unquestionably, had a major effect on the company's change of direction from a small ophthalmic business, following the precepts of "big brother" AO, to the major diversified business it became. Schumann is credited for bringing B&L into the arena of big business, introducing and promoting Soflens, establishing the solutions division and leading B&L to major corporate success. It is interesting to note that B&L owned three of the best-known trade names in the business: Ray-Ban, Soflens, and Soft-Lite. Gill, taking over from Schumann in 1973,

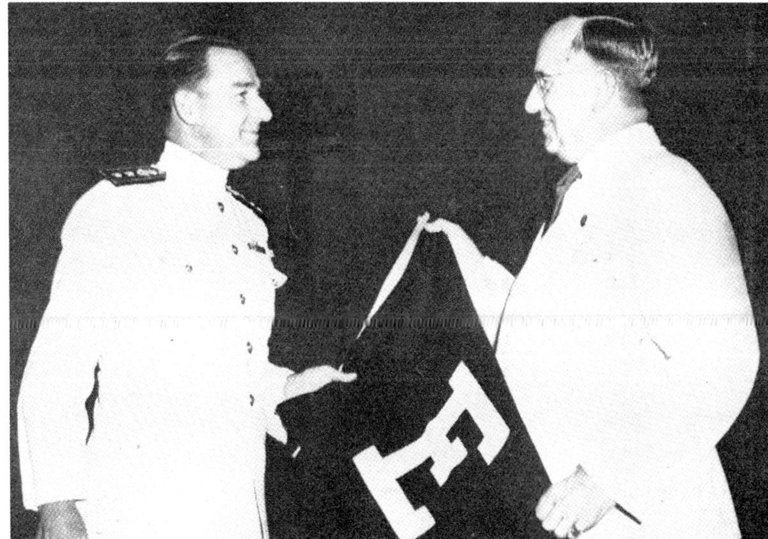

During World War II, the Navy made a habit of recognizing companies that produced war goods, above and beyond the call of duty. These companies were presented with a Navy "E" flag which they proudly flew over their plants. Bausch & Lomb earned one of the first 14 Navy "E" awards given out. B&L President Herbert Eisenhart (right) is shown receiving the company's flag from Admiral W.H.P. Blandy.

PHOTO – BAUSCH & LOMB

continued the corporate march, reorganizing the company into product divisions.

In 1973, the company acquired Bushnell and entered the competitive binocular arena. They also acquired a major plant at 1400 North Goodman Street *(formerly a clothing factory),* finally moving out of the St. Paul Street facility after almost 100 years. They expanded their contact lens capacity with the acquisition of a contact lens plant in Sarasota, Fla., in 1979 and construction of a plant in Waterford, Ireland, in 1981. That same year they divested their ophthalmic business by selling their laboratories singly, in groups or closing them. After selling off inventories of lenses and frames, all manufacturing facilities devoted to their production were shut down.

More Acquisitions

They continued on their acquisition program, acquiring Polymer Technology Corporation, producer of the new gas-permeable contact lens material in 1983 and completing a solutions manufacturing plant in Greenville, S. C., the same year. In 1985, Bausch & Lomb Pharmaceuticals was created after acquisition of Medical Technology Development Corporation. The industrial instrument division was divested. In 1986, the glass plant was closed, marking the end to an era and Dr. Mann Pharma was acquired, continuing the company's diversification.

In 1987, B&L acquired Pharmafair and introduced ReNu, a new line of contact lenses and solutions. The ophthalmic instruments and photogrammetry business was sold to Cambridge Instruments who had already purchased American Optical's instrument division, which had stayed with Warner-Lambert when the rest of AO was sold. In 1988, B&L entered the dental field with their Oral Care Division, acquiring Dental Research Corporation. In 1989, primarily as a result of these

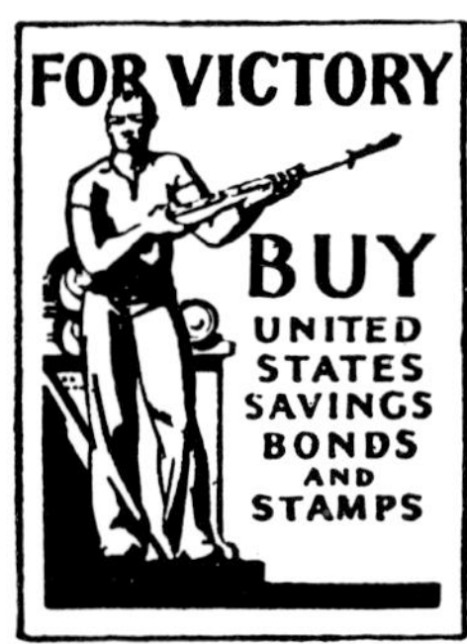

acquisitions, the billion dollar mark was reached. In 1990, B&L reentered the ophthalmic market by introducing ophthalmic frames as part of their Ray Ban line. This line was primarily sourced from international factories and capitalizes on the Ray Ban name.

The old Bausch & Lomb doesn't really exist today.

Except for the company's reentry into the frame market *(still in a fledgling stage),* B&L is no longer in the lens, instrument, glass, or optical machinery business. Their billion dollars in sales comes from businesses entered or started since 1971, the time they first entered the contact lens field.

Shuron Optical Company

Shuron was considered the third of the "majors" *(after AO and B&L)* but the company never compared in size or influence with the other two. In 1948, when AO sales were $60 million and B&L's $40 million, Shuron sales totaled $5 million. Shuron had patents in both lenses and frames, but none of them were capable of influencing the industry in any meaningful way. Shuron never had a viable instrument division other than the Genoptic line acquired in 1930 along with General Optical and it was ultimately discontinued. They were never in the wholesale or retail business although the company's predecessor, the original Kirstein Optical Company, a leading laboratory in its day, phased out of lab work in favor of manufacturing.

From the 1920s through the 1950s, Shuron promoted themselves as the "independents' factory". They were the alternative source of products for independent laboratories, whereas AO and B&L felt free to compete directly with their customers at both wholesale and retail. New wholesale laboratories opening business could almost never obtain a B&L or AO listing. Their only choices for

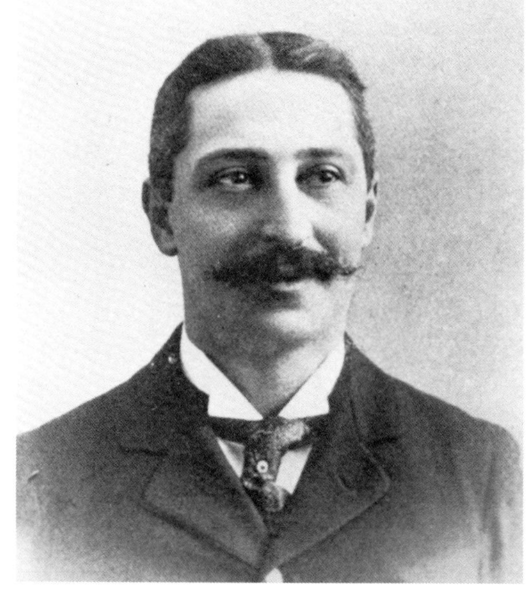

Henry E. Kirstein (above). It was his father, Eduard, who founded E. Kirstein and Sons, the company that would become Shuron Optical. The Kirstein company produced the spring-loaded finger-piece mounting that was so secure on the nose, it was called Shur-on, a name the company later adapted for its own. OLA OPTICAL INDUSTRY MUSEUM

lenses were Shuron, Continental and Titmus and those manufacturers were generally approached in that order. First choice was Shuron and, as a result, Shuron became the primary line for many independent labs during the '30s, '40s and '50s.

Company Origins

The company that was to become Shuron was started by Eduard Kirstein in 1866. Working from his home, he sold steel and silver frames throughout the eastern states. Expanding into lab work, he started selling prescription service in an ever-expanding area. Subsequently, he was to manufacture steel rim pince-nez eyeglasses with lenses processed in his laboratory. Kirstein's wholesale business, located in Rochester, N.Y., extended its area to cover more of the United States. Eduard's two sons, Henry and Louis, joined the company in 1891 and the company became E. Kirstein and Sons. Both Henry and Louis had worked as apprentices for Bausch & Lomb before joining their father. Kirstein became a major

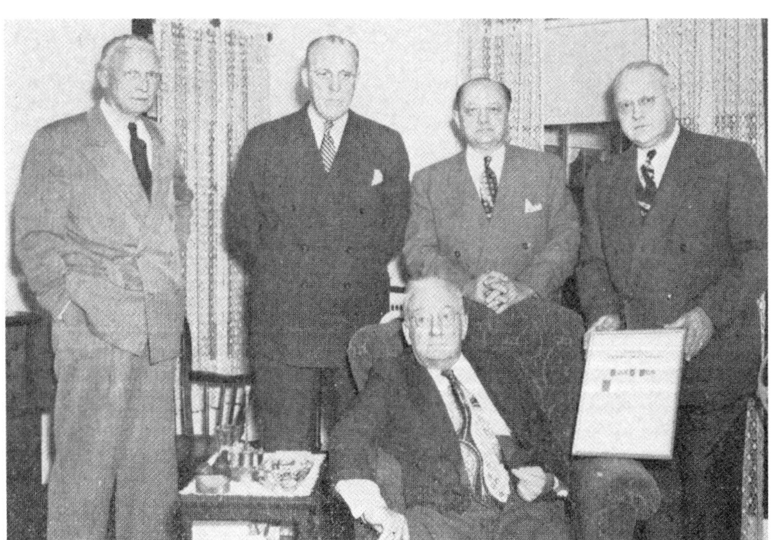

Harold J. Stead (seated) *had once manufactured lenses but spent his last years overseeing Shuron's Statistical Services and was highly respected by every lab owner in the country. In 1952, the A.I.O.W. presented him a plaque of appreciation. Seen in the photo are, left to right, Don Southgate, Shuron secretary* (later president), *Beverly Chew, Shuron Board Chairman, Jack Rohrbach, Shuron president* (father of the Browline) *and Art Hager* (Central States Optical) *who made the presentation for the A.I.O.W.*

ILLUSTRATION - OLA OPTICAL INDUSTRY MUSEUM

prescription laboratory as well as a major wholesaler of optical merchandise. Louis eventually left the company to become vice president of Filene's Department Store in Boston. In 1920 the company name became Kirstein Optical Company.

General Optical

The expanded company initiated mass production of lenses in Geneva, N.Y., and soon afterward acquired a Mt. Vernon, N.Y., bifocal manufacturing facility, General Optical Company, the manufacturing division of E. B. Meyorowitz. This addition gave Kirstein a bifocal product, a single vision lens line and the Gen-Optics instrument line. Kirstein was involved in frame manufacturing as well and developed a number of patented items. One such item was a finger-piece mounting, a spring-loaded eyeglass that stayed so secure on the nose it became known as Shur-On. The Offset Guard *(a novel pad structure)* was patented by Ivan Fox of Philadelphia and the flexible bridge, the mounting's primary feature, was the invention of Dr. Leo F. Adt of Albany, N.Y. Both products were manufactured and sold by Kirstein. The company then developed the Shelltex frame, a new frame style that, for a time, brought in nearly $2 million a year.

In 1920, Kirstein, buoyed by the success of his original frame *(which was the darling of his heart),* renamed the company Shur-On Optical Company. Eduard Kirstein retired in 1925 and the company consolidated with Standard Optical Company of Geneva, N.Y. They also purchased Dupaul-Young Company of Southbridge, Mass, another frame manufacturer which they promptly moved to Rochester.

Standard Optical

This was the former A.L. Smith Company, an old time frame manufacturer that had been operating since 1869 when it was founded by Smith. In 1873, A.L. Smith Company became Geneva Optical and was later incorporated as Standard Optical on January 22, 1883. A.L. Smith resigned in 1890 and moved to Chicago where he started another company, this one called Geneva Optical of Chicago, a company that was ultimately absorbed by Riggs Optical Company. One of Standard's stockholders in 1898 was A.L. Chew, whose grandson Beverly would later serve as president of Shuron for many years.

Standard was responsible for a number of industry

ROY MARKS

Here was a man who personified the mid-20th century "go-go" years in the optical industry. His name can be found cropping up a number of times in this history. While few of his contemporaries knew it, Roy was an optometrist, having studied in Chicago. His first significant position was with the Univis Lens Company where he rose to vice president. Leaving Univis, he spent the next few months with the Soft-Lite Company before moving on to Bausch & Lomb, again as vice president. B&L needed Marks to help initiate production of flat top bifocals and help recapture some of their dwindling laboratory business. From B&L, he moved to Shuron as vice president, largely on the promise of the presidency. Two years later, he became Shuron's president after that company was acquired by Toxtron.

While still with Shuron, he put together a deal in which he, Ted Uhlemann and Al Martin *(Chairman and President of Uhlemann Optical)* bought Spratt Optical, a substantial multi-branch retail dispensing operation in Los Angeles. Marks was made president of Spratt and moved to the West Coast. He then put together a package that consisted of Spratt Optical, Uhlemann Optical *(a large multi-branch retail dispensing operation in Chicago)* and Columbian Optical *(an Uhlemann retail subsidiary in Seattle)*. The companies were combined into Optimax, an organization he then sold to U.S. Industries, a fast-growing conglomerate with eyes on the optical business.

Roy eventually left Optimax to purchase a retail drug store chain in California. It turned out to be one of his less successful ventures and he soon dropped it. He then set up an industrial consulting business with an office in San Francisco's Cannery Building. The author remembers calling on Roy Marks in that office in the late '70s and being told that Marks was advising 3M on optical applications of some of their products. From that initial work came 3M's "Surface Saver" tape which undoubtedly led to development of their lens scratch coating that was eventually taken on by Armorlite and given the name "RLX". This relationship led to 3M acquiring Armorlite, which may have been Roy Mark's last big deal. During that same time, Marks served the California Optical Laboratories Association *(COLA)* as executive director. Roy Marks died in 1978.

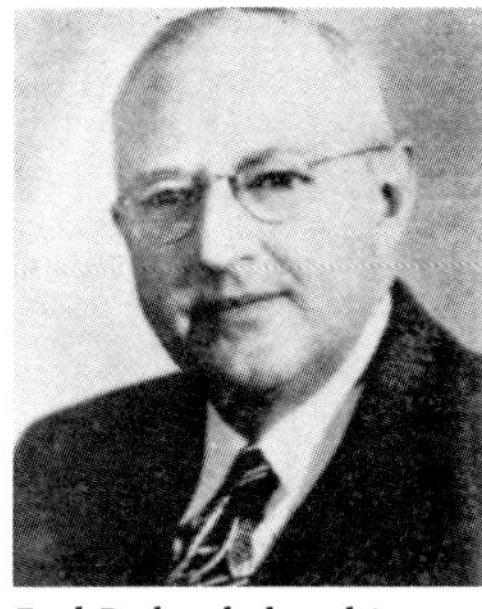

Fred Dryburgh, based in Chicago, was Shuron's Midwest regional manager for many years and considered the "grand old man" among midwest wholesalers. Many prominent optical personalities earned their spurs working under Dryburgh, including Egil Ruud, John Carnavelli, Joe Bruneni, Cal Stryker and Don Ellefsen.

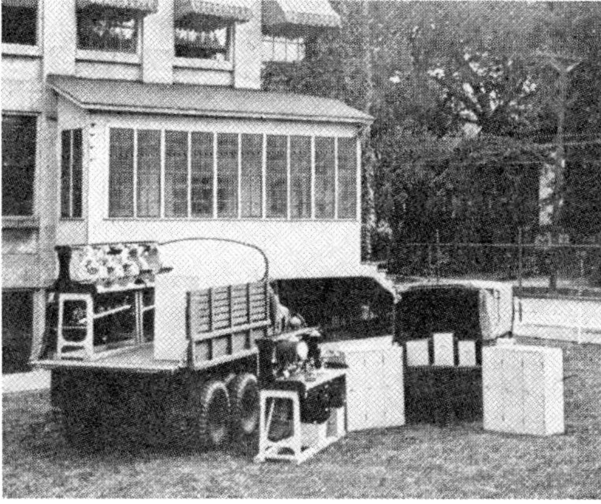

During World War II, Shuron produced many Mobile Optical Units for the U.S. Army. Mounted on a 2 1/2 ton truck, the unit consisted of 3 77-A edgers, 2 handstones and a workbench with an 82-A cutter, an axis marker, lensometer, grinder, buffer, soldering kit and a complete assortment of hand tools and repair parts. The equipment could be powered by a special generator on the truck or in a tent or building.

"firsts":

1899   Maynard Long, inventor of many Stoco *(Standard Optical Company)* machines produced the Standard Lens Drill, the first prescription machine to be sold to the trade.

1901   Introduced their first Lens Edger. The Hercules Toric Lens Grinder, forerunner of the later Tor-Cyl cylinder machine, introduced in 1906.

1908   Began grinding lenses.

1909   United States Lens Company formed with C.E. "Pop" Wilson, President.

1910   First Electric soldering introduced, based on work by Professor Bacon of Hobart College.

1913   Four members of the Chew family serve on the Board of Directors, including Beverly Chew, later elected President in 1921.

1916   66A Rx Edger introduced, a heavy duty rimless edger that became a laboratory workhorse for many years.

The first generation of the Browline was the Stag for men (pictured here) along with the Senora and Fiesta models for women. With heavy paddle temples, the frame was reasonably successful, but when Jack Rohrbach redesigned it with an all-metal chasis and metal bridge, it took off and started a trend that spread around the world. This style was later called Browline I.

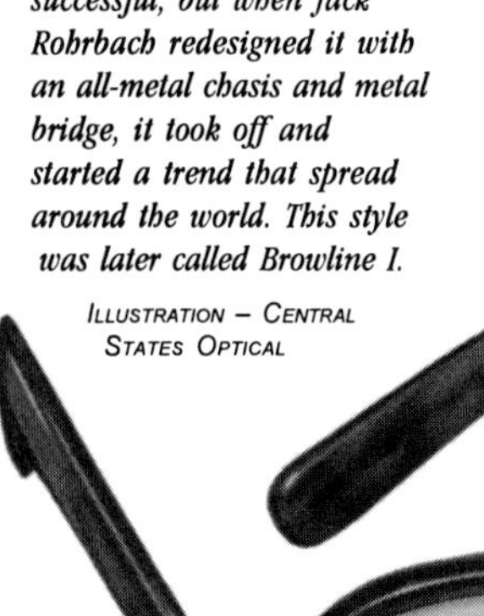

1919   Introduced the industry's first Bevel edger.

1924   Merger of U.S. Lens Company with Standard Optical

1925   Merger of Shur-On Optical and Dupaul-Young Optical with the new company acquiring an interest in General Optical, manufacturers of fused bifocal lenses and Genothalmic Equipment. Company is renamed Shur-On Standard Optical Company and becomes exclusive distributor of General Optical lens products.

1931   Name changed from Shur-on Standard to Shuron Optical Company.

The newly merged company also manufactured machinery. One of the company's more important contributions to the industry was the Oldfield lap cutter, the first successful machine for cutting toric surfaces *(cylinders)* on grinding laps and named for famed race car driver Barney Oldfield. They also produced early Tor-Cyl polishers which was one of the first machines enabling laboratories to fine and polish cylinder lenses with the desirable figure eight movement. Shur-On was also responsible for the development and manufacturing of several early, excellent edgers and introduced the first viable lens generator.

Frames

In 1949, a major facility was set up at Culver Road and Atlantic Avenue in Rochester to house an expanded frame facility. Jack Rohrbach's Browline *(this was a zyl/metal combination frame with gold-filled eyewires appended to a plastic browbar)* had, with its third design, revolutionized the frame business. In the first two designs the frame's construction was faulty but Rohrbach, then a Shuron Vice President, persisted in the face of substantial internal opposition. The frame he finally succeeded in producing took the industry by storm, along with its successors, Ronsir, Ronbelle, etc. This metal/combination styling was quickly copied by competition that included B&L's Bal Rim, Artcraft's Art Rim and many others. The Browline type of frame became the style and sales leader of the industry through the 1950s and the original Ronsir style is still made today.

In 1958, Philadelphia-Reading *(a former railroad company converted into a small conglomerate)* acquired Shuron from Manufacturers Hanover Bank, which had owned the company for some years after the Kirstein family withdrew. Beverly Chew, who had been Shuron's president for many years *(representing Harvey Gibson of Manufacturers Hanover)*, stepped down. Philadelphia-Reading held the company for exactly six months, the minimum time required for long term capital gains. They became generally disillusioned with the whole industry and happily sold the company to Textron, a Providence, R.I. conglomerate. Textron made former Vice President Don Southgate the new president and, a year later, appointed Roy Marks *(former Vice President at Univis and B&L)* in his place. Marks stayed two years. Textron acquired Continental Optical Company in 1963, merged it with Shuron and made Continental's President, Tom Hood, president of the newly named Shuron/Continental. Continental was a lens manufacturer in Indianapolis, successor to Dugbees' One-Piece Bifocal Company, which had been assigned to produce the Ultex lens, then controlled by the Kryptok Company *(or E.B. Meyrowitz)*. At one time, Continental had owned New Jersey Optical, a metal frame manufacturer, as well as other manufacturing companies.

Lenses

Shuron set up a modern lens factory in Barnwell, S.C., in 1960 and, in 1970 built a major manufacturing plant in Tampa, Fla, to produce lenses and machinery. Company administrative offices were moved to a new two-story addition to the Rochester, N.Y., facility at 40 Humboldt Street in 1965. The historic Geneva lens facility was finally closed in 1970 when the Tampa plant became operative. The Indianapolis factory closed in 1976. The Tampa facility was sold in 1978 when the machinery division was sold to CMV International, a division of De Beers Diamond Co. of Belgium.

The newly named CMV-Interamerica Company moved to a new plant in Miami. Production of plastic lenses was discontinued and all glass lens production centralized in Barnwell, S.C.

After Tom Hood's death in 1966, Egil Ruud became president. Ruud had started as a regional salesman in St. Louis, became sales manager and when Hood died, he became president. He subsequently was promoted to a group vice president at Textron, and a succession of presidents followed. In 1975, to publicize Textron, the name was changed to Shuron Division of Textron, Inc. In 1981, John Quealey was promoted from vice president sales to president.

By 1978, after discontinuing plastic lenses and centralizing all lens production in Barnwell, Shuron was producing only glass lenses. Except for semi-finished, production of single vision lenses ended. Utilizing various suppliers, Shuron continued to offer single vision lenses, but at noncompetitive prices. Eventually, the lens division produced only glass bifocals *(flat tops, Kryptoks and barium segments)* trifocals, semi-finished single vision and Executives.

In 1985, Textron sold the Shuron division to Quealey and Charles R. Whitehill, then vice-president-finance, on

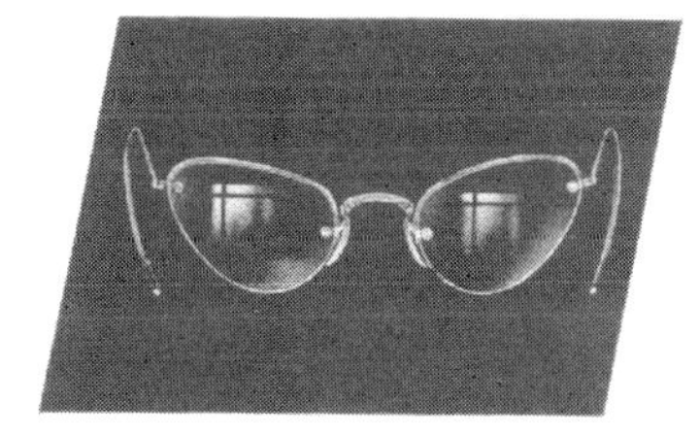

a leveraged buy-out and Whitehill became president of the new Shuron, Inc. In 1986 the frame plant was consolidated with the lens plant in Barnwell, S.C. In 1987, following the sale of the Humboldt Street location, the corporate office relocated to 20 Carlson Street, Rochester, N.Y. and was subsequently consolidated with the Barnwell, S.C. location in 1991.

Environmental Problems

From May to November 1987, there was an unsuccessful attempt to unionize the Barnwell lens and frame plant. During the organization attempt, an "anonymous" complaint was filed with the EPA Regional Office. The complaint alleged that during Textron's ownership in the 1960s, containers of "degreasing" residue containing the toxic chemical trichloroethene were buried on Shuron property, contaminating the soil and ground water. Although the current operation was proven nontoxic, the EPA cited Shuron and demanded remedial action.

In 1987, Whitehill acquired Quealey's stock and became sole owner of Shuron, Inc. and continued operations until Dec. 1991. Although the current operation did not discharge toxic material and the company was attempting to identify the extent and remedial costs of the 1960s contamination, Marine Midland Bank withdrew their line of credit, forcing the company to file for protection under Chapter 11 Bankruptcy in Nov. 1990. Production stopped in December, 1991 and assets were liquidated in January, 1992.

During the liquidation of assets in January, 1992, the company name and most of the physical assets, trademarks, patents, etc., of the frame business were purchased by Whitehill. The frame business was reorganized as Shuron, Ltd. in Columbia, S.C. where frame products continue to be available without interruption. As of August, 1994, Shuron is once again a viable frame company. In addition to new frame products, including a line of sunglasses, the company is investigating reentering the lens business with a Shuron brand of CR-39 and/or polycarbonate lenses.

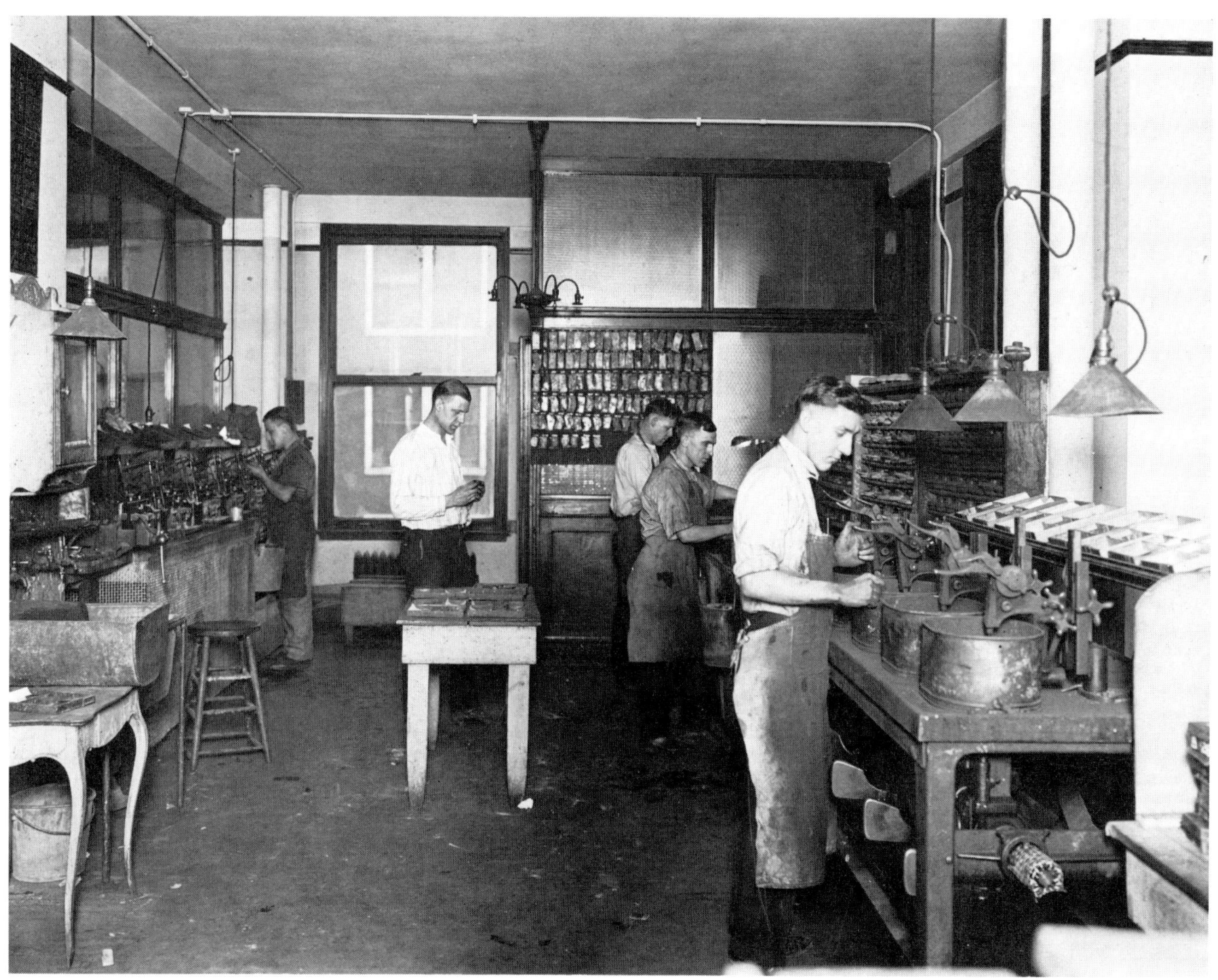

This exceptionally clean laboratory (for that time) was Uhlemann Optical's surface room, photographed in 1917. Notice the rack of tool gauges hanging on the back wall to the right of the window. These gauges are used to check the curves of grinding laps and this method of checking curve accuracy is still used today. What is noteworthy about the laps shown here is how flat the curves are. Most lenses were still flat which accounts for the flatter gauges shown here.

The machines on the left wall appear to be Shuron Torcyl cylinder machines. The men at the right rear are grinding in the curves by hand and the young man at the front right is fining or polishing. The man running the cylinder machines in the left rear is Henry J. Birch, later to found his own laboratory in Chicago, known today as Birch Optical, a member of the OLA. Standing in the center checking everyone's work is another well-known Chicago optician, Peter Swachta. Additional details on Birch Optical can be found in Chapter 18.

Uhlemann Optical became one of the industry's more successful wholesale/retail chains with many branches throughout the Chicago area. They were an early member of the A.I.O.W. and were eventually acquired by U.S. Industries as part of the Optimax Division.

Photo, courtesy of Dennis and Paul Birch and Birch Optical.

Chapter 5
Early Laboratories

Their Origins and Development

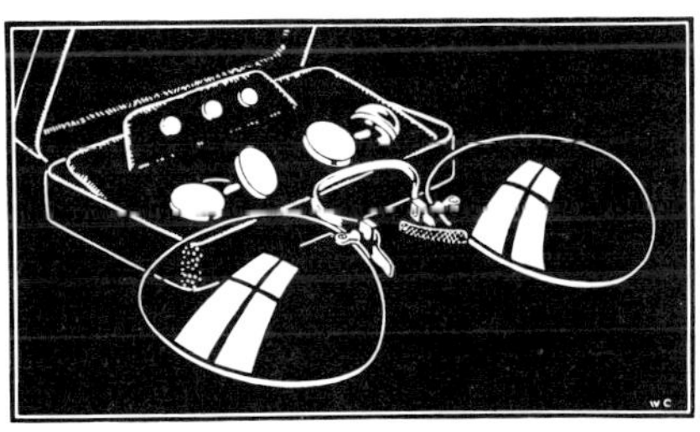

Exactly when the first optical laboratory came into being is shrouded in the mists of time. It is known, however, that the first trade association for optical laboratories was formed in 1894 when the fledgling American Association of Wholesale Opticians was founded, making it the first trade association in the industry. The AAWO would eventually become today's Optical Laboratories Association.

To understand how a need for optical laboratories came about, it helps to consider the eyeglass product being sold in the mid-1800's. Most eyewear in the United States at that time was produced in finished form by manufacturers *(almost all of it imported)* and purchased "ready-to-wear" by retail sellers. Eyeglass retailers might be hardware stores, drug stores, jewelry stores, optical stores or, as one moved away from the large population centers, itinerant peddlers traveling from town to town and farm to farm selling eyeglass goods. However they sold their wares, they all used the same method of determining what power lenses were required for each customer. The wearer simply tried on one after another until a pair was found that provided reasonable vision *(mostly for reading or close work)*. The only lenses were spheres, so the variety of lenses was comparatively small. There were few refractionists and no need for optical laboratories. All processing was done at the factory. Even when American frame manufacturing started in the mid-1800s, lenses were still imported from abroad.

Prior to 1900, wholesaling of optical goods was conducted primarily by large retailers or optical divisions of jewelry wholesalers. These companies purchased their materials, still mostly imported, at lower prices because of their volume. Toward the turn-of-the-century as U.S. lens manufacturers began to appear *(including American Optical Co., Bausch & Lomb, Kirstein Optical and Spencer Optical Manufacturing Company)*, they also sold direct to retailers and no one found fault with this

During the last twenty years of the nineteenth century, retailing of eyeglasses began to change from drug or jewelry stores to individuals specializing in selling eyewear. Calling themselves opticians, the fledgling profession eventually diverged into two distinct factions — opticians who refracted and those who did not. Many early opticians were nothing more than traveling peddlers, purchasing ready-made spectacles in the big cities and traveling the countryside selling their wares. Eventually many itinerant opticians would settle down in smaller towns and rural areas and establish businesses.

Opticians who refracted continued to refine their techniques and as manufacturers began to produce more sophisticated lenses that included cylinders, opticians began using more advanced refraction techniques to take advantage of the new lens technology. This broadening range of lens powers *(spheres combined with cylinders)* made it more difficult for simple ready-made spectacles to meet the needs of the public. Slowly but surely, refracting opticians began to use personal skills to determine and advise the customer on what lenses they should wear. The previous system of having the customer select from an assortment of ready-made glasses was gradually replaced by more scientific *(and, hopefully, more accurate)* methods.

A few opticians settled down into shops or jewelry stores and began to order edging equipment so they could edge stock lenses as needed. Large wholesalers sensing a need, began to carry finished stock lenses already edged *(and sometimes predrilled)*. Since the range of shapes and sizes was limited, this was a practical way to fill orders. When an Rx was received by the wholesaler, they picked edged *(and drilled)* lenses out of stock, assembled them in the frame ordered and immediately returned them to the retail customer.

Few retailers had surfacing facilities and as opticians became more skilled in "refracting" customers, a need began to develop for a wider range of lenses to meet the requirements of opticians and their newly developed refracting talents. This is how the need for "custom" eyeglasses arose - glasses with lenses made to the individual needs of the patient instead of adapting the patient's needs to what was at hand in factory-made glasses. Factory-produced eyewear no longer answered the needs of a more advanced marketplace. It was this increasing demand for a greater variety of lenses that led directly to the need for wholesale optical laboratories.

As this began to occur, large wholesalers *(and some lens manufacturers)* responded by installing surfacing equipment and establishing elaborate and, for that day, sophisticated laboratories. Ordering prescription lenses from lens manufacturers or large retailers in major cities, however, took time. Local laboratories began to spring up to serve areas the factories or big city wholesalers were unable to properly service, even though frames and lenses sold by these early local labs often came from the same factories they competed against. Meanwhile, some of these early labs, requested by their medical accounts, began servicing the public directly. Labs did not refract, so they were not considered competition by refracting opticians.

During this early period, it was common for large wholesalers and some manufacturers to offer instructional courses to opticians and oculists who wanted to learn the new art of refracting. These budding professionals began to grow in number until manufacturers like American Optical and Bausch & Lomb realized they needed a better way to distribute their frame and lens products to this growing market. More and more frames and lenses were being ordered in ever increasing numbers by these new "professionals" and AO and B&L, to their dismay, discovered that much of this new business was captured by independent laboratories who didn't necessarily do business with AO or B&L. For this reason, starting in the 1920s, these two dominant manufacturers embarked on aggressive programs to develop factory-owned laboratory networks to better control products used at the retail level.

In Chicago, F. A. Hardy started a wholesale supply and laboratory business in 1884 and by 1896 this successful company was processing as many as 700 prescriptions per day and giving customers two and three day service. Their lab turned out as many as 150 prescriptions an hour. The company eventually occupied 20,000 square feet and employed 150 people. This was one of the more successful wholesale laboratories and the company continued to grow until the inevitable happened. They were absorbed into the American Optical laboratory network in 1923.

Other early optical wholesalers *(laboratories called themselves "wholesalers")* included Julius King, owned by an oculist in Cleveland, Ohio, with branches in New York City and the midwest. Spencer Optical Company had their headquarters in downtown Manhattan. This was probably the largest wholesaler in the country. Nearby could be found a proliferation of other laboratories including M. E. Stern, L. Friedlander, L. H. Kosh, and Max Zadek. Further uptown were Hygrade, Unique, Potter & Schnackenburg *(later to become part of AO)* and August Neuse. These laboratories gradually replaced earlier wholesalers who had supplied the needs of retailers mainly from imported finished goods when prescription services were neither available nor needed.

Multi-branch laboratories started to develop late in the 19th century and, by the time AO and B&L began acquiring wholesale laboratories in the 1920s, a number of large independent wholesale chains existed. Many of these, such as N.P. Benson and Walman Optical in Minneapolis, Minn., sold high quality products at relatively high prices to the public on oculists' prescriptions while, at the same time, selling lenses and frames to their optometric competition *(neither Benson nor Walman refracted)*.

Most leading optical wholesaler supply houses had disappeared by 1925, either out of business or absorbed by AO or B&L as they accomplished their goal of building national distribution chains. Spencer Optical Company was one of the more successful wholesalers.

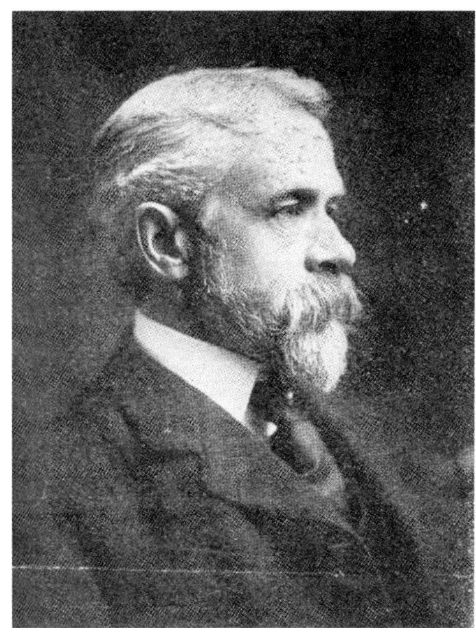

F.A. Hardy left a job as an optician in Boston to come to Chicago in the 1880s. He opened a retail store on the site of the present Marshall Field store. His company grew into one of the largest wholesale operations in the country before it was acquired by American Optical. Hardy served as the second president of the AAWO in 1896, following Julius King.

Their Newark, N.J. factory wholesaled directly to retailers. Spencer employed 2,500 people in 1898 and by 1905 they were broke. They continued operations for several years under the ownership of their original owners, John and James E. Spencer, but in a very reduced form and eventually the company vanished. Why such a prosperous company failed has never been explained.

Members of the original optical wholesale organization, founded in 1894 as the American Association of Wholesale Opticians included F. A. Hardy (Chicago), Julius King (Cleveland and New York), Johnston Optical (Detroit), D. V. Brown Optical (Philadelphia), and L. Black Optical (Detroit). A year later, these companies were joined by Geneva Optical (Chicago), E. Kirstein Optical (Rochester, NY), Globe Optical (Boston), and Levy-Dreyfuss Company (N.Y.). The original purpose of this association, as stated by a founding member, was to "protect us against deadbeats". The AAWO ultimately became the Optical Wholesalers National Association (OWNA). As American Optical and Bausch & Lomb began acquiring laboratories to distribute their own products in the 1920s, they were permitted to join this association.

As the lab distribution networks of American Optical and Bausch & Lomb grew in numbers and influence, independent laboratories found it increasingly difficult to compete against companies that existed primarily to distribute products manufactured by a factory parent. Since company profits were generated at the manufacturing level, company-owned laboratories were not saddled with the need to generate profits at the distribution level. Few independents had the courage (or *foolhardiness*) to price their goods higher than the two factory chains and the results of this market domination was that prescription prices for many years were determined primarily by American Optical and, to a lesser degree, by B&L. In highly competitive territories, independent lab owners all believed that the giants' Rx prices were often established to destroy independent laboratories.

The competition grew fierce and some independent labs began to believe that the manufacturers were dominating the association set up to help laboratories (OWNA). As a result of this political situation, a number of independent labs split off from the OWNA in 1939 and formed a new group called the Central States Optical Wholesalers Association *(COWA)*. Manufacturers were banned from membership in the new association so the group could truly represent the interests of "independent wholesalers" *(i.e. those not controlled by AO or B&L)*. The name was later changed to the Association of Independent Wholesalers *(AIOW)* to indicate the national aspect of the organization.

Eventually American Optical and Bausch & Lomb were forced to divest themselves of their retail operations in 1950 *(by court order)* and their retail stores sold to local managers of AO or B&L branches. Later, when AO and B&L shut down their laboratories, there ceased to be a need for two wholesaler organizations and the two organizations merged in 1962 to form the Optical Wholesalers Association. Since the members' core business was fabrication of eyeglasses, it was decided the name Optical Laboratories Association was a more appropriate name and the association became the "OLA" in 1977.

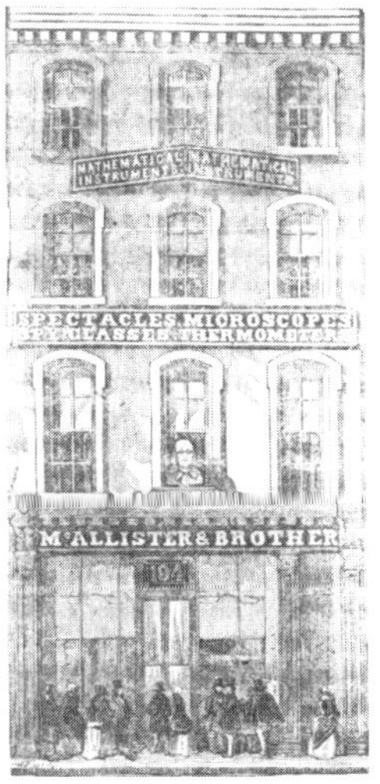

The famous Philadelphia manufacturing opticians were located at 194 Chestnut Street in 1853.

Early Laboratories

The more prominent wholesale laboratories that developed during the 19th century no longer exist, mostly because the successful ones were absorbed by Bausch & Lomb and American Optical during the 1920s and less successful ones failed or were absorbed by others. When American Optical and Bausch & Lomb exited the lab business, it was a dismal end for many profitable laboratories started by clever and innovative founders. A brief review of some of the more interesting of those vanished companies follows.

ARTHUR FRANK & COMPANY

In 1896, a 13-year-old youngster started a job with Joseph Friedlander & Brother, a prominent wholesale operation in New York City. The boy's name was Arthur Frank and nine years later, at age 22, he started his own company called Arthur Frank & Company. He began by renting desk space only but the company soon sold enough merchandise to survive and even grow a little. He took in a partner named Earl Connet, changed the name to Frank & Connet and started giving private tutoring courses in optics. They continued this until 1907 when they moved and set up their own laboratory.

Earl Connet died in 1911. Six years later in 1917, the company was incorporated under the name Arthur Frank and Company, Inc. Arthur Frank served for a number of years as president of the New York Optical Wholesalers Association and Optical Board of Trade. He also headed a clinic where, in four years, 32,000 people were provided with free optical service. Frank worked closely with Optometric groups in an advisory capacity and in 1921, personally organized the American Optometric Convention at the Waldorf Astoria.

BAUSCH & LOMB AFFILIATES

SOUTHEASTERN OPTICAL CO.

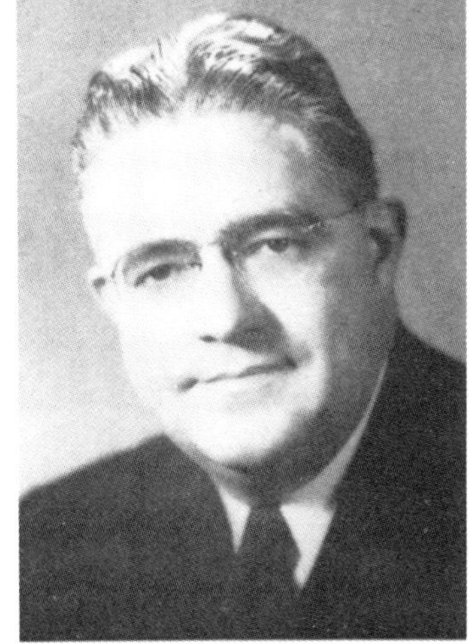

The Dempsey brothers owned a wholesale laboratory in Dayton, Ohio called Dempsey Optical. Their company belonged to both the AIOW and the OWNA and Phil Dempsey (below) attended AIOW meetings and Bart (above) attended the OWNA. They hold a unique position in the industry because each brother served as president of their respective association.

Bausch & Lomb purchased the wholesale department of S. Galeski Optical Company on August 1, 1929. This added laboratories in the following cities to B&L's growing network:

Virginia	Richmond, Norfolk, Roanoke
North Carolina	Raleigh, Winston-Salem
South Carolina	Greenville
Florida	Miami

These laboratories were combined and given the name Southeastern Optical Company. As this was done, B&L also added the just purchased C.B. Smith Optical of Petersburg, Va. The following White Haines branches were later added to the Southeastern network:

Virginia	Roanoke
Georgia	Atlanta
Florida	Tampa
Alabama	Chattanooga, Knoxville

A new laboratory was opened in Augusta, Ga., giving B&L's new laboratory division a total of 14 laboratories. Walter S. Galeski served as president of the B&L affiliate Company. By 1941, the company had grown to 24 branches. The Augusta lab was moved to Columbia, S.C. and new labs were opened in:

North Carolina	Wilson, Asheville, Charlotte
Georgia	Macon
Florida	St. Petersburg Jacksonville
Mississippi	Hattiesburg, Jackson
Tennessee	Memphis, Nashville

RIGGS OPTICAL COMPANY

This major laboratory organization began when a wholesale lab calling itself "The Omaha Optical Company" opened at the corner of 14th and Douglas Streets in Omaha. The company started with a total capital of $4,500. Theodore Roosevelt was president and work was progressing nicely on the Panama Canal. The year was 1907.

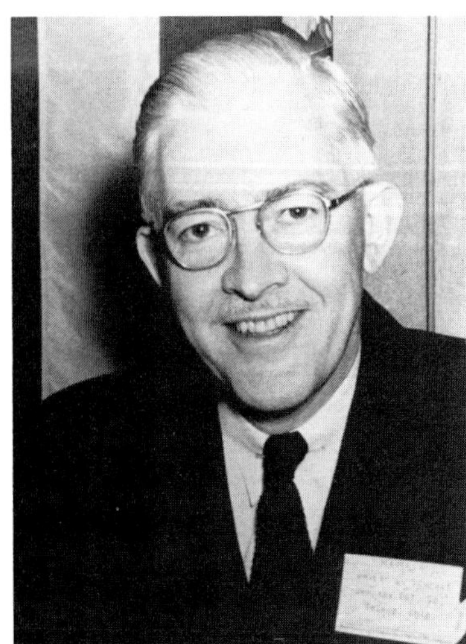

Omaha Optical ground the first cylinder lens ever produced in Omaha. The company's official day was from 7:30 am to 6:00 pm. They had a firm rule that all work received in the morning had to be completed before the day ended so it was normal for employees to work as late as midnight.

There were not many wholesale labs in the country and this kind of dedication paid off because the company grew rapidly, moving twice to larger quarters in the first few years. Two years after its founding, the company's name was changed to Riggs Optical, named for founder Elwood Riggs. The reason for the name change was the opening of a branch in Sioux City, Iowa. Iowa natives didn't take kindly to "big city" boys from Omaha so it was felt a name change would be judicious. Shortly after this, company headquarters moved to Chicago on West Superior Street. By 1932, the company's main office was relocated to the Merchandise Mart, becoming the seventh largest tenant in the largest building in the world.

Elwood Riggs was another graduate of the spectacle peddler fraternity. Early in his career, he traveled all over the West fitting glasses. He was also one of the first graduates of the Northern Illinois School of Optometry in the 1890s. Prior to starting his own company, he joined Colombian Optical in 1897 and became manager of their Kansas City store in 1899. After a difference of opinion with owner A.I. Agnew, Riggs spent several years with American Optical in Southbridge as manager of their order department and produced the first catalog AO ever published. He left AO in 1906 to move back to Omaha to start his own business.

Riggs Optical opened a branch in Sioux City, Iowa in 1912, Lincoln, Neb. in 1914, Cedar Rapids, Iowa in 1915 and Fargo, N.D. and Quincy, Ill. in 1917. The company acquired a number of smaller labs over the next few years. These included:

Omaha	Taylor-Jenkins Optical
Salina, Kan.	Quinton-Duffens
St. Paul, Miss.	Irving-Heard
Green Bay, Wis.	Northern Optical
Denver, Colo.	National Optical
Fergus Falls, Minn.	Fergus Falls Optical
Chicago	Geneva Optical
Minneapolis	Geneva Optical
Des Moines, Iowa	Geneva Optical
St. Louis	Geneva Optical
Davenport, Iowa	Geneva Optical
Minot, N.D.	Geneva Optical
Chicago	Central Optical
	Scott Optical

Little Rock	Mitchell-Harper Optical
Tulsa	Davis Optical
Fond du Lac, Wis.	Fond du Lac Optical
Rockford, Ill.	Uhlemann Optical branch
Portland, Ore.	Davies Optical, Woodward Clarke Optical
San Francisco	Johnson Optical
Kansas City	Columbian Optical
Oklahoma City	Columbian Optical
Texas	Associated Optical branches

On February 25, 1925, Elwood Riggs met with Bausch & Lomb representatives and by the end of the day, sold his company to B&L. From that point on, the company was a wholly-owned affiliate of Bausch & Lomb. By their 25th anniversary in 1932, the company had 65 branches in 24 states.

COLONIAL OPTICAL COMPANY

Based in New York City, this B&L affiliate absorbed a number of independent laboratories, including:

Boston	G.M. Smith, Bowen Optical
Providence	Hope Optical
Albany, N.Y.	Mohawk Optical
Rome, N.Y.	Mohawk Optical

Other independent laboratories were also added to the Colonial chain.

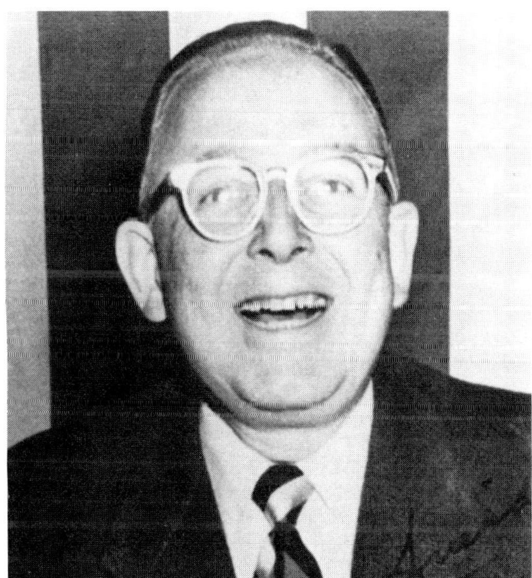

Dalton W. Bradley. His son, Bill Bradley, also participated in many activities of the OLA before retiring.

BRADLEY OPTICAL

Bradley Optical, a Los Angeles laboratory, was founded by D.W. Bradley. He began his career working for the Lincoln, Neb. branch of Omaha Optical in 1917 shortly before the company name was changed to Riggs Optical. He was moved to Omaha and made city salesman, later stock manager and eventually sales manager. Later promoted to manager of the Riggs branch in Kansas City, Bradley later moved to Chicago to manage Riggs' main branch.

In 1932, he and his wife Opal spent a vacation in California. Falling in love with what they found there, they packed up everything they owned and by August had moved permanently to the west coast. A friend named Jim Sweeney had told Bradley he had a little wholesale business in Los Angeles called Trojan Optical. Without ever seeing the business, Bradley bought it, deciding it would be a nucleus or, as he said, "a place to hang our hats". D.W.'s brother Edgar followed several weeks later and took over the shop while D.W. went on the road selling. By 1941, they had 37 people on the payroll in Los Angeles, 8 more in a Long Beach branch and 9 in Glendale.

Eventually, Bradley Optical was sold to Chicago's House of Vision. D.W.'s son Bill, who was sales manager when the company was sold sensed the industry was ready to convert to plastic lenses. He opened an all-plastic lab, a daring innovation at the time. He named the company Opalite in honor of his mother, Opal Bradley. Bill Bradley has since retired but Opalite is still going strong.

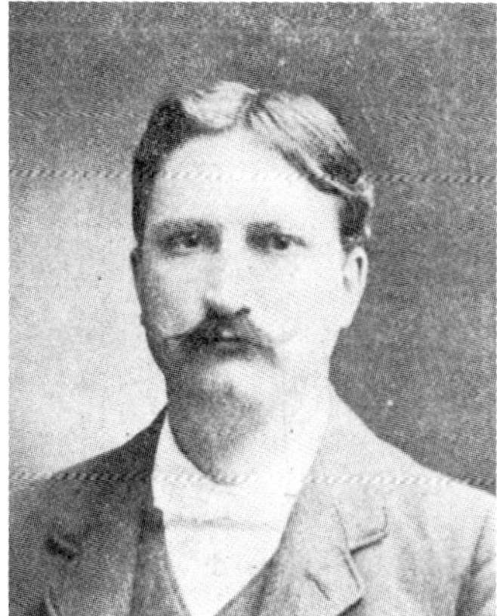

Charles C. Inskeep developed the first self-illuminating Retinoscope and ophthalmoscope.

CHAMBERS-INSKEEP COMPANY

The Chambers-Inskeep Company was a pioneer laboratory that merged in 1903 with F.A. Hardy Company, which in turn, was taken over by American Optical. It was founded in 1887 as the Ottumwa Optical Company in the sleepy little town of Ottumwa on the banks of the Des Moines River in Iowa.

In the late '80s, the town included a small drug store owned by David Chambers whose nephew, Charles Inskeep, was the prescriptionist. An optician visited the store from time to time, fitting and selling spectacles to the patrons. The more Chambers observed the optician and his work, the more it appealed to him. He and his nephew were bored with the drug store, but how were they going to get involved with this fascinating new world of optics? At that time, there were no schools of optics and the only answer seemed to be to teach themselves. They bought every optical book they could find and

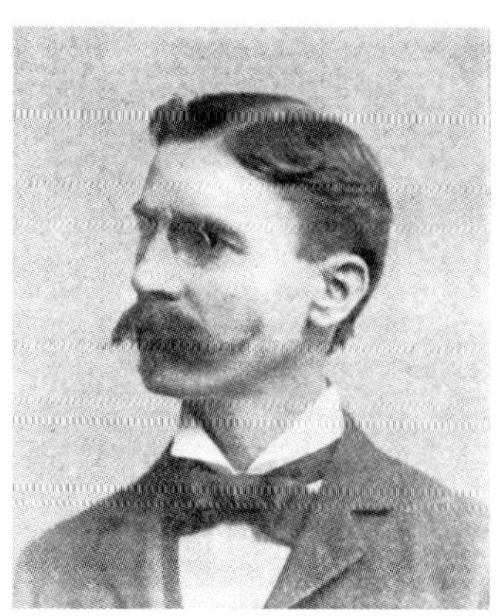

David Chambers owned a drug store but decided the optical business had more appeal to him.

studied theoretical optics while continuing to run the drug store. Gradually, they started selling eyeglasses. In 1887, the first pair of compound lenses ever fit in Ottumwa were bought and edged to a frame for a patient named McKelvie. Charles Inskeep edged them himself while 16-year-old Harry Smith turned the grindstone by hand.

Starts Wholesale Business

Chambers was determined to go into the wholesale optical business. Leaving 17-year old Harry Smith in charge of the drug store, he took off for Southbridge, Mass., then considered the country's optical center. Later that year, David Chambers returned from Southbridge, sold the drug store and launched the Ottumwa Optical Company. Harry Smith became his first traveling salesman, making his first trip in 1888. The company was a partnership that included David Chambers, Charles Inskeep, E.A. Chambers *(David's brother)* and Carey Inskeep, banker father of Charles.

The company moved to Chicago in 1888 and the following year changed their name to Chambers-Inskeep. By 1892, the year of the World's Fair in Chicago, E.A. Inskeep *(known as Ned)* left his job with an Ottumwa bank and joined the company. The company continued to grow and moved to larger quarters on Wabash Avenue directly across from famed Marshall Field's department store, and remained there until Chambers-Inskeep was sold to F.A. Hardy in 1903.

Innovations

Chambers-Inskeep introduced a number of innovations. Charles Inskeep decided it was possible to design a Retinoscope and Ophthalmoscope that would be self-illuminating instead of using reflected light as existing models did. Their work was successful and these two important instruments were introduced to the industry. The next development was the C-I Ophthalmometer. Javal in France had introduced the ophthalmometer to the world, but it was Chambers-Inskeep who introduced the first one with illuminated mires. They also developed an early lensometer.

When the company combined with F.A. Hardy Company in 1903, Charles and Edward Inskeep exchanged their stock for Hardy stock and stayed on. The Chambers all took cash and left the company. David Chambers moved to Portland, Ore. where, for a while, he operated a wholesale and retail optical business. Later he concentrated on retail and was active in it until his death. In 1905, E.A. "Ned" Inskeep moved to Denver where F.A. Hardy had a small branch at 1622 Arapahoe Street over the retail store of Paul Weiss. When AO took over F.A. Hardy, Ned Inskeep became branch manager and later was AO Mountain States zone manager until his

retirement in 1939. Ned's daughter married Paul Rinkle who also worked for American Optical, calling on independent AO distributors until his retirement.

COLUMBIAN OPTICAL COMPANY

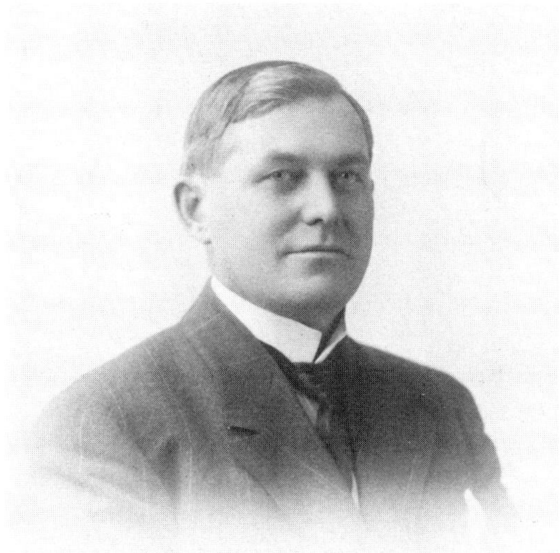

A.I. Agnew was one of the original Kryptok stockholders. An offshoot of his Columbian Optical became today's Columbian Bifocal Company.

OLA OPTICAL INDUSTRY MUSEUM

The company was founded by Aretas I. Agnew who worked for Geneva Optical in Chicago and had been in charge of Geneva's exhibit at the Chicago Columbian Exposition in 1893. Geneva Optical operated a booth during the fair and sold thousands of eyeglasses at a very substantial profit.

Agnew opened the first Columbian Optical Company office in Denver in 1895, another in Omaha in 1896, and Kansas City in 1897. Subsequent branches were established throughout the Midwest and west coast. Basically a retail operation, they also conducted an extensive wholesale business. They ground their own lenses and became one of only two manufacturers permitted to process Kryptoks in the early 20th century, the other being E. B. Meyrowitz.

Roy Wahlgren *(AAWO president, 1924-25),* an employee and later president of Riggs Optical, described Agnew this way. "He was not only a genial, friendly character and a wonderful mixer, he was a man of business ability, a shrewd operator, who before his death, amassed a considerable fortune." Agnew opened a Portland branch in 1905 and another in Klamath Falls in 1938. Sid Noles established their Seattle office in 1916 and later would buy the Seattle and Klamath Falls branches.

Elwood Riggs *(later of Riggs Optical Company),* joined Columbian in 1897 and ran the Kansas City store until a difference of policy with A.I. Agnew, caused him to leave the company in 1901. An automobile accident in 1912 led to A.I. Agnew's death and his widow continued operating the company. As an original investor, Agnew owned stock in the Kryptok Company but never got to see the astounding profits his investment produced.

Some years later, William Riggs purchased Columbian's Kansas City office, later selling it to Riggs Optical Company. It was reported that Columbian's Omaha store was purchased secretly by Riggs Optical and operated under the Columbian name. That office ultimately became part of Kindy Optical Company.

The Denver office was purchased in 1925 by Tommy Thompson *(who had been with the company since 1905)*. By this time, the name of that branch had been changed to Columbian Bifocal Company.

D.V. BROWN COMPANY

Daniel Vinton Brown *(AAWO president, 1898)* was born in 1850 at Wilmont, N.H.. Shortly after, his father moved to Southbridge, Mass. In 1867 after graduation, young Dan started work for R.H. Cole Company before they merged with American Optical. In 1880, he left AO to become a founder of the Southbridge Optical Company and when they moved to Boston, he went with them. Shortly after that, he went to work for James W. Queen & Company in Philadelphia. The first thing he did on arrival in Philadelphia is open a savings account with enough money to get him back to Southbridge in case things went bad. He never had to fall back on his nest egg. He next went to work for the Philadelphia Optical & Watch Company but left them several years before they failed. In 1890, he founded the wholesale house of D.V. Brown which became one of the major wholesale optical houses in the country. He was a prominent member and served as president of the American Association of Wholesale Opticians *(the early OLA)* in 1898. Following his retirement, the company was run by his son Andrew V. Brown *(AAWO president, 1909, 10)*. D.V. Brown died on December 7, 1915 and many leading figures from the optical industry attended his funeral.

D.V. Brown was ultimately acquired by American Optical.

GENEVA OPTICAL COMPANY

A.L. Smith started making frames in Geneva, N.Y. in 1869 and four years later, formally adopted the name Geneva Optical Company. By now he was manufacturing and wholesaling optical goods. In 1890, Smith resigned and moved to Chicago where he founded Geneva Optical Company of Chicago, Minneapolis, Des Moines, Denver and Cincinnati. This company would eventually become part of Riggs Optical in 1929 when Riggs was an affiliate of Bausch & Lomb.

Meanwhile the parent company in Geneva continued growing and in 1893, the wholesale and manufacturing functions separated. William Smith, president at that time, built a large factory on his nursery farm near the city limits and established the Standard Optical Company. James Brown and Theo Smith took over the wholesale business and incorporated it in 1900 as Geneva Optical. Jack Brayton *(AAWO president, 1904)*, the inventor of the Geneva Lens Measure, was associated with Geneva Optical for many years. Henry De Zeng, an inventor of many optical instruments also worked for Geneva before founding his well-known De Zeng Optical Equipment Company. Geneva also had a large display at the Chicago World's Fair in 1893 where they demonstrated lens grinding in the Machinery Hall.

LOUIS FRIEDLANDER, INC.

The firm was started in New York City in April, 1906 by Louis Friedlander. Their wholesale laboratory did business in all the New England territories and New York, New Jersey and Pennsylvania. Louis passed away in 1939 and was succeeded by his nephew Maurice Friedlander. By 1942, the company had 30 employees. What happened to the company is unknown.

PEERLESS OPTICAL

Homer White *(AAWO president, 1917-18)* graduated from Muskingum College in New Concord, Ohio. He had been attending college so he could follow his father in the medical profession. His father was in general practice and young Homer had spent many nights driving his father around the countryside calling on patients. That was when he decided to specialize in eye, ear, nose and throat work, a decision that led him to the optical business.

His father died unexpectedly, leaving small children at home and making it necessary for Homer to leave Ohio Medical College to help support the family. Still having his eye on the optical business, he took a job on the road selling optical goods, meanwhile taking a course with Dr. Thompson of South Bend, Ind. He continued working in the optical business until his family no longer needed his support. In January of 1907, he married and in the same year organized the Ohio Optical Company in Columbus, Ohio.

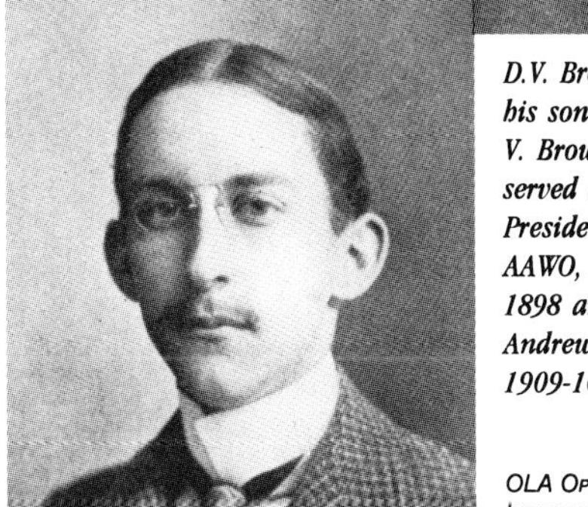

D.V. Brown and his son Andrew V. Brown both served as President of AAWO, D.V. in 1898 and Andrew in 1909-10.

A young Andrew Brown who would later serve two terms as president of the AAWO.

He joined the American Association of Wholesale Opticians and was active in the group, eventually being elected to the board of directors. He served as president for two terms and represented the optical industry on the Service Committee during World War I. The optical industry was in turmoil following the war. Homer consolidated his Ohio Optical Company with the George S. Johnston Optical of Chicago. The resulting company was then sold to American Optical. Homer was appointed zone manager for AO with headquarters in Columbus but, after two years, resigned and accepted a position with White Haines, remaining there until January, 1932. Deciding conditions were right for a new wholesale laboratory, White, Harry Stewart and Edwin Sheehy opened the Peerless Optical Company in Columbus, Ohio on August 1, 1932 with Homer White as president.

Association Work

White was a strong believer in organizations. Early in his career, he helped organize and promote the Ohio State Optical Association, later to become the Ohio Optometric Association. After entering the independent wholesale business, he and a number of colleagues formed an independent wholesale organization with Homer White as its first president. He was president when N.R.A. *(National Recovery Act)* went into effect and he represented the association on the N.R.A. Committee which formulated the code for the optical industry. The Federal Government later appointed him a member of the Code Authority.

When the N.R.A. was abolished by the Supreme Court, an all-inclusive association was organized by consolidating the AAWO and the Independent Association. This took place in Rochester, N.Y. with the name Optical Wholesalers National Association *(OWNA)*. Homer White was elected to the board of directors, a position he held for a number of years. He also helped organize and served as president of the Ohio Valley Wholesale Association. He died in April, 1954.

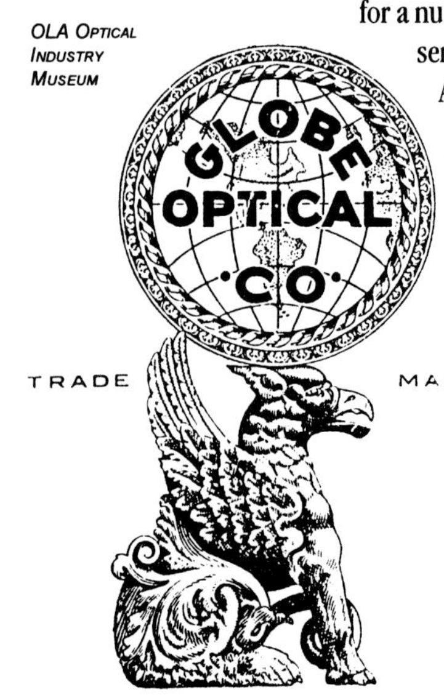

GLOBE OPTICAL COMPANY

In 1888, an optical retailer in Boston named J.W. Sanborn started doing some wholesale optical work. By 1892, deciding there was a need for an exclusive wholesaler, he organized the Globe Optical Company. This company became a major wholesaler/laboratory, selling their goods all over the country. The company was acquired, along with the Federal Optical Company by American Optical on June 1, 1923.

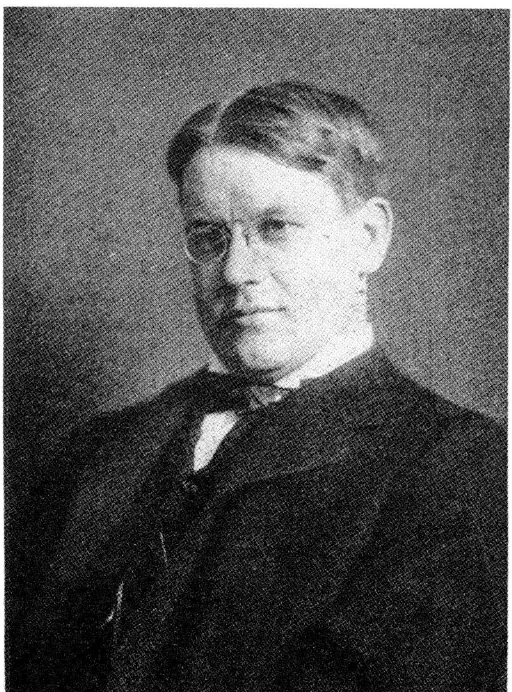

John Hardin was F.A. Hardy's protégé and ultimately bought his company. He later sold the company to American Optical and became a vice president of AO. OLA OPTICAL INDUSTRY MUSEUM

F.A. HARDY COMPANY

F. A. Hardy *(AAWO president, 1896)* was in charge of the optical and material department at Otto Young & Company. Almer Coe was one of his associates and both young men left Young about the same time. Hardy started examining eyes and supplying glasses at retail but eventually decided his interest was in the wholesale end of the business. The year Mr. Hardy set up his new company was 1884. American Optical only distributed their goods through independent wholesalers so it wasn't difficult to buy AO goods for the new company. As a side line, he added Whitcomb Jewelers Lathes which the company distributed for years.

John Hardin

In 1890, Hardy hired a young man named John Hardin *(AAWO president, 1904)* as an assistant shipping clerk. Hardin gradually worked into the stock room and then to the materials department. Hardy took to young Hardin and made it possible for Hardin to acquire stock in the company with money he borrowed at the bank. By 1908, Hardin was running the business, enabling Hardy to join the Diamond Rubber Company of Akron, Ohio, where he later became president. Diamond Rubber was taken over by B.F. Goodrich Company and Hardy later served Goodrich as president. Hardy retired from F.A. Hardy in 1910 and John Hardin became president. The company was now a corporation and Hardin made it possible for a number of employees to become stockholders in the company.

An example of how successful and well-run the company was is illustrated by an account that ran in an 1897 issue of THE OPTICAL JOURNAL. On three successive days the previous fall, F.A. Hardy had received, aside from stock orders, over 2,200 prescriptions on Saturday, Monday and Tuesday, October 10, 12 and 13. By Tuesday evening, they had shipped out over 2,000 of the jobs with errors of less than one-half of one percent.

Merger with American Optical

F.A. Hardy was probably the largest distributor American Optical had by 1921 so it seemed natural, as AO determined to form their own distribution network, to turn first to the F.A. Hardy Company. They purchased the company and immediately put John Hardin to work setting up their new distribution network. Hardin helped them acquire five more labs. John Hardin was made a trustee and vice-president of American Optical, along with Fred Merry of Merry Optical. Other wholesalers exchanging their company stock for AO stock were the Julius King Optical Company, Globe Optical, Boston Optical and D.V. Brown.

IMPERIAL OPTICAL (CANADA)

Percy Hermant arrived in St. Johns, Canada from Russia with $3 in rubles in his pocket. An orphan with no experience in optics, he was placed in the home of a high class peddler *(high class peddlers had a cart)*. During a summer holiday, he went to Boston and attended Kline's School of Optics. Returning to Canada and his cart, he was now equipped to sell glasses. For prescription work, his orders had to go back to Boston. He decided the glasses should be made in St. John's so Percy and a friend opened a small two man shop. By 1904, he had shops in Hamilton, London, Ontario and then in Toronto. During the first World War when lens blanks were impossible to obtain, Hermant purchased a small lens plant in the United States and moved it to Canada.

By the 1970s, the company was operating 105 wholesale laboratories and over 400 retail stores. They manufactured frames and lenses and had eight instrument depots and were Canada's largest contact lens distributor. Unfortunately, this optical conglomerate suffered financial reverses caused, according to rumor, by real estate reverses. The company went into bankruptcy in 1993 and no longer exists. With Imperial Optical out of the Canadian market almost overnight, independent wholesale laboratories were called on to successfully fill the sudden void created when so many laboratories vanished overnight.

JOHNSTON OPTICAL COMPANY

Johnston Optical was one of the earliest wholesalers, opening in 1876 in a small shop in Detroit. George Johnston *(AAWO president, 1897)* had worked as a salesman for L. Black & Company and decided the optical business had a great future. His brothers, John Milton and Aaron C. joined him shortly after the company opened. They remained until 1892 when George bought them out and John and Aaron moved to Chicago. One of the salesmen George hired was W.D. Fennimore who represented the company in California, later retiring to start his own business under the name California Optical Company.

George's nephew Paul Johnston *(son of John Milton Johnston)* recalled the period between 1886 and 1889. It was at Johnston Optical that he saw his first telephone, as well as the first electric light bulb. Johnston Optical was always first to adopt new and better devices. The company, by this time, covered the entire country from coast to coast and from Mexico to Canada.

Continuing Education

They published a bimonthly optical Journal called "The Johnston Eye-Echo". It was aimed at *"Opticians who have or seek an established reputation for skill in fitting the eye"* and carried an annual subscription rate of 50 cents a year. Anyone purchasing $5 worth of goods would receive it free. Each issue contained lessons on vision and refracting plus questions and answers regarding previous lessons. Little advertising and almost no illustrations were included. This was a time when education was vital to anyone attracted to the new professions. Each issue included a section called "Correspondents' Views". The November/December issue of 1889 had comments from readers such as, *"Send me back issues. I cannot do without it, C. Scofield, Optician"* or *"I cannot afford to miss anything. The Eye Echo is the Boss."* or *"Please send five years of the Eye Echo. C.P. Pengra, Ph.D., M.D."*

By 1897, the company had 6,500 accounts and claimed "the sun never ceases to shine upon goods manufactured by them." They also used a clever marketing technique for their catalog. They put all prices on the back side of

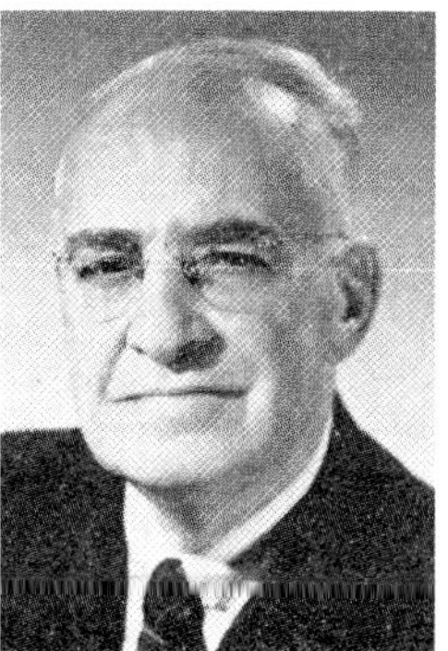

Homer White (Peerless Optical) was president of the AAWO in 1917-1918.

OLA OPTICAL INDUSTRY MUSEUM

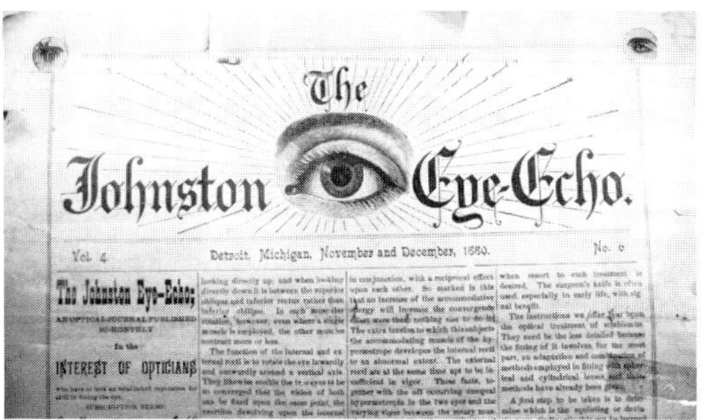

The Johnston Eye Echo was a widely distributed continuing education journal for aspiring optometrists and opticians.

OLA OPTICAL INDUSTRY MUSEUM

each sheet. In this way, the retailer could show the photos in the catalog to patients without revealing wholesale cost figures. The company also published two prices for each product. They showed the stock price *(most items were less expensive when ordered in multiple units)* as well as the Rx price.

George Johnston died in 1920 and his son George Oliver became head of Johnston Optical. George had graduated from Yale and served as an ensign in the Navy during the first World War but quickly learned what he needed to know to run what had become a major wholesale operation. The company focused on the laboratory business. Because lab work required fast, local service, they concentrated their efforts on the state of Michigan, establishing 12 branches there. The company was acquired by American Optical in 1923.

J.M. & A.C. JOHNSTON OPTICAL

This company was started by brothers of George S. Johnston *(see Johnston Optical, Detroit)*. Both brothers had worked for George in Detroit but left, moving to Chicago to start their own wholesale operation in 1892. A.C. Johnston had interests outside the optical industry and eventually J.M. bought out A.C.'s interests. The Drs. McFatrich were associated with J.M. for a time until they left to start their own school, Northern Illinois College of Ophthalmology and Otology.

Follow the Bouncing Ball

The story now grows a little complicated. In 1903, J.M Johnston decided to retire and sold the company to F.A. Hardy with the arrangement that the name would be changed to Peerless Optical and be operated by J.M.'s son George S. Johnston. This arrangement lasted until 1909 when Hardy sold his interest in F.A. Hardy to John Hardin. Hardin decided to merge the Peerless Optical operation into the F.A. Hardy Company. At that point, George S. Johnston left and set up a new company he chose to call the George S. Johnston Company of Chicago.

George built his company to 17 branches. The year was 1923 and American Optical acquired George S. Johnston Company. Following the consolidation, George Johnston moved to San Francisco and took over management of American Optical's Pacific coast territory *(see R. Mohr & Sons)*.

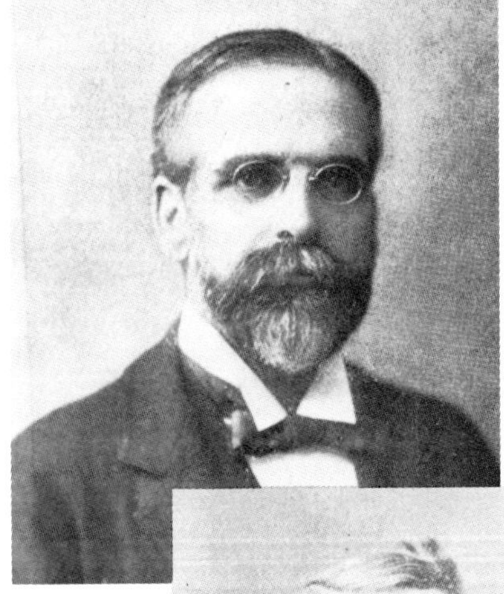

George Johnston served as the third president of the AAWO. His brothers left him to start the J.M. & A.C. Johnston Company.

OLA OPTICAL INDUSTRY MUSEUM

J.M. Johnston (pictured here) eventually bought out his brother's interests in their company.

OLA OPTICAL INDUSTRY MUSEUM

KING OPTICAL COMPANY

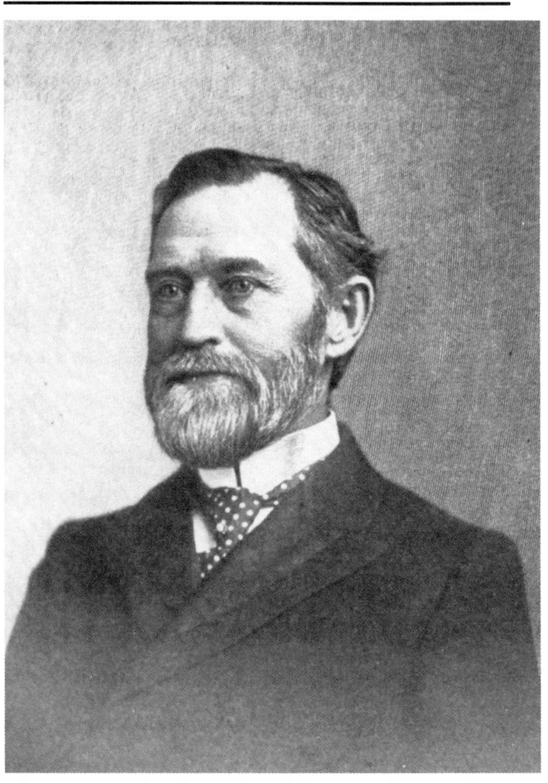

Julius King was elected president of the AAWO during its first two years (1894-95).

OLA OPTICAL INDUSTRY MUSEUM

Julius King *(first AAWO president, 1894-95)* completed his education at Duff's College in Pittsburgh and, following graduation, joined his father in his jewelry business in Warren, Ohio. The company sold optical goods on the side and young King quickly became more interested in optical than jewelry as he worked out better ways to fit glasses. In those days, spectacles could not be adjusted. The same width frame was used in every case, regardless of the patient's face size. King saw the desirability of making an adjustable frame and conceived the idea of a sterling silver bridge combined with a steel front. The frame could be bent to any required width and King came up with the uninspired name "Patent Combination Spectacle" for his invention. To help dealers sell the new frame, retail customers were told that the next time they purchased eyeglasses, they would receive a 25 cent allowance towards the cost of a new frame.

Another of King's important accomplishments was a wall chart he developed for testing vision. It was two by four feet in size and so successful, it was still being sold in a smaller size in the 1940s. The chart featured different size letters to assist in determining the proper correction for glasses.

Advertising

Julius King learned early the value of advertising. Here are several examples taken from his scrapbook titled "Advertisements from 1866 to 1870":

> *"TEN THOUSAND EYES!*
>
> *Are being constantly injured for want of a little common sense precaution. Is it a little difficult to see to read by day? You need spectacles. Go to Julius King's and let him measure your eyes with his magnificent Eye Measurer and you will get a pair of spectacles that can't be beat. King has the only Eye Measurer in the county."*
>
> *"PEBBLES COLD, GLASS WARM"*
>
> *There is no need of being deceived in buying spectacles. Genuine pebbles being made of stone are cold when touched by the tongue, while glass is warm. Pebbles are clearer and harder, keep the eye cool and cannot be scratched, which is not the case with glass. King on Main Street, Warren, Ohio, has just received his first assortment of genuine pebbles and will sell them $1 a pair less than they sell the same kind in Cleveland."*

The invention of "King's Combination Spectacle" together with improved test charts enabled King to establish agencies with other dealers, resulting in a wholesale business in addition to his retail operation. Another example of Julius King's marketing sense is illustrated by how he used a new employee named Rodney Pierce. Pierce was hired straight off the farm in 1872 and paid $8 a week, plus board, to do a house-to-house canvas of King's home town, Warren, Ohio, soliciting customers to have their eyes tested by Julius King. Rodney Pierce would later set up his own wholesale laboratory called Rodney Pierce Optical *(later acquired by AO).*

Education

In Cleveland, King had came to the conclusion that somebody in the optical profession should study medicine with the intention of teaching those interested in optics to fit eyes scientifically. Deciding he should be that person, he registered at the Western Reserve Medical College in Cleveland and ultimately received his M.D degree. Still not satisfied, he took a postgraduate course in the New York Eye & Ear Infirmary under Dr. St. John Roosa.

Returning to Cleveland, he worked up a course of instruction for opticians. He developed a practical course of "Instructions on Refraction", designed as an intimate course that would give sound and practical information on elementary optics. It was 1887 when he started his school for opticians. King didn't charge for his lectures. He invited King Optical customers, jewelers, watchmak-ers and druggists to come to Cleveland. This school was so successful and practical that optometrists and opticians from every part of the country — 1,200 of them — at one time or another, took the instruction course. These were jewelers and optical dealers who wanted to learn how to refract. Many of the most successful optometrists and opticians of this century's first 50 years attributed their success to the training received from Dr. King's course. When King Optical moved to its New York headquarters, the courses continued with L.L. Furgeson as chief instructor. The course lasted two weeks, after which the students were sold Dr. King's Elite Test Case and sent on their way *(fully informed on how to order goods from King Optical).*

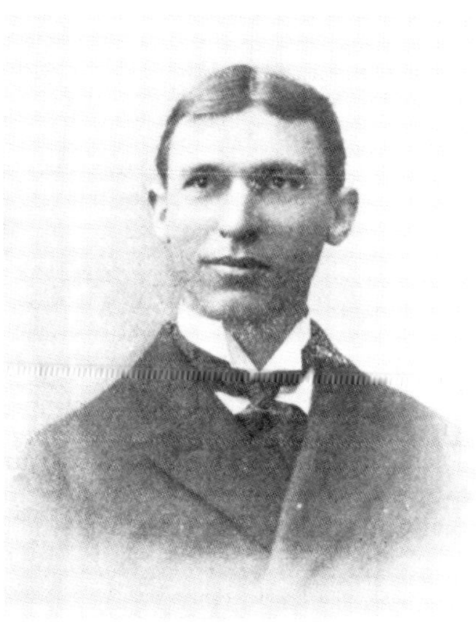

Burnham W. King was a younger son of Julius and also served as AAWO president in 1919/20.

King Optical Founded

King's success had prompted him to sell his interest in the jewelry business in 1870 and open a wholesale optical business. He immediately hired Rodney Pierce and made him their first traveling salesman. The company grew rapidly and by 1875 it was necessary to move to Cleveland. By 1885, the "House of King" was so successful, they sent their best salesman, Leo Wormser *(AAWO president, 1906),* to open a company branch in New York. Meanwhile, Julius King's inventive mind constantly worked on better ways to fit eyeglasses.

Trade-Off

In December, 1920, an agreement was reached between the F.A. Hardy Company and the Julius King Optical Company. Hardy agreed to sell their New York City factories and salesrooms to Julius King in exchange for King selling his operations in Chicago and Davenport to F.A. Hardy.

In 1891, King sent his son Burnham King *(AAWO president 1919/20)* to open a branch office in Mexico City called "Opticos de King". They later developed a successful export business with Cuba and South America.

Safety Eyewear

In 1908, Dr. King became aware of the number of industrial eye injuries. He had learned that 650 eyes were lost in one year in

Walter G. King (Julius' son) was president of the AAWO in 1901 and later headed up AO's Safety Division.

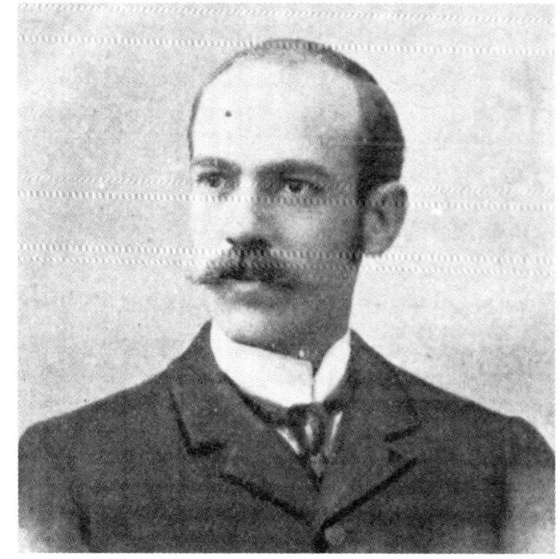

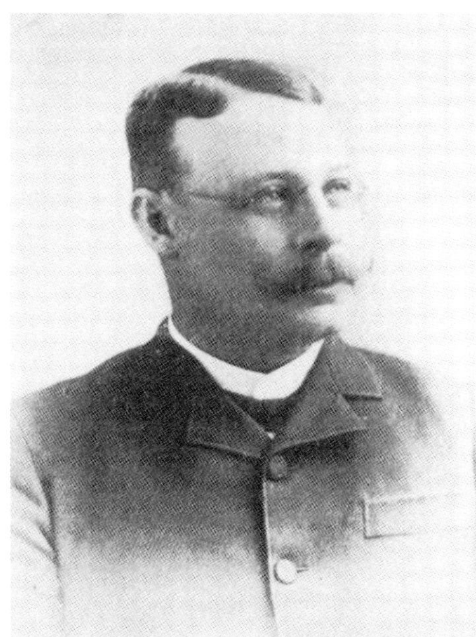

Rodney Pierce was Julius King's first employee and would later, with King's aid, set up a new wholesale laboratory called Rodney Pierce Optical.

the state of Pennsylvania. He also determined that 50,000 artificial eyes were imported every year. He became one of the first to enter the "Safety First" field and his company had a large department devoted to industrial safety and eye protection. He designed and produced a goggle known as "King's Saniglas" with large round lenses. The first lenses were made of thick plate glass, but complaints of distortion led the company to grind front and back surfaces, eliminating this complaint.

American Optical had developed a process of hardening by heat treating the glass lenses. AO called these lenses "Super Armor-Plate". The following quotation comes from a bulletin from the General Safety Agent for the New York Central Railroad:

> *"We are arranging to supply every man whose duties require him to do metal chipping with a pair of goggles known as the Julius King Saniglas Safety Goggle, which is the goggles adopted by the International Harvester Company and used by many plants of the United States Steel Corporation."*

Julius' son Walter played a prominent role in developing industrial eye safety in this country. In 1901, Walter was elected president of the American Association of Wholesale Opticians *(His father, Dr. King had been the first AAWO president, serving two terms in 1894-95).* Walter was president of the National Safety Council in 1926 and served for 15 years on their Executive Committee.

Alumni

Julius King spawned a number of other prominent optical wholesalers. In 1896, the Julius King Optical Company joined Rodney Pierce in establishing a new company called Rodney Pierce Optical Company with Pierce as president. Another key employee was Frank N. Kreisel who became sales manager for King. He left the company in 1907 to establish Sioux Optical Company in Sioux City, Iowa. This company was acquired by American Optical and Kreisel eventually became general manager of AO's Chicago office.

Willie Dow started as a messenger boy in King's Chicago office at $6 a week. He advanced rapidly to manager of the Prescription and Sales Department. When this office was sold to F.A. Hardy, Dow left and started Dow Optical Company, eventually becoming a leading Chicago wholesale laboratory. William R. Uhlemann was a gold worker in the Chicago office, but left in 1912 to start Uhlemann Optical, ultimately becoming one of the larger retail/wholesale laboratories in the country. Julius' son Fred worked for his father until 1912 when he started his own business, the F.W. King Optical Company of Cleveland, Ohio which specialized in sporting glasses and safety goggles.

In 1923, Julius King Optical Company was acquired by American Optical. Following the acquisition, Julius' son Walter G. King *(AAWO president, 1901)* helped AO develop and set up their Safety Division and served as director of safety for a number of years. Dr. Julius King was a prominent figure in the development of the optical industry. His constant endeavors to elevate the educational standards of his chosen field had much to do with the rapid advance of the optical professions. He was the first teacher of optics in the United States. He enjoyed a long and intimate friendship with AO's George W. Wells. Dr. King died in 1925.

MERRY OPTICAL COMPANY

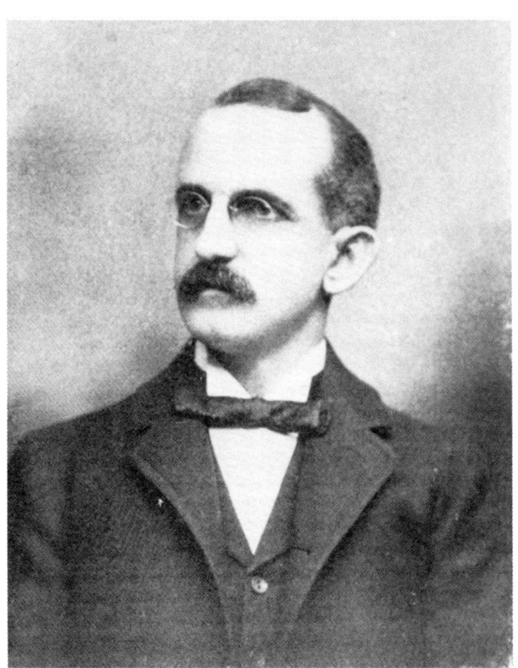

C.L. Merry served as president of the AAWO in 1902.

C. L. Merry *(AAWO president, 1902)* was a retail jeweler and optician for 15 years in Norwalk, Ohio before being hired as a salesman by the Julius King Optical Company in 1884. He spent 200 days a year on the road, receiving $1,200 plus traveling expenses. His job included calling on jewelers, instructing them in the use of trial lenses and convincing them to give more attention to their optical departments. Based on information he gained on the road, he convinced Dr. King to open a Kansas City branch in 1890, which soon became very profitable for King. Merry, determined to go into business for himself, purchased the Kansas City branch and renamed it the Merry Optical Company in 1895. It became one of the largest wholesale labs in the country. C.L. Merry died in 1920.

Fred, son of C.L. Merry, joined the Julius King organization in 1888 and went on the road. He joined the Merry Optical Company when his father bought it from King. Merry Optical was purchased by American Optical in 1922 at which time, Fred became vice president of AO. Fred Merry died in 1934.

MICHAELS OPTICAL COMPANY

In August of 1904, two young men named Lou Michaels and Sylvan Pollak opened Pollak & Michaels, a wholesale company in New York. They sold only optical merchandise and the business was successful. In 1906, they moved to 51 Maiden Lane to set up a small laboratory. Pollak contracted an illness and spent less and less time in the business and eventually died in 1918.

By this time, the company had grown considerably. Michaels incorporated the company as Michaels Optical and moved to West 46th Street and opened branches in Brooklyn and Harrisburg, Penn. The company continued to grow until June of 1930 when it was sold to Bausch & Lomb and became part of Colonial Optical Company. Lou Michaels was transferred to Richmond, Va. and became vice president of Southeastern Optical Company, another B&L affiliate.

MCINTIRE, MAGEE AND BROWN COMPANY

It was on October 1, 1884 that a skinny kid named A. Reed McIntire *(AAWO president, 1907, 1913, 1928, 1929)* started work in the optical shop of Queen & Company, probably the most progressive optical wholesaler of the day. The company had been founded by James W. Queen who had learned his trade at the McAllister firm. Queen & Company had built up a very substantial wholesale and retail business. McIntire wrote his memories in 1938 and the following is excerpted from that account:

> *I wish it were possible to make you see the picture of that old shop as I have it in my mind. There was a line of work benches along the windows on Chestnut Street and a line of grindstones set at right angle along the wall. The grindstones consisted of rough stones similar to the ones found in the barn yard of every farm [along with] the fine Creighlith stones imported from Scotland. There were two lines of spherical surface grinding*

lathes, a crude machine for grinding cylindrical surfaces, a turning lathe and work bench. Some of the surfacing machines were turned with a foot treadle.

The machine for drilling lenses was on a separate bench. The drill had a vertical shaft which held the diamond point and a table with an upright point on which the lens was set. There was an arm under the table which was pressed down to bring the lens in contact with the drill. There were no gauges of stops to control the position of the hole or the distance it would be drilled from the edge of the hole.

You must remember there were no toric (6 base curved) lenses nor were there any fused or invisible bifocals, only the old Split or Franklin bifocal and the solid or ground type. Incidentally, the Split bifocal was the first merged image bifocal made. In making it, a biconvex lens with the distance strength was cut horizontally along the line of the optical center and a lens of the reading strength treated the same way. When these lenses had been edged flat along the horizontal line, the optical center of the distance lens was below the edge and the optical center of the reading portion was above the edge. We doubt very much whether old Ben Franklin had any ideas about merged images when he invented the bifocal.

Flat Lenses

Nothing but flat lenses were used. The English inch system was used in all refractions, so all lenses were ground on curves computed on the radius of the circle giving the proper strength. All lenses were imported, principally from France. We had nothing to check the work with except test lenses. The test sets used were made by Nachet and Company of Paris. The focal power of these was not always correct and I well remember the trial set in our shop. Incorrect lenses had been replaced in this set so that, when any question

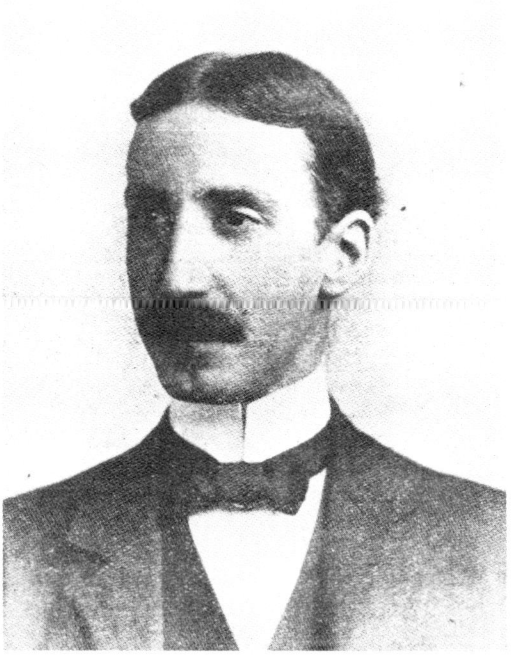

Reed McIntire, a four-time president of the AAWO (1907, 1913, 1928 and 1929) took great pride from his role in helping establish the American Association of Wholesale Opticians.

OLA OPTICAL INDUSTRY MUSEUM

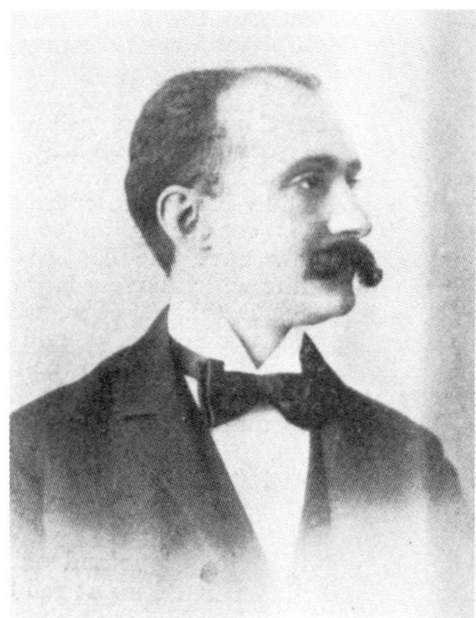

Leo Wormser was Julius King's best salesman and served as president of the AAWO in 1906.

arose regarding the focal power of a lens, that particular set was the standard.

In those days, all rimless lenses were edged by hand on the side of the Creightith stone. The face of the stone was used for bevel edging and the edge of the stone for grooving, for we still used fine steel frames, the eye wire being made of a slender round wire which was inserted in a groove in the edge of the lens. All frames were made with very small eyes in those days. I remember we had a job to make a blue steel octagon-shaped frame one time. The eyes were only 5/8th of an inch high and about 1 3/8" inch long. They were worn by a very stout man who had puffy cheeks.

Frames were made in solid gold, silver, German silver and bronze or blue steel. The eyes were very small and there was very little attention paid to pupillary centers or other measurements. The temples were usually straight, although the curved or riding bow temple was coming into use. Hardly any rimless glasses were worn, but were beginning to be sold. Opticians were giving some thought to astigmatism and prescription lenses were made up. Generally speaking, people did not get a pair of glasses until they grew old and needed something for reading.

Machine Power

We had a gas engine in the basement. There was a long belt connected with the main shaft which was on the floor of the third floor shop which we had to step over in passing. Once in a while that long belt from the basement would break or run off the pulley. Billy Hartnett and I would chase down stairs, lift a trap door on the first floor, go down a ladder, and replace the belt. I often think of the power that was wasted in that long drive from the basement to the third floor, but I suppose the gas engine was too heavy to be put up in the shop.

I started out receiving $2.50 per week but every six months or so I got a raise of 50 cents. Under the NRA (the depression's National Recovery Act) we were compelled to pay a boy $16 per week after he had been employed for six months. As a boy is really not of much value for a couple of years, this seemed rather a hardship. When I started, we worked from 7:00 am to 6:00 pm every week day except Saturday when we stopped at 4:00 pm. This made 58 hours per week.

Sales

The methods of handling the wholesale business were just as simple as the methods of manufacture. Salesmen made three or four trips a year, taking with them two large sample cases. Opticians anticipated their needs and placed orders for supplies that would last until the salesman came around again. There was no thought of having branch offices as a means of giving service to customers. Today (1938), the wholesale optical house has branches in every strategic point, thereby increasing the service to their customers.

In 1888, Mr. D.V. Brown became President of the Philadelphia Optical and Watch Company and hired me to take charge of their shop. In 1892, D.V. Brown retired and my responsibilities increased. For this I received the munificent sum of $20 per week.

In 1894, the Philadelphia Optical and Watch Company failed due to bad financial management. McIntire had worked there with Edgar Brown and these two, along with Harry Ulmer and an ex-Queen & Company employee, George Magee, formed a partnership called McIntire, Ulmer and Company. Bausch & Lomb extended credit and they started what turned out to be a very good relationship.

Wholesalers Association Formed

That year was momentous to McIntire for another reason. He continues with his story:

There was one event of great importance to the wholesale optical business that occurred in the spring of that year. That was the formation of the American Association of Wholesale Opticians (AAWO). Henry Kirstein, George Magee and I are the only men still living who attended the organization meeting in New York City. As neither Mr. Kirstein or Mr. Magee is active in business today, I claim the distinction of being the Dean of that organization.

Harry Ulmer left the business in 1895 and in 1907, the business was incorporated as McIntire, Magee and Brown Company. In 1912, Magee withdrew due to ill health but returned after the death of Brown in 1917.

World War I

The first World War was tough on the company. Some of their workmen volunteered for service and others were drafted and finding replacements became difficult. Lenses were also hard to get *(most lenses were imported at that time)*. Bausch & Lomb had started manufacturing glass but their factory was doing so much government work it was difficult to get lenses for civilian use.

Bausch & Lomb Affiliation

McIntire continues:

> *July, 1930 was an eventful time for us. We had moved to new larger quarters. We announced our affiliation with the Bausch & Lomb Optical Company and took over the branch of the Michaels Optical Company in Harrisburg and the branches of Bohling & Gibbs in Washington, DC and Philadelphia.*

Reed McIntire concluded his reminisces with the comment, *"The young people may not be interested in the past, but to those of us 'who are but children of an older growth' we are happy in our memories, for after all, it has been a tremendously interesting era in which we have lived."*

QUEEN & COMPANY

This business was started in 1853 by James W. Queen *(who had received his training at McAllister's during the 1830s)* and W. Y. McAllister, a McAllister grandson. The new company was named Queen and Company and later James W. Queen & Co. in 1858 when young Samuel L. Fox joined the firm as a partner. This company was scientifically oriented and among the very first to grind lenses in the United States, including the difficult cylindrical lenses. They may have been the first to manufacture cylinders in any quantity. They sold instruments as well, including trial sets and ophthalmoscopes, invented by the German ophthalmologist, Dr. Helmholst, in 1855.

It was at Queen & Company where many future leading lights of opticianry, optometry, wholesalers, and machinery manufacturers received early training. The company became the largest scientific optical house in the United States, selling all over the country. Queen was a leading optician in Philadelphia before retiring because of ill health in 1885. The business continued under Fox.

Queen had major financial problems in 1893 when the company went through bankruptcy after incautiously expanding in 1892, just before the 1893 business depression. The company emerged under the direction of John G. Gray as president and Sam Fox as vice-president. They never again, however, achieved the same level of prominence as in the late 19th century and eventually went out of business about 1910.

R. MOHR & SONS

Harry and Selby Mohr opened a wholesale optical business in San Francisco in 1906 called R. Mohr & Sons *(named after their father Rudolph Mohr).* Harry learned the optical business working for Standard Optical, starting in 1896. Their new company opened on April 8, 1906 and 10 days later was completely wiped out by the earthquake and fire that followed. A month later, they reopened in a basement, the only location available. Later they moved to the Jewelers Building. The company grew over the years and became one of the largest wholesalers on the West Coast, with laboratories in San Francisco, Honolulu, Stockton and Sacramento.

They were also one of the largest importers of optical goods and were leaders in the development of "ground and polished" sunglasses. Until that time, all plano sunglasses were made with cheap "drop" lenses of highly doubtful quality. Mohr believed a discriminating public would buy better sunglasses with quality ground and polished lenses if they just had the chance. They produced thousands of sunglasses, using AO frames and inserting ground and polished sun lenses in them. Many were sold in drug stores *(also a prime market for American Optical).*

In 1914, a young man named Ray McChesney started work as an errand boy *(ending up as west coast zone manager for AO).* Also working there was Harry Katz who would later form a partnership with Russell Klein, Branch Manager for Riggs Optical in Sacramento and open Katz and Klein laboratory in Sacramento. Other alumni of R. Mohr included Alec Rhine who left in 1919 and started Rhine Optical Company and Elliott Shane.

Shane worked there from 1936 until he went in the Army during World War II, rejoining R. Mohr after his army service. He left the company in 1947 to start Shane-Michael Optical, a major frame and lens importer in San Francisco. Shane tells the story that, even though American Optical acquired R. Mohr in 1928 *(for $750,000),* the AO connection remained a secret for years. Even the employees didn't know they were part

Samuel L. Fox joined Queen & Company as a partner and eventually took over the company when Queen retired in 1885.

Elliott Shane served in the 48th Evacuation Hospital during World War II in the China-Burma theater. He operated a field optical shop and is seen here cutting a lens in 1944. When a G.I. broke his glasses in the field, the soldier had to hand-crank the edger as Shane edged the lenses.

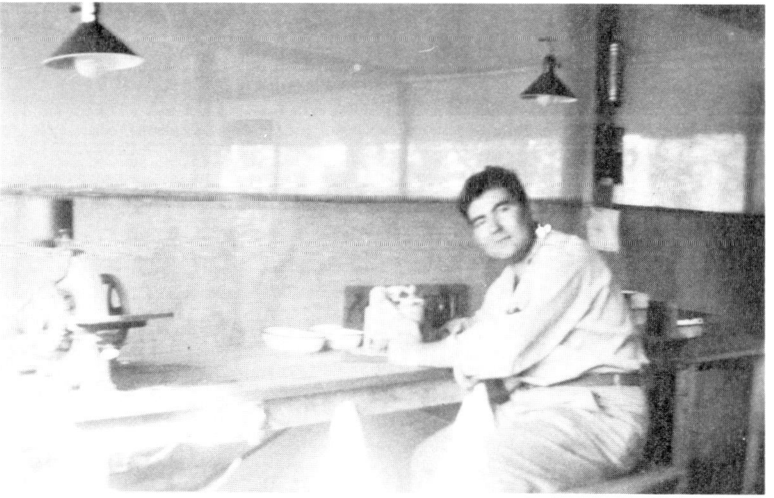

of American Optical. R. Mohr salesmen were out competing fiercely against AO every day. The truth came out in 1940 in a strange way.

By this time, Univis had introduced the flat top bifocal. Following the lead of Kryptok and Ultex, Univis would only sell to franchised laboratories. American Optical did not have a Univis franchise and independent laboratories made the most of this. At a general sales meeting held by American Optical in San Francisco in 1940, someone chided George S. Johnston, AO's zone manager, about AO not having a Univis franchise. This made him sore and he popped up and said, "What do you mean, we don't have a Univis franchise. American Optical owns R. Mohr & Sons and they have one". This was the first anyone learned of the AO connection.

The company grew to 50 employees with 6 salesmen covering every state from Denver west. Harry Mohr retired in 1938 after 40 years in the optical business

REYNOLDS OPTICAL

E. W. Reynolds had been in the jewelry business in Connecticut when he took sick and went to California to regain his health *(1888)*. He took a quantity of watchmaking tools and supplies with him and sold them from store to store in Los Angeles. Most jewelers in those days also sold glasses so Reynolds also took orders for ready-made glasses. They came in boxes - one dozen to the box - and sold under the "inch number" system.

As jewelers became more proficient at selling glasses and

began to write prescriptions, Reynolds Company added a laboratory. Roy Wetmore was manager for a number of years until he left in 1930 to go with B&L where he ultimately headed up the Central Division of Riggs Optical *(His son Jerry later would later serve as president of Superior Optical)*. The business continued to grow until the entire optical business of Reynolds was sold to American Optical.

RIGGS OPTICAL OF OREGON

In January, 1916, Elwood Riggs purchased the optical department of Woodard-Clarke, the wholesale business of Spokane Optical, Standard Optical of Spokane and the E. Lalonde Company in Helena, Mont. These companies became the nucleus of Riggs Optical of Oregon. A variety of other companies were added, including National Optical of Salt Lake. In 1925, Riggs Optical was purchased by Bausch & Lomb. The Riggs division bought eight northwest branches of Davies Optical in 1927 and five branches of Associated Optical in California and Arizona. The western division of Riggs ultimately had 45 labs in eight western states.

SPENCER OPTICAL

James E. Spencer became an apprentice to an optical firm in New Haven when he was 16. Several years later, the owners retired and, at age 20, Spencer rented their factory and started producing optical goods. The year was 1859. In 1861, his brother John joined as an apprentice, later becoming a traveling salesman. The

Photo was taken during the early '20s in Merry Optical's Houston, Texas lab, later purchased by American Optical

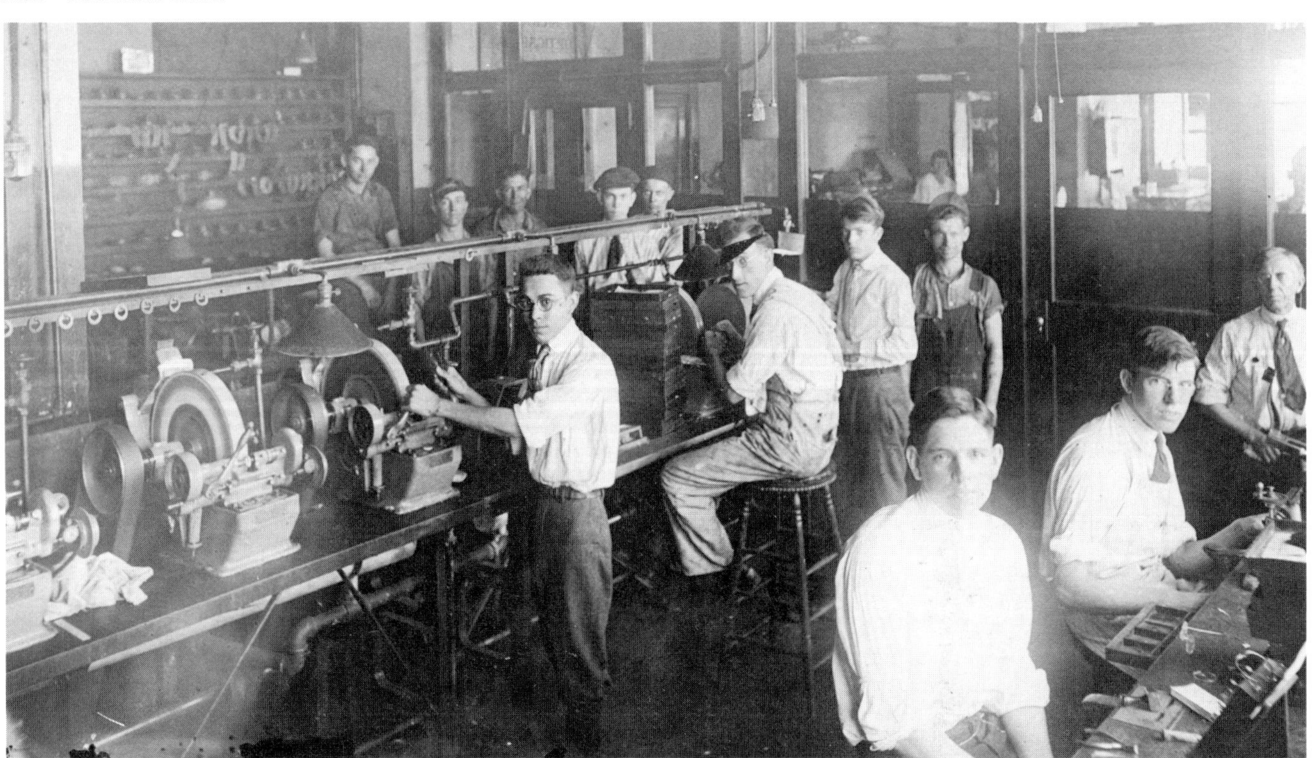

business grew enough that, a few years later, John became a partner and the company was renamed Spencer Optical Manufacturing Company. During his business career, John took out 19 patents. By 1897, Spencer Optical occupied almost a city block and employed over 2,500. They were located near the Pennsylvania Railroad system with access to shipping all over the country.

Wide Product Line

They manufactured frames, lenses, instruments and tools. Their trial lens department was an important part of the company. They had an extensive lens grinding department and carried over 8,000 tools of different curves to produce all the lenses they sold. They paid particular attention to interchangeability of their goods, a rarity at that time. Customers buying lenses and frames from Spencer could be sure that any of the lenses would fit any of the frames by merely removing a screw. Magnifiers, reading glasses, opera, and field glasses were a large part of their sales, most of which were manufactured in their Paris factory. Spencer was the first company to make an aluminum alloy eyeglass frame.

Spencer also set up a teaching facility called the Spencer Optical Institute. Classes were formed on the first Tuesday of each month and continued for two weeks. Students were taught refraction through a clinic system. The course was $15 with board and nearby lodging available at reasonable rates.

SPRATT OPTICAL

George W. Spratt started his optical career in 1913, working in a Vancouver, Wash. lab. Three years later, he

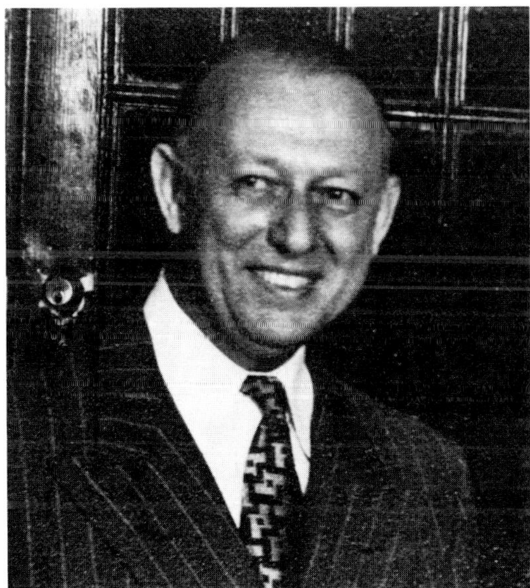

George W. Spratt was president of the AIOW in 1956-57.

formed a partnership with Tommy Llewellyn and opened a wholesale lab in Los Angeles. A year later, Spratt sold out and opened Spratt Optical. He bought his first equipment from Shuron Standard Optical and spent $800 more than he had. After doing everything himself, surface, finish, bookkeeper and anything else that came along, he sold his brother Raymond a half interest in the business. They took on a salesman named Leonard Manes, a salesman for American Optical, and in 1928, Manes bought a third interest in the company.

They opened their first branch in Long Beach with others following in the Westlake area of Los Angeles, Santa Barbara, Santa Ana, Beverly Hills, Phoenix, Huntington Beach and a second one in Long Beach. They were a wholesale/retail operation serving primarily medical accounts. In the 1960s, Roy Marks, Ted Uhlemann and Al Martin formed a small chain by combining Uhlemann Optical (Chicago), Columbian Optical (Seattle) and Spratt Optical (L.A.). Roy Marks was made president of the new company which ultimately became Optimax and was sold to U.S. Industries.

PACIFIC COAST LABS

Henry Kahn opened a wholesale business in San Francisco in 1874 which was the first wholesale and manufacturing company west of the Rocky Mountains. This company eventually became retail only. Butterfield Brothers opened a combined watch material, jewelry findings and optical business in Portland in 1887. W.D. Fennimore had opened an office for Johnston Optical in San Francisco, but later left to open the California Optical Company, also in San Francisco.

Cooperative Optical Company was started in 1916 by George E. Pryor who for years had been manager of the E.B. Meyrowitz store in Paris, France. Cooperative was eventually sold to Elwood Riggs in 1922. Walter Diederich left the Merry Optical Company to move to Chicago where he became manager of the Julius King Optical Company. He left there to go to Los Angeles as manager of Riggs Optical. In 1928, he opened the Diederich Optical Company in downtown Los Angeles, a company that became a major wholesale laboratory in Southern California.

TRIANGLE OPTICAL COMPANY

The Rodney Pierce Optical Company was founded in 1896 and, while quite successful for a time, eventually went out of business in 1922. A young man named Louis Tucker was working for Rodney Pierce Optical when it was purchased by American Optical. In 1924, Tucker left AO to join Triangle Optical, a company started in 1920 by Ralph Grodstein. Grodstein had also worked for Rodney Pierce Optical.

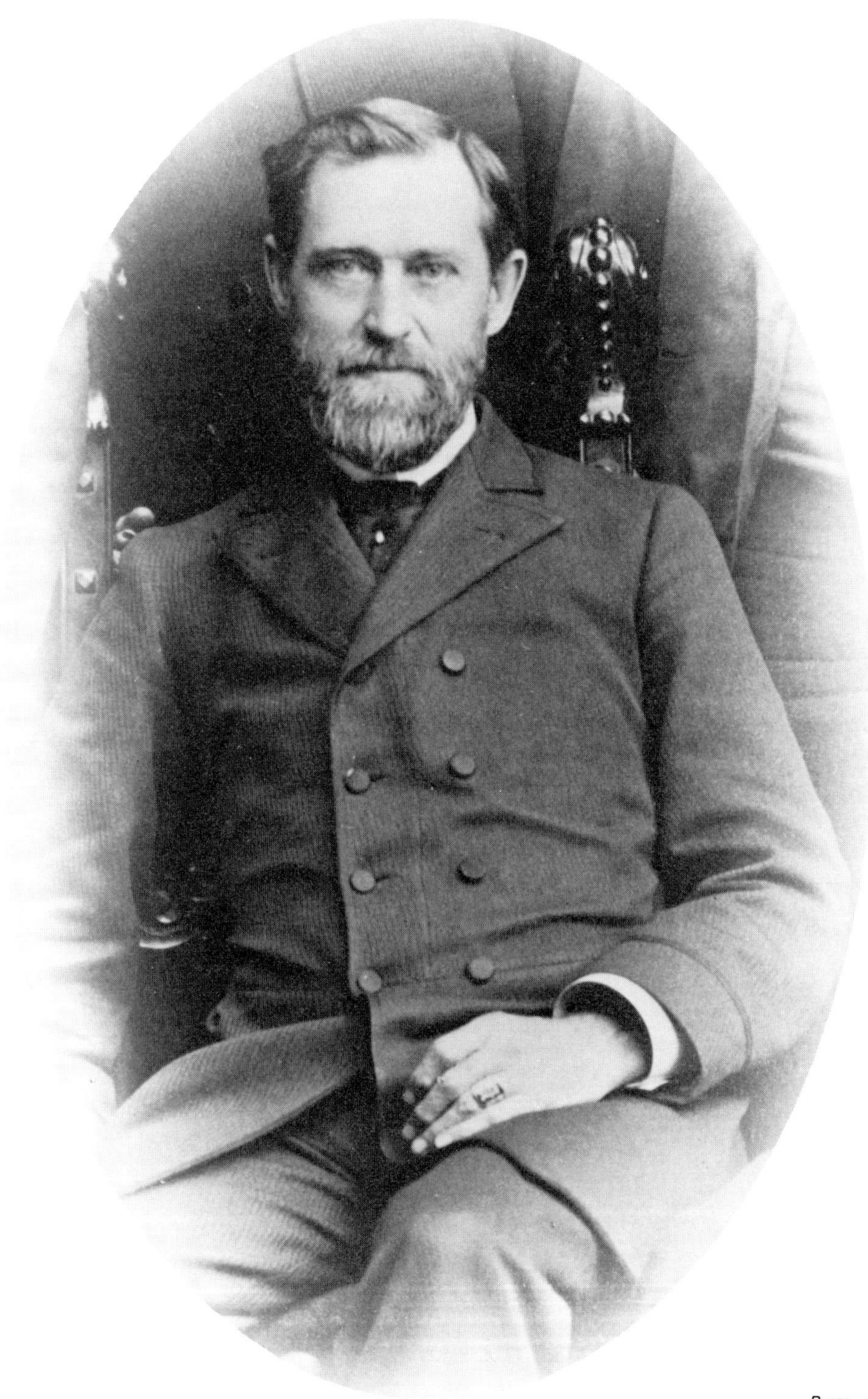

At the first meeting of the new AMERICAN ASSOCIATION OF OPTICAL WHOLESALERS (today's OLA), lab owners chose Julius King, M.D. as their first president (1894-95). This remarkable lab man started working in his father's jewelry shop but left as eyeglasses consumed his interest. He founded King Optical in 1870. He studied medicine with the intention of teaching those interested in optics to fit eyes scientifically. He registered at Western Reserve Medical College and received his M.D. degree, taking a postgraduate course in the New York Eye & Ear Infirmary. In 1887, Dr. King started his school for opticians and invited jewelers, watchmakers and druggists to come to Cleveland and become opticians/ optometrists. Many of the most successful optometrists and opticians in this century's first 50 years attributed their success to training received from Dr. King's course. Illustration was taken from a group photo of students attending his lecture course in Cleveland in 1891.

** This group became today's OPTICAL LABORATORIES ASSOCIATION (OLA).*

Chapter 6
OLA Family Tree

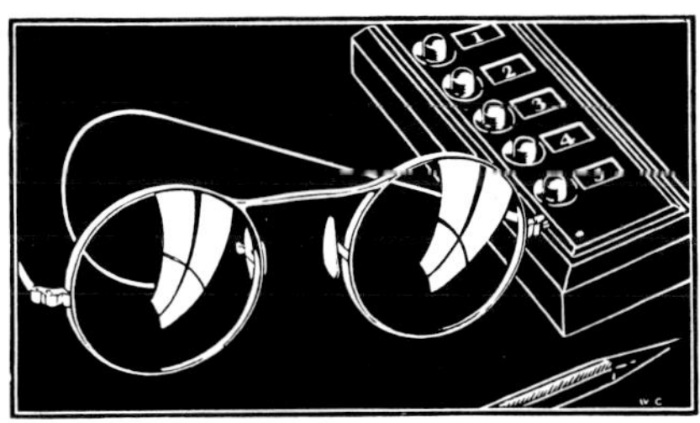

The Optical Laboratories Association is the oldest of all optical associations and considered one of the oldest national trade associations in the country. Early meetings were informal in nature and no records of them have been found. Some information from those earliest years is available, gleaned from personal letters written more than 40 years ago by a few of the men involved in the creation of the lab association *(at that time they called themselves wholesalers)*.

A preliminary meeting was held in Niagara Falls in 1893 to determine what interest there was in forming a trade association for optical wholesalers. A complete list of everyone present at that meeting doesn't exist, but it is known that, among those involved in that fateful first meeting, were F.A. Hardy and Fred Smith from Chicago, Dr. Julius King and James Spencer from New York, Henry Kirstein, Rochester, N.Y., George Johnson, Detroit, Edward Fox of Philadelphia's Queen & Company, James Brown from Geneva, N.Y. and Mr. and Mrs. Lansberg of L. Black & Company, Detroit. These were some of the country's leading wholesalers and they show up in other chapters of this history.

The suggestion to form a trade association must have been favorably received because, as a result of the Niagara Falls meeting, an organizational meeting was scheduled for the old Astor House in New York City in March or April of 1894. In addition to those from the earlier meeting, A.G. Barber from Boston, Leo Wormser of New York and Philadelphia's D.V. Brown, A. Reed McIntire, George Magee and Edgar Brown *(Philadelphia was then an important optical center)* were also present at the meeting. A number of those present would later serve as association president. The name chosen for incorporating the new group was the American Association of Wholesale Opticians *(AAWO)*. Dr. Julius King was elected president and would serve two consecutive terms.

Credit Exchange

The swift agreement to form a trade association resulted from an event that happened just prior to these meetings. A surgical instrument house in Pennsylvania had methodically placed virtually identical orders with almost every wholesaler in the country. These orders were for trial lens cases and other optical merchandise, including glazed goods. The company then collapsed and every wholesaler who had shipped to them lost everything they had shipped. It was an effective demonstration of how much the optical industry needed a credit information source in a rapidly growing market. Exchanging credit information would continue to be a major activity for the newly formed trade association. The present wholesalers' association *(Optical Laboratories Association)* has not been involved in credit exchange for many years but during the first 50 years, credit information was a primary membership benefit.

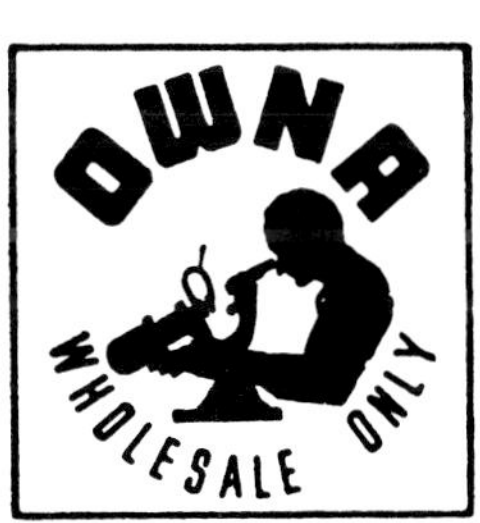

This logo identified laboratories belonging to the Optical Wholesalers National Association.

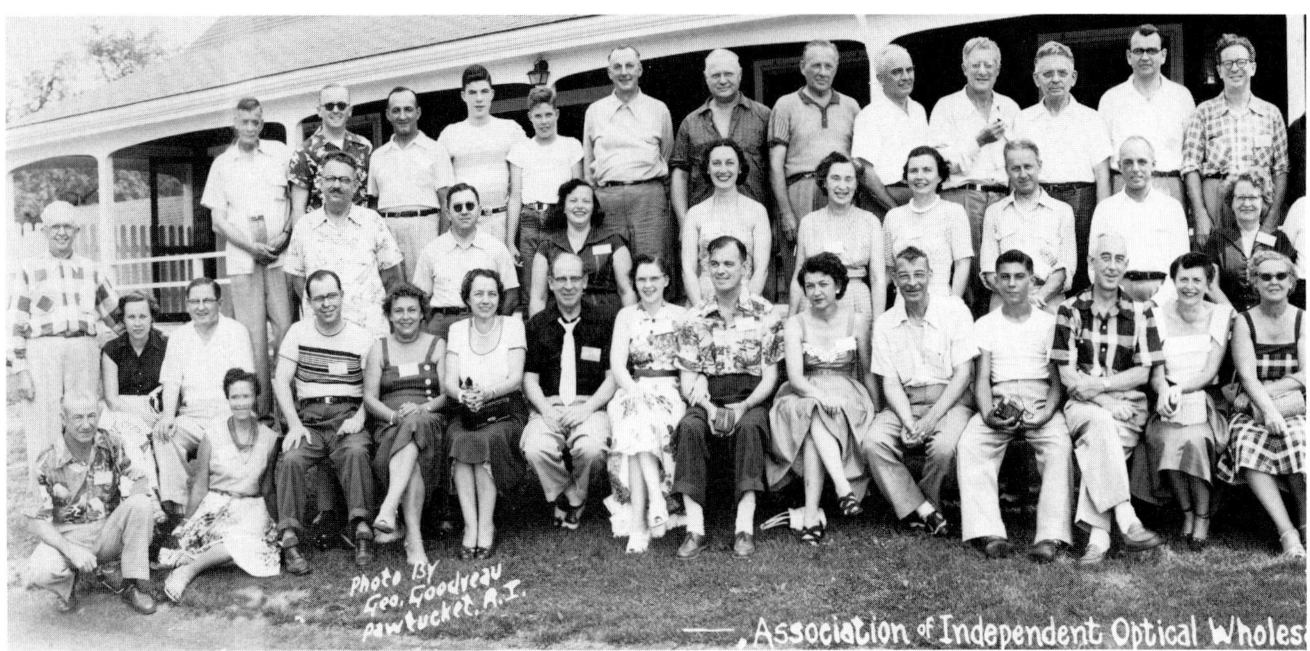

This very active group made up the Association of Independent Optical Wholesalers in 1952. Sitting near the center in the front row (page 69) is R. F. Duffens (holding sign in lap). In the back row behind him (in dark shirt) is young Fred Soderberg. Many other notables appearing in this history can be found in this photograph. It is suspected that some of the young people sitting on the ground may be active members of today's OLA.

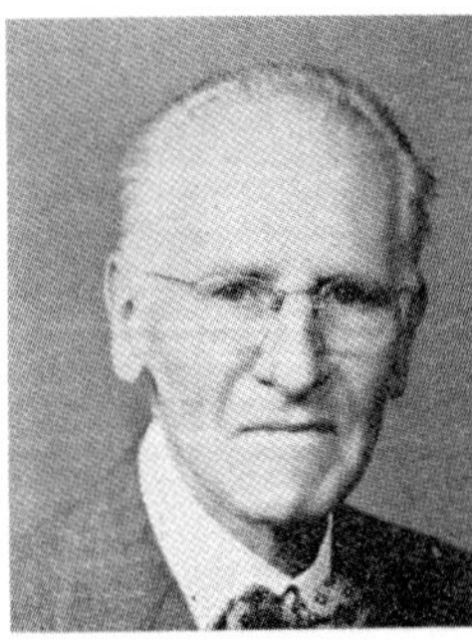

Guy Henry served as president of the OWNA in 1915-16 while he was working for F.A. Hardy before they were acquired by American Optical. He later served the OWNA for many years as secretary-manager until his retirement in 1952.

OLA OPTICAL INDUSTRY MUSEUM

Wholesaler Officers

The list of men serving as president of the AAWO reads like a "Who's Who" of the fledgling optical industry and is worth listing here:

1894-95	Dr. Julius King *
1896	F.A. Hardy *
1897	George Johnson *
1898	D.V. Brown *
1899	E.P. Wells *
1900	F.H. Smith
1901	Walter G. King *
1902	C.L. Merry *
1903	A.G. Barber *
1904	J.H. Hardin *
1905	J.T. Brayton
1906	Leo Wormser *
1907	A. Reed McIntire *
1908	J.B. White
1909-10	Andrew V. Brown *
1911-12	R.C. Thompson
1913	A. Reed McIntire *
1914	W.G. Wilkins
1915-16	Guy Henry *
1917-18	Homer E. White *
1919-20	Burnham King *
1921	V.R. Irvin
1922-23	Dan Hubbell *
1924-25	Roy Wahlgren *
1926-27	Samuel Dempsey
1928-29	A. Reed McIntire *
1930-31	Wm B. Jones
1932-34	Roy M. Martin *

These men's stories appear elsewhere in this history

The office of association secretary/treasurer was originally an elective office rotated among members until 1920 when it became a paid position and Guy Henry was selected for the permanent position. Henry would fill the position until the association changed its name in 1935.

First Convention Exhibits

The AAWO held their annual meeting at New York City's McAlpin Hotel on May 18, 1918. This was the first time optical manufacturers were invited to the meeting. Wholesaler Arthur Frank was president of the New York Wholesalers Association and arranged what he called a "fake exhibition" for the convention. Each manufacturer was invited to set up exhibits of a comical nature and more than 60 exhibits resulted from his efforts. American Optical displayed a potato knife with a sign claiming "it had been used by Sir William Crooks in cutting out ultra violet rays" *(Crooks tinted lenses were a staple of AO's lens line)*. Bausch & Lomb displayed a glass and iron treasure chest with six lenses labeled *"Meniscus Lenses, members of the cuss family. These lenses are found in great abundance in the Genesee Valley (Rochester, N.Y. area). Rumor has it a few of these are found in the vicinity of Southbridge, Mass. (home of AO)."* The optical industry was being investigated at this time by the federal government for alleged price fixing. Mr. Guiler was U.S. Attorney at the time and one display claimed to be *"Mr. Guiler's brain"*. The display featured a small peanut mounted under a high power magnifying glass.

Admission to the exhibits cost 25 cents. Receipts of $163 were collected and sent to France to buy cigarettes for

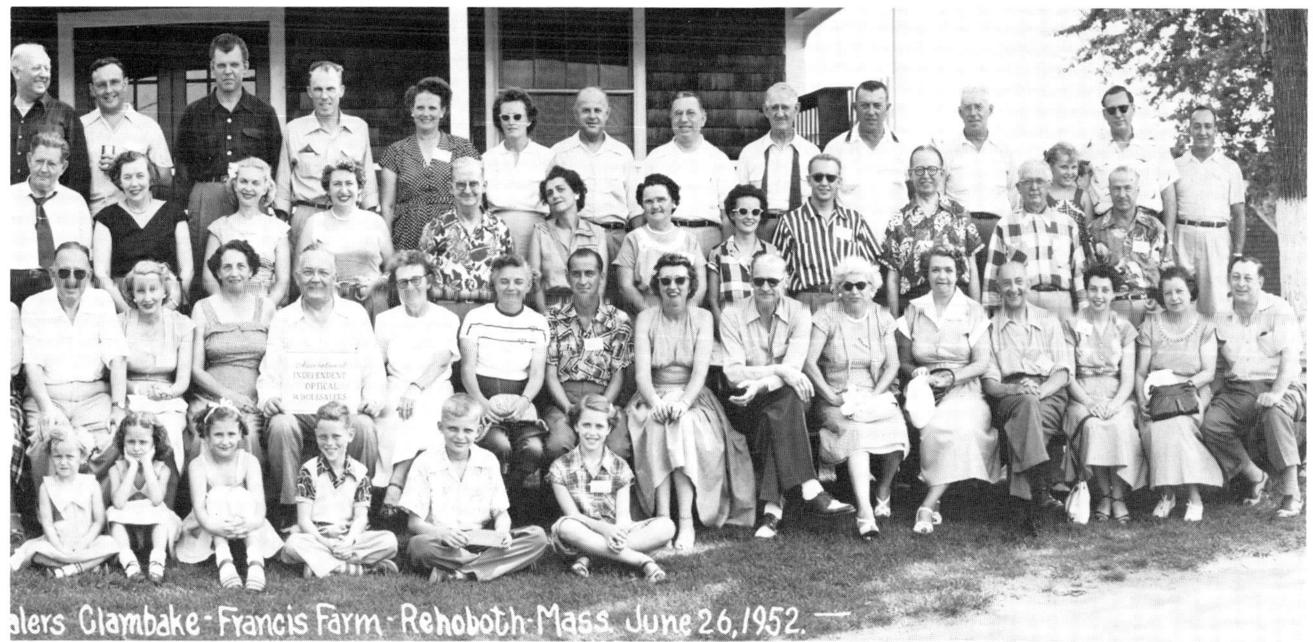

the boys "over there" *(World War I was still being fought)* Providing cigarettes for service men was still considered a patriotic gesture in 1918.

Optical Wholesalers National Association

In January, 1933, a group of wholesalers organized a group they called the Independent Optical Wholesalers Association. None were affiliated with a manufacturer and, in the fall of 1935, the group decided to join forces with the AAWO and create a new group which would be called the Optical Wholesalers National Association *(OWNA)*. The AAWO ceased operations at the end of 1935 and was reorganized in December, 1935 as the Optical Wholesalers National Association, Inc. *(OWNA)*.

Guy A. Henry was hired as secretary-manager of the newly named association and held that position until he retired. Henry was an interesting man who played an influential role in the industry. His first optical job was as an assistant to an oculist before the turn of the century. Later he worked for Chambers-Inskeep and when the company was sold to F.A. Hardy, Henry took over the ophthalmology equipment department. Part of his job was instructing professional students in using the equipment. He retired from the OWNA in 1952 and was replaced by his assistant, William Tellefsen.

The association met twice a year during those years and the first convention of the new association was scheduled for the Congress Hotel in Chicago on May 15-16, 1936. At that meeting, President William Dow proudly announced that 90 percent of all eligible labs were presently members of the OWNA *(they had 133 members at the time)*. The program included extensive discussions regarding credit information, a primary concern of the members. During that meeting, Guy Henry stated he was reviving the system of having wholesalers report their sales to the OWNA each month and the accumulated information would be passed back to those who participated. This information gathering was objected to by many independent lab owners who believed their confidential information was shared with manufacturers, primarily AO and B&L.

Robinson-Patman Act

Pricing policies of the manufacturers were a vital concern of wholesalers during the '20s and '30s. OWNA secretary-manager Guy Henry commented on this sensitive subject in a letter he wrote on April 24th, 1941.

> *"There had been a good deal of criticism on the part of different wholesalers on account of the tendency of the factories to extend more and more of their wholesale terms to the larger retail buyers. This was the situation that grew and grew and in evil mounted until finally, in 1936, the Robinson-Patman law was enacted and now an optical manufacturer who classifies accounts and allows a differential to optical wholesalers is regarded as violating that law if he extends that same differential to retailers. If we had had the Robinson-Patman Act some ten or fifteen years back, the optical industry, in some respects at least, would not be in the awful mess it is. I do remember a very apt remark that George S. Johnson made along about that time when he gave as his definition that an optical wholesaler was one who eked out a precarious livelihood selling those accounts left by the manufacturers for wholesalers to sell."*

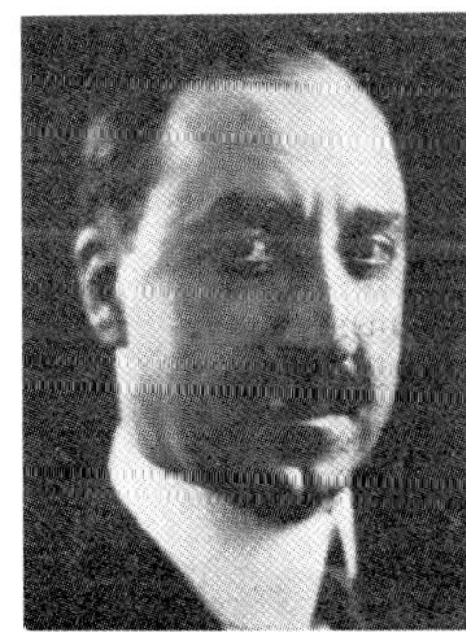

A. Reed McIntire was present when the AAWO was originally formed and served four times as president of the association. His story can be found in Chapter 5.

OLA OPTICAL INDUSTRY MUSEUM

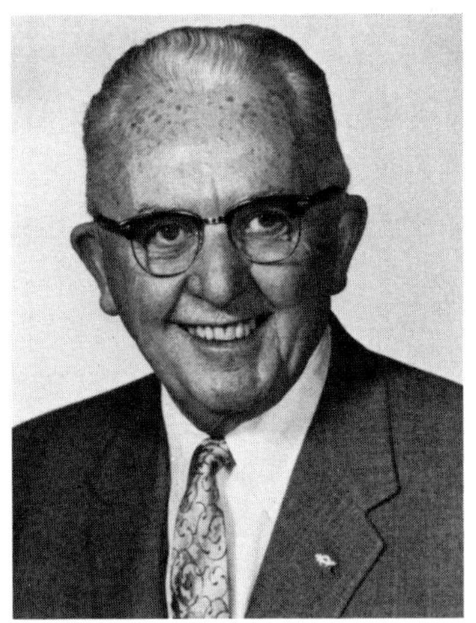
Gig Wright served the A.I.O.W. for many years as Executive Director with an office based in Chicago.

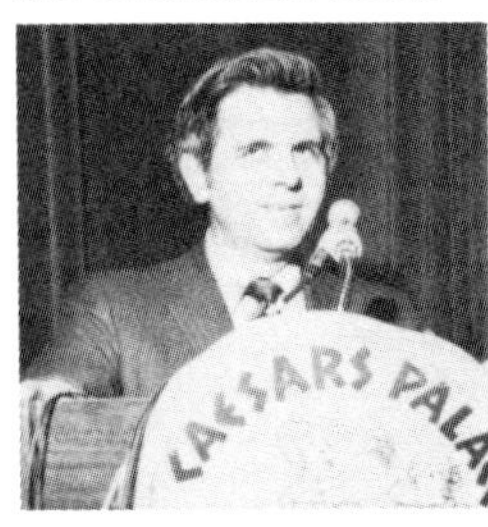
Irby Hollans, the present Executive Director of the OLA, is seen addressing the first of his many association conventions in 1973.

Wholesale Pricing

In another letter dated May 14, 1941, Guy Henry answered a question regarding wholesaler discounts from manufacturers.

"The terms "A-jobbers" and "B-jobbers" have no meaning at this time. I believe that a few years back Bausch & Lomb used these terms to differentiate between wholesalers who had men on the road selling merchandise (these were indicated as "A-jobbers") and those who did not have road men and whose business was generally restricted to Rx work in local territory ("B-jobbers"). As I understand it, these designations are no longer employed."

OWNA Membership

Asked how the OWNA classified members at that time (1941), Guy Henry wrote:

"In the OWNA there are three classes of members according to the following:

Class 1 - Optical wholesale dealers whose business is not controlled by or affiliated with any individual, partnership, association or corporation engaged in the manufacture of optical merchandise.

Class 2 - Optical wholesale dealers whose business is affiliated and controlled by stock ownership with any corporation engaged in the manufacture of optical merchandise.

Class 3 - Optical manufacturers who are engaged in business as wholesale dealers of optical merchandise."

Members such as Riggs Optical, a mostly-owned affiliate of Bausch & Lomb, therefore would be a Class 2 member. A laboratory like Winchester Optical would be a Class 1 member and a manufacturer like American Optical would be a Class 3 member.

Association of Independent Optical Wholesalers (AIOW)

This group would strongly influence what ultimately became the Optical Laboratories Association *(OLA)*. The AIOW came into being when 20 independent lab owners met on October 19, 1939 at the Pickwick Hotel in Kansas City. Sixteen of the 20 went on to join the new association. Among those charter members were many present-day members of the OLA, among them Barnett & Ramel, Central States Optical, Columbian Bifocal, Quinton-Duffens *(now Duffens Optical)*, Twin City Optical and Walman Optical. The 20 labs were there to determine if there was interest in setting up a co-operative association for exchanging ideas and problems of mutual interest. The formal establishment of the association took place one year later in Chicago.

This was at a time when the two industry giants, AO and B&L, were fierce competitors at both wholesale and retail *(many wholesale labs were heavily involved in retail dispensing for their medical accounts)*. Independent laboratories felt themselves greatly disadvantaged because of the clout and competition posed by the two manufacturers who, between them, had more than 600 branches. Independent labs also felt they had little voice in the affairs of the national laboratory association *(OWNA)* because that group permitted manufacturer membership. The general feeling was *(with a good deal of justification)* that B&L and AO's "one branch, one vote" clout gave them effective control of the OWNA.

It was with this background that the AIOW was created as a forum to address issues of primary interest to laboratories not owned or controlled by manufacturers. The group met twice a year for a number of years and many present-day members of the OLA came out of the AIOW. The Association was headquartered in Chicago and run by a very capable executive director named Gig Wright. Their members included wholesalers who dispensed and those who did not. At least half the membership was involved in some form of retail dispensing. Many members ran what was then called "dual" operations. They owned and operated multiple retail branches, soliciting patient referrals from oculists and also solicited wholesale Rx business for their labs. Some dual operations solicited wholesale business primarily from medical offices *(House of Vision, Spratt Optical, Uhlemann Optical)* while others like Benson called on both O.D.'s and M.D.'s for lab business.

As one might imagine, it wasn't easy for retail companies such as Benson Optical to get business from optometrists who usually considered any dispensing office as competition. Benson did it very effectively with a clever story that they somehow seemed to make work. Their story to the optometrist went this way, "Doctor, you're fortunate that Benson has a retail branch in town because our high retail fees enable you to collect higher fees than you could if we weren't here." Benson was also a good marketer and offered services unique to their company, many produced by Precision-Cosmet, their wholly-owned accessory manufacturing company.

An idea of lab owners' concerns 50 years ago can be gained by reviewing the program at the November, 1944 Annual Convention. The overriding concern at that time was gearing up for the end of the war. The allies had landed in Europe and were running roughshod over the Germans on their way to Berlin. Included in the AIOW audience were guests Dr. E.B. Alexander *(Optometric Extension Program)*, Maurice Cox, Editor of The Optical

Journal and Review *(now Review of Optometry)* and Martin Topaz and his sister Mae from the Professional Press.

Subjects on the 1944 AIOW program included:

- Selection, training and compensation of salesmen
- Suggested Tolerance Code
- Inventory control and its importance to the independent wholesaler
- Panel on dispensing
- How a Vision Program helps production, quality and safety in industry
- Panel on labor relations
- Panel on postwar merchandising

With the end of the war in sight, lab owners were more than ready for peacetime selling. U.S. industry had learned to live with thousands of wartime control boards set up to harness *(and harass)* industrial production. Joe Ramel *(Barnett & Ramel, Kansas City)* addressed the audience that year on the subject of "Post War Merchandising and Planning".

He included this warning to his fellow lab owners,

"How do we get universal answers to our many Federal rules and regulations? These thousands of different Boards and Directors are not going to fold up and look for a job when the war ends. So it's your business and my business they are going to pry into. For that reason, we should prepare ourselves in advance, because it's coming just as sure as taxes and death."

"How are we going to meet the new trend of the O.D.'s now on foot? The best way of explaining that trend is to quote from resolutions recently adopted by state Optometric associations. I quote first from the ARKANSAS OPTOMETRIC ASSOCIATION:

Whereas, there are many unethical practices . . . in permitting supply houses to deal directly with their patients and collecting what is erroneously known as a retail price. We consider such practices by our members as contradictory to the ethical standards set up by this Association."

In a similar resolution the NEBRASKA OPTOMETRIC ASSOCIATION in April urged -

"That optometrist be urged to discontinue, wherever feasible, such laboratory work as surfacing and edging of prescription materials.

That all supply houses be urged to discontinue, wherever feasible, dispensing directly to the public.

Resolved that advertising and/or supplying to the public of all ophthalmic materials by trade name
be discontinued, both by our members and manufacturers and that manufacturers advertise value of professional service and need of visual care, rather than products in publications or public matter."

Ramel addressed other pertinent issues of postwar planning. "In the past several months, I have talked to quite a number of wholesale men and asked them, 'What is the labor cost per surface in your grinding room?' Some did not know and some guessed. Some said 35 cents per surface; some said 22 cents. The highest was 43 cents per surface and the lowest was 22 cents per surface for labor alone. Thus, if you take your pencil and take the lowest figure I have quoted, it will show that to grind 4 surfaces, which is necessary on a pair of +.50 spheres, the labor alone would be 88 cents. *(Editor's note: Wartime production had rationed semi-finished lenses to such an extent that labs were often forced to use rough blanks, surfacing both front and back surfaces, even for simple spheres).* Now if you visualize that many Rx houses sell +.50 spheres as low as 50 cents a pair to $1.00 a pair finished, it just doesn't make a proper answer."

Ramel ended his presentation by referring to all the increased costs labs would experience at war's end, such as increased labor costs, collection of taxes for the state and federal government and shorter work weeks *(cut*

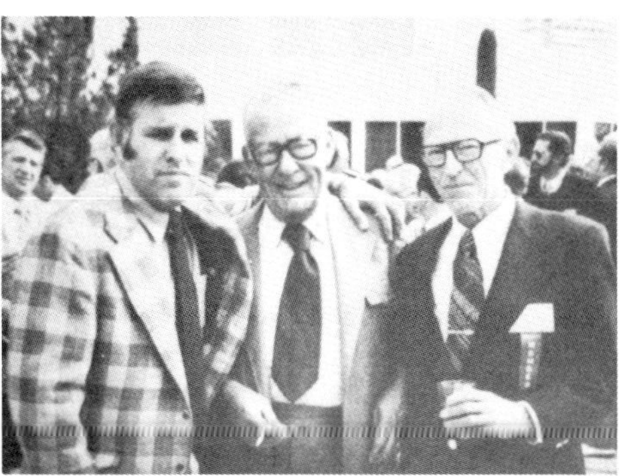

A scene from the 1973 OWA convention. Zyloware's Henry Shyer (then known as "Hank"), *left, is seen with Oklahoman Tom Brown, center, and Fred Reed of Albuquerque.*

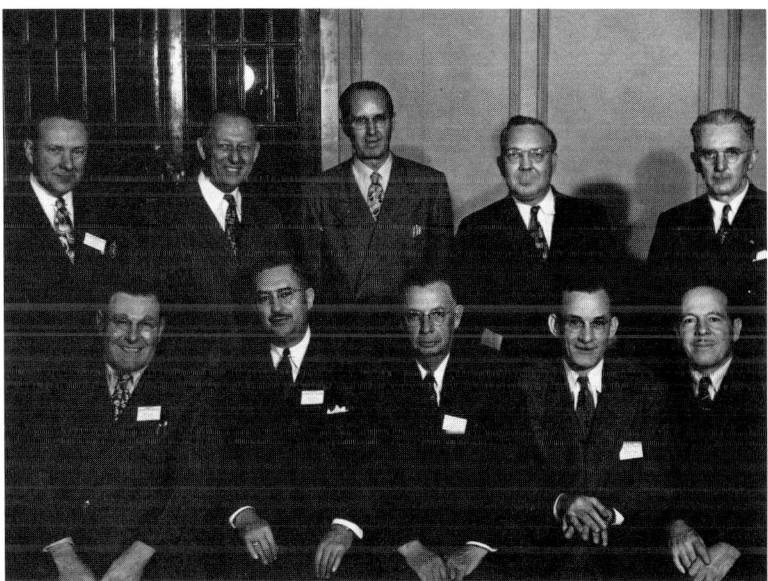

These were the officers and directors of the A.I.O.W. in 1944. In the front row are, left to right, Joe Ramel, Les Meyers (A.I.O.W. president), *Charlie Fehr, Norm MacLeod and Ralph Lanious. In the back row are Earl Lewis, George Spratt, Chelsie Ray, R.F. Duffens and Gig Wright.*

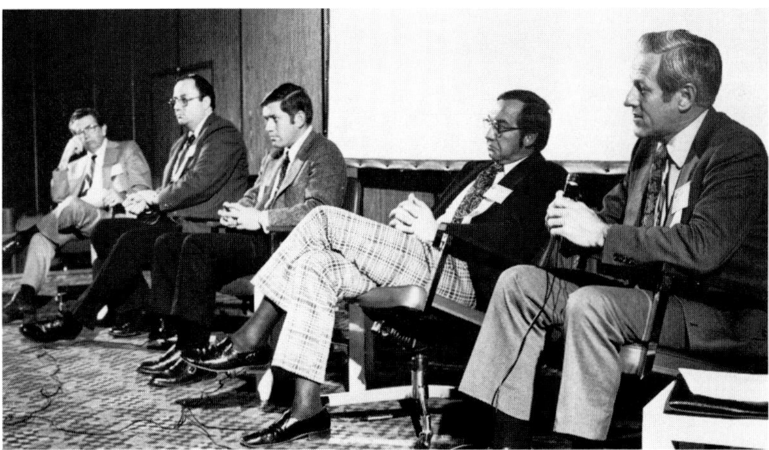

from 48 hours). He concluded his talk with the poignant question, "Where are we going to get the $500 per month per man to travel?"

A number of wholesalers belonged to both the A.I.O.W. and the O.W.N.A. An interesting side-note to this was Dempsey Optical of Toledo, Ohio. Run by two brothers, Bart and Phil Dempsey, Bart attended O.W.N.A. meetings and eventually became president. Brother Phil went to A.I.O.W. meetings and also served as president of that association.

Regional Groups

By 1941, a number of regional area wholesale groups had sprung up, mostly informal in nature. Some would continue to meet for years and two still meet on a regular basis. These regional groups included:

> *Cincinnati Wholesale Optical Association, organized in 1924.*
>
> *Michigan Wholesale Optical Distributors Association, organized in 1939.*
>
> *Minnesota Fellowship Club, wholesalers located in the Twin Cities area.*
>
> *Ohio Valley Association of Wholesale Opticians, organized in 1937.*
>
> *Optical Wholesalers Association of Eastern Pennsylvania organized in 1936.*
>
> *Optical Wholesalers of New York, first regional group, organized in 1908.*
>
> *Optical Wholesalers Association of Northern New York, organized in 1936.*
>
> *Philadelphia Association of Wholesale Opticians, founding date unknown.*
>
> *Southern Optical Wholesalers Association reorganized in 1938.*
>
> *Western Association of Wholesale Opticians, date unknown.*
>
> *Central Optical Wholesalers Association organized in November 1940.*
>
> *Independent Optical Wholesalers Association founded in 1933 and merged into AAWO in 1935.*
>
> *Southwest Association of Optical Suppliers organized about the same time as MOWA. The group is no longer active.*

California Optical Laboratories Assoc.

The first organizational meeting of a California laboratory association was held in 1956 in a San Luis Obispo bar. Attending were John Martin, who owned Martin Optical in Modesto, Bill Hartzell *(Hartzell Optical)* and Art Johnson *(California Optical)*. The meeting was prompted by the difficulty smaller labs had in getting on factory distributor lists. John Martin had purchased a Bausch & Lomb lab so he had a B&L listing, but it was tough to get better factory listings and COLA founders felt an organization could speak up for smaller independent labs and would have more clout with the manufacturers.

The next meeting was in Fresno at the California Hotel with a larger group. Art Collard and Ed Rose were there along with Lynn Houghton, Katz, Klein and a number of others. Ed Rose was selected to be the first president *(1957)*. John Martin became president in 1970 and led a drive to get larger independent labs such as Bradley Optical and Watts Optical into the group. The group was successful in reaching their original goal of better understanding and relations with the manufacturers. They began inviting factory representatives to their meetings and the organization has been successful ever since. No exhibits are presented and the twice-a-year meetings are strictly educational and social.

Art Johnson *(Bill Hartzell's brother-in-law)* served as COLA president in the late '60s. At the end of his term of office, COLA met at Yosemite Park for an annual meeting and election. Johnson loved the Torcyl cylinder machine and had a garage full of them. He couldn't throw one away. The machine was manufactured by Shuron and was considered a workhorse in surface rooms during the '20s, '30s and '40s. Like Ford's tin Lizzie, they ran forever. Johnson told his friends that when he died, he wanted a Torcyl machine as his headstone. John Martin had his brother chrome plate an old Torcyl and COLA presented it to Art Johnson as a gift.

John Martin and his son Ken are the only father and son team to serve as COLA presidents. Ken Martin is again serving on the COLA Board. The first executive director was a non-optical person named Jack Haugen from Modesto. Later, COLA decided they needed an experienced optical person for the position. Roy Marks had just left U.S. Industries *(Optimax)* and was looking for something to do and applied for the job. Roy served the group until he died in 1978. He was succeeded as executive director in 1979 by Maurice Giss who presently runs the association.

Midwest Optical Laboratories Association

In November, 1950, a number of Kansas City optical men attended an OWNA meeting in Toledo to hear Trade Practice Rules discussed. The concerns of wholesale laboratories at that time were coupons, discounts, rebates, spindling of orders *(to get the maximum quantity discount)* and other profit-destroying marketing evils of the day.

The first meeting was held at the Phillips Hotel in Kansas City on March 17, 1951. The original name chosen was MOWA, using the term "wholesalers" rather than "laboratories". E. H. Sutherlin, Sutherlin Optical, was elected president and Harold Thompson, Rite-Style Optical, became the first vice president. One of the speakers at that first meeting was Henry Lehrich, legal counsel for the Optical Wholesalers National Association *(OWNA)*.

When the OWNA changed their name to OLA, MOWA changed their name to MOLA. The group still meets each year and, in addition to educational seminars, they also present manufacturers' exhibits.

A Name Change

In September, 1975, when Ben Lynch was president of the Optical Wholesalers Association, a special Industry Forum was organized and sponsored by the OWA. This was the first time such a comprehensive group of lab and industry leaders had ever gathered together and there has been nothing else like it since that time. People from both within and outside the OWA were invited. Participants were divided into three work groups and three sessions during the two-day meeting. Some important questions facing laboratories and the industry

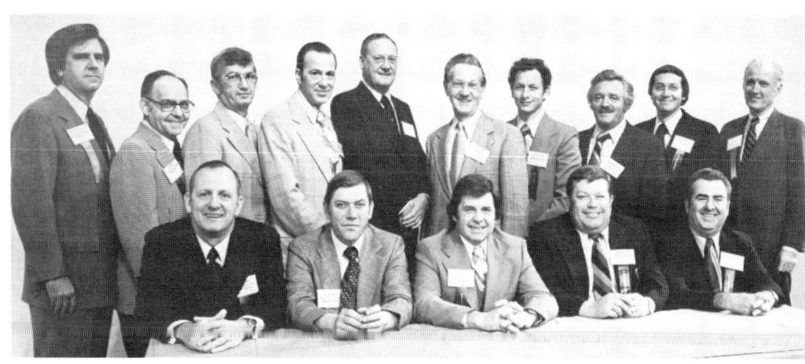

Newly elected OWA officers and directors are seen here in 1977. Left to right (seated) are Robert Hines, Keith West, President Robert Mueller, Ed Sutherlin and Walt Daniels. Standing, Irby Hollans, J.P. Waring, Phil Eichelberger, Rolf Sulzberger, Howard Underwood, Robert Honsa, Tom Sloan, Herb Ackerson, Robert Wheelon and Legal Counsel Joe Gill.

were discussed by the groups. What inadequacies are there in the eyewear delivery system? What changes are taking place? Can the laboratory industry have a meaningful voice and how does it need to change? Third party eyecare was discussed as well as proposed ANSI standards. Most important, what should the role of a national association be? There was talk of the federal government setting up a national standard for producing eyewear and there was great concern in the industry that standards might be established that existing lab technology would be unable to meet.

Thirty-five people participated in the Lab Industry Forum. These were industry leaders of that day and included many people mentioned elsewhere in this history, such as Bill Benedict, Ed. Dietz, Jr., Gerald Dougher, Roy Duffens, Joe Gill, Irv Greenberg, George Grotelueschen, Irby Hollans, Bob Honsa, Ellis Katz, Norm MacLeod, Sr., Robert Mueller, James Negaard, Richard Palmer, Dr. Stanley Pearl, Sylvan Ray, Victor Rogers, Franklin Rozak, Ed Sutherlin, Keith West and President Ben Lynch.

From the detailed notes of the work sessions, a 117 page management study for the OWA Board of Directors was prepared by a management consultant named John Evans. Using this study as a guide, the OWA Board revised the association bylaws and sent them out for a membership vote on November 23, 1976. Most obvious among the proposed changes was an increased emphasis on the laboratory as the keystone of the association. For that reason, a name change to Optical Laboratories Association was proposed. Increased educational and regulatory duties for the Association were proposed and to support the increased budget these necessitated, a substantial increase in dues was proposed.

The proposed changes must have struck a responsive note with OWA members because, on January 3, 1977, Hollans sent the membership a notice reporting the bylaws had received an 85.6 percent approval. In every sense of the word, those momentous events led directly to the outstanding international reputation and status of today's Optical Laboratories Association.

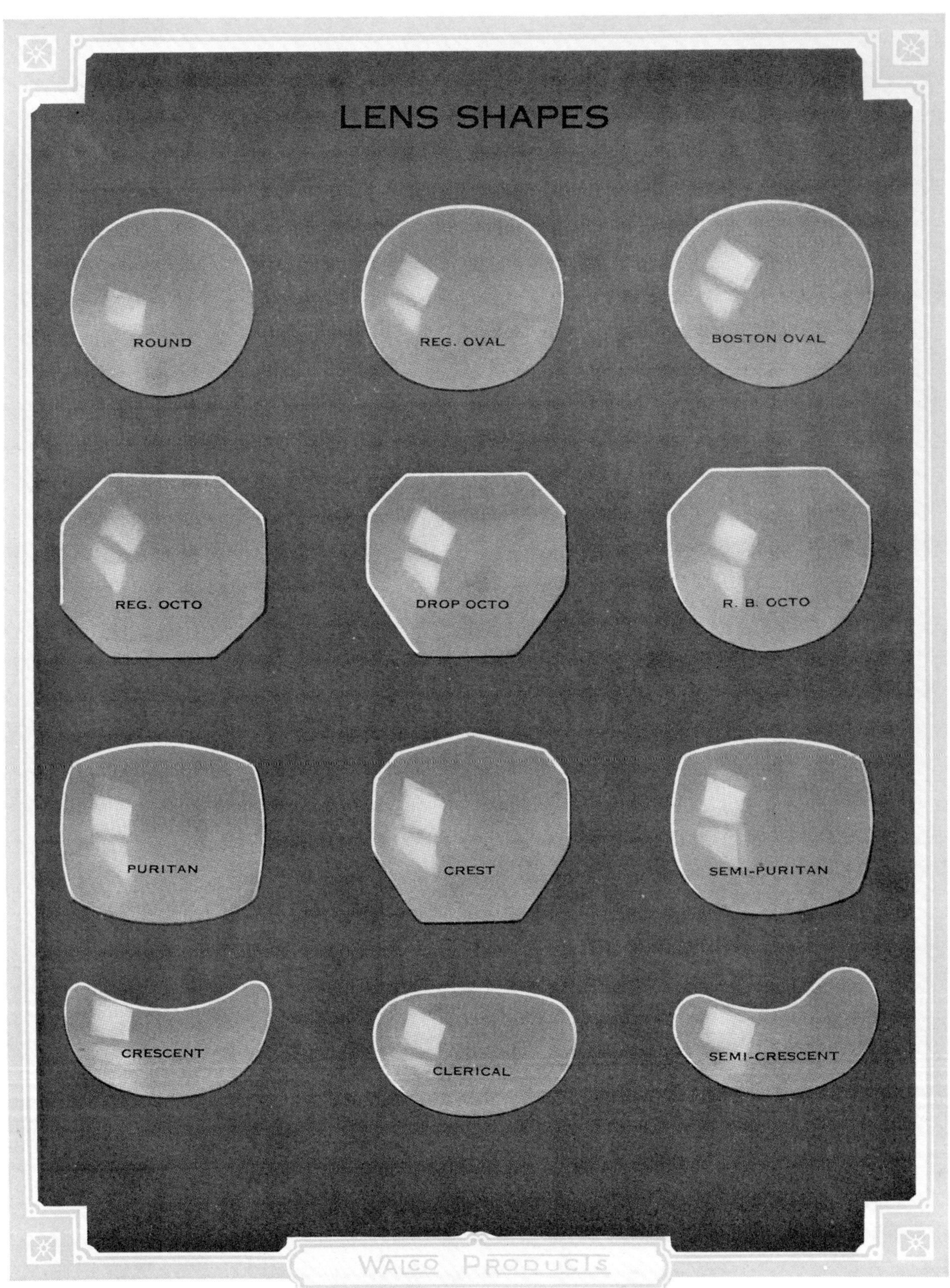

This chart represents all the shapes used in a modern lab in the year 1917. Life was a lot simpler when 12 patterns covered every frame coming through a laboratory. This chart appeared in Walman Optical's 1917 price list.

Illustration — Walman Optical

Chapter 7
Lenses

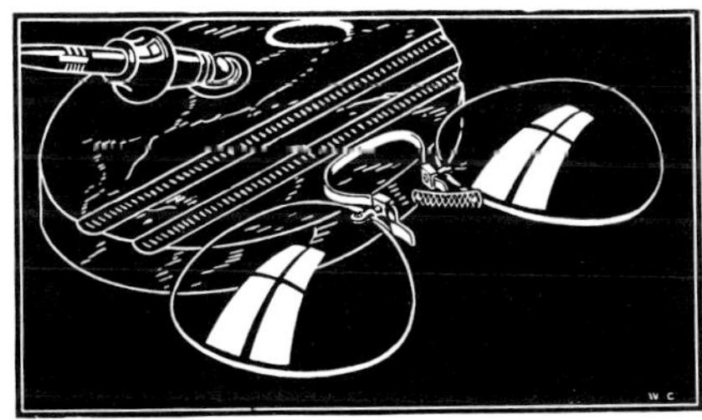

The word "lens" comes from the Latin word "lentil", a species of bean that resembles the shape of a lens. Single pieces of glass or rock crystal, convex shaped like a lens have been dug up in ruins dating back thousands of years. They were probably used as magnifiers but never combined in the shape of spectacles until the 13th century. The very earliest spectacle lenses were made of quartz crystal, sometimes called "pebble lenses". The first glass lenses were made from hand-blown glass. The term "crown" comes from the shape the glass assumes at a certain stage of the blowing process. As the industry grew, hand blown glass was replaced by lens blanks formed from flat sheets of glass. These blanks were called "dropped" lenses from the process in which flat sheets of glass were heated until the material softened and dropped into cavities that would shape the blank to a desired curve.

The first lenses were all convex *(plus)* lenses, primarily used for magnification by older people. The first concave lenses (minus) were first mentioned in 1461 in private letters of the Medici who suffered from hereditary myopia. Concave lenses weren't used much until the late 1800s.

Bausch and Lomb and American Optical were the first U.S. companies to initiate mass production of glass lenses. Prior to that period, most lenses were imported from Europe, either as rough blanks or in uncut form. No optical glass was manufactured in the United States until World War I cut off traditional glass sources for the country.

EVOLUTION OF LENSES

Pebble Lenses

Lenses of rock crystal were first introduced in England under the name of Scotch Pebble and later as Brazilian Pebble, names that indicate their country of origin. Crystals were found all over the world but only in a few places were they large enough to make into eyeglass lenses *(lenses at the time of pebble lens popularity were not much larger than a half dollar coin)*. The best quality crystals were found in Brazil and, strangely enough, no rock crystals in paying quantities were ever found in the United States. Pebble lenses normally carried a considerably higher cost than glass lenses *(see story on early counterfeiting)* because they were much harder than glass and more difficult to grind to curve and polish. The harder surface of pebble, however,

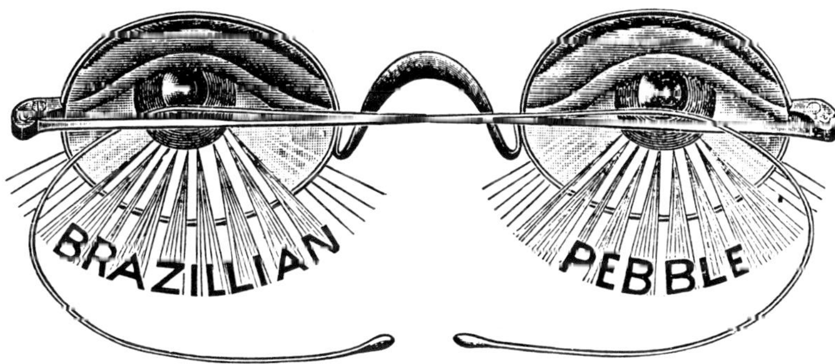

Lenses made of rock crystal were first introduced in England under the name of Scotch Pebble and later as Brazilian Pebble, names that indicate their country of origin. The best quality crystals were found in Brazil. Pebble lenses normally carried a considerably higher cost than glass lenses because they were much harder than glass and, as a result, more difficult to grind and polish. Even as glass lenses became plentiful, pebble lenses were still sold as superior lenses because of their longer wearing qualities. Their price kept rising as the supply of rock crystal diminished. Pebble lenses were still being sold in the 1920s.

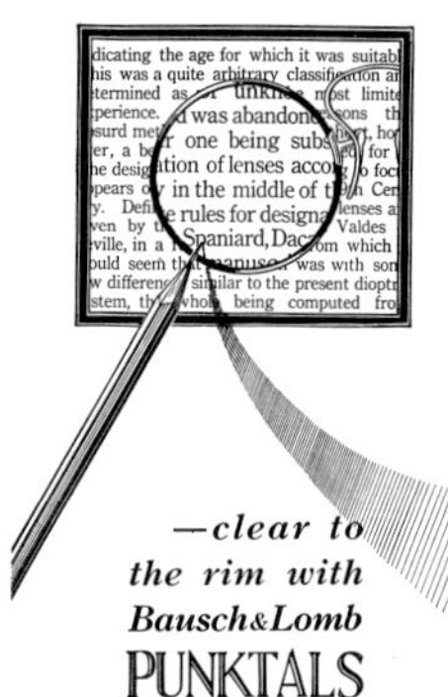

—clear to the rim with Bausch&Lomb

PUNKTALS

The first brand name corrected curve lenses were manufactured by Germany's Carl Zeiss Company and imported by Bausch & Lomb.

made them last longer without accumulating scratches. Even as glass lenses became plentiful, pebble lenses were still sold as superior lenses because of their longer wearing qualities. Their price kept rising as the supply of rock crystal diminished. Pebble lenses were still being sold in the 1920s.

Flat Lenses

The first lenses produced, whether pebble or glass, were all biconcave *(minus power)* or biconvex *(plus power)*. Flat lenses were the easiest to produce and no one gave much thought to making them any different. Flat lenses were the only lens form available until periscopic or meniscus lenses were devised in the late 1800s. Flat lenses were still widely used into the 20th century.

Meniscus Lenses

The next objective step in the evolution of lens design was to attempt to eliminate problems created by the biconvex or biconcave design. Eventually it was determined that if lenses were ground with a concave curve on the back side and convex on the front surface, the lens would be positioned further from the eye providing wearers with a considerably wider field of vision *(see below)*. This had the additional advantage of positioning the lens further from the eye and avoiding contact between the lens and the wearer's eyelashes which had always been a problem with flat lenses. Meniscus lenses were described as early as 1645 but were not available until the periscopic lens was invented in 1804 by an Englishman named Wollaston. These had a standard -1.25 back curve on all powers. Conventional meniscus lenses became available around the 1890s but flat lenses were still being used well into the '20s. As 6 base meniscus lenses slowly replaced flat lens inventories, retailers and manufacturers ended up with large stocks of unsold flat stock lenses. Rumor had it that many of these overstocked inventories of flat lenses were sold to Third World countries where they were still being used in the '40s and '50s.

Lens Tints

Early in the evolution of ophthalmic lenses, manufacturers began looking for lens options that could increase their profits. The first lens "add-on" was adding color to the glass. The earliest use of color included treatment of disease and improvement of vision. In the early 19th century, blue, pink or green lenses were introduced. Later, Dr. William Crookes, the eminent British scientist, developed a lens color that filtered infra red rays and came to be called "Crookes". It was a cool blue/gray shade that was quite effective. Unfortunately, it tended to give wearers a somewhat ghastly look because of unattractive shadows cast beneath the eyes. American Optical included Crookes lenses in their line for years but Dr. Tillyer eventually came up with a more attractive pink shade he called "Cruxite". Various shades of Cruxite became the primary tint for American Optical. Between the two World Wars, pink lenses in a variety of shades were very popular. Soft Lite Lenses, manufactured by Bausch & Lomb and distributed by Soft Lite Lens Company, became the top-selling premium-priced lenses on the market. For sports and sun use, B&L developed and sold Ray Ban *(green)* or G15 and G30 *(Gray)*. AO's gray was called Tru Color.

Between 1916 and 1920, American Optical produced a lens they called "Pfund". This was a special lens for industrial use that had gold deposited on the front surface for heat deflection. It was used for people working in high heat environments such as steel mills, glass manufacturing, etc. Later, AO's Calobar was developed to screen out IR and UV rays and the Pfund lens became a thing of the past.

TORIK OR DEEP PERISCOPIC LENSES.

The advantage of Torik or Deep Periscopic Convex Lenses lies in the larger field of vision afforded by them as illustrated in the accompanying figure, in which the difference between them and double convex is plainly shown. Their peculiarity is that the surface next to the eye is deeply concave, so that the field of view is much enlarged. They are particularly useful also, where a patient has long eye-lashes which are liable to come in contact with the lenses in ordinary glasses. The demand for Torik Lenses is increasing every day, the only drawback heretofore, being their great expense. However we have succeeded in hammering down the cost to such a reasonable price, as to bring them within the reach of all, as shown by the following low quotations:

				Sample	Per Doz.
No. 36.	Gold Filled Rimless Spectacles, 10 Year, Torik Lenses			$1.00	$10.50
No. 37.	Gold Filled Rimless Eye Glasses, 10 Year, Torik Lenses			.75	8.00
	Torik Lenses—Bevel Edge (for frame) or Rimless Style		per pair	.50	4.80
	For Cement Bifocal, add 60 cents per pair.				

Corrected Curve Lenses

Then came the next major shift in lenses. Lens designers discovered that merely changing a lens design from biconvex or biconcave to a 6.00 diopter base curve provided wearers a wider view. They also found that other inherent distortions cropped up as lenses grew larger. The coined term for these inherent distortions was "marginal astigmatism". The first effort to solve the problem was attempted by Punktal lenses, made by Germany's Carl Zeiss Company. Zeiss had determined that carefully changing the front curve of each lens power could minimize marginal astigmatism and, indeed, almost eliminate it. These excellent lenses were state-of-the-art for that day *(developed in 1908 by Zeiss' Dr. M. Von Rohr and introduced to the American market in 1913)*. They were imported into the United States by Bausch & Lomb. B&L enjoyed a very close working relationship with Zeiss, both companies routinely exchanging technical data. This budding relationship ended abruptly with World War I.

Punktal lenses had one major drawback. Every correction required a slightly different base curve so laboratories had to stock hundreds of variations of semi-finished blanks in order to fill orders for Punktal lenses. There was widespread interest in Punktal lenses but they were never commercially successful for that reason and the war ended their availability. Punktal lenses did accomplish one thing, however, that would eventually dramatically impact the optical world. They demonstrated that simple meniscus lenses did not provide the best possible acuity and this led directly to the development of corrected curve lenses.

American Optical had a superb lens designer named Dr. Edgar Tillyer and he was given the project of finding a compromise between the Punktal approach and the basic 6 base lenses then being sold in the United States.

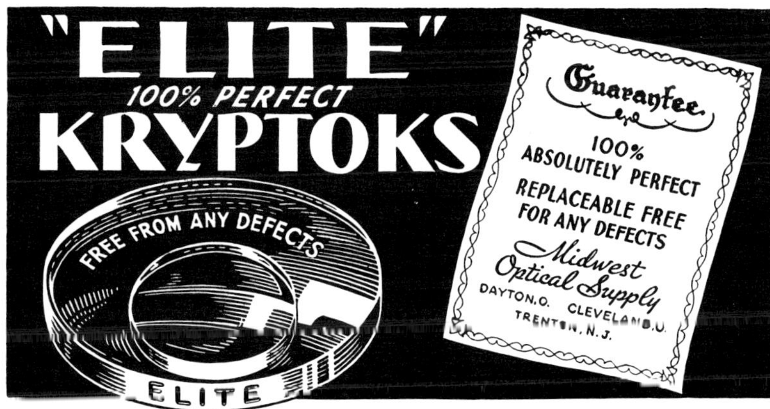

Ad from 1937 Midwest Optical catalog

ILLUSTRATION – MIDWEST OPTICAL

He ultimately developed a line of corrected curve lenses *(the term used to differentiate lenses corrected for marginal astigmatism)* that changed base curves for every one to two diopters of lens power and limited the number of semi-finished blanks required to grind corrected curve lenses to less than 10 variations. In honor of their designer, the name chosen for AO's corrected curve series was "Tillyer", patented in 1919 and named for their designer. American Optical's 6 base toric lenses, from that point on, carried the trade-name "Centex". Ultimately, AO produced and promoted a complete range of lenses in both series.

Bausch & Lomb quickly followed suit with their own corrected curve lens series called Orthogon. It wasn't long before almost every lens manufacturer offered standard 6 base lenses *(which the industry called "toric")* and their own variation of corrected curve lenses.

Then came the tough part - convincing retailers to prescribe corrected curve lenses instead of the old-fashioned and less desirable toric lenses. To give an idea of the difference in costs between toric and corrected curve, AO's 1935 price list showed a +0.50 +0.50

EARLY SAFETY LENSES

During the '30s and 40's, a clever lens was developed that was advertised as "a non-shatterable lens". It carried the name Motex and consisted of two thin glass lenses with a soft plastic inner film holding the layers together. Safety windshields in automobiles at that time were constructed in the same manner, and Motex advertising stressed the similar safety advantages of Motex lenses. Every pair of lenses came with a $15,000 insurance policy. It should be noted that this construction did not keep the lens from breaking. It only kept the glass particles from entering the eye. In practice, because of the thinness of the glass wafers, Motex lenses were easily cracked.

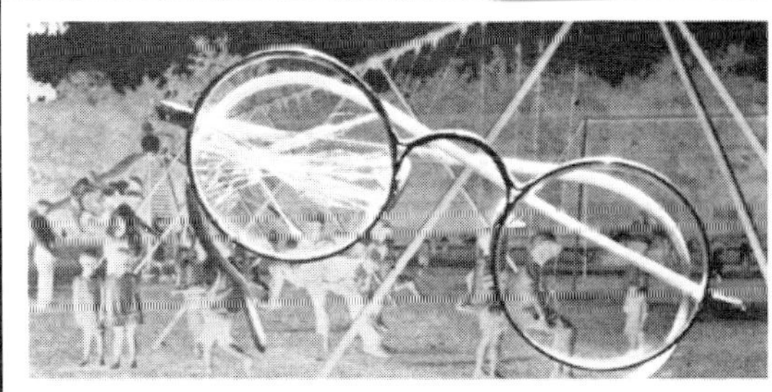

Broken but **INTACT!**

Above, a school boy's spectacles after "head-on" collision with another child during play. MOTEX SAFETY LENSES used for the correction undoubtedly saved the boy from painful laceration and perhaps serious eye injury.

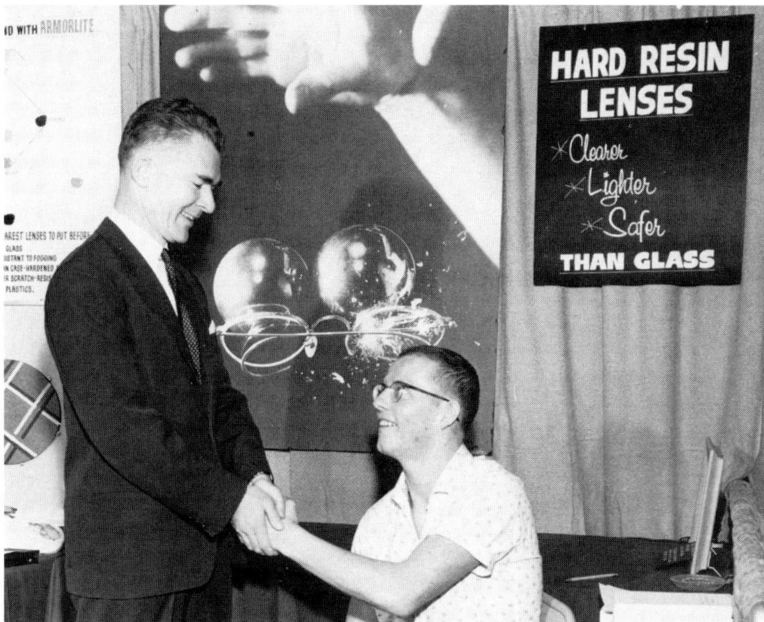

Photograph shows Dr. Robert Graham, left, exhibiting his new plastic lenses at an early trade show.

Following the requirement of tempering of all glass lenses, heat treat units like the one pictured here became a common sight in all labs.

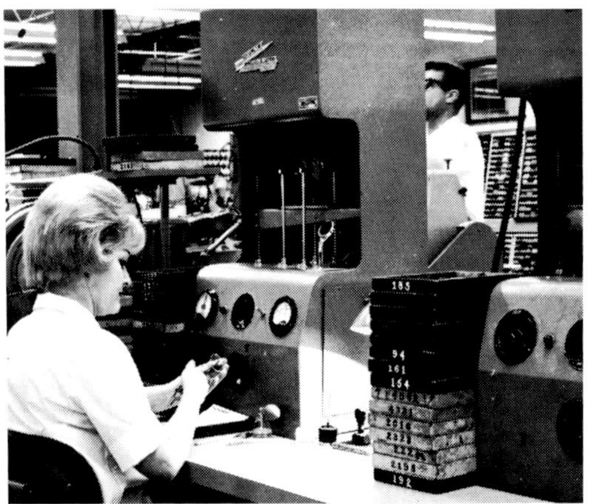

compound Tillyer uncut lens priced at $1.80 a pair. The same power in AO's Centex *(non-corrected curve)* was $1.55 a pair, a difference of only 25 cents.

Converting to Corrected Curve

Today, a 25 cent add-on would be an easy sale but the struggle to convert the industry to corrected curve lenses ended up taking more than 30 years. For example, on December 29, 1952, a bulletin of the Association of Independent Optical Wholesalers *(one of the organizations that became the OLA)* was sent out over the signature of member Gus Schrader *(Bell Optical, Denver)*. Schrader urged labs to start on their 1953 Corrected Curve program. His message included, *"When the automotive industry introduced four-wheel brakes, they discontinued the use of the old fashioned two-wheel type. But when our industry introduced Corrected Curve Lenses, it continued to make Toric. Why?"*

The AIOW proposed action to eliminate toric *(the commonly used name for non-corrected curve lenses)* lenses in 1950 when they unanimously passed a resolution at a Fort Worth meeting urging manufacturers to drop toric lenses *(labs had to carry inventories of both toric and corrected curve lenses)*. Laboratories continued to fight this double inventory battle until the late '50s when manufacturers *(who had the same inventory problems)* began slowly dropping toric lenses from their lines. The battle between toric and corrected curve lenses was ultimately solved, however, by another issue altogether.

Minus Cylinders

As fused multifocals gradually took over the multifocal market *(onepiece Ultex sales steadily dwindled)*, visual inequities between single vision lenses, available only with plus cylinders *(cylinders ground on the front side of the lens)* and fused multifocals, all produced with inside cylinders, soon became apparent. As patients became presbyopic and switched from single vision to bifocals, they often experienced difficulty in adjusting to the visual differences created when switching from plus to minus cylinders.

About this same time, most labs were using bevel edgers for finishing lenses. One of the most exciting developments provided by bevel edgers was the ability to apply a "hide-a-bevel" to higher minus lenses. This put most of the bevel on the back side of the lens, hiding it behind the frame. Plus cylinders, especially in higher cylinders, left an unattractive bulge in front of the frame rim along the axis of the cylinder. Cylinders on the back of the lens, on the other hand, were completely hidden by the frame. There was, therefore, considerable cosmetic advantages to minus cylinders, in addition to the visual advantages.

Manufacturers, however, preferred producing plus cylinders in glass *(all lenses were glass during this time period)*. Plus cylinders were easier *(therefore cheaper)* to produce because they were produced in multiples. Minus cylinders are manufactured, one at a time, much the way wholesale laboratories produce prescription lenses. As a result, minus cylinder lenses were more expensive than plus. Even so, the visual and cosmetic advantages of minus cylinders were too obvious for manufacturers to continue ignoring.

Lens manufacturers, facing the heavy costs of converting production equipment to produce minus cylinders had no intention of producing these superior lenses in the old-fashioned toric form. The result was, as the industry switched from plus to minus cylinders, they in effect converted to corrected curve as well. The switch to single vision minus cylinders effectively doomed toric lenses, to everyone's relief. Today, all single vision lenses are minus cylinders and considered corrected curve.

Plastic Lenses

Before and during World War II, a great deal of work was done in England to develop lightweight plastic lenses. This resulted from work done with acrylic *(polymethylmethacrylate)*, widely used for aircraft windshields. I-Gard, a British manufacturer, produced prescription lenses in acrylic that received modest distribution in the United States before World War II and after the war by McLeod Optical of Providence, R.I. McLeod sold these advanced lenses to other labs such as Benson Optical in Minneapolis, Duffens Optical in Kansas, Bell Optical in Denver, Spratt in Los Angeles, and Dietz in Ft. Worth, Texas. The lenses were available in finished uncut form only and could not be surfaced. They had the advantage of being lightweight but proved to be brittle, subject to scratching and prone to yellowing after a few months in inventory.

Others tried to improve on acrylic materials but it was Pittsburgh Plate Glass Company *(PPG)* who eventually came up with a workable material called CR-39 - actually the 39th experiment produced in cast resin by their subsidiary, Columbia Resin Chemical Company. This formula ultimately became the standard monomer for producing hard resin lenses. Combined with IPP *(Isopropyl Peroxide, an extremely volatile catalyst in its native state)*, CR-39 lenses produced lightweight, Ultra Violet absorptive, non-shatterable lenses which scratched less than acrylic, and were easier for laboratories to handle. The learning curve for processing these lenses lasted for more than 10 years with both manufacturers and laboratories experiencing over 50 percent reject rates. As a result, prices for CR-39 remained high and volume low with minimal profits for everyone handling them. The only blessing was that only a few labs were processing these new lenses.

Initially, CR39 enjoyed limited popularity for a number of reasons. The material was difficult for laboratories to process, was expensive at all levels of sale, and the quality was perceived as less than that of glass. The major lens manufacturers, AO, B&L, Shuron and Univis, each experimented with the new material but all eventually backed away - in part because they had substantial investments in glass facilities. One company was totally committed to CR-39 lenses — the Armorlite Company of Pasadena, Calif. *(later moved to Burbank)*. They suffered through a variety of financial problems while the few laboratories who were trying to process the new material also incurred severe losses connected with quality problems associated with surfacing of these lenses.

The situation changed dramatically in 1972 when the U.S. government decided, under ANSI standards, that all glass lenses would have to be case hardened and impact-tested. The test consisted of dropping a steel ball of 5/8" diameter on a lens held on a neoprene ring one meter below the ball. If the lens survived the impact, it was considered satisfactory - even though the impact undoubtedly set the stage for easier breakage in the future. The result of this mandated test was that henceforth glass lenses had to be considerably thicker to

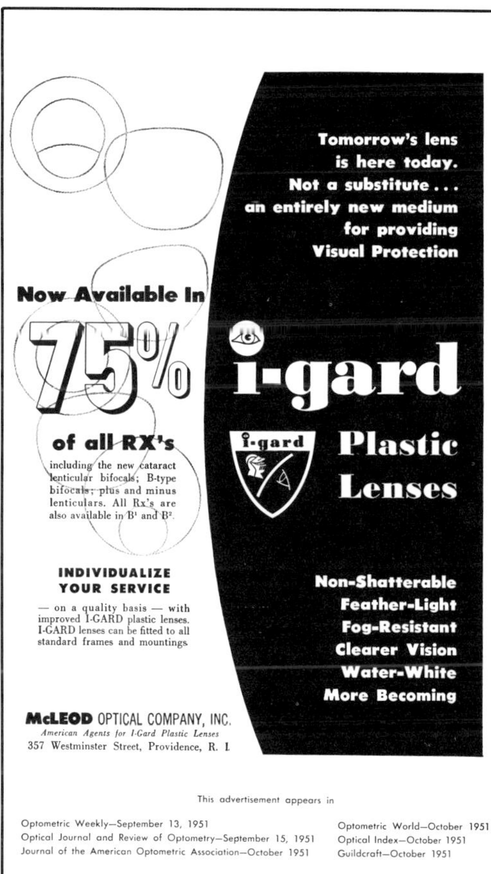

Following World War II, the first plastic lenses called "i-gard", manufactured in England, were distributed by many leading independent laboratories. They were imported and promoted by Norm MacLeod and McLeod Optical.

withstand the drop ball test. At the same time, frame styles were becoming increasingly larger which meant bigger *(and heavier)* lenses. The increased weight factor presented a cogent argument for the industry to consider changing to a lighter material *(CR-39)*.

Concurrently, labs that had been pioneering the processing of plastic lenses, in association with equipment manufacturers, developed improved equipment and more reliable processing techniques. These advanced laboratories began specializing in CR-39 production and soon hard resin lenses of decent quality with acceptable delivery times and more moderate pricing began to appear. These new lenses were lighter

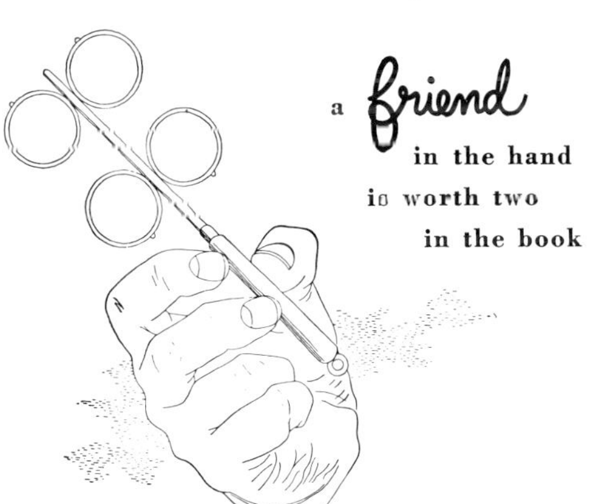

One of the most common dispensing aids found in most professional offices during the '30s and '40s was the Soft-Lite flipper. This handy tool had a pair of plano Soft Lite #1 lenses on one side and #2 tinted lenses on the opposite side. Holding it in front of the patient's eyes and asking "Which tint is more comfortable?" led to extra sales of B&L tinted lenses.

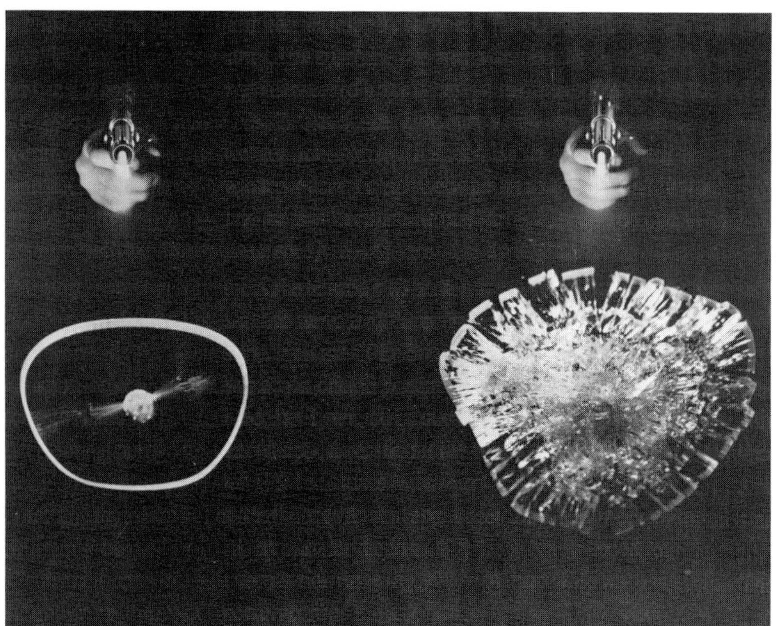

and cosmetically more appealing because of improved manufacturing techniques. Plastic lenses were more expensive than glass but this was considered an advantage because it allowed better profits for retailers. Doctors and dispensers were attracted by another feature of plastic lenses. Plastic lenses could be readily tinted to virtually any shade of the rainbow and, suddenly, this opened a new profit center for laboratories and retailers. During the next 20 years, CR39 became the standard in the American market and currently represents over 70 percent of domestic sales and increases in popularity internationally.

Photochromic Glass

Lenses that would darken automatically in the sun were a development of Corning, introduced in the mid-60's. They took the industry by storm. Suddenly, eyecare professionals had a premium single vision lens to offer and the results were immediate. Every glass lens manufacturer began producing single vision lenses in photochromic glass. For the first few years, these lenses were only available in single vision, primarily because Corning had yet to perfect a glass that would produce a fusible segment for photochromic glass.

During this prolonged period of single vision photochromic glass, an innovative company called Craftsman Lens sprung up in Los Angeles in 1974. Owned by Norman Rips, an experienced optician, Craftsman had devised a way to laminate a thin photochromic wafer over a clear glass blank *(containing a FT25 segment)*. Called "Photo-D", the result was a photochromic flat top. There were a number of drawbacks to the lens. It was quite thick. The front wafer had to be at least 1.5 mm thick to darken properly. It was very expensive but it was the only

game in town. Eventually, Corning produced a fusible photochromic glass and that should have been the end of Craftsman Lens.

But now a new need arose. Consumers liked photochromic lenses and as plastic lenses grew in popularity, a desire for photochromic lightweight lenses sprang up. Again, Norman Rips came to the rescue. By 1977, he was offering his laminated process, but this time the photochromic wafer was laminated over a single vision plastic blank. Again, it produced an expensive lens but this one was more difficult to sell because it was a single vision lens and, while it was lighter than an all-glass lens, the weight savings weren't enough to justify the added cost. There was also an additional problem of delaminating because of the expansion differences between glass and plastic materials. This lens had very limited success but it pointed the way for one more innovation from Norman Rips.

When the interest in producing eyeglasses in an hour sprang up, Rips realized his laminating process could be adapted to the production of "instant" bifocals. He spent several years refining the process *(this time, laminating plastic to plastic, a more workable system)*. Elliott Shane joined in this venture and their laminating process was eventually sold to Dicon/Vismed, who continue to market the wafer system with a reasonable degree of success.

Photochromic Plastic

Producing a photochromic plastic lens has been a quest for lens manufacturers for at least 15 years. American Optical produced one in 1981 but with little success because of limited darkening and a somewhat unattractive blue color when activated. Rodenstock also produced a photochromic plastic lens that worked reasonably well but only enjoyed marginal success in this country because of the nontraditional colors.

PPG Industries, the primary producer of CR-39 resin used in most of the world's plastic lenses, had special interest in a photochromic plastic lens, if such a thing could be produced. They spent a great deal of money and many man-years researching the subject during the '80s and ultimately developed an imbibition process that would allow a CR-39 lens to become photochromic. In July, 1990 a joint venture was formed between Transitions Optical and Essilor International. The newly formed company was named Transitions Optical, Inc. The initial product was well received and considered successful. The first generation of Transitions lens didn't get as dark as people preferred and was very temperature-dependent. Darkening in the sunbelt states was less than desirable.

In October, 1992, an improved lens called Transitions Plus was introduced with most of the shortcomings of the first lens eliminated. Transitions Plus lenses accomplished what the industry wanted - a lightweight lens that would darken in the sun. Today, most major lens manufacturers include Transitions photochromic lenses in their line.

Polycarbonate

Prototype polycarbonate lenses began to show up at trade shows in the '70s but ophthalmic lenses made of polycarbonate for dress wear didn't hit the market until the 1980s. The early product was quite primitive, compared to the present generation and many eyecare professionals who tried those early lenses were expecting the same quality as CR-39 but found that not to be the case.

These first impressions of lesser quality kept many doctors and dispensers from using polycarbonate. They were put off by the fact that minute specks of carbon could sometimes be seen in the material, even though they had no affect on acuity. Polycarbonate lenses are injection molded rather than cast as CR-39 lenses are. The common complaint of polycarbonate was the distortion created, it was believed, by the material's low "Abbe" value. Distortion could sometimes be found in the lenses but, as was later discovered, the actual cause of visual discomfort was distortion created during the molding process, not distortion from the Abbe properties. Over the next 10 years, a number of things happened. Resin suppliers of polycarbonate pellets made substantial improvements in the raw material. Next the molders *(lens manufacturers)* learned better techniques for designing their molds and distortions created by the molding process virtually disappeared. The result of all these improvements was a remarkably improved product.

Negative Lab Response

As recent as 1991, less than 15 percent of laboratories were equipped to process polycarbonate. This was a major factor holding back wider use of polycarbonate. Retailers sending a poly prescription to a lab that did not routinely process the material would, more often than not, get a phone call from the lab reminding them how bad the material was and suggesting another high index material. The biggest problem labs had in processing polycarbonate was coating the back surface after surfacing. By 1990, superb coating equipment was developed that did not require "clean room" environments and instantly cured the coating with UV light, enabling labs to produce polycarbonate lenses as quickly as convention plastic.

None of this might have been enough to overcome the initial negative impressions created by the early polycarbonate lenses had it not been for other events,

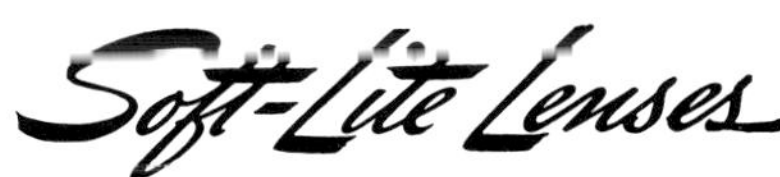

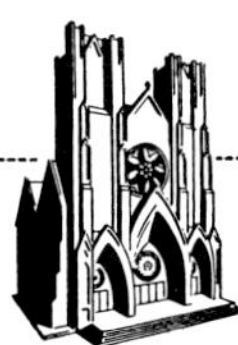

This Soft-Lite ad appeared in 1950 and gives some idea of the success enjoyed by what was considered to be a premium lens. Soft-Lite tints were exclusive to Bausch & Lomb and the prestige of this heavily-advertised tint helped in the marketing of Bausch & Lomb's entire lens line.

starting in far-off Wyoming. In 1981, a rancher wearing glass photochromic lenses suffered an eye injury when his glasses broke during a roping accident. This resulted in a law suit and the jury ruled that the accident would have been prevented with polycarbonate lenses. During the next few years, several other law suits resulted in judgments based on the fact that patients had not been warned about lens materials.

Duty To Warn

As a result of these legal activities, the Optical Laboratories Association published a "Duty To Warn" Kit in 1987, advising eyecare professionals how to fulfill their professional responsibilities in "informing" patients about impact resistance of lens materials. The kit was widely distributed during 1988 but for the next several years many doctors and dispensers, for the most part, continued to ignore the problem. In 1993, a jury ruling in Minnesota brought the whole subject back into the news. Again, a substantial judgment was granted on the basis that the patient *(and his parents)* was not properly informed regarding lens materials. The story was widely reported in the trade press and the OLA responded by updating and reissuing the Duty To Warn Kit.

Children and Sports

This time, however, many major retail chains recognized the liability problem and switched totally to polycarbonate for children. Combined with the increased interest in sports eyewear and a growing consumer awareness of polycarbonate, these lenses are suddenly in great demand. Every manufacturer of polycarbonate lenses has expanded their production facilities and most are

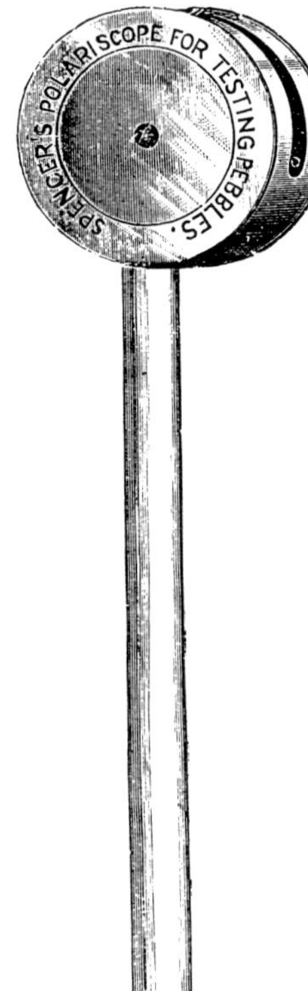

Pebble lenses were much more expensive than the more common glass lenses. Every office carried one of these Pebble Testers to show their patients they were getting the genuine article.

operating double shifts in an effort to keep up with demand. The Polycarbonate Lens Council, made up of manufacturers and labs, has launched a major public relations program to inform consumers about polycarbonate lenses. Today, the Council estimates that a majority of laboratories are now processing and promoting polycarbonate lenses. Once a lab develops their production techniques, they often promote polycarbonate because of better profit margins when compared to CR-39. Greater involvement by more laboratories, combined with increasing use for children indicates a bright future for the polycarbonate industry.

HIGH INDEX LENSES

Glass

Different indices of refraction in glass have long been available but were never widely used because of the excessive weight of flint glass. Ravenscroft in England had conceived that a higher index would produce a thinner lens in 1675 but the difficulty in producing such a lens prevented any practical applications until the 20th century. High index lenses were produced but did not gain much use. When FDA impact resistance requirements became law, flint high index glass could no longer be used. In 1973, Schott Glass introduced a titanium-based glass called High-Lite with an index of 1.70 that could be strengthened chemically. Corning later developed a 1.60 photochromic high index glass and clear glass lenses of 1.80 index are now available.

Plastic

The first high index plastic in the United States was 1.56 index, introduced at about the same time by two companies, Younger Optical and Polarlite. Younger's lens was made from Hi-Ri, a PPG material and Polarlite's was a Japanese product. Polarlite had been importing a polarized lens from Japan since 1984. Greg Daniels, with Polarlite, was making frequent trips to Japan. On his second trip there, he was shown the first prototype of a high index plastic by a company called Mikasa.

Daniels later left Polarlite. Osaka Optical of Japan wanted to set up a manufacturing facility in the United States to cast high index lenses. Daniels was hired to set up a facility called Eye One, to manufacture high index lenses in Salt Lake City, with Daniels heading it up. By the late '80s Eye One, Younger, Trusight, Polarlite, Optima were all selling high index lenses. Once the market was established, virtually every lens manufacturer added high index plastic lenses to their product line. In 1989, Optima introduced high index lenses from Japan with a 1.60 index and started a whole new craze. Today, many lens suppliers include 1.60 lenses in their line. Optima

later introduced a 1.66 index material, currently the highest index available in plastic.

This was a whole new field in chemistry, and everyone involved learned as they went along. During the early years, there were continuing changes and improvements in the high index formulations. This created substantial problems for laboratories because, each time the formula of the material changed, processing techniques had to be changed.

For example, it was not uncommon for the index to shift slightly as substrate manufacturers made changes in the resin. At a meeting of the California Optical Laboratories Association *(COLA)* in 1990, a panel of high index suppliers discussed this new field. A representative from one of the major computer programs was in the audience and asked the panel when the manufacturers were going to settle down and produce a fixed index. His company was having to reprogram lab software almost monthly in an effort to fine-tune the changes in index occurring as resin suppliers tried to improve their products.

Fortunately, this transition period didn't last too long and eventually product fluctuations settled down. The present-day product is as consistent as any other material. Compounding problems, however, is the growing proliferation of high index materials. Laboratories must stock and retailers must be familiar with high index plastic lenses in 1.54, 1.56, 1.57, 1.59 *(poly)*, 1.60 and 1.66. The industry estimates that at least 16 percent of the lens market in 1994 is high index plastic *(including polycarbonate)*

POLARIZED LENSES

The Beginning

The story of polarized lenses began in 1926 when a young 17 year old Harvard student strolled down New York's Broadway one summer evening. As he walked, he was overcome with the glare coming from hundreds of illuminated theater marquees, billboards and automobile headlights. The lights seemed to compete with one another and the resulting glare, he felt, was a real danger to pedestrians and drivers. The pedestrian was Edwin Herbert Land and, as a science student, young Land already knew that light vibrates in a multitude of planes. His stroke of inspiration that evening was that it might be possible to devise a filter that could control light so that it would emerge with all light vibrating in one direction. If he could do this, he felt, annoying glare would be eliminated.

Shortly after his New York trip, Land took a leave of absence from Harvard and moved to New York. Since he wasn't a registered student, the only way he could get in the physics lab at Columbia University was to sneak in after hours through an unlocked window. This is where his quest began for a filter to polarize light. After a three year leave of absence, Land returned to Harvard University. Harvard was sufficiently impressed with his progress to furnish him a laboratory and it was from that lab in 1932 that he announced the first man-made material to polarize light. Edwin Land was 23 years old.

Polarization of light had been understood since the 1700s when Dutch physicist Christian Huygens observed that certain natural crystals could limit the direction of light waves. Scientists, however, were never able to grow enough crystals to be of any practical value and natural crystals were as rare as sapphires. Land's early experiments used large crystals but he soon realized that this would never work commercially. He devised a way to incorporate countless needle shaped crystals in a plastic sheet which he then stretched mechanically so that all the microscopic crystals fell into parallel rows, forming a multitude of tiny crystals.

Creating a Name

Needing a name for his new material, his colleagues' first suggestion was the name "Epibolipol". Fortunately for everyone, Dr. Land decided "Polaroid" was a better name for his new filter material. "Oid" as a suffix is frequently used as a scientific term and means "likeness or resemblance". Land's primary goal at the time was to use his miracle filter for auto headlights but prior patents prevented him from completing this pet project. Instead, the first contract for his newly formed Polaroid Corporation was for $10,000 with Eastman Kodak for a camera filter Kodak called "Polascreen".

By the mid-'30s, sunglasses were becoming popular in the United States and American Optical was one of the largest sun-wear manufacturers. Most sunglasses were made of colored glass and were expensive, costing consumers as much as $5. Land decided this was an ideal application for his new Polaroid material. The company's second contract, signed November 5, 1935, was with the American Optical Company for a product called Polaroid Day Glasses, forerunner of all present-day polarized sunglasses.

Innovative marketing

The story of how Edwin Land convinced American Optical to use his material is an interesting one. Land didn't want to meet the A.O. people in his dingy basement laboratory, so he rented a suite at Boston's Copley Plaza Hotel for the princely sum of $10 a day. He bought an aquarium and some goldfish and placed the tank directly in front of a large window in the hotel suite. When AO's people arrived at noon, the sunlight on the fish tank was so intense, the fish couldn't be seen. Land apologized for the glare and said, "I imagine you can't even see what's in the tank". He then handed each person a square cut from a polarized sheet and asked them to look again at the aquarium. The glare had disappeared and the six fish could be seen gracefully swimming around the tank.

The contract was signed and the first Polaroid Day Glasses were launched by American Optical in December, 1936. Shortly thereafter, another contract was negotiated with Bausch & Lomb. Sunglasses became a major profit center for the new Polaroid Company. During the 3-D movie craze, the company sold more than five million pairs of cardboard glasses a year. Because the 3-D boom ended so fast, a rumor persists that warehouses full of cardboard glasses still exist. The Polaroid Corporation itself did not start manufacturing sunglasses until 1976.

Today the company's polarizer products play important roles in computer display filters. Linear polarizers are an essential component of liquid crystal displays utilized in laptop computers and many corporate jets feature polarized variable transmittance windows. The term "Polaroid" is a registered trade name and only lenses manufactured or licensed by the Polaroid Corporation can be called "Polaroid". The correct terminology for any other polarized ophthalmic lenses is "polarized" lenses.

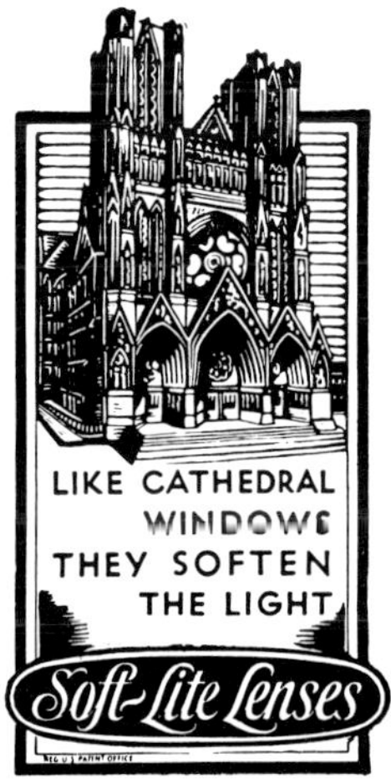

The Soft-Lite Company used a cathedral as a logo to demonstrate that their lenses softened light rays much like the pleasant light coming through a stained glass window. Soft-Lite lenses were manufactured and distributed by Bausch & Lomb.

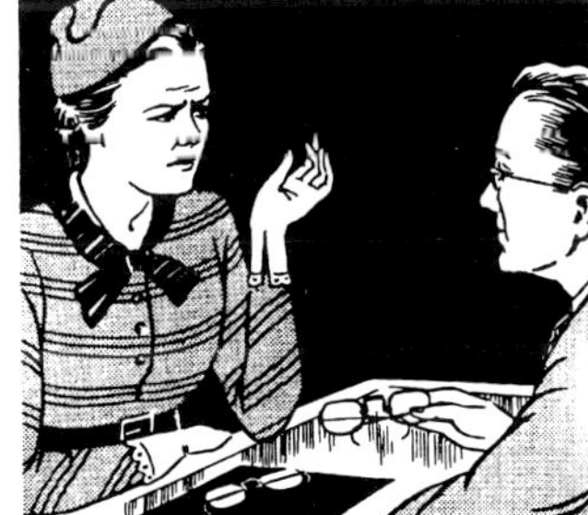

In selling Univis Bifocals there is no cut-price evil to contend with

Selective licensing and established minimum prices protect Univis lenses from demoralizing competitive tactics . . . . They are not in the hands of the chiseling element . . . . These fine identified lenses give the highest degree of satisfaction to wearers and likewise the highest degree of protection to the dealer . . . . Use Univis Bifocals, finished C. S. O. precision.

(Univis Lenses can be supplied only to licensee.)

Univis distribution was controlled by special licensing agreements between Univis and the labs handling their line. Rx prices and retail prices were all established by the manufacturer and any labs or retailers who failed to live up to the agreed pricing were dropped. Univis was proud of keeping their products out of the "chiseling element", as this 1936 ad reveals.

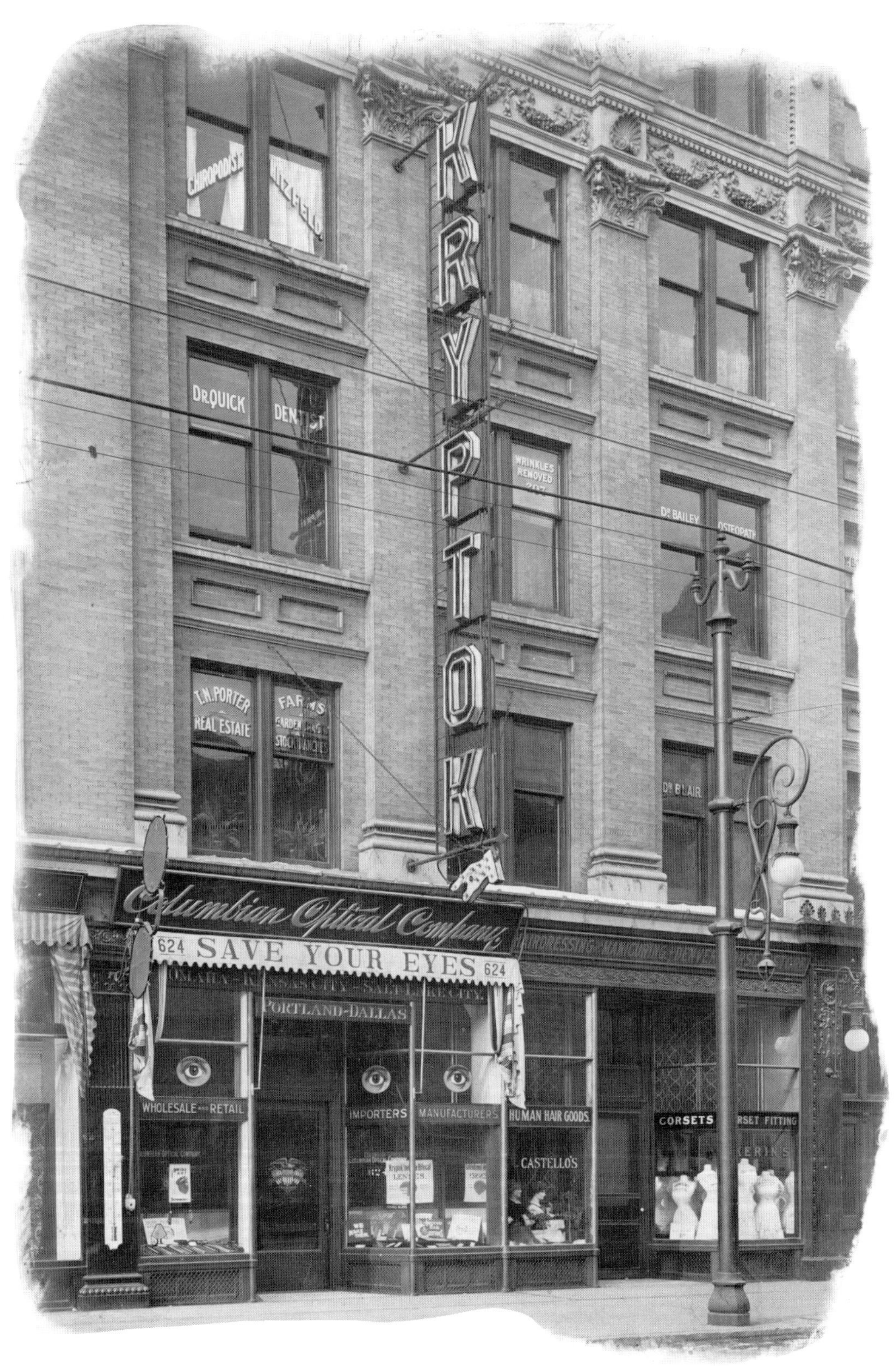

Optical retailers with a Kryptok license quickly discovered how valuable it was. Once consumers found there was an alternative to the ugly split and cement bifocals, they wanted them. Columbian Optical in Denver had purchased the marketing rights for 4 states for $8,000 from the Kryptok Company. Two weeks later they sold the California territory for $10,000. Columbian made sure local eyeglass wearers knew where to order invisible bifocals. This is how their store at 624 15th Street in Denver looked in 1904. OLA OPTICAL INDUSTRY MUSEUM

Chapter 8
The Kryptok Story

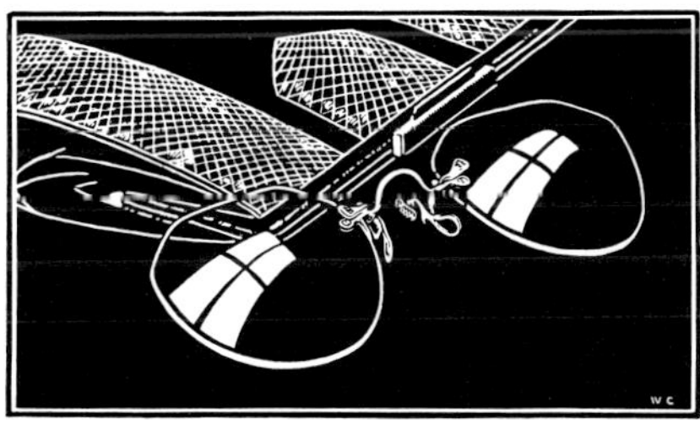

It was January 21, 1909 when Dr. John L. Borsch, Jr. introduced the first fused bifocal to the world. The new lens was to become the biggest thing to ever happen to the optical industry. This single product would produce profits never before seen in the optical business. It would also herald a new public awareness of the importance of quality in eyeglass lenses and usher in an era of $12 to $20 lenses at a time when most lenses sold for a mere fraction of those figures. The new lens also created some of the fiercest court battles the young industry had ever known.

The story of how the Kryptok bifocal evolved—the years of planning, the experimenting, the predictions of defeat, the bootlegging that followed and the innumerable litigations it caused—make one of the most interesting stories in the history of the optical industry.

The Beginning

This story starts with Dr. Borsch's father, a pioneer dispensing optician in Philadelphia, takes us to Paris, France and covers a period of twenty-six years, from the time the first patent was issued in 1899 to the death of the Kryptok Company *(but not the lens)* in 1925 when all patents covering the manufacture of Kryptok lenses expired.

John L. Borsch, Sr. was a descendant of four generations of optical workers. He had invented the original cemented form of Kryptok bifocal, a lens called "Invisible Bifocal". A patent for his early bifocal was issued on November 21, 1899. In its original form, it consisted of two pieces of glass cemented together with Canadian Balsam. In the lower section of a distance lens, a circular depression would be countersunk. In this concavity was cemented a circular glass disc of the same diameter but made of glass in a higher index. The depression would usually have a -10.00 to -12.00 diopter curve.

Grinding of the segment involved a delicate procedure. One side of the segment was matched to the curve of the depression and the opposite curve selected to match the front curve of the distance lens. The glass segment was then cemented into the concave depression. The cemented segment was exposed and this was the chief drawback to the lens. Segments were easily dislodged, dirt accumulated in the juncture and their visual performance was poor. This suggested a need for improvement to John Borsch. His answer was a three part Kryptok lens. In this new form, a carrier lens would be cemented over the entire front surface, covering both the distance and near portions of the lens. This 3-piece improved bifocal was covered by a new patent issued to Borsch in 1899.

Harold Stead Remembers

Harold Stead, a well known optical personality and author, still remembered by old-timers in the

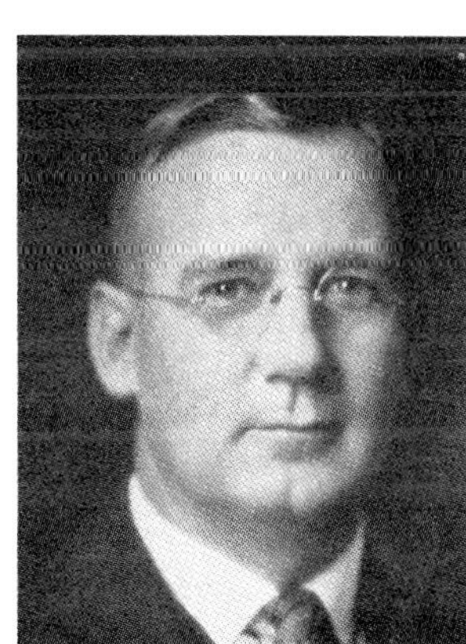

Harold Stead

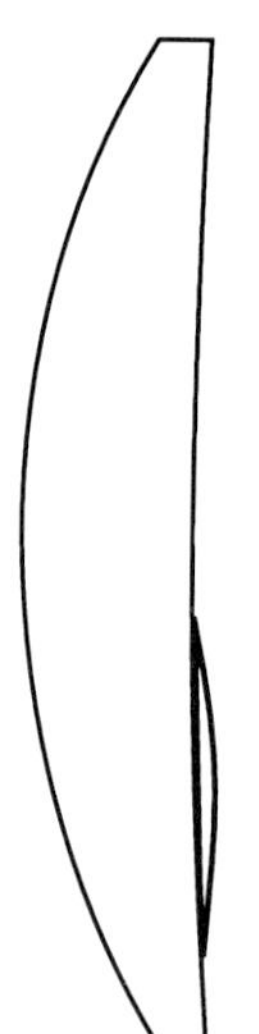

Cement bifocal was usually applied to back surface of lens.

OLA OPTICAL INDUSTRY MUSEUM

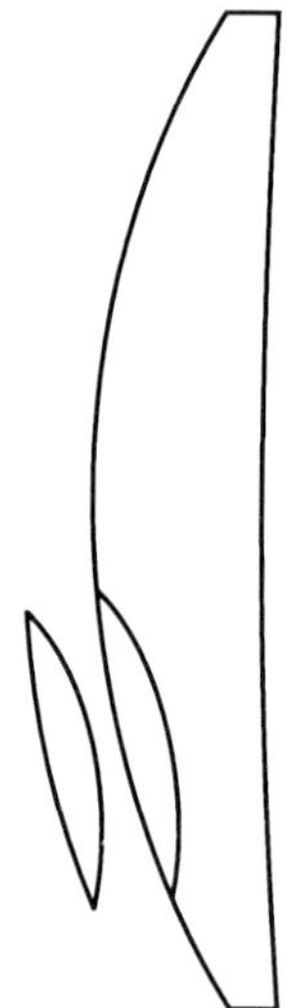

Original Borsch Kryptok. Flint segment button was cemented into the cavity after being ground and polished.

OLA OPTICAL INDUSTRY MUSEUM

industry, gives a graphic description of the first pair of invisible bifocals he ever saw.

"In about the latter part of 1899 or the first of 1900, when I was working at lens surface grinding with the Geneva Optical Company, Geneva, New York, a pair of glasses came in for the replacement of one lens which was broken. Now, we were all familiar with all of the different types of bifocal lenses way back to Benjamin Franklin. but never had we seen anything like this one. It was an object of curiosity for everyone in the establishment because while it apparently was a bifocal—that is, it had two fields of vision, there was apparently no segment exposed on the surface, and a lens measure indicated power curves only for the distant vision portion. We wondered why anyone would go to all that trouble to make a bifocal lens.

The reading field was circular, about 16 mm or 18 mm. in diameter and appeared to be imbedded within the glass comprising the major lens. It could be readily observed that this was composed of two sections, because the lenses were of the rimless type and one hole was broken out, which shattered the glass so as to expose the construction. Then too, the edge indicated that it consisted of two thin lenses cemented together. The application of heat soon disclosed the actual construction and permitted the separation of the two parts exposing the reading section, which in turn appeared to be cemented in a cavity in one of the pieces comprising the major lens.

It was at once obvious that the lens could not be replaced because we had no knowledge of the existence of such an article on the market, and inasmuch as none of us knew the specifications required, it was returned to the customer. It did seem to be the consensus of opinion that the glass forming the reading section must be of greater power or "index" to effect the increased optical effect required for reading, and just to try this out I experimentally reproduced the lens using a piece of "window" glass.

This resulted in a slight increase in power, but, of course, served only to demonstrate the effectiveness of the idea for we still lacked the formula for determining the proper kind of glass, index of refraction, curvatures, etc."

Kryptok Licenses

Almer Coe, a prominent optician in Chicago saw the cemented Borsch Bifocal for the first time in about 1905. Dr. Swan, a Chicago eye physician showed him the first pair he had seen and he became wildly enthusiastic. The Invisible Bifocal he saw *(the name was about to be changed to "Kryptok" at about this same time)* was the new 3-piece version of the Kryptok. Coe saw tremendous possibilities in the lens. In those days, it was difficult to get patients to wear bifocals because of their appearance. Here was something truly different - invisible bifocals at a time when bifocals were generally being shunned by the public. Learning that John Borsch, Sr. was the inventor, Coe went to Philadelphia to see him. Unfortunately, he didn't get along with Borsch. He thought him a "queer sort of person".

A few months later, a representative of Borsch came through Chicago on his way to see F.A. Hardy, at that time, Chicago's leading wholesale laboratory *(ultimately to become a key acquisition for American Optical)*. Hardy, however, had turned him down. Borsch's representative crossed town to drop in on Almer Coe. Coe promptly offered him $1,000 in cash for the manufacturing rights in certain Midwest states. Later, Coe arranged to go to Atlantic City to learn from Borsch how to make the lenses. He came back from this visit with slabs of flint glass that were four inch square and one inch thick. These slabs had to be sawed by hand with a diamond wheel into small segments two or three millimeters thick. Each of these segments would then be carefully ground to shape. This tedious procedure was just to make the reading segments. The cover glass was only one to two fifths of

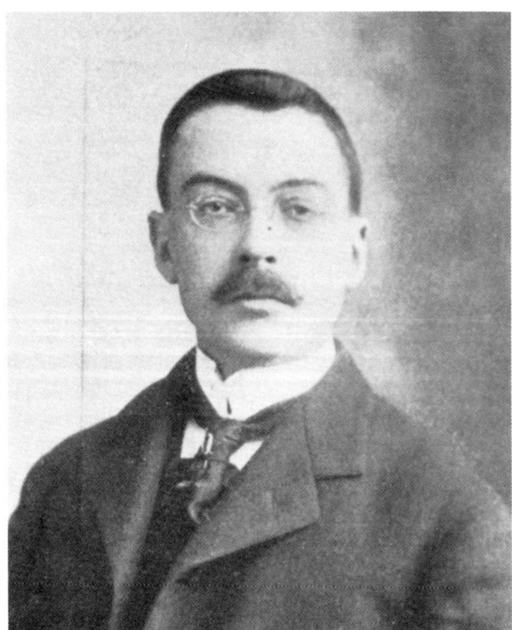

Almer Coe, a prominent Chicago optician was one of the first to see the possibilities of the fused Kryptok.

OLA OPTICAL INDUSTRY MUSEUM

a millimeter thick. These thin cover sheets were easily broken and the balsam cement had a tendency to fail. All in all, this was a tedious way to make a pair of lenses, but they were able to sell every pair they made and the profits were enormous. Coe was getting $12 a pair when he first began selling them.

Marketing Rights

In spite of their desirability, wholesale labs did not have much to do with these new bifocals. The manufacture and sale of cemented Kryptoks was confined exclusively to large retail dispensing opticians in various parts of the country. Borsch sold the marketing rights in almost every state. As an example of how these state rights were snapped up, the Columbian Optical Company paid $8,000 for the exclusive rights to market Kryptok lenses in Colorado, Kansas, Nebraska and California. Just two weeks later, they sold the California rights to Chinn-Beretta for $10,000.

There was, however, a great deal of territory overlapping. Someone in Indiana would hear about the lens and write to Almer Coe in Chicago even though John Wimmer owned the rights to the Indiana territory. To avoid this type of confusion and for their mutual interest, this group of Kryptok-licensed opticians formed the Kryptok Association to solve any problems that might crop up. The thirteen original licensees were:

Andrew Lloyd & Co.	Boston
E.B. Meyrowitz	New York
John L. Borsch	Philadelphia
Charles A. Euker	Baltimore
Frank Edmonds	Washington, DC
John L. Moore & Sons	Atlanta
Almer Coe	Chicago
John Wimmer	Indianapolis
Southern Optical Co.	Louisville
A.S. Aloe Company	St. Louis
Columbian Optical Co.	Denver
Chinn-Beretta Optical	San Francisco
J.C. Freeman & Co.	Worchester

And, to be sure, problems did arise. Manufacturing these complicated lenses was not easy. The distance lenses *(called "blades")* were thin and delicate and the disc forming the reading section was razor sharp. All the manufacturing problems would be magnified when holes had to be drilled for rimless jobs. When frames were too tight, the blades would separate and often fracture. Everyone agreed there had to be a better way to "fuse the parts together" and a number of patents

were issued to Brown, Wimmer and others for new and different processing methods.

The Fused Kryptok

This brings us to the most dramatic part of the story, the development of the fused Kryptok, a dramatic improvement in the Kryptok bifocal. This was invented in 1904 by Dr. John L. Borsch, Jr. The new process was finally patented in 1909 after years of litigation. Young Borsch grew up in the optical business, working in his father's optical shop in Philadelphia. He obtained his professional and technical training at the Jefferson Medical College of Philadelphia and at the University of Paris. He received special training at the General Hospital for Diseases of the Eye in Vienna and was assistant and later chief of the Paris Clinic for Diseases of the Eye.

In September 1898, however, young Borsch was 25 years old and still studying for his degree at the University of Paris while working at the Eye Clinic under Dr. deWecker. It was during this time that he conceived the idea of making "invisible" bifocal lenses by welding two pieces of glass of different indices of refraction together without the use of any foreign substance. The circumstances of how he achieved his idea are somewhat uncanny. The senior Borsch family were in the habit of making frequent trips to Paris while young Borsch was studying there. On this occasion, they had booked passage on the French Line steamer Burgoyne. Two days before it was to sail, Mrs.

Borsch's improved 3-piece Kryptok featured a cover lens which was cemented over the carrier lens and cemented segment. This was the lens that so mystified Harold Stead and his fellow workers in 1900.

OLA OPTICAL INDUSTRY MUSEUM

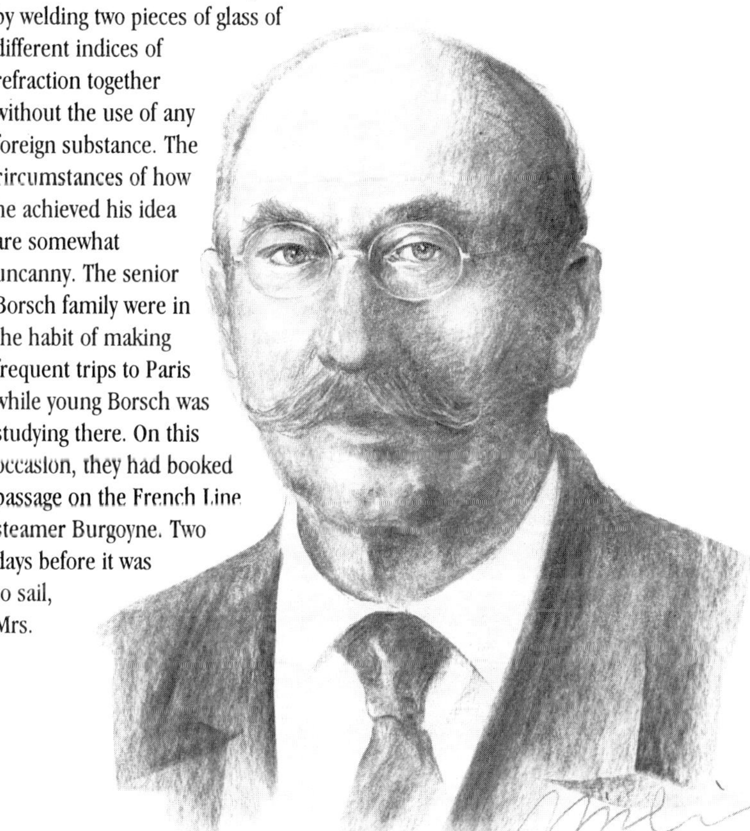

John L. Borsch, Sr., inventor of the cemented and 3-piece Kryptoks. His son John, Jr. improved his father's design by fusing the segment to the distance lens, eliminating all cementing and producing what was advertised as an "invisible lens".

DRAWING OLA OPTICAL INDUSTRY MUSEUM

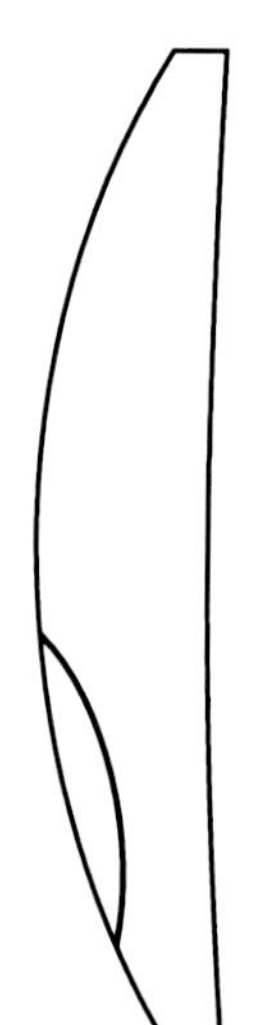

The fused Kryptok, a nearly invisible bifocal when compared to earlier bifocals.

Borsch, Sr. had a dream that the ship was going to sink. They canceled their trip and, strangely enough, the ship did sink. As a result of this unusual episode, young Borsch decided to go to Philadelphia instead. During this visit, as he watched workmen in his father's shop cementing bifocals in accordance with his father's invention, he formed the idea he was to doggedly pursue during the following years.

The Experiments Continue

On his return to France, he set out to achieve his goal. Early experiments, conducted in his kitchen where he constructed a crude brick furnace, proved to be fruitless. In 1899, his mother's death necessitated a trip back to America. On returning to Paris, he continued his experiments while working at the Clinic and completing studies at the University. Letters to his father during this time indicate he still hadn't given up —

"What is new in the optical line at home? Here things are about as they were in good old Ben Franklin's time. Speaking of Franklin reminds me to tell you I have been working on that solid bifocal idea of mine. I made some experiments in welding different lenses. Result: succeeded in cracking them and burning my fingers besides making a botch of the welding.

I need three things to develop my idea - time, money and an intelligent workman to carry out my ideas of a furnace. I have very little of either of the former and if you ask a French workman to do anything for you, you are lucky if he does it for you before your hair turns gray."

To this letter, Borsch, Sr. replied -

"I advise you to let that fused bifocal idea of yours alone. You only waste your time and it can't be done. Tend to your doctor business. That will please me much more."

Apparently his father's advice did not impress the young man for in his next letter to his father on February 14, 1900, he wrote -

"I have been trying to get to Mantois' to see them make their glass. The last time I was there they seemed very reluctant to allow anyone in their factory and gave me to understand that they allow no one to see it.

You see I have not given up my idea of making bifocals by welding the flint and crown together instead of cementing them. I spoke to deWecker about it but he said it is impossible to make them that way and so does Mantois' man.

I have been reading some books on glass

making but can find nothing bearing on the welding of glass for optical purposes such as I want. A few days ago I tried to weld two lenses (a concave and cx. one) over a Bunsen burner in the laboratory; they stuck together on one edge but cracked to pieces. What I need is an electric or gas furnace or oven made of magnesia such as I spoke to you before I left. Just as soon as I can, I am going to try and make one. I know you are laughing at my idea but somehow I feel it can be done."

It's interesting to note that during the same time this correspondence was going on, Borsch, Sr. was getting patents on his own inventions for the cemented form of Kryptok bifocals. In 1900, after receiving his French degree, J.L. Borsch, Jr. returned to America. In 1902, he must have attained some degree of success, for in a letter to his fiancee in France, he wrote -

"I have been very much occupied these last few days. I am continuing the work on my solid bifocal lens when I have the time succeeded yesterday in making one in a fellow's furnace. This glass is not perfect, of course, but enough to demonstrate that they can be made to adhere by means of heat, as I have stated. The old gentleman is not very enthusiastic."

Success

It was in the latter part of 1902 when young Borsch finally succeeded in producing a good lens. On October 10, 1902, he produced a solid welded bifocal lens in a small gas furnace that had formerly been a jeweler's furnace for melting gold. This demonstration took place at his home in Philadelphia and he was to describe it as follows:

"I took a piece of glass, being the major lens, and therein made a depression. Then I took

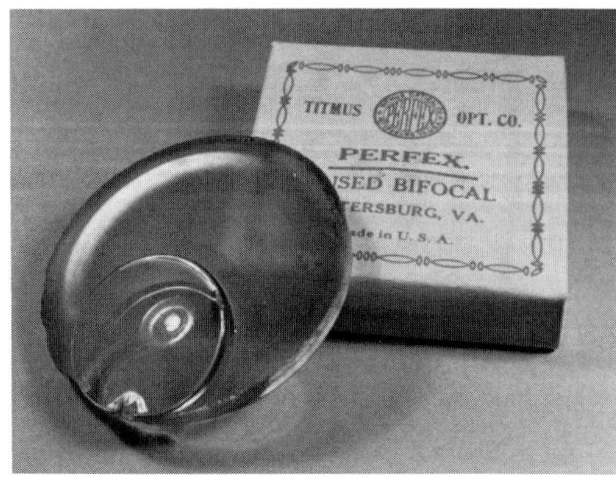

In the early days of fused Kryptoks, labs were required to finish both sides of lens blanks. Photo shows fused blank as it came from the factory, before the front surface was ground and polished.

another piece of higher index of refraction - a smaller block of glass - and ground and polished it convex on one surface. I introduced this smaller piece of glass into the depression in the larger portion, arranging it in the furnace and applied the heat"

This first successful blank was then ground and polished in the Senior Borsch's shop and was immediately followed by several other fused blanks. As more and more blanks were successful, Dr. Borsch, Jr. applied for a patent on January 23rd, 1904. After some litigation, the patent was ultimately issued to him on January 21, 1909, which officially became the legal birthday of the fused bifocal and the birth of the final form of Kryptok lens.

Bootlegging Kryptoks

There were two reasons for the widespread bootlegging that followed development of the Kryptok lens. The first reason was the stringent restrictions set up for the sale and manufacture of Kryptok bifocals. The second, of course, was the huge profits made possible by this exciting new technology. Many of those excluded from Kryptok licenses started to market "Kryptok-type Bifocals". Some of these companies operated under the protection of what came to be called the "Brown Patent". Others operated under the "Seymore Patent". Harold Stead developed his own process and established the Stead Lens Company in Kansas City. And so it went. All these patents, however, antedated the patent application of the younger Borsch on January

23, 1904. As a result of these developments, the Kryptok Association was to take on hundreds of litigation suits in efforts to restrain others from entering their lucrative new field.

At the beginning of the Kryptok proposition in 1906, Meyrowitz Manufacturing Company was one of the 12 retail licensees who were stockholders in control of the Kryptok Company. They owned the patents. The function of the company was to furnish Kryptoks to the 12 stockholder retail licensees and any other organizations they might later franchise, such as large jobbers like F.A. Hardy. Only a few of the stockholders would manufacture their own blanks, among them Almer Coe, Mason, F.A. Hardy, John L. Borsch and others.

The question of where the name came from is up for debate. The word was coined from the Greek "krypte" *(hidden)* and "tok" *(eye)* or in other words, "hidden eye" or "eye in a crypt". While Mr. Meyrowitz was alive, he claimed he had coined the name. It's reported that the public had great trouble with the name but, in spite of this, Kryptok ultimately became the most widely consumer-recognized optical name. Retailers authorized to sell Kryptoks would prominently feature the name on the front of their stores and in all their advertising. In 1918, one daring company began national advertising of a bifocal they chose to call "Crip Tock".

Harold Stead, a man who was to play an important part in the optical industry tells his version of the Kryptok story in a personal letter he wrote on May 12, 1941.

Denver's Columbian Optical was one of the few companies permitted to both manufacture and sell Kryptoks and they proudly acknowledged this throughout the lab. Old time opticians will recognize the blocking bench covered with pitch in the foreground. Circa 1907.

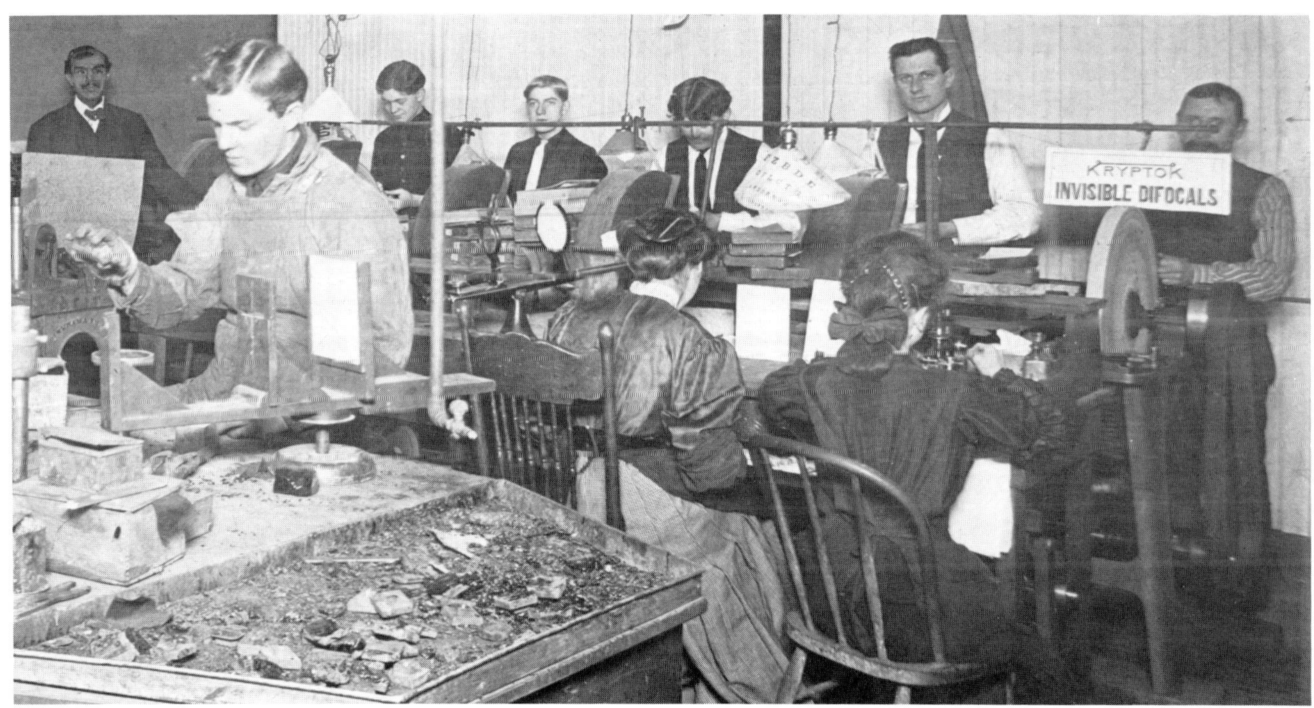

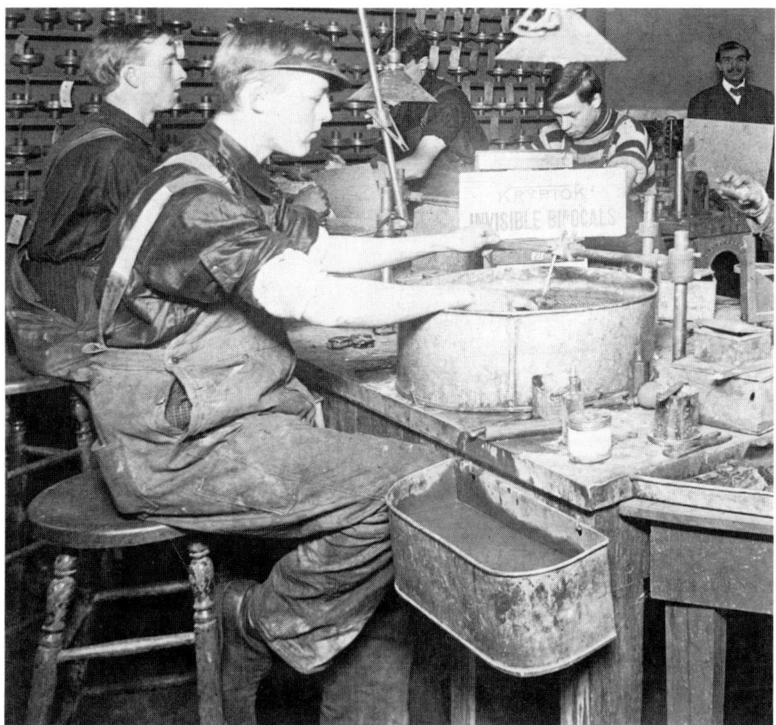

After fusing the segment to the distance blank, the front side had to be ground and polished. This was accomplished in roughing pans as shown in this photo taken in Columbian Optical's lab. Circa 1907.

OLA OPTICAL INDUSTRY MUSEUM

"About a year later (1901), my attention was called to a circular published by E.B. Meyrowitz of New York City describing and offering for sale bifocal lenses called "Kryptok". They were priced at $12.00 to $18.00. The matter seemed more like a curiosity, for we wondered how the trade could ever expect anyone to pay that much for a pair of lenses. It seemed like a lot of grinding to do to secure a double vision lens.

It was not long thereafter, in fact, in June 1904 that I became connected with the Rx shop of E. B. Meyrowitz in New York City. In the meantime, of course, the trade had learned quite a lot about Kryptok bifocals, but here for the first time I was brought in close association with their manufacture. It appears that the wholesale optical trade were not acquainted with the marketing of these bifocal lenses - in fact, they could not handle them commercially because it was confined exclusively to large retail dispensing opticians prominent at that time in various parts of the country. This came about through the fact that the lens was invented by John L. Borsch, one of the pioneer dispensing opticians of Philadelphia. The patent was filed March 18th, 1899 and issued November 21, 1899 and in its original construction consisted only two pieces of glass cemented together with Canadian balsam.

The exposure of the "segment" made the use of such lenses rather precarious, which in turn, suggested a further improvement later forming the subject of another application for patent by Mr. Borsch covering the construction of a "three part lens". This patent was filed February 25, 1899 and issued May 23, 1899.

The second invention of Mr. Borsch called for the enclosure of the segment portion entirely within the lens—that is, to the original form was added a third member covering the entire distant and reading surfaces. On these two portions were ground the curves required for distant vision.

A representative of Mr. Borsch solicited all of the prominent retail dispensing opticians in the United States at that time and was successful in selling rights to manufacture the lens under the Borsch patents in various states and territories. For mutual interest this group was formed into what was called the "Kryptok Association', and all of these concerns made the lenses in their own Rx shops. Naturally, considerable difficulty was experienced in the manufacture because the "blades", as they were called - that is, the distance sections, were extremely thin and delicate, and the discs forming the reading section were razor edge. There was not only technical difficulty in grinding the parts but there was further trouble in securing them together with Canada Balsam - and keeping them together, because when holes were drilled for rimless jobs, or even when frames were too tight, the "blades" would separate and quite often fracture.

For these reasons, naturally, the thought of securing them together by some more substantial means than with cement was current in all of the establishments engaged in production. This resulted in a number of inventions for methods or processes of "fusing" the parts together; and of record, there are a number of patents to Brown, Wimmer and others, covering processes of manufacture. but not before an application had been made by John L. Borsch, Jr. , a son of the Philadelphia optician, who had been outstanding as an oculist and was practicing his profession in Paris, France. On January 23, 1904 he applied for patent on the present form of Kryptok lens and on April 29, 1904 he applied for a patent on a process of making it. These patents were issued on January 21, 1908 and May 5, 1908, respectively. It was not long before all of the retail (members of the Kryptok Association) were attempting to *work out Borsch Jr.'s process patent. It was a most involved and difficult undertaking and not at all as successful as would appear today, because of the fact that then there was no definite information on the various properties of optical glass utilized in the construction - that is, Crown and Flint glasses. Annealing was the most trying operation. Hundreds of lenses were fractured in an attempt to perfect the annealing process and it was found that the annoying factor was the illusive element of the "coefficient of expansion", that little thing involved when glass is heated and cooled.*

Because a number of the retail licensees could not make the lenses to meet their requirements, the Meyrowitz Manufacturing Company, a subsidiary of E.B. Meyrowitz of New York City, formed to produce various articles of manufacture for his then extensive business, was constituted the first manufacturing licensee and began to supply a number of retail members with the rough product which was later finished according to Rx in individual grinding shops.

Because of the increasing popularity of Kryptok lenses through the authorized retailers' promotion, wholesalers, and even manufacturers, became intensely interested in distributing the product, but it seemed the Kryptok Association had little interest to extend sales or manufacturing rights to these groups. Consequently, a number of concerns, principally the Globe Optical Company of Boston, the Toric Optical Company of New York, and the F. A. Hardy Company of Chicago, began to market similar products, operating under what was then called the "Brown patent".

Then because of the development in processes of manufacture by various member licensees, the Kryptok Association was abandoned in favor of a stock corporation called the Kryptok Company by which development all of the licensees controlling territories turned in their rights and obtained shares of stock. E. B. Meyrowitz was the first president and Almer Coe was vice-president. It was then that the Kryptok Company acquired the John L. Borsch, Jr. patents and a number of other patents, including the Brown patent.

All of this was not without some litigation in an attempt by the Kryptok Association to restrain manufacturers such as Toric Optical Co. and others from invading this new field. However, on a threat of other large manufacturers who seemed confident of over-riding legal obstacles and acquiring a new field of business operation, the Kryptok Company finally granted manufacturing licenses to the American Optical Company of Southbridge and to the Bausch & Lomb Optical Company of Rochester, New York. The result of these negotiations ended the litigation over the Brown patent, and the lawsuit for infringement brought against the Toric Optical Company in New York City was compromised by the signing of a consent decree acquiescing in the validity of the Borsch patents.

Long before that - in 1905 - I went to Kansas City, Missouri, and became associated with the Merry Optical Company. This was one of the large wholesale concerns who were anxious to take part in the commercialization of Kryptok

Retailers with a Kryptok license made sure their community knew they carried this exciting new bifocal. Here is how one optometrist modestly displayed Kryptoks in his office window. Circa 1910.

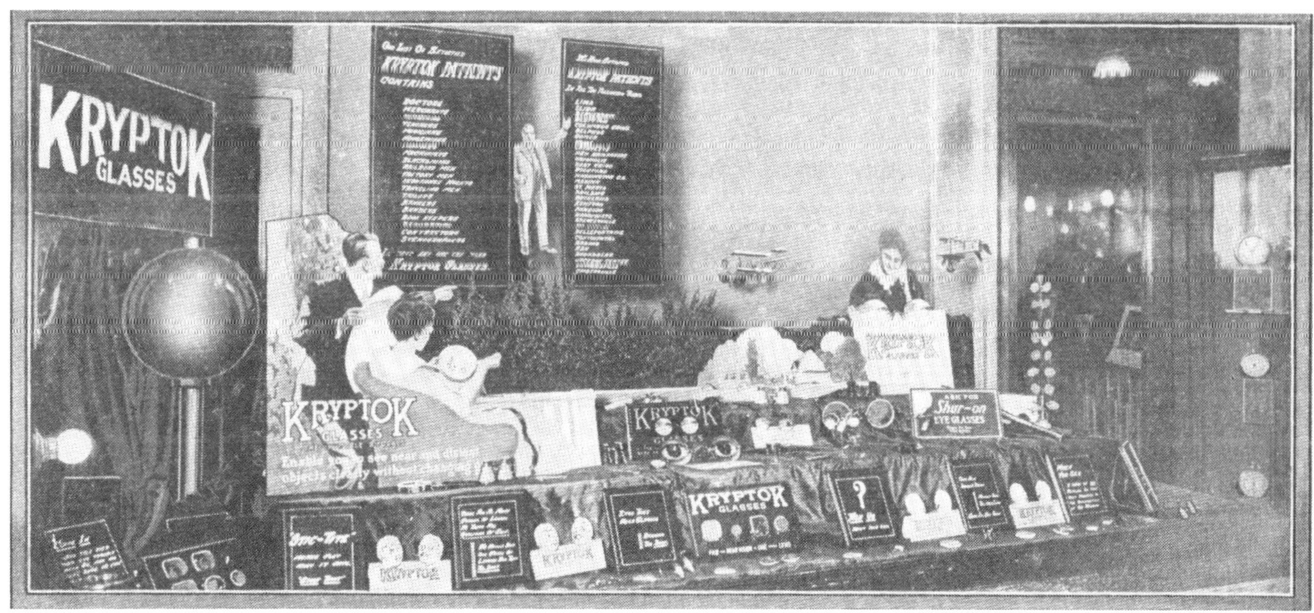

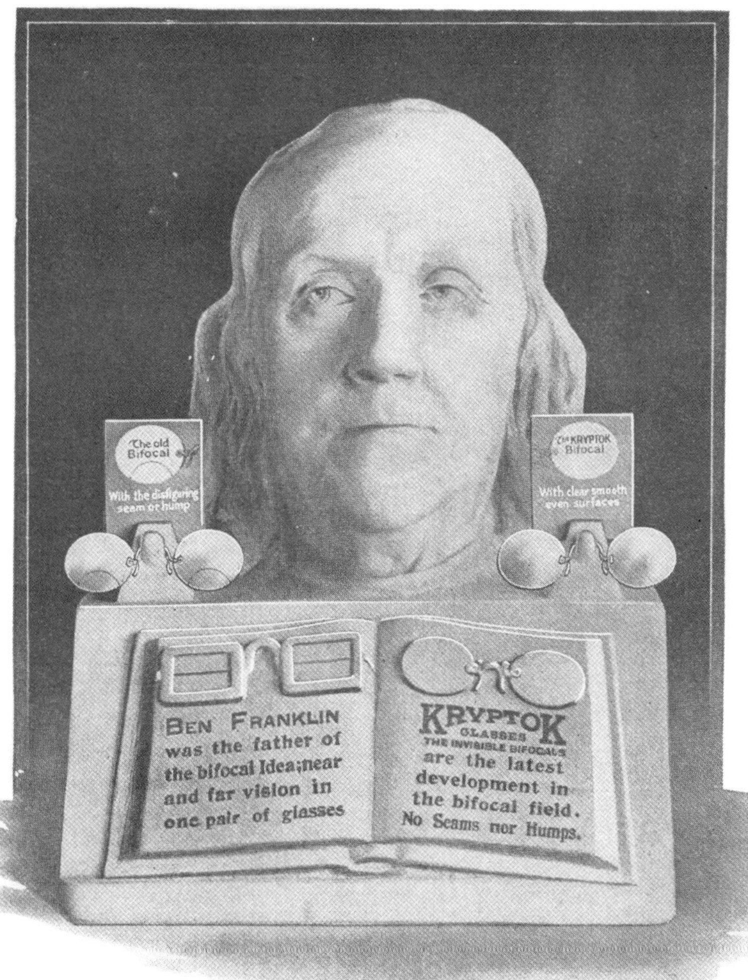

*The Kryptok Company
controlled the Kryptok patent
until it expired in 1925. They
offered many advertising aids
to licensed retailers. This
plaster-of-paris bust of
Franklin could be ordered for
$6. Dealer could hang actual
eyeglass samples on the two
mounting posts. Circa 1910.*

OLA OPTICAL INDUSTRY MUSEUM

*York City and Geneva New York, comprising J H.
Harris, H. B. Graves and W. W. Page, who
formed the United Bifocal Company and located
a plant in Toledo, Ohio.*

*It was not long after the establishment of my
business in Kansas City in November 1907 that
suit for infringement was brought against me by
the Kryptok Company who claimed infringement of the Borsch patents. This litigation ended
adversely for me in June 1914. Although suit
was brought in 1909, it was not finally tried
and decided until July 1913 in the U. S. Circuit
Court in Kansas City. The Borsch patents
covered the article itself and because I could not
obtain a manufacturing license from them, it
meant that my patent was worthless, and the
business that I had built up in five or six years
of work was destroyed.*

*Of course, there is much more to it than this.
There was the litigation with the United Bifocal
Company and the Standard Optical Company,
which was finally compromised. There were
literally hundreds of instances, some of which
would make books in themselves. However, I
thought this might serve your purpose."*

The Company

Once Kryptok blanks were being manufactured, the
Kryptok Sales Company was formed as a subsidiary of
General Optical. The name was registered with the
County Clerk of New York and was owned by Meyrowitz
Manufacturing Company. Manufacturing was by
General Optical and when Shuron-Standard merged
with DuPaul-Young and Company, a selling agreement
from General Optical was given to Shuron-Standard, as
the company was then known. A gentleman named
Harry C. Ulmer became the first representative of the
Kryptok Sales Company with a territory that extended
from New York to San Francisco and from Winnipeg to
the Gulf. His first year's work was calling exclusively on
wholesalers of the country *(Tiring of full-time
traveling, Ulmer was to later join the Merry Optical
Company in Louisville, Kentucky as branch manager.
Merry Optical was purchased by American Optical
and in 1941, Ulmer celebrated his 24th anniversary
as Louisville branch manager).*

The quality of those first blanks was nothing to rave
about. The fusing technique was primitive and there
were difficulties caused by poor fusing and improper
annealing. Other problems involved color in the
segments and a great deal of breakage, often with no
apparent cause. The Kryptok sales rep's first duty was
to get the wholesaler to sign a contract. This included a
clause that bound the signer to acknowledge the

*lenses but were unable to do so because of
patent restrictions. Through the interest of Mr. C.
L. Merry, a man by the name of J. I. Seymore
introduced some experimental developments
and later obtained a patent on a process of
manufacturing lenses of the "Kryptok type". This
process involved blowing or forming molten
glass in molds as a major part of the process.*

*As a result of these developments I became an
inventor on my own account and on July 12,
1907 applied for a patent for a process of
manufacture of a "Kryptok-type bifocal" using
in part a method of blowing or molding the
glass. This reached such a development that I
left the employ of C. L.. Merry and started the
Stead Lens Company in Kansas City for the
purpose of manufacturing the product of our
patent.*

*The Seymore patent and process was sold by the
Merry Optical Company to a group from New*

validity of all Kryptok patents. This was a serious concern to wholesalers and most initially refused to sign. They had to have the product, however, and by the end of the first year, most had signed the contract. Only three declined to acknowledge the validity of the patents and even those companies later became authorized Kryptok jobbers.

Kryptok Wholesalers

It was Mr. Ulmer's opinion that there were never more than ninety Kryptok wholesalers. He readily acknowledged that there was a definite system of price fixing which covered, not only the price paid by the wholesaler, but the price the wholesaler charged the optometrist or retailer and even retailers were required to charge their customers a fixed retail price for these modern bifocals.

An idea of lens pricing in those days *(1910)* can be understood by itemizing how Kryptoks were priced. Wholesalers paid $2.50 a pair for flat blanks *(most lenses in those days were flat)* and $3.50 for torics *(6 base curve)*. Labs were required to charge the retailer $7.50 for finished lenses and the retailer was required to sell them to the public for $13. These prices were closely adhered to since wholesalers or retailers who cut price or rebated were immediately dropped from the authorized list. During this same period, several companies that infringed on the Kryptok patent were taken to court.

In 1910 Bausch & Lomb and American Optical Company were granted licenses and, in spite of their added competition, sales of the Kryptok Sales Company continued to soar. All manufacturing licensees, namely the Kryptok Sales Company, AO and B&L each paid royalties to the Kryptok Company which was located in Boston and owned the patents.

Many labs at that time were afraid to grind Kryptoks because of their high cost. Perhaps as a way of addressing that fear, the Kryptok Company issued labs a guarantee that promised, in case of breakage, if the broken pieces were sent back to the manufacturer, they would be replaced with new blanks.

Kryptok was also the first optical product advertised in a full page ad in the Saturday Evening Post, the leading magazine of that day. This was the first optical consumer advertising that ever appeared.

Kryptok Sales

During the effective life of the Kryptok patents, the courts ruled that any fused bifocal conflicted with the Kryptok patent and this, in effect, gave the fused bifocal market to Kryptok. By 1924, the company was selling 1,000,000 pairs of blanks annually. In the last year of operation, royalties alone generated over one half million dollars. Seventy-five thousand dollars represented the original capital and the company never paid out less than that amount in the form of dividends in any one year. The last Kryptok patent expired in 1925 but by that time, Kryptoks had become the largest selling single item in the entire optical business. The company's growth was encouraged because of the comforting protection of a product patent *(J.L. Borsch, Sr. Patent #637,444, Nov. 21, 1899)* and a process patent *(Dr. J.L. Borsch, Jr. Patent #876,933, Jan. 21, 1909)* and when those patents expired in 1925, so did the Kryptok Company. With the death of the patents, everyone could - and did - make Kryptok lenses.

Kryptoks continued to be the most-used bifocal for many years. The author remembers Kryptoks still widely used in the 1950s when they sold to laboratories for $1.50 a pair. As lens manufacturers began introducing nokrome seg bifocals, similar in appearance to Kryptoks but with much less color in the seg, marketing efforts were concentrated on these and other new bifocal designs. Today, almost one hundred years from the time the first Kryptok lenses appeared, one company still provides a finished stock glass bifocal carrying the Kryptok name.

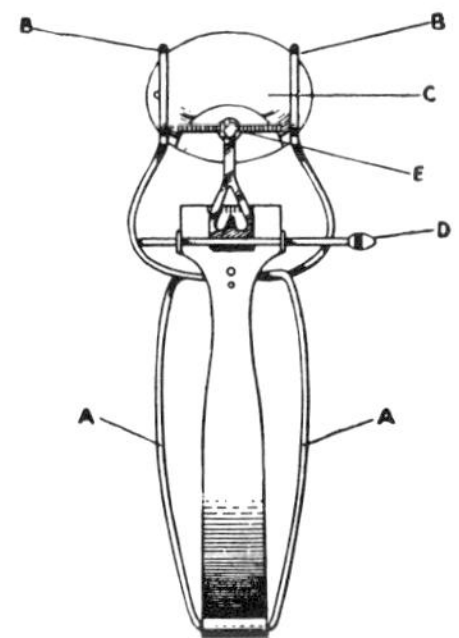

This clever tool was used when applying cement segs. After the cement was heated and applied to the wafer, it was placed on the distance lens held in the clamp. By turning wheel "D", pressure was applied to the seg, squeezing out any bubbles.

ILLUSTRATION, MARK MATTISON-SHUPNICK

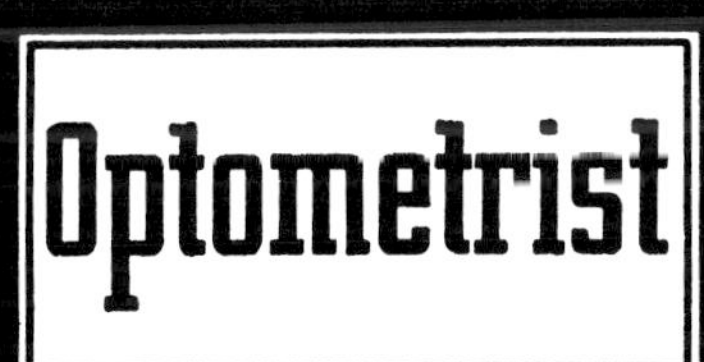

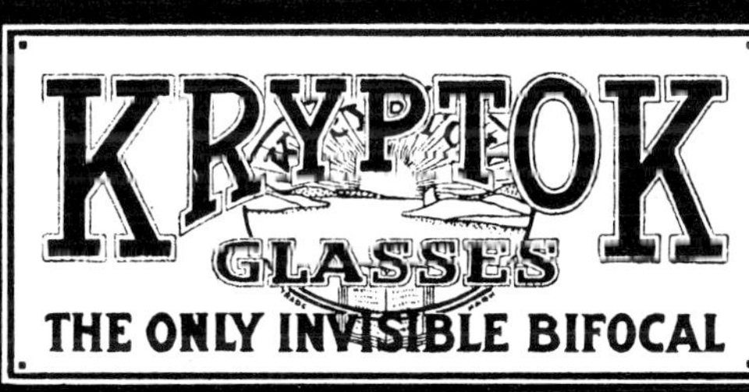

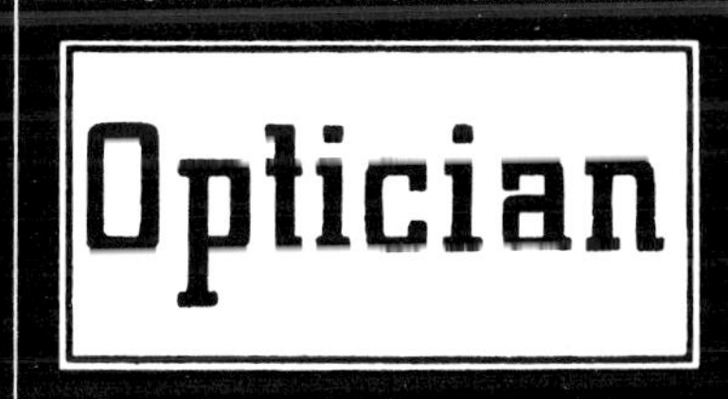

KRYPTOK 3-PANEL TRANSLUCENT SIGN
TO ATTACH TO THE UPPER PANEL OF YOUR DISPLAY WINDOW

THE MANUFACTURING STAGES FOR A FUSED BIFOCAL LENS

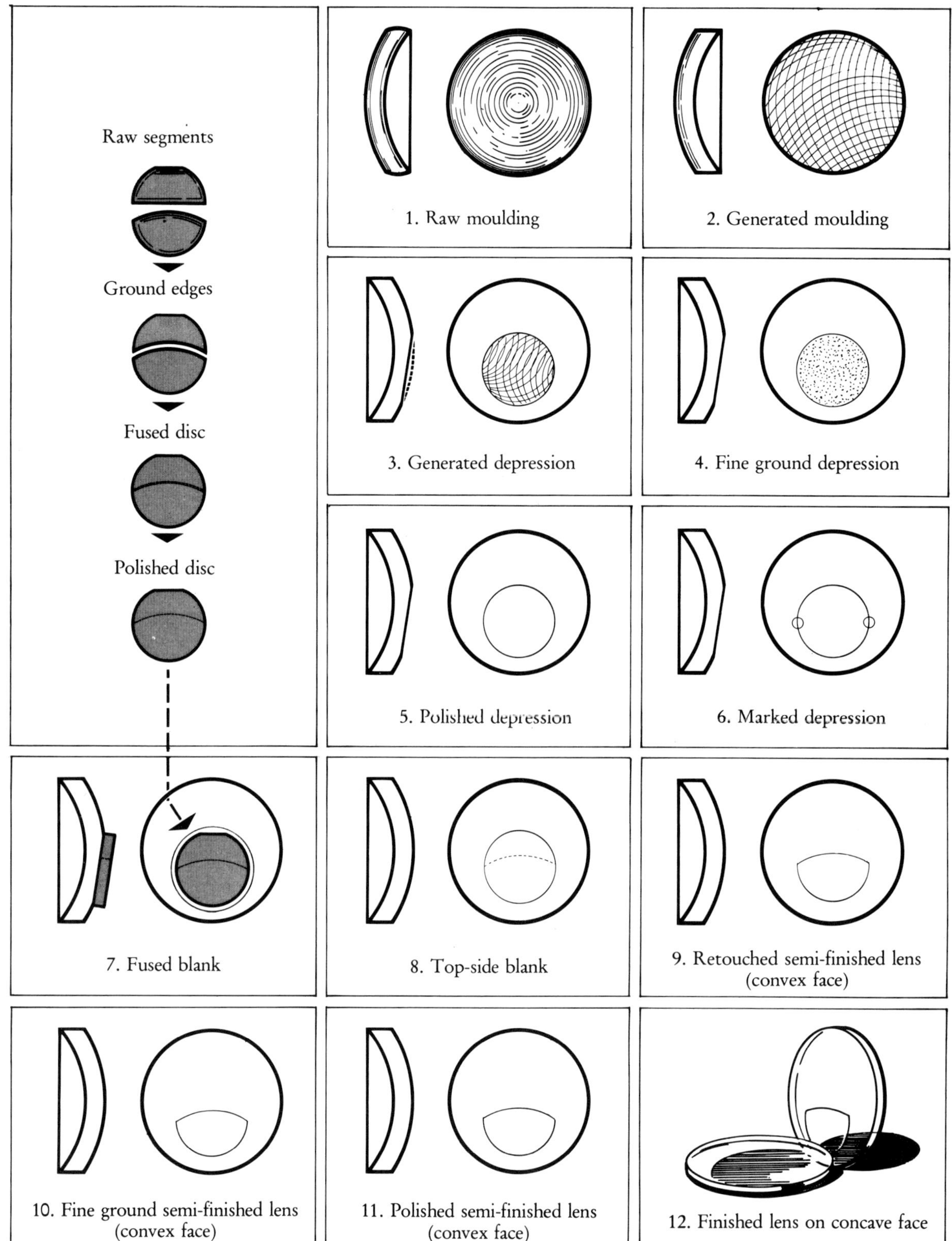

This chart illustrates the process used in producing fused glass multifocals. The same process is still used today for glass lenses. All plastic multifocals have reading segments produced by cavities in the mold so that no fusing is required. ILLUSTRATION, COURTESY CORNING, FRANCE

Chapter 9
The Evolution of Multifocals

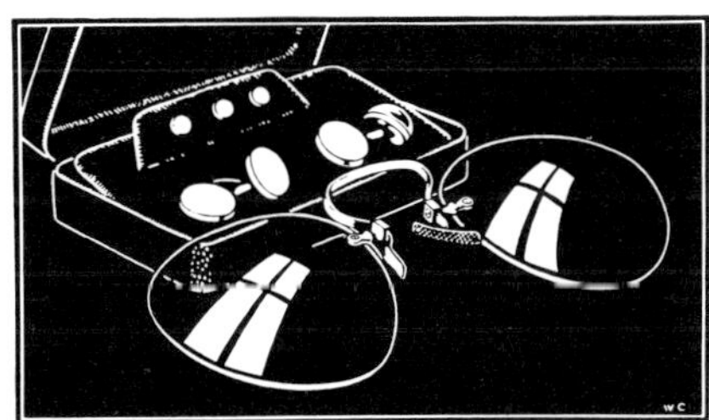

This review of how bifocals *(multifocals)* evolved includes the more significant bifocal designs developed over the past two hundred years. There were many attempts to find more effective ways to provide vision for presbyopes but most of them dropped by the wayside, either because they were ineffective visually or because they were simply too difficult or expensive to manufacture.

Franklin Split Bifocal (1785)

Most present-day opticians consider the Franklin or split bifocal to be a crude, makeshift attempt to provide near and distance vision for eyeglass wearers. In practice, however, these primitive bifocals worked reasonably well. Since both sections were made of the same glass, they presented no color fringe problems, an inherent problem with fused glass bifocals. There was no cement holding the lenses together, allowing them to slip and slide on hot days. The primary problem was the unsightly line across the lenses with its accumulation of debris, accompanied by the fact that when the frame screw holding the frame together loosened even a little, wearers ended up with two half lenses falling in their laps. Another minor problem was overhead light reflecting off the top edge of the bottom half, creating an annoying visual nuisance for wearers.

As laboratories grew more sophisticated, they began to carefully position the Franklin individual halves so the optical centers of each section were carefully aligned horizontally and positioned exactly at the cutoff line. In effect, this eliminated "jump" as the patient's eyes moved from the distance half to the near half. Their appearance may have been crude, but they were visually correct and, at a time when cosmetics of eyewear was seldom questioned, they served their primary function very well.

Solid Upcurve Bifocal (1836)

The first commercially successful improvement of the Franklin bifocal was created by a man named Schnaitmann. He created his design by "slabbing off" the top portion of a reading lens, in effect reducing the plus power of the lens for distance use. This improved bifocal was less visible than earlier lenses but had a severely restricted distance field of view, as well as another drawback that eventually killed it. As one might suspect, the distance portion induced a strong base down prismatic effect. These clever lenses must have surely produced some splendid headaches for their wearers.

Cement Bifocals (1884)

The cement bifocal is sometimes credited to George W. Wells *(American Optical)* although a patent for a cement bifocal was granted to B. M. Hanna in 1884. These consisted of thin reading segments cemented to

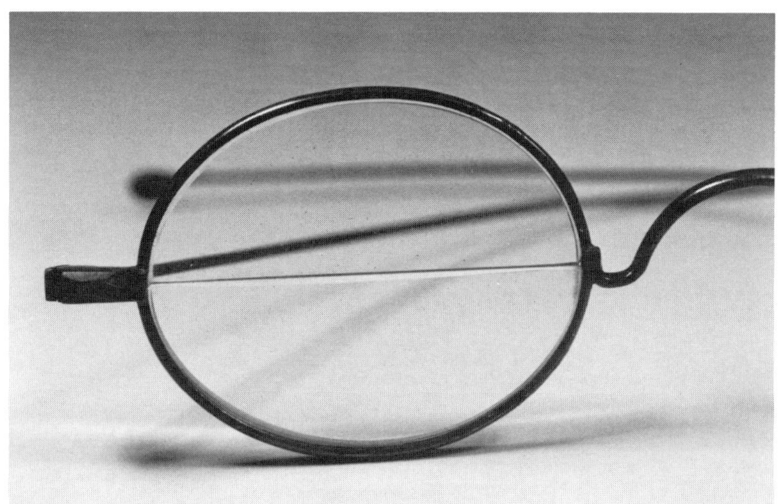

This Franklin Split Bifocal is mounted in a blue steel frame. Notice the debris-collecting ledge where lens halves meet in center. (Marked "N" in cover photo.)

Early Kryptok ad.

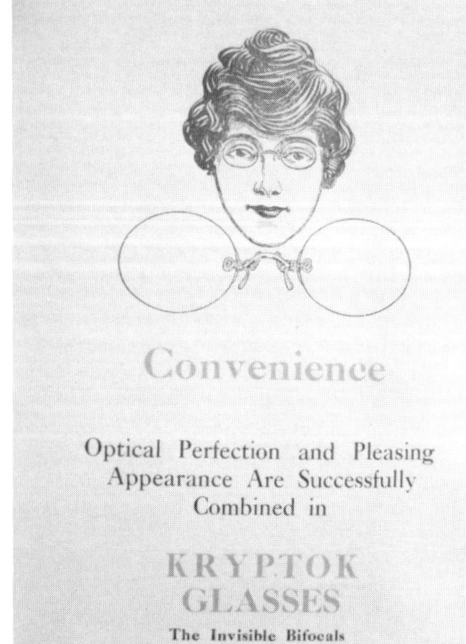

the inside surface of the distance lens. Optically, the lenses worked rather well, but they had the familiar problems of collecting dirt around the edge of the segment where debris would stick to exposed adhesive. Cleaning the dirt dissolved the cement, leaving even more space for dirt accumulation. On a hot day, it was also common to experience the segments sliding or shifting position. Conversely, on cold days the cement became brittle and the slightest jarring could detach the segment or cause a rainbow separation. They were inexpensive to produce, the only requirement was a lot of hand work, so almost any lab could create the lenses from scratch. In spite of other advancements in bifocal designs, cement bifocals were still widely used up to the mid-'20s.

The Perfection Bifocal / Perfection Grooved Bifocal (1886)

It took a long time for someone *(B.M. Hanna)* to develop a way to modernize Franklin's concept. In Hanna's version, instead of merely cutting lenses in half, the reading section was produced in a half moon shape with a corresponding cut out in the distance lenses. Some versions of this bifocal had the junction between the lens sections edged flat while more sophisticated designs went to the extra trouble *(with incredible handwork)* of beveling the edges of the reading section and grinding a groove in the matching edge of the distance lens. While much more attractive, this form of bifocal still collected dirt in the groove and, of course, if the frame screw loosened, the sections fell out.

Hanna's original design for both "Cement" bifocals and his "Perfection" bifocal featured a small round segment. Later designers made the reading segment larger and more "moon" shaped. Hanna, however, is given credit for being the first to inset the reading segment for convergence reasons, a greater visual advancement than anyone realized at the time.

Looking at photos of these early split bifocals, it's apparent that there was little subtlety to the lenses. They announced to everyone that the wearer needed bifocals. Since nothing else was available, other than switching between two pairs of glasses, the world endured the stigma of such obvious *(and ugly)* bifocals. This, however, was about to change and when more attractive bifocals became available the optical world was turned upside down.

Cemented Kryptok (1899)

The first successful attempt to create an invisible bifocal was the effort of John L. Borsch of Philadelphia *(The complete story is told in Chapter 8)*. Borsch created a reading segment made of flint glass and countersunk a depression in a carrier lens made of conventional crown glass. The segment was held in position with balsam cement. This lens, although virtually invisible, still collected debris at the edge of the segment. Borsch took his design a step further by cementing a thin wafer of crown glass over the entire assembly. This made a superb bifocal with few of the earlier problems. The bifocal was relatively invisible but still had the usual problems of cemented lenses in hot or cold weather, compounded by the lab having to grind and polish six surfaces *(see diagram)*. To keep the lens from becoming too thick, the cover wafer had to be extremely thin, not an easy accomplishment in the days before generators. This lens carried the name Kryptok but was made obsolete with the introduction of fused Kryptoks.

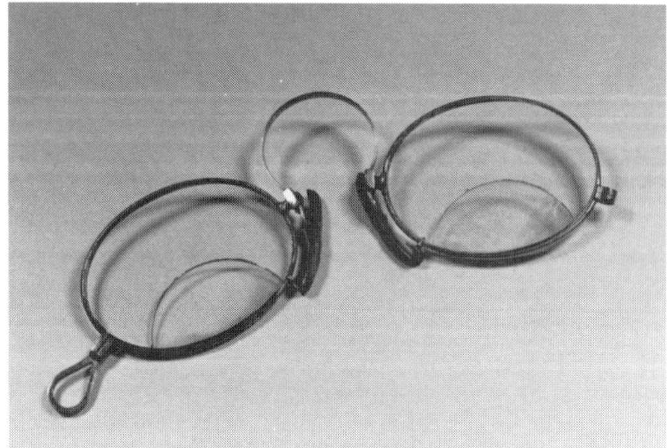

Early Pince-nez frame with cement segs. These glasses are more than 100 years old, yet the segments are still firmly attached, although the cement has yellowed and partially separated. (Marked "O" in cover photo.)

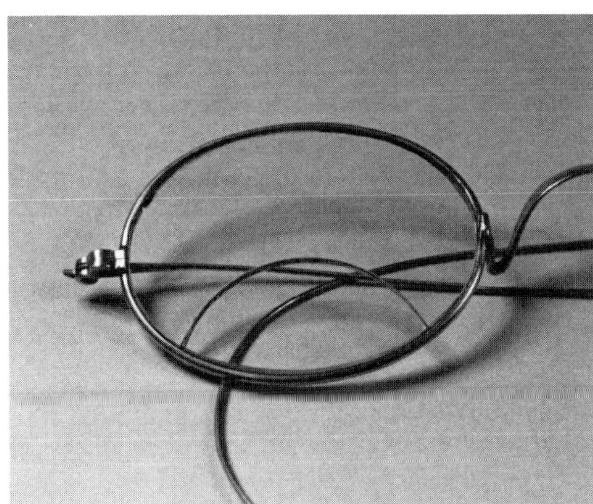

Perfection Bifocal shows the half-moon shaped bifocal segment carefully positioned in the distance lens. Manufacturing these early bifocals required great skill and precision by the laboratory. Notice there is no inset to the segments. It was the custom to position all lenses with no inset, varying the bridge and eye size to match the patient's P.D. (Marked "K" in cover photo.)

EYEGLASSES FROM DR. WM. ROSENTHAL COLLECTION

The Opifex Bifocal (1905)

Patented in 1905 by Albert Bowers, this was simply a minor improvement on the cement bifocal. It was produced by grinding the wafers thinner. They were considerably more expensive but really not much of an improvement. They were promoted by a group of large laboratories called the "Big Five" - Globe Optical, Julius King Optical, F.A. Hardy, D.V. Brown and Merry Optical. Release of fused Kryptoks spelled the end of the Opifex bifocal.

Kryptok (1908)

One basic fact had been established by the awkward and expensive cemented Kryptok — there was a viable market for a less visible bifocal. John L. Borsch, Jr. (son of the original designer) applied for a patent on a lens that welded the segment in place by heating both blank and segment to more than 1000 degrees Fahrenheit. This eliminated the cementing process as well as the thin glass cover of the original Kryptok. With a fused blank, grinding the front surface of the fused blank finished the front of both segment and carrier blank. It solved most problems of previous bifocals and set the stage for substantial growth of a lens design that would continue as the industry standard for almost 50 years.

The Kryptok lens also influenced the young industry in a more subtle way. Fusing bifocals required a greater investment in equipment and technical skill and, for this reason, was more suitable for large-scale manufacturing than in small-scale, one-at-a-time prescription shops by individual opticians. This basic fact would eventually substantially alter the fledgling industry.

Bi-Sight Bifocal (1905)

This was a one-piece bifocal developed and patented by Benjamin Mayer. Patent litigation, however, later granted the patent rights to C.W. Connor (see ULTEX ONEPIECE BIFOCAL).

Ultex Onepiece Bifocal (1910)

For years opticians attempted to make a bifocal lens out of a single piece of glass and avoid the prism problems evidenced in the Solid Upcurve Bifocal. Finally an optician in Indianapolis named Charles W. Connor achieved this goal. To do it, however, he took a different approach than anyone else. He replaced the normal size glass blank with a large oversize blank. The outer rim of the lens contained the distance correction while the center section had a stronger curve on the back side to create increased power for close work. Once both curves had been ground and polished, the oversize blank was cut in half, producing two semi-finished bifocal blanks that could then be surfaced on the front side to the patient's correction.

One major difference between Ultex and fused bifocals was that Ultex lenses had the bifocal portion on the inside (later a front surface Ultex would be developed but was never commercially successful). Fused multifocals, on the other hand, had the segments on the front side of the blank. Labs received orders for both types and, as a result, had to carry inventories of surfacing laps for both convex and concave grinding. Because they were made from one piece of glass, Ultex lenses produced no color fringe in the reading segment but suffered from two drawbacks. The segments were very obvious in appearance, leaving little doubt that the wearer wore multifocals. In addition, their basic design

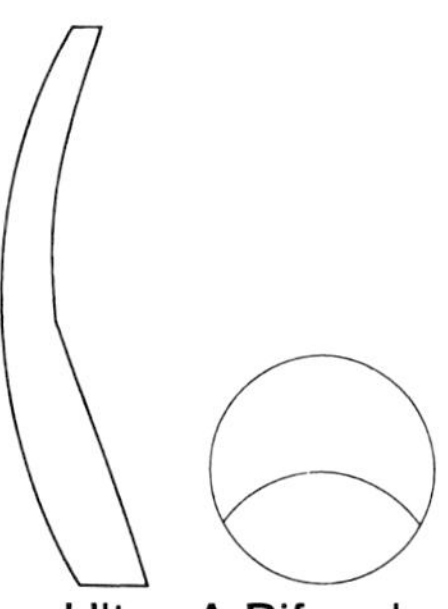

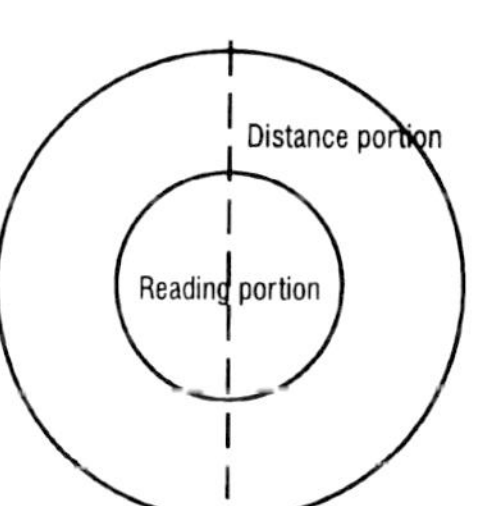

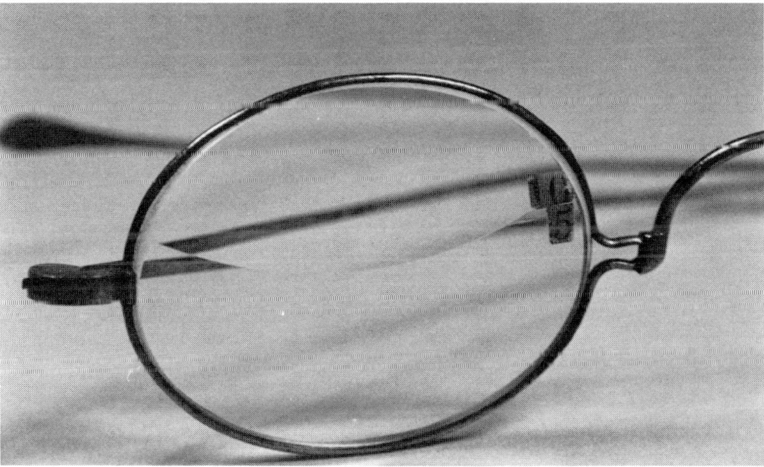

The Solid Upcurve bifocal was an attractive lens but as seen in this photo, the prism it created is obvious. These lenses were produced at the factory and sold ready-made. This pair still has factory stickers on the lens, indicating the focal length of the lens is 10 inches in the distance and 5 inches for near.

ANTIQUE EYEWEAR FROM DR. WM. ROSENTHAL COLLECTION

created base down prism in the seg which made them less suitable for minus corrections. Wise refractionists restricted their use to plus corrections. An Ultex "K" bifocal was developed, identical in shape to the Panoptik. This was a one-piece bifocal with the "K" segment on the inside surface. It provided satisfactory vision but received only marginal acceptance.

Taking a lesson from the Kryptok Company, the Ultex bifocal was controlled by a tight patent *(following extensive litigation)* and only authorized labs and authorized dealers were permitted to sell the lens during the life of the patent. It's interesting to note that when AO and B&L started purchasing independent labs in the 1920s, they often had to continue operating the labs under their original names until their Kryptok or Ultex licenses expired.

The original Ultex was called Ultex A. Later an Ultex E with a smaller diameter segment was developed, followed by two others with even smaller segs, the "B" and the "D". When an extra high seg was desired, Ultex "AL" was ordered. A special Ultex with a minus segment at the top of the lens was called "RedeRite". A trifocal and a "baseball" double seg occupational lens were also produced. These gave retailers a wide range of choices in Ultex but created a monstrous inventory problem for laboratories. A front side Ultex design was developed but moving the segment to the front side increased the vertex distance, making the lens impractical.

Eventually the industry converted to minus cylinders *(see Chapter 7)* and this, combined with one other event, marked the end for Ultex multifocals. The other event was the expiration of the Kryptok patent. When that happened, anyone who wanted to make Kryptok bifocals, could do so. The Kryptok was a relatively easy *(and inexpensive)* bifocal to make and the lens worked quite well. The industry was tired of restrictive licensing agreements and Kryptoks *(the name became generic)* soon became the most-used bifocal in the world. Labs were delighted to get away from grinding front curves and these events helped eclipse Ultex lenses.

Steadfast (1910 approx.)

This one-piece bifocal was developed by Harold Stead *(who later joined Shuron Optical)*. He had been knocked out of the Kryptok market by fierce patent litigation *(which he lost)*. This lens design was his attempt to reenter the bifocal market. His bad luck continued, however, when Connor's Ultex patent forced him out of this market as well.

Nokrome Seg Bifocals (1921)

Technically, Kryptoks were a marvelous improvement

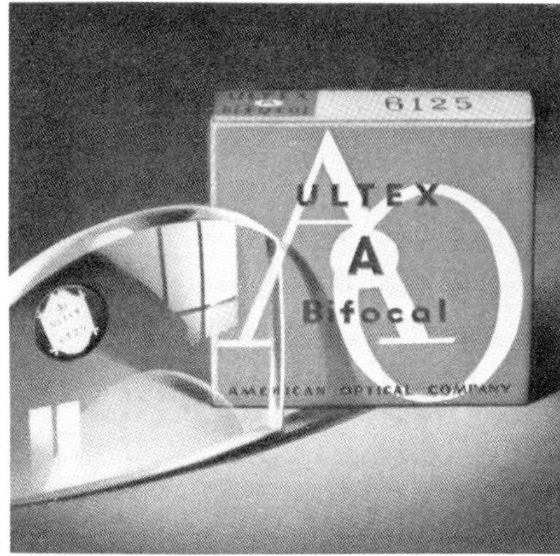

Most major lens manufacturers included Ultex lenses in their line. Notice the shape of the lens blank. Ultex blanks were manufactured by grinding a large, oversize blank and cutting it in half to produce 2 blanks.

OLA Optical Industry Museum

over all previous bifocals but they exhibited one drawback that every patient noticed immediately. Every lens has the capacity to form color to some small extent but Kryptoks tended to form a colored rainbow fringe around objects viewed through the reading segment. Instrument lenses *(binoculars, telescopes, camera lenses)* eliminate this problem by making their lenses "achromatic" by combining a concave flint lens of weaker refracting power with a stronger convex crown lens, thus eliminating any color fringe. Kryptok lenses, however, accomplish just the opposite. They combine a strong convex flint lens with a weaker concave crown lens. By their basic design, therefore, Kryptoks became "color-making" lenses rather than "color-eliminating" as are lenses used in instruments and cameras.

A patent for color elimination in bifocals was issued to a man named Bugbee, Sr. *(the Ultex man)* in 1921 and to Drescher *(Bausch's son-in-law)* in another patent issued in 1924. Both patents, however, required special optical glass unlike anything currently available. Ted Drescher was a Bausch son-in-law and the problem of producing the special glass was turned over to Bausch & Lomb's new Glass Plant, the only plant in America producing optical glass in commercial quantities. After a great deal of experimentation and research, B&L solved the problem. The result was a new achromatic fused bifocal named "Nokrome", a color-free bifocal produced in four base curves.

In 1928, B&L had introduced an Orthogon "corrected-curve" lens. It was a corrected curve bifocal that had the fused segment on the inside surface. Responding to demand, B&L developed a corrected curve Nokrome

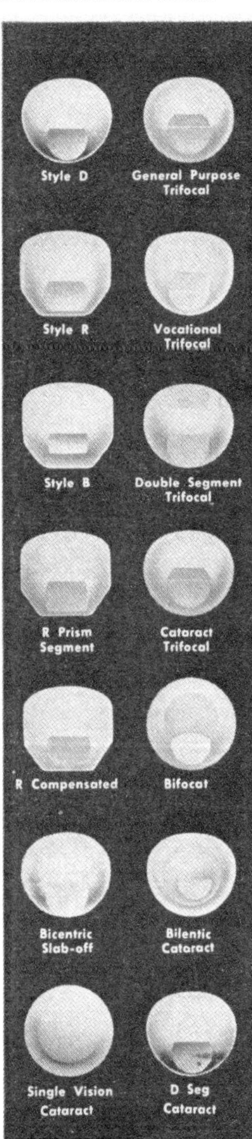

A Univis Ad in a 1950 issue of OPTICAL INDEX showed all the multifocals in the Univis line. Univis had become the premier bifocal manufacturer by this time.

OLA Optical Industry Museum

CEMENT BIFOCALS

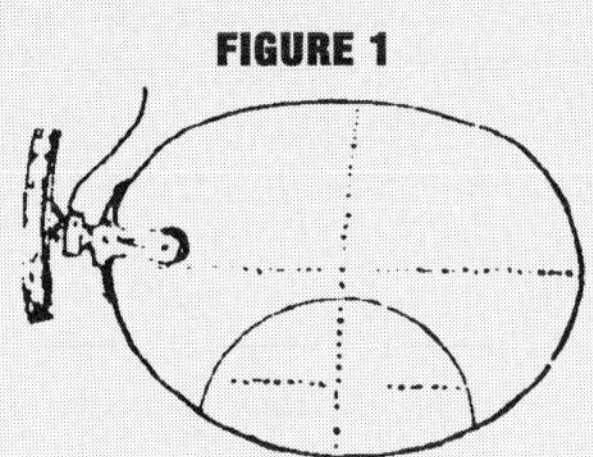

FIGURE 1

In October, 1896, an optician named L. M. Kaiser in San Francisco wrote a paper published in THE OPTICAL JOURNAL. The bifocal of choice at that time *(Kryptoks were some ten years in the future)* was the cement bifocal, considered to be a modern improvement over the old "franklin" or "perfection" split bifocals. To fit frames, the patient's PD was taken and a frame selected of the same width as the PD. Lenses were positioned with optical centers "on center".

Understanding how lenses were ordered then *(second half of the 19th century)* may explain this simple system. Most lenses used were simple spheres. Manufacturers, accustomed to selling complete eyewear *(frame and lenses complete)* found opticians beginning to customize eyewear they dispensed. Since frame styles were limited, manufacturers began supplying pre-edged stock lenses. A retail office could produce a wide variety of prescriptions from a basic inventory. Stock lenses were even supplied with pre-drilled holes for rimless mountings. To use these factory-edged stock lenses, opticians or optometrists merely varied the frame size to keep lenses centered before the patient's eyes. If it was a rimless mounting, optical centers were controlled by varying the lens diameter. It was a crude system that worked reasonably well.

During this time, it was customary to glue cement segs directly below the mechanical center of the lens. In his paper, Mr. Kaiser expressed indignation that most opticians were ignoring decentering of cement bifocal segments. He wrote;

FIGURE 2

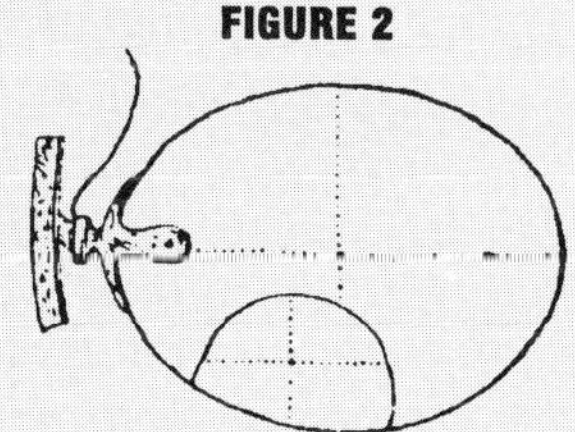

"An optician fitting a frame 6mm wider than the interpupillary distance would be deemed incompetent, yet that is what is done *(for the reading point)* when cement bifocal lenses are fitted as they are usually furnished. See Fig. 1. Many persons who after repeated trials could not accustom themselves to the use of bifocal lenses wore them with perfect comfort after decentering the reading segment 'in' 3mm in each eye. See Fig. 2. The slight additional work entailed by this decentering will not be considered when the noticeably greater comfort of a client is apparent "

---

bifocal called "Orthogon D" in 1931 with the segment on the front side. Within a few years, most bifocal manufacturers were producing Nokrome bifocals *(American Optical's was called "Tillyer D")*. By industry tradition, all Nokrome seg bifocals were produced with corrected-curve front surfaces. Nokrome seg bifocals soon became "state-of-the-art" and Kryptoks were relegated to a second class "economy" bifocal. In spite of this and perhaps because of the depression about to hit the world, Kryptoks continued as the most used bifocal.

Quintex Trifocal (1932)

This unique fused trifocal was developed by Dr. Otto Haussman of Philadelphia and incorporated five separate focal areas. The name was coined from "quinque" meaning five and "texo" meaning to weave. The blanks were usually sold in rough form so labs could produce any size transition field, depending on how far down the lab ground the front surface. This was an innovative approach to producing what Haussman considered a universal multifocal "age lens". His early advertising reads remarkably like ads for present-day progressive addition lenses. In a paper he wrote for the 1940 Year Book of Optometry, Dr. Haussman wrote, *"The ideal multifocal lens, I grant you, would be the one in which the fields would be so gradually blended that there would be no dividing line."*

Univis D (1926)

This bifocal design was considerably more difficult to manufacture but, because the segment's flat top positioned the segment's optical center closer to the top edge, wearers experienced less "image jump" as they dropped from distance into the reading area. The design was produced in Great Britain by United Kingdom Optical *(previ-*

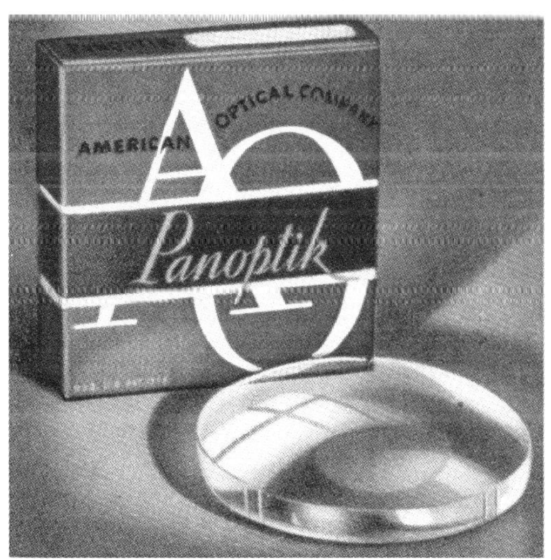

American Optical produced Panoptik lenses for a time but eventually dropped them because of the manufacturing expense, leaving Bausch & Lomb as the only supplier.

OLA OPTICAL INDUSTRY MUSEUM

ously known as Zeiss-England until appropriated by the British government during World War I). Shortly after that war, M.H. "Bunt" Stanley, who owned an optical shop in Dayton, Ohio, visited England with his wife. Mrs. Stanley broke her glasses and when they visited a local optician, they learned of this new bifocal. Stanley obtained exclusive rights for the United States and arranged to begin importing flat top bifocals. Returning to Dayton, Stanley sold his retail business and organized the Univis Lens Company in 1926. When World War II broke out, Stanley obtained manufacturing rights.

When the war ended, the Univis Lens Company established a large sales force and set out to convert the industry to flat top bifocals, with obvious success *(See Chapter 14, Lens Manufacturers).* Eventually, every bifocal lens manufacturer was producing their own flat top bifocals. The first flat tops featured a 20mm segment. By the '50s, a 22mm segment had become the industry standard. By the '70s the standard was 25mm and today 28mm is probably the most-used size. Segments as wide as 45mm can now be ordered. As the industry gradually switched to plastic lenses, flat tops became the standard bifocal and few round segs are used in plastic lenses. Today, the increasing use of progressive addition lenses is reducing flat top usage.

Fulvue Bifocal (1931)

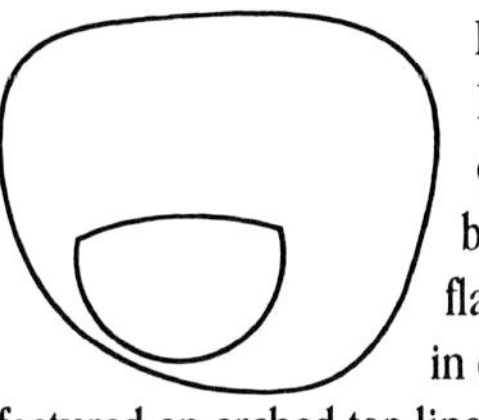

Like the Panoptik, the Fulvue was designed to compete with flat top bifocals without infringing on flat top patents. It was similar in every way to the flat top but featured an arched top line rather than the straight top of the flat top. This was produced by a number of manufacturers with modest success. It was more expensive to produce than the flat top, and as the variety of tints and bifocal forms increased, it gradually faded into obscurity.

A few laboratories such as White Haines promoted Fulvue bifocals to their retail customers for years as a way to insure their patients came back for Fulvue replacements rather than having a budget optical shop replace the lenses with "cheap" flat tops.

Panoptik Bifocal (1929)

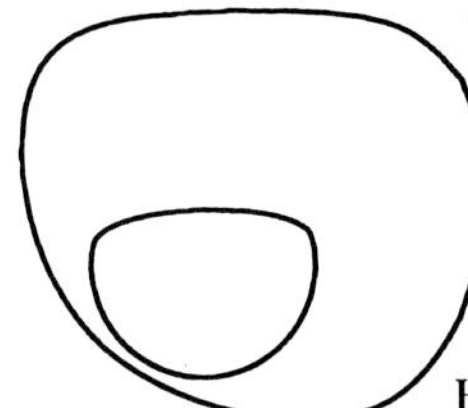

This innovative approach to a flat top design was developed by an Optometrist named Jim Hammon from Vincennes, Indiana *(Hammon also played some part in development of the earlier 3-piece cement Kryptok and the fused Kryptok).* A few crude samples were produced in 1929 but it took B&L the better part of a year to develop the manufacturing processes for this complex lens. The first salable lenses were produced by Baush & Lomb for Perfected Bifocals, Inc. in 1930. Perfected marketed the bifocal until the Panoptik Company was organized in 1932 *(this company would later be taken over by Bausch & Lomb).* Both AO and B&L were given manufacturing licenses to produce the lens. A trifocal had been developed by 1940.

The Panoptik was a handsome lens, basically a flat top with rounded corners that became the bifocal's major selling point. Panoptik advertising stressed how this unique shape conformed to the round shape of the pupil *(whatever logic there was in that).* An inherent feature of the design was that it permitted prism to be incorporated in the segment while maintaining the familiar shape. The lens was extremely difficult to manufacture which meant competitors had little interest in "knocking it off". As a result, AO gave up manufacturing it early on and the Panoptik became B&L's flagship multifocal for many years. There is

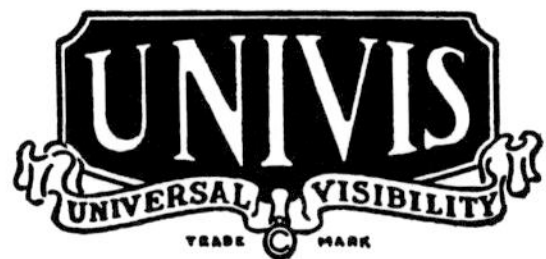

The Bifocal Service That Is Most Comprehensive and Completely Protected

Univis provides the most comprehensive variation of styles for people requiring lenses of more than one focal power, in order that the individual requirments of each patient may be met with exactness. This is important to the patient and to the practitioner whose prestige is enhanced by success with difficult cases . . . . . All Univis lenses are made with utmost precision, and their distribution is definitely protected by the strict Univis licensing policy.

(Univis Lenses can be supplied to licensees only)

An early Univis advertisement from a 1936 newsletter.

considerable doubt whether Panoptik was ever a profitable product for B&L because of the high costs of manufacturing such a complicated design.

Progressive Addition Lenses

The concept of a progressive power lens was first patented in 1907 by Owen Aves in Europe. The first patent in this country was issued to A. Estelle Glancy and American Optical in 1924. The first practical progressive addition lenses were introduced in Europe in 1959, giving Europeans a considerable lead over this country. This probably accounts for the higher percentage of progressive lenses used in Europe.

A list of the early progressive lenses and their release dates would include:

Varilux I	1959 - Essilor
Omnifocal	1965 - Volk
Varilux II	1972 - Essilor
Ultravue 25mm	1976 - AO
Ultravue 28mm	1978 - AO
Younger 10/30	1978 - Younger Mfg.
Super No-Line	1979 - Essilor
Unison	1980 - Univis
Progressiv R	1981 - Rodenstock
CPS	1982 - Younger Mfg.

The first major industry-wide marketing of a progressive lens in this country occurred when American Optical released their Ultravue lens. The lens was relatively crude compared to today's designs, but it was the first by a major manufacturer and AO launched a massive marketing promotion, conducting hundreds of detailed fitting seminars all over the country.

Progressives were a totally new concept to most dispensers and doctors attending these seminars. Compounding the problem for these neophyte fitters was the wild system AO's technical people conceived for taking measurements. Recognizing that determining pupil placement for progressives was considerably more critical than dispensers were used to, they decided the Grohman Device was the best way to determine PD and pupil placement. This was a Rube Goldberg contraption with all sorts of movable fingers which attached to the frame with clamps. Approaching the patient with that device attached to the frame must have been a frightening experience for the patient.

Varilux's original design was soon replaced by an improved design called Varilux II *(known today as Varilux Plus)*. This was superseded by their Infinity lens and that was again succeeded by a newer design called Comfort. Similar design improvements have been experienced by most of the major lens manufacturers. The OLA publishes an identification chart of progressive lenses and the number of progressive brands sold in this country today is well over 50 and continuing to grow.

Conclusion

One of the major changes that has taken place during the last 25 years has been the erosion of brand identification for lenses. During the period from 1930 to 1970, brand identity for all lenses *(single vision and multifocal)* was important to the practitioner. Most retailers knew exactly which brand of lenses they were using and would often specify the desired brand by name. Today, few offices have any idea which manufacturers' single vision or bifocal lens they are dispensing. The exceptions are progressive lenses which are still almost always ordered by brand name.

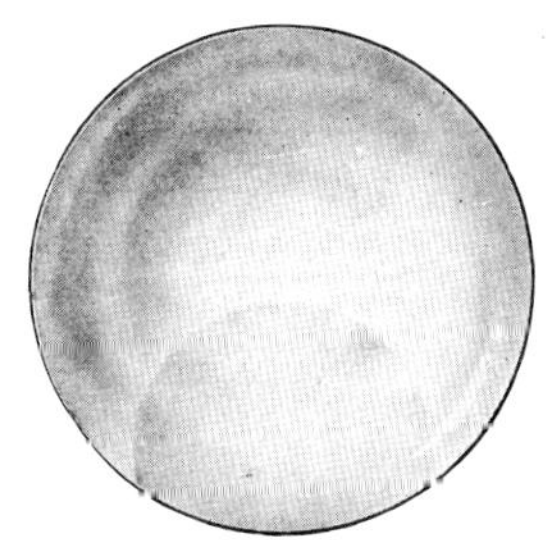

This advertisement was created by one of the lesser-known manufacturers, using a very lyrical copywriter. The lens in question featured nokrome segments, thus eliminating color fringes associated with Kryptok lenses.

OLA Optical Industry Museum

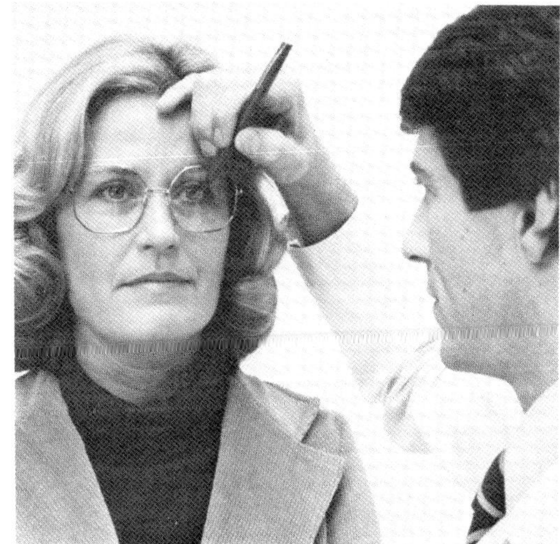

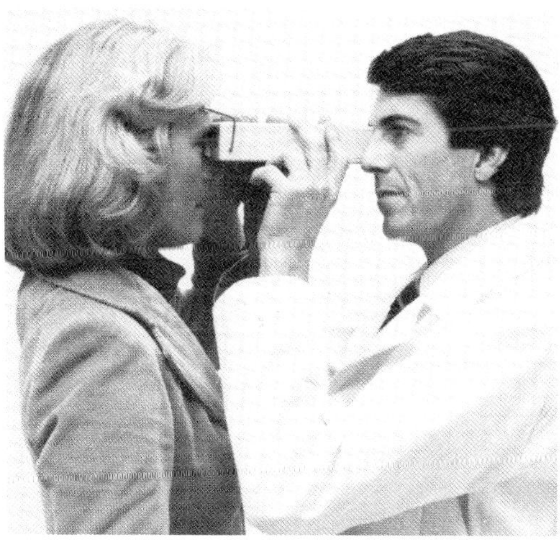

With the advent of progressive lenses, positioning the reading area became much more critical and led many offices to use an electronic pupilometer instead of the familiar millimeter rule. Top photo shows marking the pupil height on adhesive tape positioned over the patient's frame.

Photos — Varilux Corporation

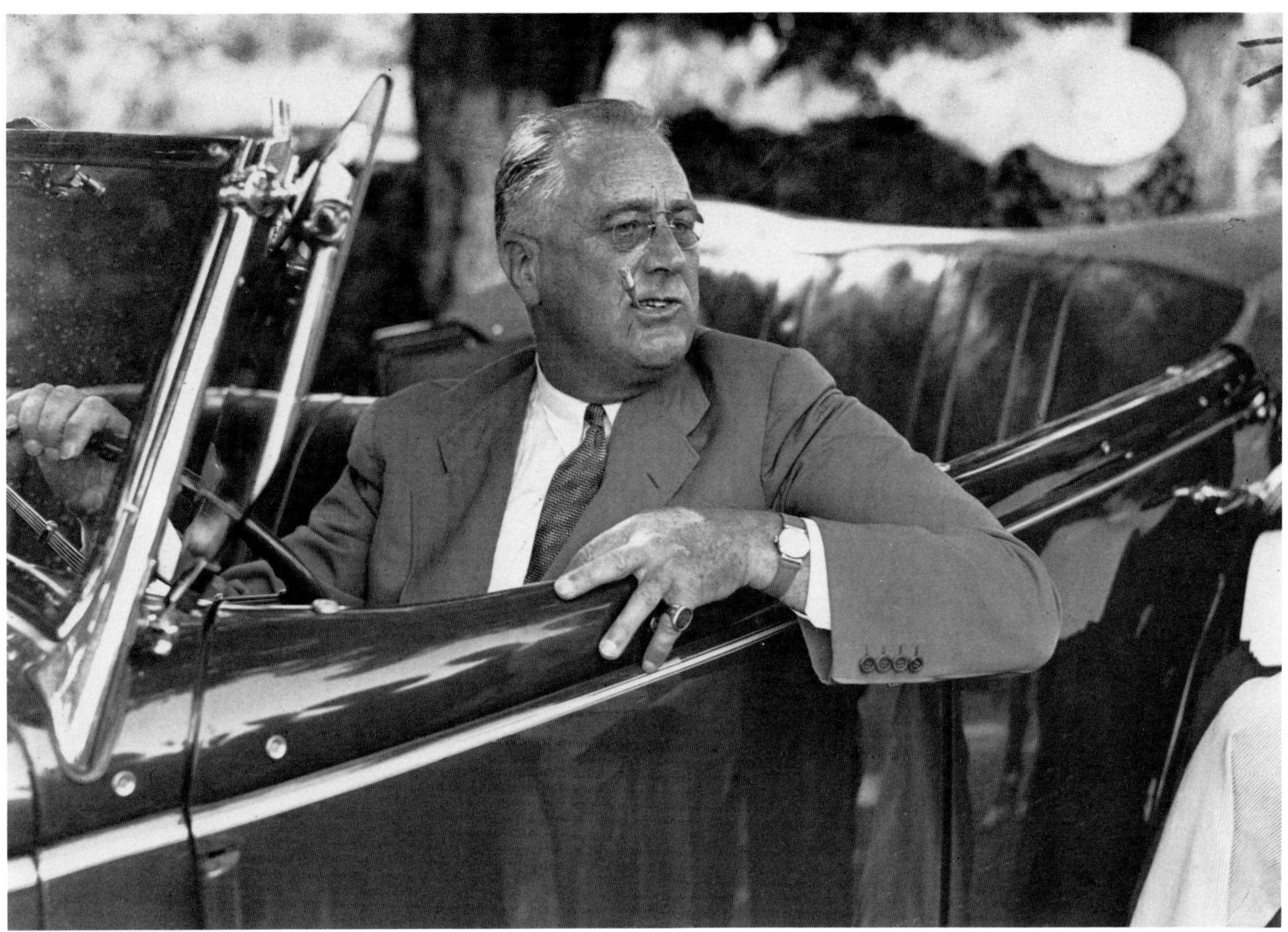

Pince-nez frames or mountings today are looked on as fads or affectations, but they were immensely popular for many years and were worn by both sexes. They provided wearers with the lightest eyewear possible and, in many cases, the least conspicuous. Because pince-nez lenses were always edged "on center" with no decentration, they also produced the thinnest edges because the outside and inside edges of the lens were uniform. Franklin Delano Roosevelt, 32nd President of the United States, (1932-1945) was one of the last public figures to wear pince-nez eyeglasses. His eyeglasses and cigarette holder were included in every political cartoon in which he ever appeared. Trying to picture Roosevelt wearing a more conventional frame or mounting simply boggles the mind.

It's important to remember that, in those pre-FDA days, there was no minimum thickness for lenses and glass lenses such as President Roosevelt wore (he was near-sighted) were often ground as thin as 1.0mm. One of the author's first jobs was hand edging lenses and it was a common experience to push a thumb through the center of a high minus lens while beveling it. All of which should remind us that eyeglass wearers appreciated lightweight, thinner lenses long before the current crop of high index and polycarbonate lenses was conceived.

Chapter 10
Frame Evolution

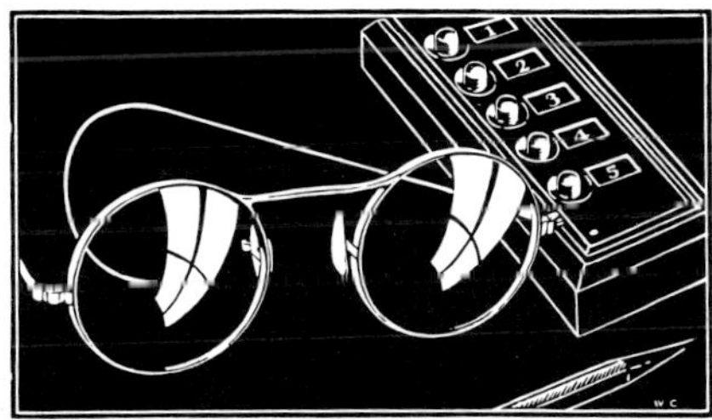

Eyeglasses date from late in the thirteenth century and since that time, a great variety of materials and construction methods have been tried in the effort to position a pair of lenses in front of the eyes *(explained elsewhere in this history)*. The concern of this chapter is to trace how frame design, construction and distribution evolved from 1840 to the present time.

American Optical

American Optical started in 1833 by searching for a way to mass-produce metal eyeglass frames. This was a natural transition for founder William Beecher who had left the family farm in Connecticut to finish a jeweler's apprenticeship in Providence. Moving to Southbridge, Massachusetts in 1826, he opened a jewelry and watch shop and began producing metal frames seven years later. The materials commonly used for eyeglasses at that time were gold, silver, and steel. Other materials, such as bronze, nickel, horn and tortoiseshell were used but were imported from Europe or manufactured individually by artisans who were primarily jewelers or watchmakers *(only the wealthy could afford eyeglasses)*. Beecher's distinction was his development of innovative machinery for producing his silver frames. In 1843, Beecher expanded his production to include steel-rimmed frames. This started a fashion trend that was to last for sixty years.

Bausch & Lomb

In 1853, John J. Bausch established his retail optical store in Rochester, N.Y. and expanded operations in 1864 to include frame manufacturing. The story goes that one day Bausch bent over and picked up a piece of hard rubber as he crossed the street. He began experimenting at home on the kitchen range. Persevering, he eventually created a rubber frame. By 1866 he was manufacturing hard rubber frames under the name "Vulcanite Optical Instrument Company", having been granted an exclusive license to manufacture optical instruments *(including frames)*. His company was renamed "Bausch & Lomb Optical Company" in 1872.

Eyeglasses or Spectacles

In just such hit-or-miss ways mass manufacturing of eyeglass frames was introduced in the United States. Frames fell into two distinct categories: "Eyeglasses" was the term applied to eyewear with no temples that were positioned on the nose by spring action on the bridge of the nose. Oxfords, for instance, were a variation of the eyeglass, appearing at the turn of the century. These stylish glasses featured a long, flat spring attached to the rim tops and usually dangled from the neck on a classy ribbon, giving the wearer an elegant look. "Spectacles" was the term used for frames that featured temples extending over the wearer's ears. These were somewhat more comfortable and more secure than the "torture chamber", as eyeglasses with spring-loaded bridges were often called. Literally hundreds of patents were issued for variations of the spring action bridge. Ads for these innovative designs often bragged about eliminating the usual indentations or red bruises that were the hallmark of an "eyeglass" wearer.

Whatever fashion aspects eyewear had in those early days came from the lens shape. Shapes might be round, or oval, or a variety of geometrical shapes *(square,*

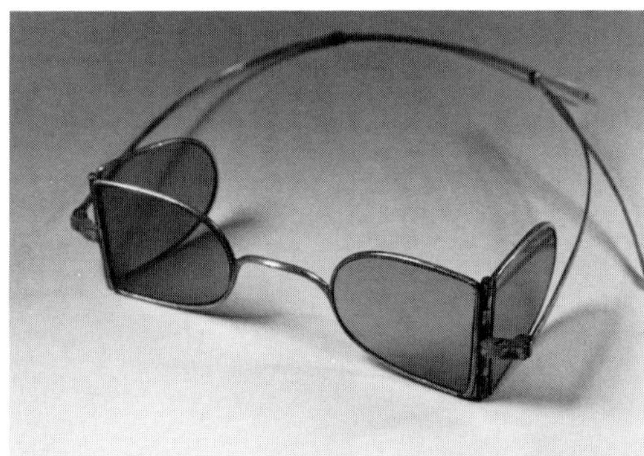

The "horseshoe" glass, named for its distinctive shape, was sometimes called "railroad double" glass because it was often worn on trains or stagecoaches to protect passengers' eyes from flying cinders, a common hazard when riding early railroads. Sometimes the front lenses would be clear with sideshields mounted with sun lenses, providing a double-function eyeglass. Sometimes the sideshields held clear plus power lenses providing "quick-change" reading glasses (This frame is marked "C" in cover photo. Circa 1820).

rectangular, hexagonal, octagonal). Sizes were minuscule by today's standards, yet functioned reasonably well since frames of that day usually fit close to the eyes. Until the turn of the century, frames featured spherical lenses to correct simple hyperopia, myopia or presbyopia. Sizes were designated by code numbers, "0" being 41 x 32mm in size down to "5" which was a discrete 32 x 23mm oval shape. Later "00" and "000" sizes became available. "Pulpit" glasses, as half eyes were called, permitted far-sighted patients to peer over the top of their reading lenses. Most eyeglasses were for close work and the smaller oval frame styles made it easy to look over them for distance vision.

Lens blanks were sized 43 to 47mm in diameter at the turn of the century. Frame fashions changed and blanks gradually increased in size until the late 1980s when they reached today's diameters of 80+mm. Now, interestingly enough, frame fashions are smaller and several lens manufacturers are bringing out smaller blank sizes to ease the strain (and waste) of edging oversize 80mm blanks down to today's small shapes.

Endpieces (i.e. hinges) during the 1800s were almost always located at the mid-point of eye shapes. Since most shapes were symmetrical, there was little reason or advantage to raising the endpiece above center. Bridges for metal frames carried special codes to designate their design. Some were coded as "K", a bridge shape where the flat part of the letter represented the top of the bridge. "X" bridges had a symmetrical shape. Imagine the letter lying on its side. This shape permitted the lenses to "teeter" as the head was moved. "Curl" bridges were designed to sit easily on prominent noses. These were later replaced by the more practical "saddle" or "Liebold" bridge which accomplished the same purpose but fit a wider variety of noses.

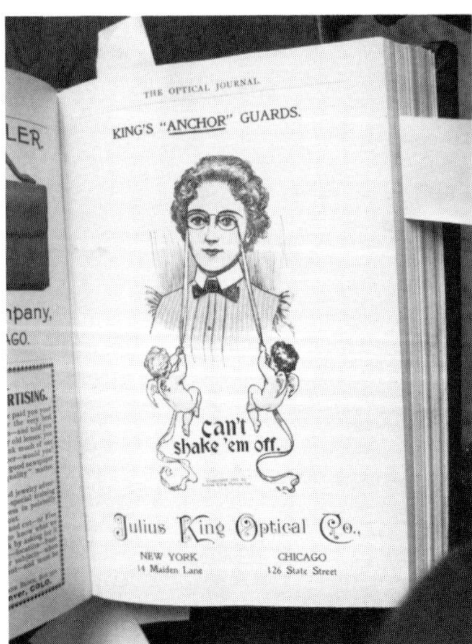

Fingerpiece mountings that were secure on the nose were greatly appreciated. Hundreds of patents were issued for novel ways of holding fingerpiece and pince-nez glasses in place.

Metal Frames

Metal frame color (except for karat gold frames) was normally white since most quality frames were made from silver. Gold colored frames were more desirable but gold was prohibitively expensive. When a method of making frames in a gold color was developed through the process of "rolled gold plating", gold colored frames for the masses suddenly became possible. This exciting development is attributed to Bay State Optical Company in 1885. "Gold filled" was a method of reducing the cost of true karat gold which was inexpensive by present day standards. Solid gold frames meant charging prohibitively high prices.

"Pure gold" is 24 karat, but gold of this purity is much too soft to use in any wearable product. Pure gold is almost always alloyed to a fraction of its original gold content (i.e. 12 Karat gold is 50 percent pure). An 18 karat frame in the early days, fitted with lenses, would sell for about $10 but this price must be translated to today's value. The true cost can be better understood by considering that people then worked happily for fifty cents a day. Ten dollar glasses could represent a month's wages.

In many written descriptions of frame making in those days, it was explained that when a frame maker needed gold to make frames, $25 gold pieces were melted down. This was the easiest way to obtain raw gold. "Rolled gold plate" involved a process that took a layer of karat gold and adhered it to a base metal, generally 18 percent nickel silver. Gold wire, used in temples had the gold wrapped around the core; in the case of flat stock, used for bridges or eye rims, the gold was adhered to one or both surfaces of a sheet of base metal. This "clad" material was then "rolled" to its final thickness, maintaining the same gold/base metal ratio even when rolled out to produce miles of slender wire. The final product would be designated by its gold content by

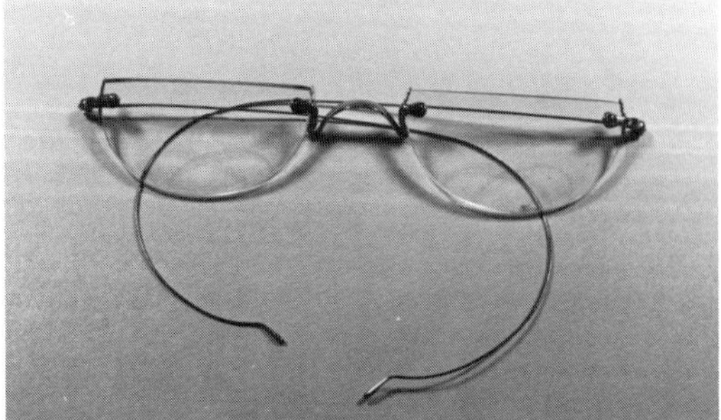

Today's half eye styles were once known as "pulpit" glasses. This pair of rimless pulpit glasses are novel in that the lenses are Kryptok bifocals. The logic in prescribing bifocal lenses in a pulpit mounting is somewhat difficult to understand today (Marked "A" in cover photo).

volume *(i.e. 1/10 12 K gold-filled was 5 percent gold: 10 percent of the frame was 12 K gold which is, by definition, half gold).*

By the time gold-filled materials for eyeglass frames were developed, a process for plating the material with different colors was also achieved. Thus, to make white gold-filled, the normally yellow material would be plated first with an inexpensive heavy nickel plating and then with a light layer of rhodium, which was costly. All gold-filled, and, indeed, karat gold frames had to be plated once the manufacturing was completed. Soldering operations at the endpiece or where the pad arms were joined invariably left blackened areas caused by the heat of the soldering operation. Gold color frames were, therefore, electroplated with a thin gold layer as a final finishing operation.

Less expensive steel was widely used but ultimately proved to be less satisfactory because of discoloration with wear. Nickel silver was used, but this also discolored when left unprotected. So, with the increasing costs of gold by the time of World War II, the industry adopted a standard of 1/10 12 karat gold-filled *(i.e. 5 percent gold content, later modified to 4.5 percent, allowing for loss of gold in the manufacturing process - excluding screws, nosepads, hinges, joints, and temple tips).*

With the freeing of the previously government-controlled gold price after World War II and the meteoric rise in value from $32 per ounce to its present $350 plus, the optical industry reduced the standard to 1/20 12 K, then 1/20 10 K, and even 1/50 10 K, roughly equivalent to the gold content of a well-electroplated frame. During the 1930s, 40s and 50s, most rimless frames still utilized 10K solid gold bridges in addition to the 1/10th gold filled used for the rest of the frame. It was common practice during those years for retail offices to save old metal frames to send in for reclaiming the old gold. This provided a "slush fund" for many offices. When the United States went off the gold standard and the price of gold soared, a few individuals in the optical business realized a small fortune by selling obsolete metal frames for their gold content, worth many times the original value of the frames.

Meanwhile, manufacturers of cheaper frames resorted to electroplating nickel silver frames. This proved unsatisfactory though because the plating was inferior caused by manufacturers' attempts to over-economize. Plated frames quickly developed a bad reputation in the industry. Imported frames, on the other hand, even though plated, often proved quite satisfactory. Eventually the American industry came to realize that it was possible to produce well-plated frames that would satisfy the marketplace. Further, good plating processes produced far more exciting colors and combinations of colors than the good old American standbys of

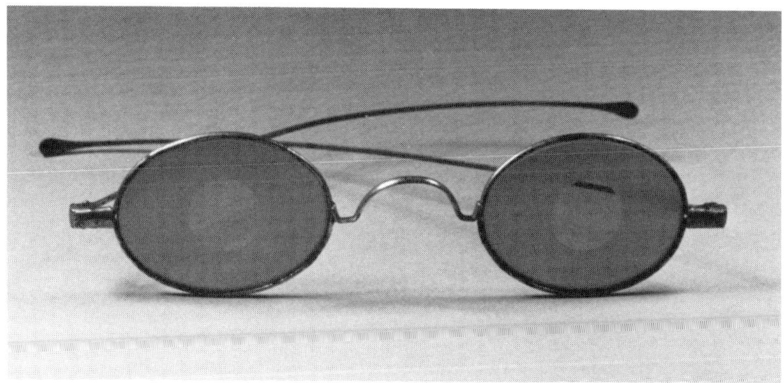

Landscape shooting glasses are described elsewhere in this history. This pair features amber lenses (marked "K" in cover photo).

Eyeglasses from OLA Optical Industry Museum

yellow, white, or gunmetal. Modern plated frames often receive a final coating of thin durable veneer of plastic that fully protects the gold color during normal wear.

Rimless Mountings

Rimless mountings, also made of metal, could not be truly called "frames" since they did not encircle the lens. Fingerpiece mountings were among the first rimless mountings to win acceptance by the public in 1905 or 1906. This was a spring loaded mounting that was invented by Jules Cottet in Morez De Jura, a little optical town in the Juarez Mountains in the east of France. Cottet sold the rights to his design to Rafael's of London. They turned it over to the Julius King Company who apparently asked American Optical to manufacture it.

The first fingerpiece mounting of any prominence was the "So-Easy" mounting produced by American Optical. They produced it with different types of guards for the Globe Optical Company, Julius King *(So-Easy)*, F.A. Hardy *(Anatomical)*, Merry

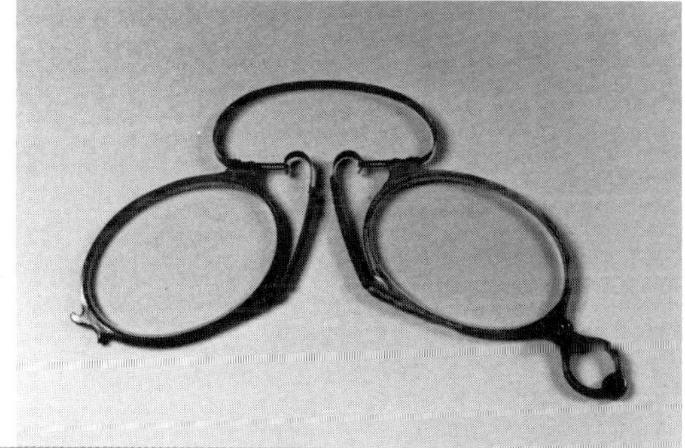

This is a typical tortoise pince-nez frame manufactured by Bausch & Lomb, circa 1895 (Marked "O" in cover photo).

Eyeglasses from Dr. Wm. Rosenthal Collection

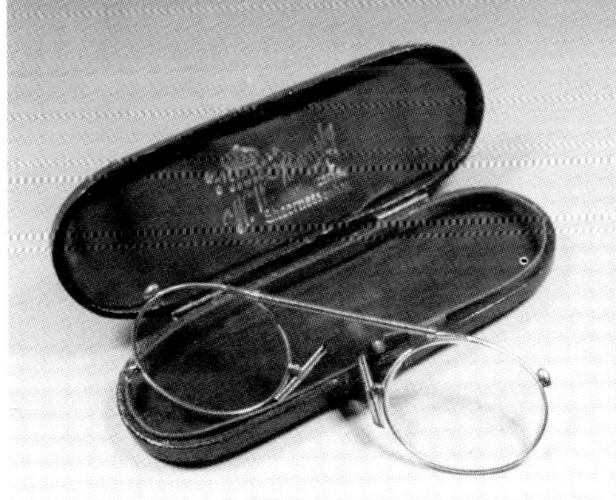

Cylinder lenses began to be used in the late 1800s, at the height of the pince-nez period. Because pince-nez frames tended to teeter on the nose, making it difficult to keep cylinder axis correctly aligned, a spring bar version of the pince-nez was developed specifically for patients wearing cylinder corrections. This frame is marked "F" in cover photo. (Circa 1885).

Eyeglasses from Dr. Wm. Rosenthal Collection

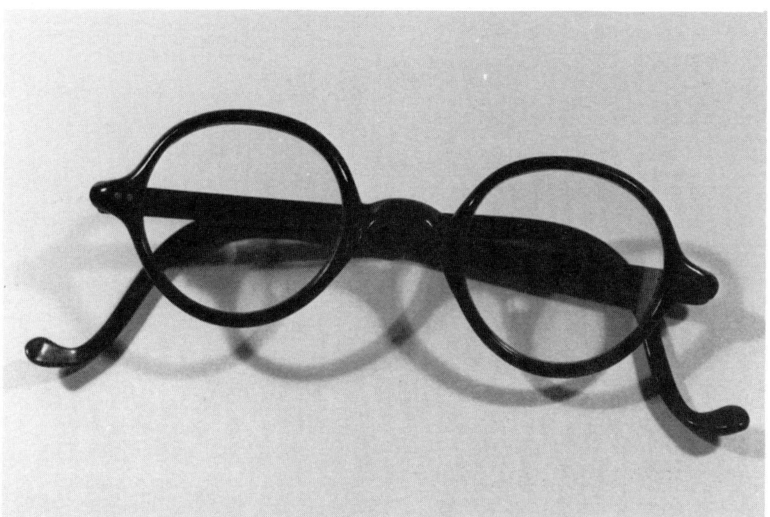

Here is an example of a zyl fingerpiece mounting carried by Walman Optical in 1917. Many fingerpiece mountings had no provision for attaching a chain or cord, so keeping these delicate eyeglasses firmly attached to the nose was important.

ILLUSTRATION – WALMAN OPTICAL CATALOG

Optical *(Real Comfort)* and E.B. Brown. In 1908, New Jersey Optical introduced a model called the "Rockanlock" because the bridge could be locked or left as a rocking guard. Kirstein introduced a model featuring a guard with studs and a spring carrying the name "Shur-on". This was the first fingerpiece advertised to the public and the name was widely used for all fingerpiece mountings.

The craze for fingerpiece mountings lasted from 1906 to 1930. During that time, they were the most-used rimless mounting. It might be assumed that with almost everyone wearing the same rimless mounting, the doctor's frame inventory would be minimal. To the contrary, retail offices carried fingerpiece fitting sets that included twelve to eighteen mountings. This variety was necessary to properly fit every patient. Lenses with strong cylinders or bifocal corrections required rigid guards with rocking pads. Narrow bridge mountings were required for those with narrow faces or narrow PD's. If the patient had a very wide face, a mounting with lens straps farther apart was necessary to avoid large *(and heavy)* lenses.

A peculiarity of those days was that optical centers were seldom decentered for rimless mountings. The basic procedure required the dispenser to carefully determine which mounting best fit the patient's nose. The width of that mounting was carefully measured and that distance was deducted from the patient's P.D. The difference would indicate the size of the lens to be ordered. One advantage of this system, of course, was that edging all lenses "on center" kept the nasal and temporal lens edges uniform.

The fingerpiece craze gradually diminished and other types of rimless mountings began to replace them. These newer mountings held the lenses by means of screws or rivets, passed through a hole at the edge of the lens and then secured to a "strap" which protruded over both sides of the lens. Bausch & Lomb devised a clever process called "Loxit" to hold rimless lenses in place. In place of screws, a slim lead cylinder was placed through the strap and lens. Placing the assembled lens and rimless mounting in a Loxit machine, heat was applied electrically to the strap, melting the lead and locking the lens securely. A neat little gold plug was inserted in the melted lead, effectively sealing the plug of lead. It was the most sophisticated method of mounting lenses in rimless mountings.

Uhlemann Optical developed an attractive design for a rimless mounting, using no screws, called "Willsedge". A special "keystone" edge was applied to the top rim of the lens, utilizing a special designed edger for grinding the keystone edge. The lens then slipped into a keystone groove in the top rim of the mounting. "Willsedge" cement held the lens in place. It was an attractive design at a time when other rimless had distracting unattractive screws and straps protruding into the lens area. Most labs did not have a Willsedge edger and lab people went slightly crazy trying to apply this "Willsedge" keystone groove by hand.

The new rimless eyewear was attractive. All the wearer had to worry about was keeping the lens from breaking too quickly. All lenses were glass and, in those pre-FDA days, most were less than 1.5mm thick. Rimless mountings are still popular today but most rimless in this country use plastic lenses, often with a nylon string extending around the bottom of the lens and knotted at both ends to the metal top bar.

Nonmetal Frames

Hard rubber remained the standard for nonmetal frames for many years but the color range for these practical frames was limited. Other materials *(horn and tortoiseshell)* were also available, but at higher prices because they were mostly produced by artisans rather than mass produced. The entire frame business changed, however, when the "plastic" world was created.

The first use of a man-made "plastic" for eyeglass frames in the U.S. was by Spencer Optical in 1876 with frames made of Celluloid. Their first catalog boasted *"Celluloid was lighter than rubber, horn, shell or any other previously used material. The rims are stronger and more durable than others. They are not affected by atmospheric changes and stand equally well in hot or cold climates."* John E. Spencer, Spencer's vice president, obtained a patent for Celluloid frames in 1879. By 1885 Spencer was producing large numbers of eyeglass and spectacle frames made from Celluloid.

Another early company making frames from this man-made material was the Wagner Comb Company. Making frames from Celluloid must have been easy for a comb manufacturer.

Shell Frames

Plastic frames were created originally as an inexpensive substitute for frames made from tortoise shell, most of which were made by hand and imported from Europe. Many of these were imported by Andrew J. Lloyd of Boston and E.B. Meyrowitz of New York City. In 1890 Trenkmann Brothers became the first to make tortoise shell frames in this country. As plastic frames grew in popularity, they were called "shell" by the public and the trade.

At the end of the 19th century, DuPont introduced "Zylonite", a thermoplastic material that could hold to any desired shape. The material was actually nitrocellulose, the same nitrate used for making gunpowder. A significant advantage of this new material was its superior dimensional stability, assuring frames would stay in adjustment. A wide range of colors became available, far superior to anything available in hard rubber. This new material also would not fade with use.

The trade began to call all plastic materials "Zylonite" and then shortened the name to "Zyl". Before long Monsanto Chemical Company and Celanese Corporation offered similar materials, as did Nixon Nitration Works. The big demand for shell frames was started by a popular movie actor named Harold Lloyd. College students followed his lead and began ordering eyeglasses with dark shell frames. Optical Products Corporation (O.P.C.) made the frames worn by Lloyd on the screen. He would order six at a time and constantly lose them. OPC's Lou Grossman reported in a letter written in 1941, *"I can remember one instance when Harold Lloyd lost the only frame he had left and production on an important picture was held up until we could supply a new one."*

Zyl frames took a while to catch on but, as metal prices continued to climb and fashion factors were recognized, plastic frames came into vogue. It was easy for opticians to insert lenses, they merely heated the rim over an open flame and snapped the lens in place. Plastic frames offered a wider color choice, were easier to adjust than the increasingly complex pad arms of metal frames, and were less expensive than metal frames. After World War I, plastic frames gradually took over more than 50 percent of the frame market. Anyone ignoring the trend paid the price. M. H. Harris, a large optometric chain in New York failed to survive this change in frame fashions because they flatly refused to show plastic frames.

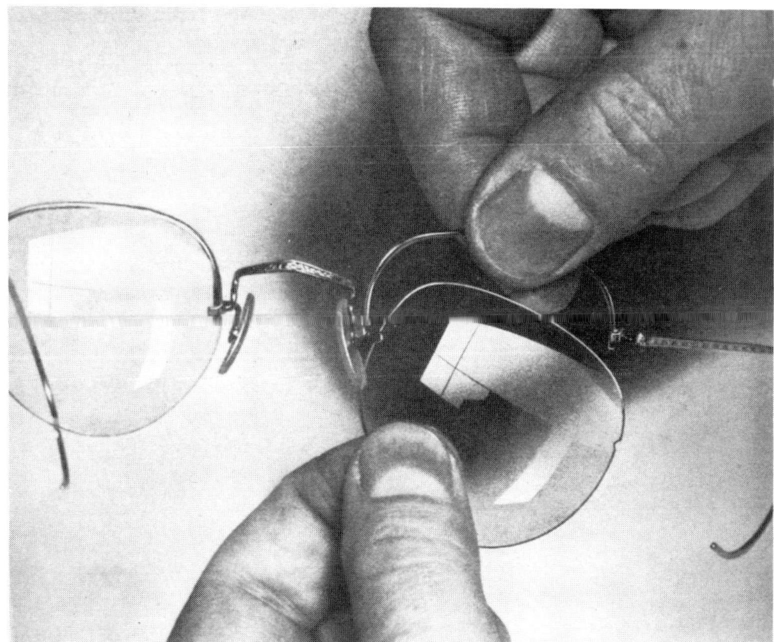

Bausch & Lomb introduced a novel and quite popular rimless mounting called "Balgrip" in the 1950s. Similar to rimway but without distracting screws. The bar behind the lens was stiff and spring-like, providing the tension required to hold lenses firmly in place. Every lab had a special Balgrip machine for notching lenses.

Manufacturing the plastic sheets from which the frames were made was complicated and lengthy. First, plastic flakes were formed into a 51 inch block or cube through the use of solvents such as acetone and, as this was done, color dyes were added. This block was then "cured" for several weeks to several months, permitting the solvent to dissipate. The length of cure time determined the quality of the material and the price to be charged for the sheets. The less solvent remaining in the plastic, the more stable the plastic. When multi-colors were desired, the block was sliced into thin sheets. These sheets were interlaced to form a new block which would be treated with solvents and put through the same complex curing process. This process was repeated at least four times for the finest quality demi-amber *(a tortoiseshell equivalent)*, demi-blonde *(a lighter, yellowish version of the darker demi-amber)*, or verdal *(a green version of tortoise)*.

Colors

In addition to these colors, the most used colors until the 1950s, were flesh and basic black. Black was the easiest material to produce since it was basically an amalgamation of all waste materials, although "virgin black" could also be produced. Non-virgin black had one drawback. It invariably shrank more quickly than other colors, resulting in a smaller frame.

With all of its admirable characteristics, nitrocellulose had one small defect: it was highly flammable. A favorite trick at many frame factories was played on fire extinguisher salesmen who came to demonstrate their wares. They would be taken into the parking lot and asked to prove the efficacy of their product by extin-

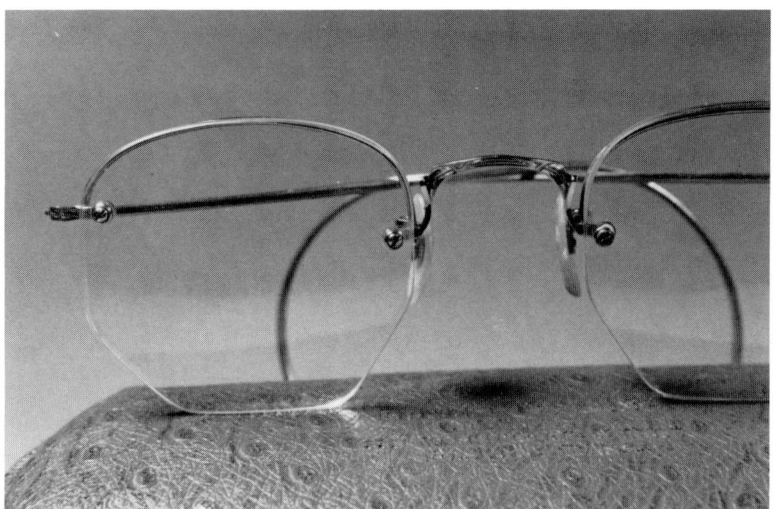

Here is the famous rimway mounting, this one manufactured by Shuron. Rimway lens screws had plastic sleeves and were usually locked in place with a lock nut, providing sturdy and practical rimless eyewear. Most metal manufacturers produced rimway mountings with 3 or 4 different bridge styles. (This frame marked "D" in cover photo).

This schematic drawing illustrates the ease with which the browbars of Shuron's Browline frames could be switched, a distinct advantage for inventory purposes. Labs carried a basic inventory of chassis (in yellow and white gold) and would assemble the ordered color as they were sold.

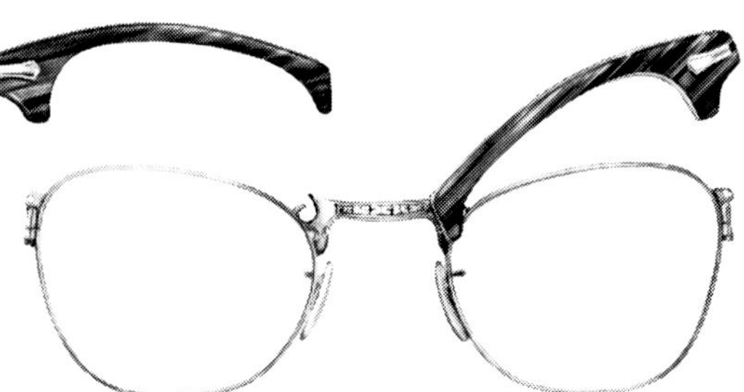

guishing a pile of plastic scraps *(nitrate)* lying on the ground. The salesman would touch a match to the pile and, before he could raise his extinguisher, the nitrate would vanish in a puff of smoke. In the frame factory, everyone kept a close eye on the operator responsible for spinning out the center of the lens openings using a steel blade inserted into a small, drilled hole. It was quite common for the heat generated during this operation to start a fire. The factory would empty of workers in seconds while the operator doused the flame with a sand pail prominently positioned next to the machine.

The federal government banned the use of nitrate in the optical industry in 1950. It seems strange now that the last use of nitrate was for eyeglass frames. Nitrate toilet seats were banned years before but the flammable material continued to be used on the face for years. No explanation has ever been given why the government considered bottoms more important than faces. It should be noted, however, that DuPont employed hundreds of workers at their plant in Arlington, N.J. to supply the optical industry so there may have been reluctance to end all those jobs.

By 1947, Celanese was promoting a newer material called cellulose acetate. It was similar in many ways to cellulose nitrate but did not have dimensional stability. Acetate had actually been available during the time that nitrate was being produced and was produced in much the same manner as the nitrate block method. Celanese, however, developed a new extrusion method for producing the material. The end product was somewhat more stable, less expensive and nonflammable. Production of this new material was accomplished by loading a hopper with acetate particles, heating the particles and forcing the molten material through apertures in a nozzle of any desired width or thickness.

At first extruded sheets were 51" wide and 51" long, the same size as sheet stock produced by the old-fashioned block method. It soon became apparent that substantial economies could be accomplished by extruding the plastic in the exact width and length required for frame fronts and extruding a different size for temple stock. In this way, waste material was minimal.

Less than 20 percent of plastic material purchased by frame manufacturers actually ends up in the finished frame. The balance was eye cutouts and outside borders after the fronts and temples had been cut. Since the scrap value of leftover plastic was pennies per pound compared to several dollars per pound for new material, frame manufacturers were always attempting to dream up ways to utilize scrap *(key rings, poker chips, etc.)* but with little success. As a result, optimizing the size of the new extruded plastic material produced important savings for frame producers.

Fashion for Eyewear is Introduced

Until the end of the first World War, eyeglasses were simply a device to hold a pair of lenses in front of the eyes, allowing people to see. By 1920, the industry belatedly began to recognize that sales might increase if the manufacturer produced better looking frames, stressing the cosmetic aspects of eyeglasses. With the advent of nitrate, a wide selection of colors became available *(solid colors of all hues, in addition to many mottled colors)*. Frame manufacturers started using gold filled metals and offering colors in metal as well. Suddenly a whole new fashion world opened up for frame producers.

American Optical had the foresight *(or luck)* to take out a basic patent for a rather simple frame design feature called Ful Vue. This all-encompassing design patent covered, according to AO, any frame that featured a hinge located more than 3/4 of the way up the side of the frame. Once the public saw this new feature, they wanted it. Before long, manufacturers were no longer able to sell frames with on-center endpiece construction. Adding this simple design change to any new frame, however, forced the manufacturer to take out a license from AO under their Ful Vue patent. To be fair, American Optical did give them a choice. They could take out a license or get out of the frame business.

Shortly after this, a "Numount" patent was issued to Uhlemann Optical Company, a prominent Chicago wholesale-dispenser. Uhlemann authorized AO to issue licenses and collect royalties for them under this patent. The Numont design was a rimless, two screw construction at the bridge with a metal bar passing behind the lens to the outer edge where the temples connected. Bay State Optical, a Massachusetts frame manufacturer, received a patent for the "Rimway", much like the Numount design except it included the added security of four screws instead of two. Bay State's patent was also assigned to AO for licensing and royalties. These last two patents came to dominate rimless frame designs worldwide. AO's arrangement with Uhlemann and Bay State Optical required that all royalties, less collection costs, be remitted to the patent holders. American Optical was content to handle the bookkeeping and administration at no charge because this gave them firm control over the entire frame market. Because of these three patents, AO dominated the industry for many years.

In the 1930s and 1940s, the vogue for rimless frames steadily increased. Numont and Rimway designs were more efficient than the easily broken rimless frames of the past and more attractive and less conspicuous. They became the most-used frames during those years. The author's first on-the-job training in lab work was drilling holes in lenses for rimless mountings. He particularly remembers most orders coming in to the lab on Monday mornings would be "lenses only" for rimless frames, replacing lenses broken over the weekend.

Resistance From the Professions

The Better Vision Institute *(described elsewhere in this history)* was formed in 1929 under the leadership of Mike Julian, an experienced advertising executive. The organization was supported by all elements of the professions and the industry, including manufacturers, wholesale laboratories, Optometry, Ophthalmology and Opticianry. For years, it was BVI's custom to have past presidents of the Optical Laboratories Association serve as president. BVI was created to promote the concept of attractive eyewear while promoting the professional and technical aspects of modern eyecare. In 1930, eyeglasses were featured in a fashion style show at the Waldorf Astoria Hotel in New York City, an historic first. This advent of frame fashions, however, created a bit of a dichotomy. Eyecare professionals guarded their prerogatives jealously and most refused to accept the concept of public advertising.

Many were even opposed to letting the public choose which frame they would wear or even the color. They believed frame selection was the prerogative of the professional fitter, not the patient. Univis Lens Company advertised trifocals to the public during the '50s as Shuron Optical did for their Browline frames. Both companies abandoned consumer advertising because of the strenuous objections from professional associations and individual members. BVI, however, encouraged both consumers and professions to regard eyewear as something more than a device to hold lenses, succeeding

in setting the entire industry on the road to making eyewear a part of the fashion world. Julian was replaced in 1960 by Gus Nelson and Larry Aasen took over the BVI reins in 1967, remaining until 1987. The Vision Council of America *(VICA)* organization eventually absorbed BVI in 1989 and currently uses the organization for much of their public relations work in campaigning for better sight.

Fashion Eyewear Group of America

In 1961, the frame industry made another grand effort to promote the concept of fashion in eyewear to the benefit of the professions and the industry. This effort was launched by a group of frame material manufacturers that included plastic extruders, hinge and screw manufacturers, and gold-filled material manufacturers. They selected Fashion Eyewear Group of America *(FEGA)* as the name for their organization. An outstanding fashion publicist, Ruth Hammer Associates, was hired to promote the fashion concept. When FEGA called a convocation of industry and professional interests at the Waldorf Astoria Hotel in 1962 to review her plans, Miss Hammer encountered a flood of problems. Forewarned about the industry's attitude regarding professional control of the frame sale and proper frame fitting, she was ready for early criticism of her projected publicity. The first complaint came from an optician who

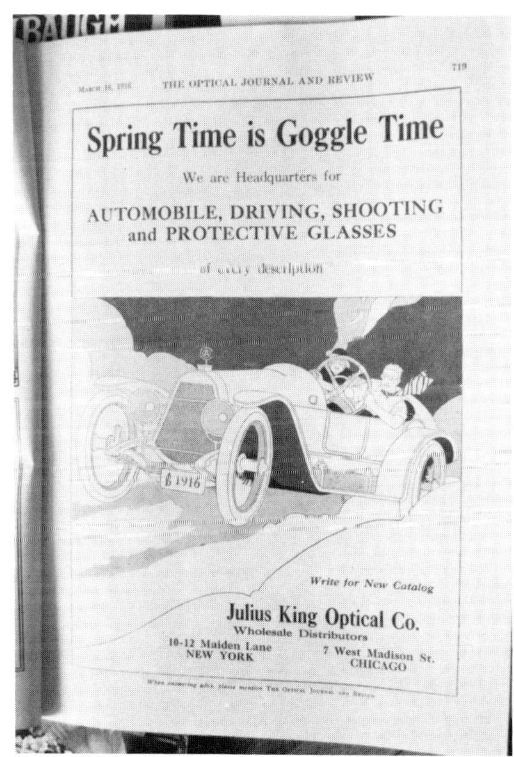

Driving glasses of all types were a staple item with wholesalers during the first quarter of this century. Early automobiles were open to the weather and driving goggles, in addition to protecting the eyes, provided wearers with a snazzy modern look when they wore them hanging around their neck.

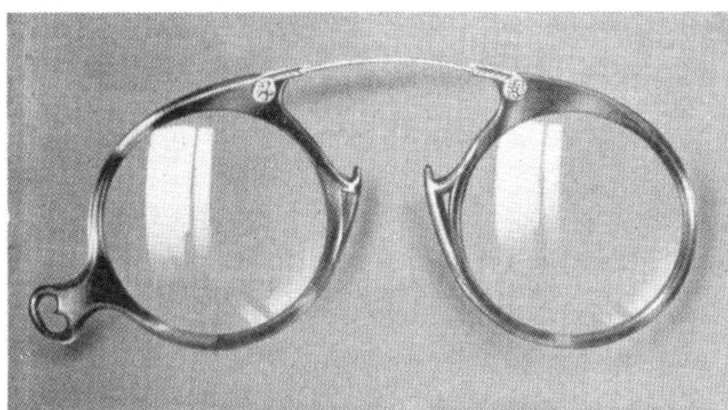

Oxfords came in a wide variety of styles. They were available in both metal and zyl but every style included that important handle at one end for attaching a cord, chain or ribbon.

Many elegant men and women attached a spring loaded reel and chain to their Oxford or pince-nez glasses. When their eyeglasses weren't being worn, they hung discretely from the reel which was usually attached to their lapel or blouse.

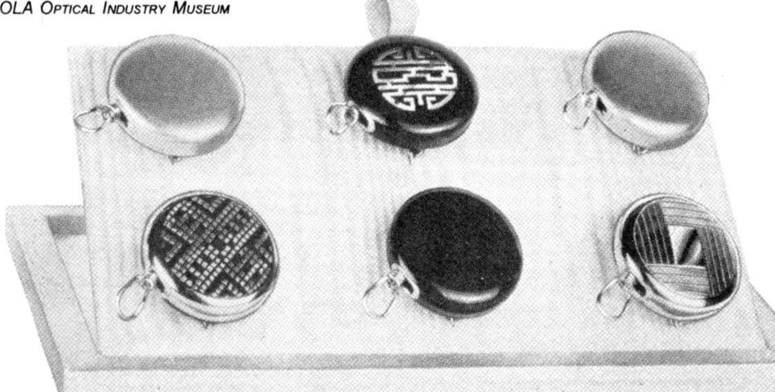

expressed grave concern that the model's neck was too long and her eyes were not centered in the frame, totally ignoring the value of consumer exposure.

Sy Newhouse, at that time publisher of Vogue magazine, was convinced by Harlequin's president Martin Singer (Nat Singer's son) to devote the entire beauty section of his July, 1962 issue to eyewear fashions. Most of their readers were over 40 and the majority wore glasses, so Newhouse was assured a new class of advertiser would be created. He asked Diane Vreeland, then editor of Vogue, for approval. Diane was attending fashion openings in Paris and her telegraphed reply was: "over my dead body". Fortunately, Newhouse was so intrigued with the concept, he overruled her and even supplied 20,000 reprints of that section at actual printing cost to the FEGA organization.

Ironically, it took massive persuasion on the part of Walt Tucker, President of FEGA and President of Nixon Nitration works *(an acetate producer)* to get his group to sponsor the beauty section and even more arm-twisting to obtain FEGA financing and approval for the 20,000 reprints.

The responses of manufacturers contacted to advertise in that issue of Vogue reveals a lot about the frame industry at that time. Bob Stewart, American Optical's vice president for distribution, accepted the idea enthusiastically. Al Marsters, a former AO vice president, serving as Bausch & Lomb's vice president for sales, first wanted to know what AO was doing and then agreed to go along. Bob Barber, vice president of Univis *(Univis had purchased a frame manufacturing company and was now in the frame business),* was disturbed that a "can of worms" would be opened giving American Optical an advantage because of their size and Univis refused to participate. Roy Marks, President of Shuron, had no interest in the idea. Vogue was successful in securing full page ads from B&L, AO and Martin-Copeland, a

relatively small and unknown frame manufacturer who went on to become an industry leader a few years later. Quarter page ads were placed by Tura and Harlequin. When Vogue attempted the same thing the following year, almost no one participated. AO and B&L had received severe criticism from the Industry's professions. It was a dismal ending for a bold, courageous attempt to take the fashion eyewear story to the public.

G.I. Glasses

During World War II, virtually all materials were scarce and many frame factories were involved in producing eyeglasses as well as other products for the armed forces. Traditionally, B&L held navy contracts and AO the much larger army contracts. Both metal and plastic frames were produced in a very simple basic style *(with Ful Vue endpieces, of course).* Gray smoke was the color used for plastic, and metal frames were primarily white in a wide range of sizes.

One interesting operation during World War II involved several of the smaller factories producing gold-filled frames. They possessed a much-coveted gold license. In the unstable economic atmosphere prevalent during the war, gold became the accepted standard for anyone with a lot of money, particularly in Latin America. These few unscrupulous frame manufacturers would sell "gold-filled" frames made of solid 12 karat gold to "customers" outside the country. The price charged to the customer on the company's books was the proper price for gold-filled frames but the balance of the real price was paid in cash. In this way, "customers" were able to ship gold out of the country with no interference from the United States or their own government. All they had to do to regain the gold was melt down the frames.

New Designs

In the late 1920s, the P-3 shape became the popular choice for the "modern" look. This was a pear-like shape with a 3mm difference between horizontal and vertical dimensions. Soon after, the perimetric shape, called P-4, was introduced. This had a 4mm difference, featuring a cutaway on the nasal side of the lens. In 1939, Altina Sanders introduced her Harlequin frame, the first fashion frame in the industry. This was a "cat's eye" severely upswept shape that is still called "harlequin". Before long Monroe Levoy *(founder of Tura)* was offering his Futura frame. This was an attractive plastic frame with a dreadful pierced metal plate wrapped around the top rim. Unfortunately, the poorly plated metal adornment discolored with wear and the frame was an absolute monster for lab technicians. It was almost impossible to insert lenses without chipping or breaking them.

Although neither of these frames were very successful,

they did pave the way for "fashion" frames. Levoy went on to develop his famous Tura frame, an all-aluminum frame in an upswept shape produced in two sizes: Levoy often described them as "too large" and "too small". They were made, however, with a bewildering array of anodized colors and featured classy adornments on the front and temple. There's little doubt that Tura and Monroe Levoy pioneered fashion eyewear. During the same period *(late '40s and '50s)* Harlequin was offering a wide variety of colors in plastic *(all nitrate, in those days)* as well as a variety of more exotic materials such as acrylic and a "bamboo" type plastic that was actually a beige acetate, hand carved, dyed, and then polished.

One of the significant frame designs was the Browline, the first-ever "combination" frame featuring plastic tops on metal rims, with plastic temples. Developed in 1947 by Jack Rohrbach, a vice president at Shuron, the frame failed with the first two designs but became a runaway best seller when produced with a metal bridge. B&L was quick to copy the style by introducing their Bal Rim. These two companies started a design trend that ultimately affected almost half of all frames sold during the 1950s.

Several frame factories offered acrylic frames, available in luminescent colors but with one small problem. They were more fragile than glass and easily broken. Experiments were attempted using cellulose butyrate. This was a decent material, but it smelled terrible as it was produced and when heated. Dispensers and labs took a dim view of this fragrant feature. Leather had been another early material for frame making but was gradually replaced by horn and tortoiseshell. Nylon had an advantage because it could be machined or milled and frames could also be molded. Molding was considerably easier, cheaper and more accurate. Fabricating nylon in traditional ways required expensive carbide tools and was difficult to accomplish. Zyloware imported the first successful molded nylon frame from France in 1959, but were careful not to publicize the fact that it was molded. The industry's experience and opinion of molding was poor. That Zyloware nylon frame *(Invincible)* is still sold today.

Molded Frames

Bay State Optical attempted to produce the first molded frame in 1948. The frame proved totally impractical. It was made of a thermosetting plastic requiring lenses to be sized and inserted like a metal frame. Celanese Fortrel, the material used, turned out to be extremely brittle. Over-the-counter sunglasses featured molded frames for many years but the prescription industry refused to accept more expensive prescription frames made in what they considered a cheap form of manufacturing.

In the early 1950s, however, the federal government gave approval to molded plastic government issue frames, giving a certain amount of credence to molding. American Optical experimented with the process, introducing certain sizes and colors into their Modern Times and Jaguar frame styles, all the while stoutly denying they were molded. It was not until polyproprionate was introduced in the 1970s, however, that molding was accepted as a proper way to manufacture frames. This material could only be used by molding and these frames proved to be lightweight, stylish and less expensive.

In the 1960s, in Germany-Austria, William Anger pioneered a remarkable new material called Optyl. This was a cast material that permitted stylists to create unusual three dimensional effects that were simply impossible with traditional hand-fabricated frame production. The material required special handling for glazing and adjusting. Two variations of the material were soundly rejected by the industry before the present third generation material was developed. The professions then had to be taught how to handle this revolutionary new material.

Recent years have witnessed the advent of even more exotic materials: carbon, stainless steel *(a throwback to those early frames made by American Optical but this time the metals are ultra-light and extremely flexible metal)*, and a variety of other machined and molded materials. The major materials in use, however, continues to be cellulose acetate and plated nickel silver.

Designer Names

In 1955, American Optical conducted a daring experiment by introducing the first "brand name" frame line featuring a dress designer named Madame

Each year the Fashion Eyewear Group of America (FEGA) judges would select the frame that represented what they believed would be in style ten years later. During the 1960s, this was one of the frames chosen as a "Frame of the Seventies".

PHOTO – PAM FRITZ

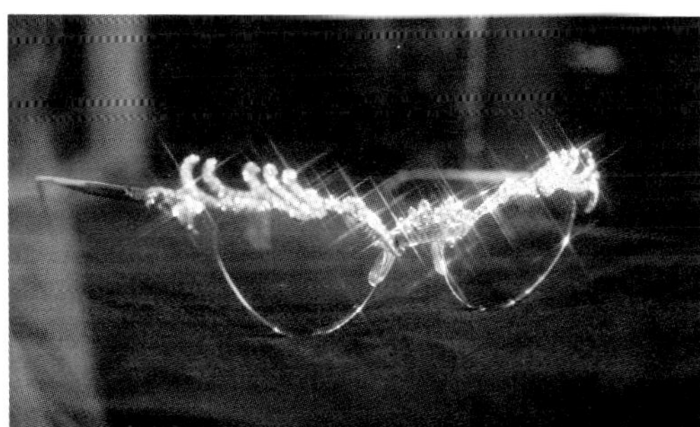

This is the famous Schiaparelli rimless mounting that is currently residing in the vaults of the American Optical Museum.

PHOTO – AMERICAN OPTICAL MUSEUM

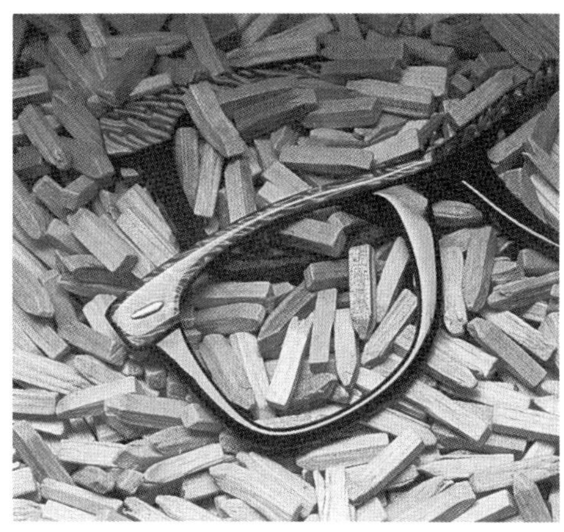

After acetate zyl frames were cut or pantographed to shape, they would spend four days in tumbling barrels in a mixture of wooden "shoe pegs" and various polishing compounds. This process smoothed the edges and produced a deep, high sheen to the surface of the frame.

Schiaparelli which they sold to selected retailers. Only those who bought the original collection were permitted to order prescription frames, which came in 36 models. The company made up four presentation models of precious metals and gem stones which were loaned out from time to time for retailers to feature in their store windows, with appropriate publicity. Local AO branches received a 10 percent commission on all Schiaparelli sales but AO branch managers soon ran into major public relations problems and convinced the company to get out of the designer business. The problem was that AO's better customers often were not authorized Schiaparelli customers. In many cases, those authorized to sell the frames were local area price cutters and this was totally unacceptable to many of AO's regular customers. Today, the American Optical Museum features the only one of those precious metal frames that still exists. It is a remarkable frame made of iridium platinum and encrusted with 201 diamonds, totaling seven and three-quarters karats. In addition to the value of the precious metals and gems, it has incredible historical value and is appraised at more than $200,000.

Today the frame marketplace features a wide variety of designer names. Adding such names to frame lines permits selling them at considerably higher prices, partly because of their fashion styling and partly because of the ready acceptance of well-known names. This has been profitable for frame sellers and the industry. Presenting frames that carry a recognized name, even if it's the name of a shoe or a motorcycle, seems to be successful.

Designer frames cost dispensers or doctors more, but brand name identity permits collecting higher patient fees. Designers Dior, Givenchy, Polo, Bill Blass, joined by personalities such as Sophia Loren, Diane von Furstenberg, Lauren Bacall, Gloria Vanderbilt and even Humphrey Bogart *(in absentia)* have been extremely successful for the frame industry. These highly-recognized individuals *(if alive)* enthusiastically endorse their products even though they may have had little involvement in their design. Whether the concept is approved or not, brand name frame products have raised the price level of the entire industry, permitting other frame prices to rise as well. Frame manufacturers have achieved excellent industry recognition and, in some cases, even public recognition of their company name. Rodenstock, Safilo and Ray Ban are just a few examples of factory *(or product)* names that command higher prices because of consumer recognition.

Frame Distribution

Of all frames sold in the United States today, well over 90 percent are manufactured outside the country. In a few cases, frame parts are manufactured abroad and assembled in the United States. Two-thirds of the frames are sold directly to retailers by foreign manufacturers or import firms. There are still a significant number of frames distributed through laboratories and stock houses, as in the past.

Frame distribution in the United States has changed greatly over the past 30 years, perhaps revealing a few things about the future. For the first half of this century, American frame manufacturers overwhelmingly dominated the U.S. market. Most frames were produced by U.S. manufacturers and distributed through wholesalers who sold frames, stock lenses and other accessories. Few frames during those years were imported.

Plastic frames in this country were produced on a mass production basis from sheet stock, formed by stamping heated sheets of plastic with steel dies *(much like cookie cutters),* creating both fronts and temples. This was a made-to-order system for frame fashions that changed slowly. Steel dies required for this mass production were expensive. This was offset by the stability of frame styles that would sell well for years. This type of production worked particularly well for the U.S. market. Tooling for new frame styles was expensive, so manufacturers tended to find a good frame design and stick with it. Frame fashions were conservative with smaller frame suppliers emulating bestselling styles developed by the major producers. And — there was no one around to rock the boat.

Frame production in Europe and the Far East, on the other hand, had just survived a devastating war. Frame factories suffered war damage or had their equipment converted to other uses. When the war ended, frame production in those countries had to start over from the ground up. Frame producers were essentially cottage industries, making their products in small quantities. The United States, on the other hand, rolled into high gear, once the war was over. Relying on an enormous market and a fast-growing population, American factories were designed primarily to mass-produce frames. Other countries were not locked into such "long-run" production methods and had, in addition, converted to pantographic production of frames. This process, using pantographs that duplicate a master model, essentially carve out frames one at a time, a simple system offering a number of advantages.

First, there are no heavy start-up costs for steel dies. Once a design is created, the producer immediately starts making frames. Second, frames could be made in small runs, making it easier to try innovative and creative designs to see how the market would respond. This was a system made to order for a world that had just gone through a devastating war and wanted a change. More important, people were tired of the same frame styles. They wanted a new life and a new look.

Selling Frames Direct

Frame producers in other parts of the world have always eyed the enormous American market with envy because of its sheer size. As foreign frame producers increased their manufacturing, it was only natural to turn to this vast market to sell their growing frame production. They were confident their styling was far advanced over what they had seen in the United States. They were confident their products would be welcomed in the states with open arms, knowing their more sophisticated manufacturing was producing frames superior to what was available in the United States at that time.

Resisting Change

When these foreign frame manufacturers sent advance scouts to the states and began calling on frame distributors *(mostly labs),* they got a surprise. First, they discovered that most labs had long-term relationships with frame suppliers and had little or no interest in adding new vendors. They also learned that most labs carried 15 to 25 frame lines. Frames were sold here in what seemed to be a strange way to them. Every new frame required attractive four-color kit boxes, usually with a different box design for each new frame. These boxes seemed to serve as nothing more than delivery boxes. Retailers would take the frames out of the kit and throw the expensive box away. Distributors seldom showed a complete frame line. Wholesale sales reps carried a jumble of kits from a wide variety of frame suppliers. Importers watched in amazement as lab sales reps called on their customers, wheeling in dollies stacked with all these odd-sized kit boxes, many containing cute trinkets such as ties, coffee cups, jewelry, or cosmetics, a "reward" for buying the kit.

Importers also noticed that most U.S. frames were sold separately as fronts and temples, creating what seemed to be a totally illogical process as well as an inventory nightmare. Imported frames were shipped completely assembled. When offshore frame producers tried to get distributors to look at what they knew to be superior frames, they experienced a complete lack of interest *(as well as a lot of complaining about "assembled" frames).* Yet, when they showed these imported frames to retailers, there was a great deal of interest.

As a result of being thus shut out of the American market, these importers proceeded to hire a few sales people in the New England area and some in Los Angeles and take their frames direct to retailers. In time, many foreign manufacturers would establish arrangements with go-getter salespeople who would import, stock and sell their frames direct to retailers. Gradually, these importers spread across the country until direct-selling frames became available in every area.

It required a number of years, but this transition enabled direct sellers to crowd out many of the existing frame distributors and manufacturers, eventually taking over the lion's share of the American frame market. Currently direct-selling frames represent somewhere in the neighborhood of 80 percent of all frame sales.

In the Meantime

Many American frame producers remained steadfast in their dedication to doing things the way they always had and ended up like Captain Smith of the Titanic. They went down with the ship. *(See Chapter 14 - Frame Manufacturers.)* A few savvy companies, however, survived this onslaught by conforming to the new frame market instead of fighting it. Today these American companies feature mostly imported products and many frames they sell are produced in the same overseas factories as those sold by direct sellers. This new generation of American frame sellers have found it still pays to distribute their products through laboratories and local stock houses, primarily because lab personnel enjoy the strongest ties with retail dispensing staffs.

The Pinnacle Group

There is a renaissance for domestic frame companies and laboratories that still handle frames. Labs and frame producers joined forces recently to organize the Pinnacle Group, aimed at promoting the advantages of "one stop shopping" for frames and lenses. Some labs that had stopped selling frames are once again doing so. A few forward-thinking direct-sellers are setting up special frame collections distributed only through labs or stock houses. This trend may indicate how frames will be distributed in the future. The logic of ordering frame and lenses with one phone call is a powerful inducement.

Relics and Survivors

One thing that shows up consistently during the past hundred years is that change is a continuing factor in the industry. As individual company histories are studied, their stories inevitably demonstrate that companies that change with the times survive. Those who don't, for the most part, no longer exist. This history reveals a number of companies that have survived the years very well and remain a vital part of the ophthalmic community.

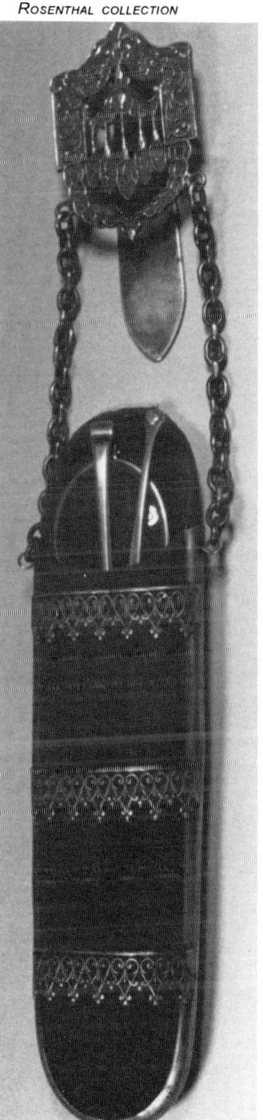

"Chatelain" cases were designed to protect eyeglasses and still be readily available when needed. The case hung from a ladies belt, giving the wearer a refined appearance (marked "I" in cover photo).

CASE AND FRAME FROM DR. WM. ROSENTHAL COLLECTION

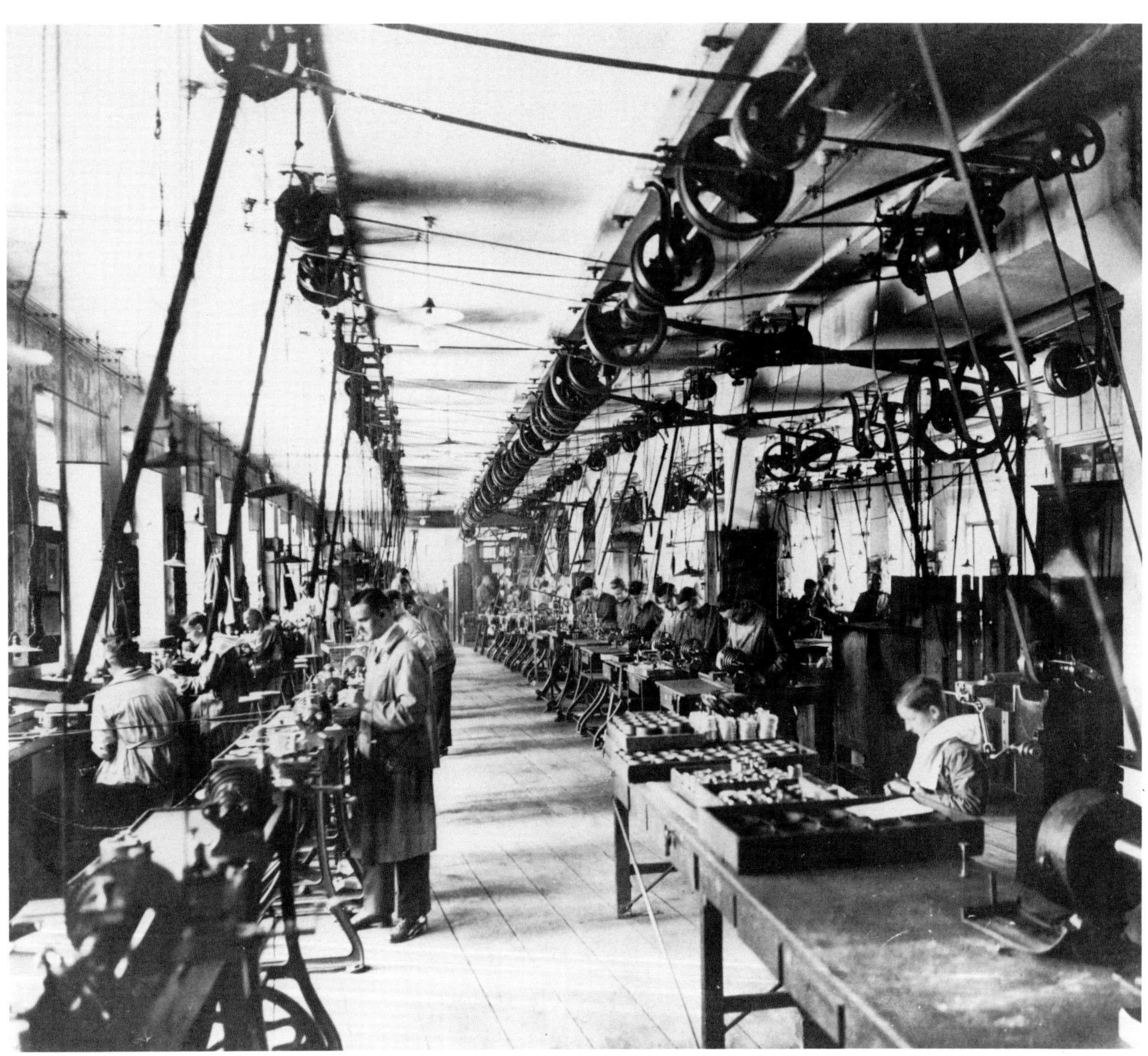

Prior to the 1920's, the power to drive frame and lens manufacturing equipment usually came from a common source. This might be a powerful, direct current motor mounted in the basement or, in earlier times, a steam engine or a powerful water wheel. In the 19th century, most manufacturing plants were placed beside rivers or streams. The amount of energy lost in the maze of belts running all over the plant was awesome. The noise produced by all those belts slapping and turning was an accepted part of the work environment.

Chapter 11
Making Lenses

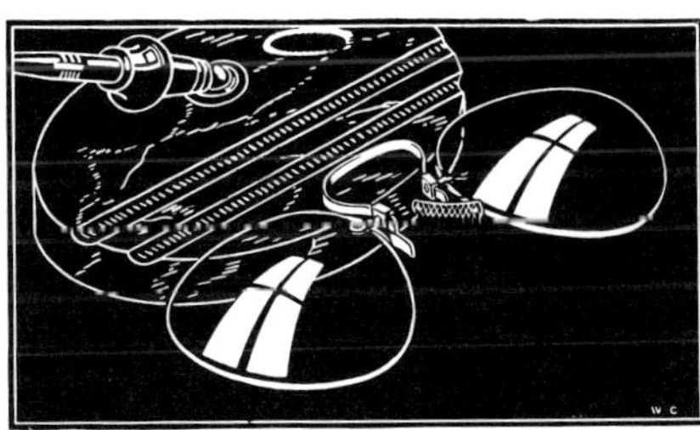

Early 19th century lens manufacturing machinery was primitive by anyone's standards. Making lenses involved a difficult hand process that could take anywhere from three to twenty hours to produce a single lens. Lens blanks were held by hand and rotated against an iron tool turning on a vertical spindle. The first spindles were driven by foot power, later by waterpower, steam, and eventually, around the turn of the century, by electric power. Demand for eyeglass lenses was minimal so this tedious process worked reasonably well for the primitive needs of that time. Lenses were first rough-ground, then taken through several fining processes, and finally a laborious hand polishing process, usually using the same tool and spindle for each step. This required skilled, dedicated workmen if the optics were to be anything more than minimal. Small wonder that the young United States relied on imported lenses for most of their needs. As the demand for eyeglasses increased and European sources proved unreliable, it soon became evident a way to mass-produce lenses was required if eyeglasses were ever to become available to the general public, not just for the wealthy.

Mass Producing Lenses

Plano-convex and plano-concave represented state-of-the-art in lenses for much of the 19th century. These lenses required flat surfacing tools for one surface and whatever curve was required to produce the desired power for the opposite side of the lens. As ways of mass producing lenses were developed, it was found that multiple lenses could be fastened to the inside or outside of a bowl shaped holder. The curve of the bowl determined the curve of the finished lenses. This system worked well for spherical lenses and the same method is still used today for producing glass lenses.

The first lenses to be "mass-produced" in the United States were produced in 1860 in New York by Charles Alt, an immigrant who had migrated seven years before from Germany. With only his wife and a French workman to help him, he was never able to turn out more than limited quantities.

As the industry evolved to six base meniscus lenses, replacing earlier flat lenses, the previous method for producing spheres was still viable. But cylinder lenses for correcting astigmatism were then introduced. Mass-producing cylinder lenses required a totally different system. Only glass lenses were manufactured during this period and to mass-produce cylinder lenses, manufacturers used round wheels to which lenses were adhered with pitch to the outside circumference of the wheel. The diameter of the wheel determined the base curve and, obviously, the flatter the base curve of a lens, the more lenses could be attached to the wheel. A controlling factor was the size of the lens blank. When lens blanks grew larger, fewer blanks could be attached to each wheel, directly affecting their price.

These wheels were then rotated in front of a concave shaped ceramic *(later diamond wheels)* which applied cross curves and created the cylinder power. The wheel full of lenses would be rotated using fine emery on fining wheels or cerium oxide on polishing wheels. Mass–producing cylinder lenses in this way required the cylinder to be on the front side of the lens. There was no way then, or today, to grind and polish multiple lenses with cylinders on the inside *(minus cylinders)*. Minus cylinder lenses, when introduced, had to be produced on single spindles, one lens at a time. This is one reason it took so many years for the industry to completely convert from plus cylinders to minus cylinders.

Fused Bifocals

Fused bifocals, once they were invented, were manufactured by grinding and polishing the front surface of a flint segment to be used for the reading segment. A concave depression would then be ground and polished in the carrier lens *(the distance portion)*. Each flint segment was carefully cleaned and temporarily held in position over the depression with small wood-like pegs. The assembly was then placed in an oven, heating the parts until they fused into one lens, burning up the wooden holders in the process. This basic method is still used today for producing glass fused multifocals. The evolution of bifocal design is found in Chapter 9 of this history.

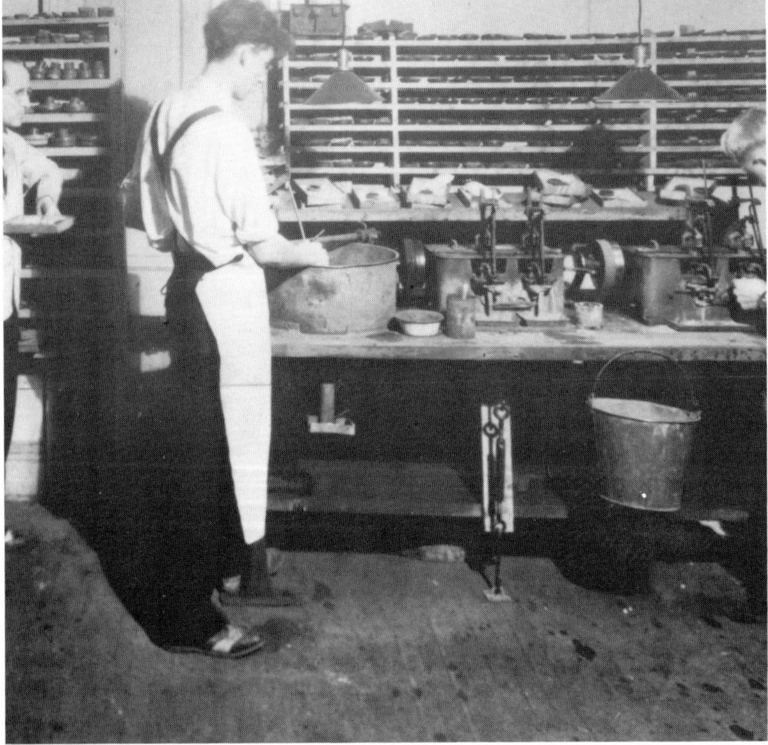

The optician standing at the left is hand-surfacing lenses while his partner fines cylinders on one of Shuron's famous Tor-Cyl machines. Photo was taken in early 1930s in Art Optical's lab in Grand Rapids, Michigan. This company ceased producing glasses in 1984, concentrating all their present production on oxygen permeable contact lenses.

PHOTO – ART OPTICAL CONTACT LENS, INC.

Lab Machinery

Much like factory lens production, laboratory machinery also started with foot pedal power or sometimes by wheels turned with hand power *(aided by large pulleys)*. These pulleys turned iron spindles on which the lenses were ground and polished. Water, steam or even animal power was used. Eventually, around the turn of this century, electricity came into the picture. The first electrical power was direct current, turning huge motors connected by overhead pulleys and great leather belts to machines all over the lab. By the '40s, small individual motors began to be substituted for earlier belt-driven systems. In the early days of electric power, a nearby water source was always essential for producing the electric power and sources for water power dictated the location of plants such as Bausch & Lomb and American Optical.

Late in the 19th century, more automated machines were developed by lens manufacturers who often produced individual prescriptions, much like a laboratory. Machinery they designed and developed was also available to smaller independent laboratories as well. This was a good system but had one major drawback. Once the labs bought the machinery, they would be obligated to buy lens products produced by the lens factory, either through contractual arrangements or because lenses produced by the manufacturer required specialized machinery available only from that manufacturer.

Roughing

Hand pans were the basic machine used by labs for producing spherical or cylindrical lenses. This was accomplished by holding the lens *(mounted with pitch on a metal lens block)* with a point fastened to the middle of a "poker arm" positioned over a revolving tool. The lens curve was roughed in using a harsh abrasive *(corundum, generally)*. To produce a cylinder surface, first the spherical curve was shaped. Then a second tool was selected that matched the desired cross curve. The lens was then held in place *(without rotating)*, by holding the ears projecting from the lens block. Holding the lens at the desired axis, the cylinder was then "rocked in" with the grinding done in one meridian, producing a second curve that created the required cylinder. It took a trained eye and years of experience to be able to "rock in" cylinders with any degree of accuracy. In the '40s and '50s, it was still possible to find surface men who were skilled at rocking in cylinders. Today, it is a lost art. Spherical lenses for most corrections are now fined and polished on cylinder machines, and most American labs use hand pans and sphere polishers sparingly, if at all.

Cylinder Machines

The first semiautomatic cylinder machine was developed in Philadelphia by Anton Wagner in 1895. This was a unit which fined and polished cylinder surfaces, using a "figure 8" motion. At the time, Wagner was employed by an optician the reader has already met — John Borsch, inventor of the original cemented Kryptok bifocal. Borsch was a progressive optician and an early user of cylinder lenses, which his workers had to make by hand. Wagner's new machine enabled two major laboratories, McAllister and later Queen Optical, to become the first serious producers of cylindrical lenses in the United States. McAllister, however, had been producing cylindrical prescriptions on demand as early as 1828 *(produced laboriously by hand)*. There wasn't much demand for cylinder lenses because refractionists knew little about checking for astigmatism. Cylinders did not come into common usage until the end of the 19th century. Even then, their use was confined to a few highly specialized refractionists who understood astigmatism.

Standard Optical produced what they called an "automated" cylinder machine *(the famous STOCO Tor-Cyl)* in 1901. This first-of-its-kind machine fined and polished a cylinder lens automatically. All that was required was a worker who would stand in front of the machine and continuously paint the lens and tool with emery or polishing compound. It was a marvelous improvement over previous methods. A good cylinder man could keep as many as eight of these machines in action but he looked like Fred Astaire as he danced up and down in front of his bank of machines, painting on emery or rouge and changing laps and lenses. It was thirty-some years before any serious attempt was made to pump the fining or polishing compound automatically. The Standard Tor-Cyl machine enabled laboratories to readily produce cylinder lenses which were beginning to be ordered as refractionists learned how to determine toric needs. STOCO's early lead was soon copied by AO and B&L, followed later by smaller machinery manufacturers.

Shortly before World War II, automated cylinder and sphere polishers were developed that used a slurry *(a watery compound of fining or polishing compounds)* automatically delivered to the lens through pumps or, sometimes by scoops that flushed the slurry from the bottom of the unit as the bowl rotated. One of the earliest of these machines was developed by R.F. Duffens and his partner Jack Quinton. Robinson-Houchin Optical Company entered the market about this time, offering their popular Greyhound machinery line.

A significant development relating to lab equipment occurred in 1963, caused by litigation known as the "Milwaukee" case. This Federal Government action forced American Optical and Bausch & Lomb to restrain their wholesale activities and eventually eliminated their retail operations. Because of this legal restriction, Bausch & Lomb eventually completely backed out of the machinery business. From that time on, they commissioned the fledgling Coburn Optical to supply machinery needed for their branches. At the same time, American Optical totally ceased selling surfacing machinery or even parts for their machines to independent laboratories. Cutting off independent sales enabled them to set much lower sales prices for machinery they sold to their own branches. This had the effect of reducing the monthly burden for AO branches and gave the company an opportunity to lower lab prices and still show the profit required by the new standards enforced by the Federal Government.

A typical surfacing setup in the 1920s, showing a surfacing pan on the left and an American Optical cylinder machine on the right (which could also be used with spheres). Notice the belt drive used to power the units.

Generators

Shortly before the second World War, lens manufacturers began to develop generators for production use but these units were much too big, too ungainly, and too expensive for laboratory use. Just after World War II, Harold Fluegge, a wholesale lab owner in Milwaukee and an excellent lab technician, began working on a laboratory generator. This author visited Fluegge Optical in the early 1950s and had an opportunity to see Fluegge's first working generator. It was not much more than a vertical floor stand drill press with a large three-foot cardboard wheel with diopter curves hand marked around the circumference. Fluegge eventually turned his ideas and preliminary work over to Shuron. His advice and consultation was so valuable to Shuron, they presented the first generator to come off the Shuron production line to Harold Fluegge.

Jack Suddarth, who also worked for Fluegge Optical, came up with his own idea for a generator while sitting in a foxhole in the South Pacific during the war. Following the war, he offered his concept to Shuron but they were already working with Cincinnati Milling Machine Company to adapt one of Cincinnati's milling machines for use as a laboratory lens generator and turned him down. Suddarth then took his design to Coburn Optical and the rest is history. Shuron's 190 generator, however, was the first practical generator introduced for laboratory use.

Many independent laboratories in the '50s and '60s used the famous Shuron 88-A Tor-Cyl for fining and polishing cylinders. Tor-Cyl was a registered trademark, dating back to the original STOCO (Standard Optical) 6-C Tor-Cyl machine, the first practical cylinder machine produced for laboratories.

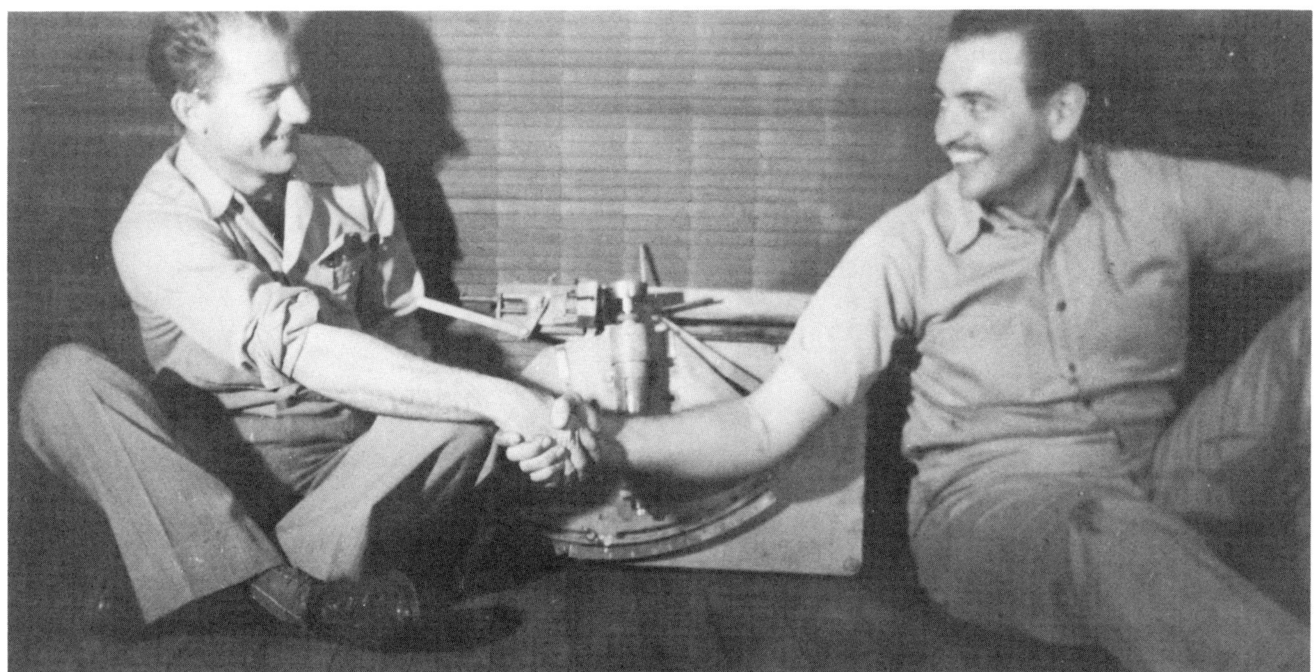

At this time Bill Coburn was selling his only product, a pitch blocker also developed at Fluegge Optical. He had purchased the patents and all rights to the Suddarth generator for $10,000 *(to be paid from future sales)*, hired Suddarth and ultimately produced a line of generators. His first generator was a desk-top model with coolant in a drawer that pulled out from the front of the machine. This primitive machine sprayed coolant in such a random way that, within minutes of turning it on, the operator would be sodden with coolant oil from head to toe. Virtually handmade, it was crude and unattractive but it worked. It was so much better than roughing by

hand, labs lined up to order them. Coburn's first model sold for $600 at a time when Shuron charged $3,600 for their more sophisticated unit.

The desk top generator didn't last long and was soon replaced by larger and more reliable models. Both Coburn and Shuron generators used diamond wheels and produced spherical and cylindrical prescriptions in seconds on either front or back surface, completely revolutionizing laboratory production. Diamond tools had been tried in a few cases, using special hand pans with high speed spindles and heavy-duty motors but the skill

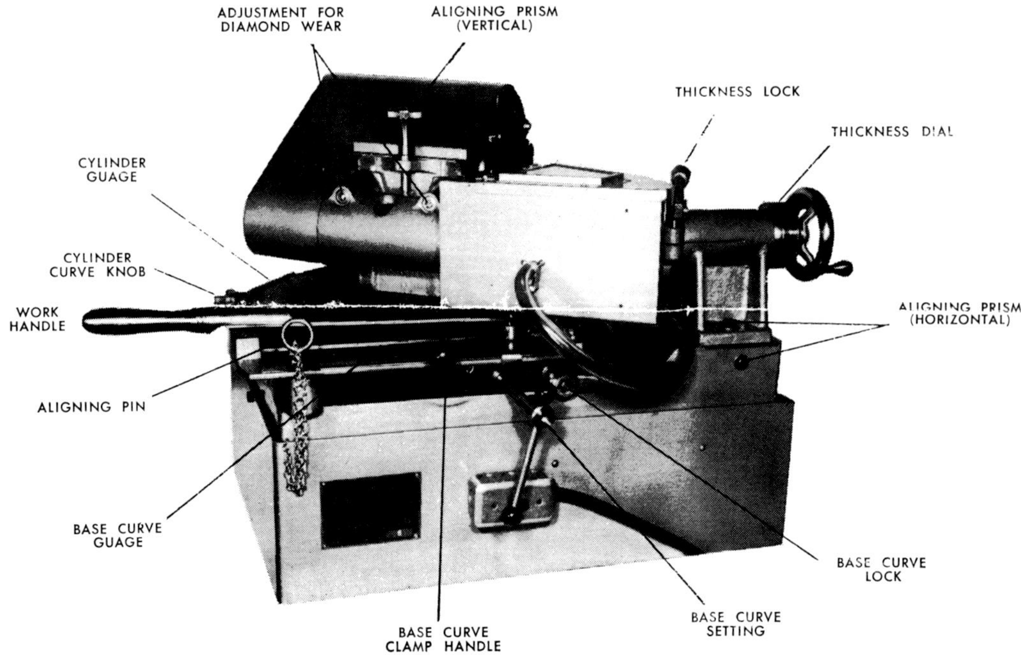

*The first generator produced
from Suddarth's design was
this early Coburn generator,
the first in a long line of lens
generating machines
produced by that company.*

OLA OPTICAL INDUSTRY MUSEUM

of a highly experienced workman was still required. Coburn promptly proved at the Optical Wholesalers Association Convention in Chicago in 1956 that his generators could be operated by anyone, in this case, young, inexperienced *(in lab work)* women. Those present at that convention will never forget the sight of four attractive young ladies, each dressed in white shorts and shirts with the Coburn Rocket emblazoned on their backs, turning out lenses on Coburn generators. Women were almost unheard of in laboratories of that day, certainly never in a surface room and, other than wives, were seldom found at lab conventions. With one dramatic gesture, Coburn established that unskilled workers could produce reasonably precise lenses. Finishing these generated lenses required nothing more than a short fining operation and a much quicker polish. Hand-roughed lenses were seldom exactly on curve *(especially cylinders)* and always required a good deal of fining before they could be polished. Suddenly all that was in the past - the modern laboratory had come of age!

What may have established Coburn's generator as much as anything was a story that was told and retold, from coast to coast. The story was that, during a meeting of the Southwest Association of Optical Suppliers held in Texas, Bill Coburn got involved in a crap game with a few lab boys. At some point during the evening, Coburn bet one of his generators against the pot - and lost! The winner was Ed Dietz, Sr., partners with Ray McLean in Dietz-McLean Optical. The generator Dietz won was sent to a Dietz & Dillard laboratory in Temple, Texas, a branch later sold to Dietz-McLean Optical. That generator is still used today and is the machine on which Drake McLean *(Ray's grandson)* learned to make lenses. Shuron personnel always claimed Coburn lost the bet just for the publicity. People who knew what an inveterate gambler Bill Coburn was claim he never lost a bet on purpose in his life.

Coburn and Shuron generators performed the same function in relatively the same manner but were able to avoid each others' patents by accomplishing the actual grinding in different ways. Coburn's generator passed the diamond wheel in front of a stationary lens. Shuron took the opposite tact and passed the lens in front of a stationary diamond wheel. Shuron's generator was built by an experienced machine tool company, Cincinnati Milling Machine and, as a consequence, was sturdier and more professionally-built. It was considerably more expensive than Coburn's and required interpretation by the operator in making settings based on millimeter scales from a set of tables supplied with the machine. Coburn's, on the other hand, enabled the operator to make direct settings, using the actual Base Curve and Cross Curve, expressed in familiar diopters. Both

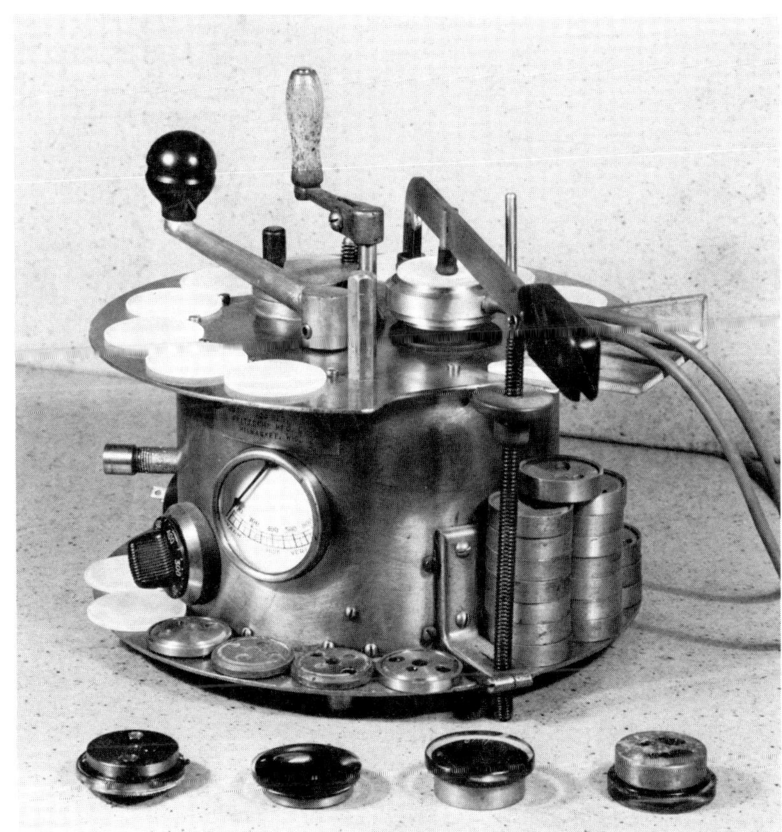

The first attempt to automate the messy and labor-intensive blocking operation was this unit produced by Fred Fritzsche of Milwaukee. The rights to this device were purchased by O.W. Coburn and this blocker served as the foundation of Coburn Optical.

machines used mechanical chucks that would hold a steel or bronze block to which the lens was adhered by pitch, later replaced by alloy.

About this same time, American Optical introduced their generator which was somewhat smaller and used a vacuum chucking system. After an initial introduction, AO generators were sold only to AO branches domestically and to international customers. B&L also developed a generator for their branches. It was a monster, filling an entire room, and was only installed in one or two branches, one of them being Chicago. It was never developed commercially.

Responding to Coburn's keen competition, Shuron developed a new, direct system of machine setting. It used a Quick-Set plate enabling the operator to set desired diopter powers on the scale, adjusting the generator to the correct power by viewing a target through a coaxial peep sight. Soon Shuron's 290B *(The "B" indicated the unit was equipped with Quick Set)* gave way to the 390 which offered an automatic sweep feature. Other, more sophisticated models, the 490 and 790, were released but were never very successful.

Coburn, meanwhile, added a semiautomatic sweep feature *(108B)* and proceeded to develop the Dial-O-

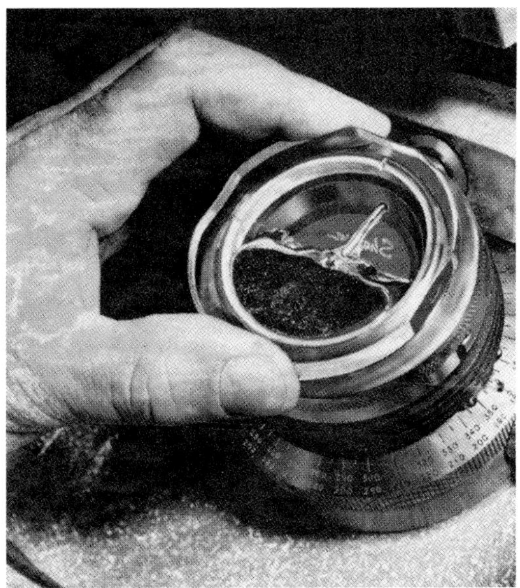

Eventually, pitch blocking was replaced by alloy blocking, using a low-melting metal alloy. Photo shows alloy being pumped between the lens blank and the block.

OLA OPTICAL INDUSTRY MUSEUM

Matic *(or 113)* generator, the first truly automated machine for optical laboratories. This unit featured potentiometers, hydraulics, and other up-to-date machinery innovations. In recent years it was followed by the 112, 120, 130, and other sophisticated, computer-operated models.

Blocking

Using pitch for fastening lenses to blocks was always a dirty job and often allowed the lens to drop off in the generator chamber, ruining the lens and sometimes the diamond wheel. A better blocking method was needed. Coburn had developed the 98 blocker as a mechanized means of applying pitch for mounting a lens for surfacing. Prior to that, pitch was heated over a flame and dripped over the lens and blocked by hand, usually burning the operator's fingers and frequently deblocking in the process. Coburn's 98 blocker enabled the user to heat the pitch in an electrically heated pot and inject it between lens and block by means of a small hand pump. This was ultimately replaced by the 99 blocker which substituted a metal alloy that melted at 158 degrees Fahrenheit, accomplishing the same thing but without the dirt and danger of pitch. Alloy blocking was considered a marvelous improvement at the time it came out and no one gave any thought to the possibility that the high lead content might be a hazard to employees. Today, the industry is searching for a viable replacement for alloy blocking because of the hazards associated with alloy.

Shuron and AO developed alloy blockers as well, producing all-alloy blocks required by their vacuum chucking systems. These blockers enabled the user to dial in any required prism. Coburn's system created prism through a series of prism rings, fiber or metal, placed between the blocked lens and the generator chuck to create the desired angle. "Prism blockers" made it easier to dial in prism but sometimes produced unwanted prism. In recent years, other suppliers have developed blockers that enable operators to block a lens so that the prescription is generated on the true optical center *(i.e. the center of all optical factors)* but is fined and polished on true mechanical center, the actual center of the lens as determined by mechanical measurement.

Tools/Laps

A requisite of good laboratories has always been properly trued lens tools. Tools, originally made of cast iron, were very heavy, and wore down quickly since they tended to be ground away by the same abrasives that ground the lenses. When only spherical tools were involved, this wear was not critical since the wear was symmetrical and only made the tool thinner without changing the curves. With an increasing use of cylindrical tools, however, tool truing became more difficult since all truing had to be done by hand, through use of files or other abrasive tools.

In 1919, STOCO discovered that a machine developed by famous race car driver Barney Oldfield for producing overhead cams for racing engines could be adapted to cut optical cylinder tools. The STOCO 10A Oldfield Lap Cutter was introduced to universal acclaim from lab operators. AO later introduced their 401 Tool Cutter and B&L developed one enabling laboratories to equip their labs with cylinder tools trued as accurately as desired. It was not until the late 1950s that Coburn introduced the 301 Lap Cutter, but this was a significant development because it reduced tool cutting time from 45 to 15 minutes. This was followed by the 302 which reduced that time to less than six minutes. Strasbaugh Company also offered two different models of high speed lens truers and other companies soon offered their own tool cutters as well.

Laps *(iron tools cut to curves that produce the desired powers)* were offered, after an initial period of confusing varieties, in two basic styles: conical base tools which everyone used for spherical tools and AO also used for their cylinder machines and flatback tools, which fit all B&L, Shuron and Robinson-Houchin cylinder machines. Adapters enabled labs to accommodate either style lap to the other type of machine. With the advent of plastic lenses, it was quickly apparent that iron tools retained too much heat that could aberrate CR-39 lenses. Aluminum tools were found to work better and also worked well for glass lenses, particularly since they could be covered during fining and polishing operations with appropriate pads to minimize tool wear. Laps were always covered with pads for polishing in any case. Aluminum tools were also easier on cylinder machines, which by this time had become fairly sophisticated with movement in the vertical spindle holding the tool as well as movement of the upper spindle - both oscillating in "figure 8" motions. Aluminum also minimized machine wear because of the tool's lighter weight. Lapping tools have become increasingly larger to accommodate today's larger lens blanks. Various plastics have also been used for producing tools *(sometimes on a throwaway basis after limited usage)*.

Cylinder machines made significant advances in 1971 with the introduction of Coburn's 504, a four spindle machine that featured movement of both the upper spindle *(holding the lens against the tool by air pressure)* and the lower spindle, decreasing time required for fining or polishing. This machine worked equally well for plastic or glass except the rubber baffles protecting the vertical spindles from the slurry were cut by glass particles and leaked badly, corroding bearings located under the spindle and rusting parts. OLA member Tom Mitchott, then with Columbian Bifocal, Portland, Oregon, decided that tilting the 504 eliminated this problem and, in this way, the 505 *(2 spindle)* and 506 *(4 spindle)* machines were created. These models, variations and copies, are industry standards today, produced by a variety of machinery manufacturers.

Surfacing Tape

A major innovation was offered by the 3M Company who had developed a pressure-sensitive tape that, when applied to a plastic lens and sometimes even glass lenses by use of a vacuum machine developed by 3M, would protect the lens from scratches during blocking and processing. This protection is used internationally today for all plastic lens production.

Layout Markers

Layout markers were designed to enable surface or finishing departments to "layout" or mark lenses for proper positioning before grinding. They started out as hand-drawn systems, then printed protractors on which each lens would be laid out, positioned and marked by hand. Soon mechanical devices were developed which backlit the protractor for easier viewing. Then markers came out that would apply the required dots or lines on the lens with an automatic inking device, identifying the optical center and the necessary axis lines for surfacing. Shuron, AO, and Coburn all offered variations on the same theme. Today's markers are more sophisticated but basically perform the same task, often aided by computer calculations which input all required information direct to the generator.

Computers

In recent years, computers have been increasingly used in laboratories for surface and finishing calculations as well as for pricing and billing. With the ability of computers to perform marketing, management, and statistical tasks, labs have become increasingly dependent on these electronic devices. Fifty years ago, only two people were essential when opening a laboratory. One for surface layout *(with the ability to rock in cylinders)* and another for finish layout. Those technicians did the

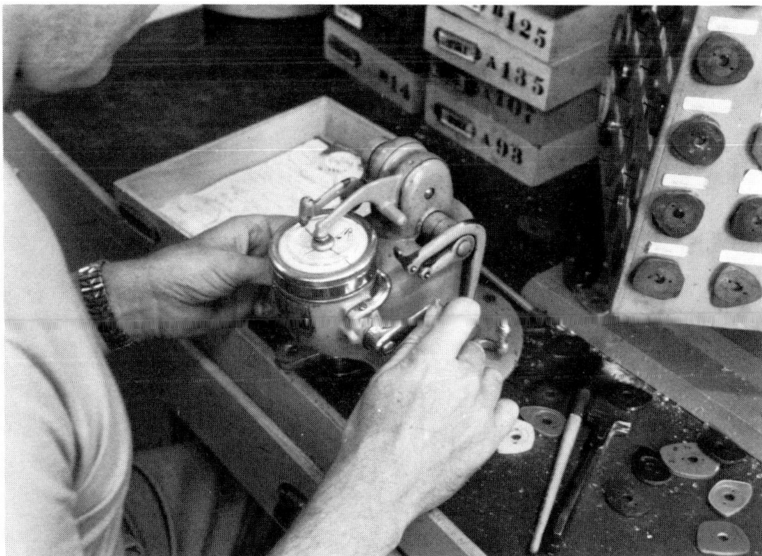

Here is the Shuron Lens Cutter in use. This simple, highly efficient unit could be found in almost every wholesale and retail lab in the country, far outselling competitive cutters.

necessary calculations in their head. As lenses became more sophisticated and equipment more technical, lens calculations required special layout calculating machines. Later a few computer companies came out with effective programs and layout computers grew in popularity. As the capabilities of computer programs improved, computers became more essential to laboratories. Today virtually every lab of any size relies on computers for billing and accounting functions as well as providing management statistical and sales information. In many labs, Rx data entered in the computer at the time the job enters the lab, controls each machine as it works on those lenses.

Lens Cutters

Uncut glass lenses were originally processed by scribing the lens by hand with the shape of the frame or mounting, using a diamond tipped tool or steel scribe. The resultant scored lens would then have the excess glass chipped away by hand, using special chipping pliers and leaving the lens slightly oversize in the approximate desired size and shape for finishing on ceramic edging wheels. Then lens cutters were designed that used a steel lens pattern to cut the lens to the pattern shape, using a diamond point or a cutting wheel, much like a glass cutter. Cutting was a vital step between finish layout and edging during the time that all lenses were glass. Plastic lenses, of course, go directly to edging without cutting to shape.

Edging Equipment

Edging of lenses originally used ceramic wheels, first turned by hand, then by foot pedals, then belt drives and eventually electric motors. Before World War I, AO, B&L, and Shuron were able to automate the edging process by including chucks to hold the lens above, or in front of,

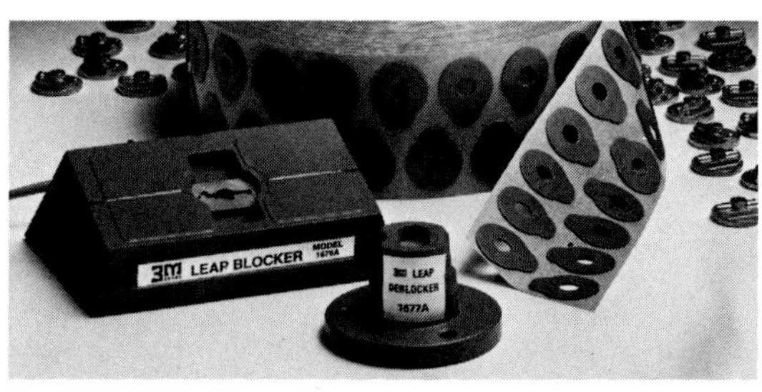

The 3M LEAP blocking system for edging, with its adhesive pads, revolutionized lens edging and eliminated one of the most common problems in edging lenses - lens slippage and off-axis lenses.

the edging wheels. These holders would rotate the lens as the wheel turned producing a finished lens of the desired diameter and shape. Shape was controlled by a pattern, or cam, placed at the end of the rotating lens spindle. Size of the finished lens was determined by a dial indicator wheel. After World War II, special ceramic wheels were developed with V grooves that would edge lenses to shape, leaving them with a beveled edge. This enabled lab technicians to eliminate most hand beveling, although metal frames still required a lot of hand sizing.

In the early 1950's, three brothers, Arnold, Irving, and Ted Stern lost interest in their father's non-optical diamond wheel manufacturing business and devoted their talents to developing an automatic diamond edging machine to replace the ceramic wheels used up to that time. They formed AIT Industries in Skokie, Illinois and introduced automatic diamond edging to the industry. Their bevel machine was easy to use and produced a finished lens from an uncut plastic lens in less than two minutes. They also produced a line of diamond wheels for a variety of other optical machines. Their edgers became so popular, they ultimately accounted for 72 percent of all American edger sales by 1980. American Optical produced an edger that simply adapted diamond wheels to its old ceramic machine. Shuron produced a ceramic bevel edger with a large, bowl shaped wheel for beveling. When that proved to be less than successful, the company began distributing machines made by Weco of Germany, a company owned by Textron, Shuron's parent company at that time.

Coburn produced a lens edger *(2001)* which effectively generated an edge curve on a slanted wheel but it was difficult and cumbersome to use. Their 202 and 203, with variations, were eventually replaced by Weco edgers when Shuron sold their machinery division to CMV. Bevel edgers are now available from a wide variety of companies, some domestic and many foreign. No one company today has ever been able to capture as large a share of the American market as AIT once enjoyed.

In the early 1980's National Optronics *(started by a former controller of AIT)* introduced a fluted carbide cutter edger that is widely used for CR39 and polycarbonate edging. Router edging has been adopted by other manufacturers in recent years. Polycarbonate lenses have captured an increasing share of the market and "router" type edgers helped make this possible.

Edging Tape

3M made another major contribution to the industry by developing a two-sided adhesive tape called LEAP for attaching a lens to an edging block for holding the lens in edgers. This system replaced the previous alloy blocking which, in turn, had replaced pressure blocking. It is interesting to note that edgers in most other countries to this day use a vacuum chucking system featuring a simple suction cup. AO tried this vacuum chucking for years but it was only accepted in their own branches.

Hand ceramic edgers are still frequently used for removing the starry edge effect created by most diamond wheels. Fine diamond hand stones are also used for this purpose.

PATTERN MAKERS

During the years up to the 1950s, most frame manufacturers provided durable steel patterns for edging lenses to their frames. As the variety of frames began to grow, less expensive plastic patterns became the prevailing custom. Frame styles continued to proliferate and, before long, the number of patterns required in laboratories became simply overwhelming. It became apparent that "bench operations" needed to be able to produce custom patterns to supplement those supplied by frame manufacturers. Dr. Ezra Novak, a Los Angeles optometrist, developed a design for the first successful pattern maker and had it made exclusively for his company, Novamatic, by Takubo in Japan. For many years, this was the only pattern maker available and it still serves as the industry standard. Shuron and Weco both developed reasonable variations of the Novamatic model. In recent years, computer-operated pattern makers have been developed but digitally-controlled edgers are increasingly being used, especially in laboratories. Frames to be used are traced, sometimes by the lab, sometimes by the customer. This digitized information is stored in the lab computer and called up electronically by the edger when the lens is ready for edging. Patternless edgers represent the future for lens edging.

Heat Treating/Chem Tempering

With the passage of the Federal Drug Administration regulations in 1970 which mandated tempering of all glass lenses, every finishing lab was required to install heat-treating ovens. These were produced by Coburn, Shuron, Precision-Cosmet and by Kirk who offered a less expensive version. Other units became available as well and, before long chemical tempering units began to appear. Chemical tempering required a 16 hour process *(as opposed to just a few minutes in a heat-tempering oven)* but enabled labs to put a whole day's production

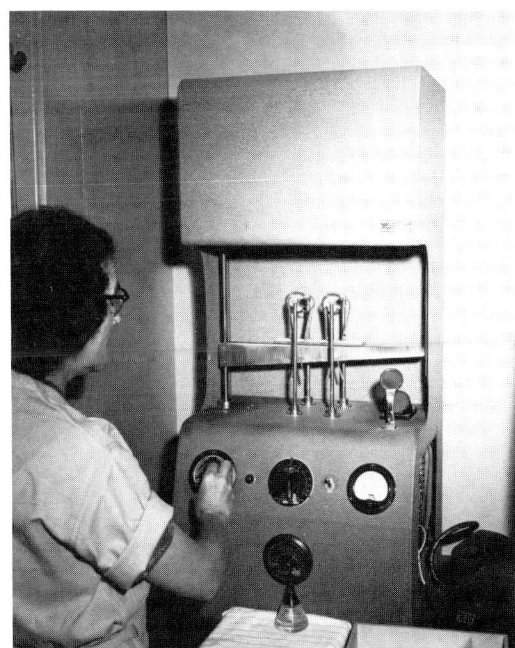

Most labs had long used heat treating units for tempering industrial eyewear, but once the FDA rule went into effect, they were mandatory for all glass lenses. Units like this model, produced by Precision Cosmet (a subsidiary of Benson Optical) were soon added to every lab's equipment. Eventually, a chemical tempering process was developed and labs switched over to this more efficient process, reserving heat-treating only for rush jobs.

worlds apart from the lenses produced in labs just 50 years ago. Their optics are more precise and the new substrate materials for ophthalmic lenses are producing lighter, thinner and more protective eyewear. One hundred years ago, eyewear was only for the wealthy. George Washington Wells' vision was eyeglasses for the masses. He was largely responsible for making that happen but even he would be amazed to see how far we've come in the past 100 years.

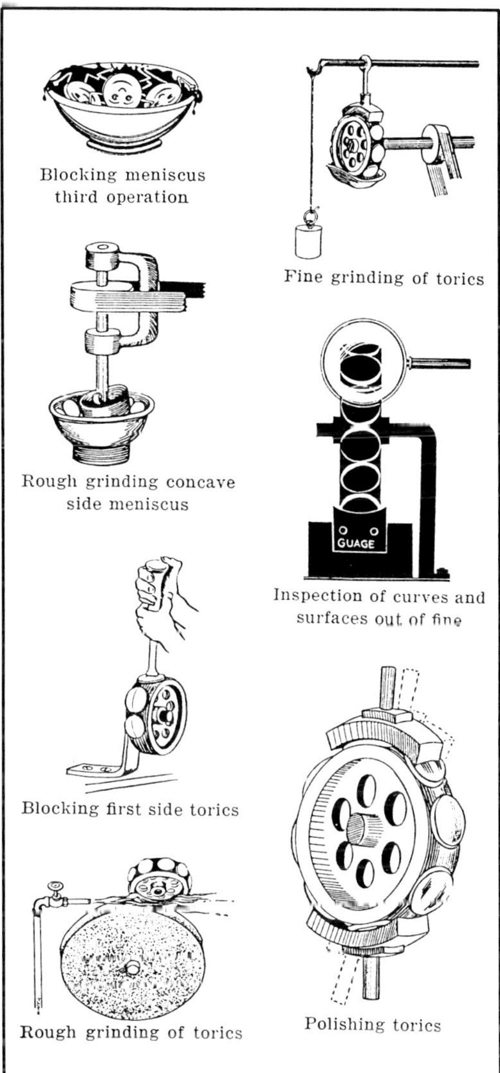

Mass Producing Glass Lenses

The system developed to mass-produce glass lenses was relatively crude but created reasonably accurate lenses. To grind the inside spherical curve, lenses were blocked in a bowl whose radius matched the desired curve. The first lenses were basically flat because many more could be placed in each bowl. Converting to six base reduced the number of lenses in each bowl and increased cost (drawings show meniscus lenses). A reversed bowl was used for the other side of spherical lenses. Cylinders required a huge grind stone, shaped to the desired cross curve. The radius of the wheel holding the lenses determined the base curve. Producing lenses this way was a slow, labor-intensive process that worked reasonably well. Eventually, in the 1940's, generators replaced the rough grinding process.

in one or more units. Chem-tempering also generally produces a stronger lens than heat-treating. Photochromatic glass required special time cycles in both tempering and chemical ovens. This meant at least two chemical *ovens (or dual units)* but the same tempering unit could be adjusted for any type of glass required. The chemical process was complicated by litigation based on a patent which required royalty payments by anyone using the process.

The future of optical machinery may be indicated by several new processes. One was introduced by Gerber, a stranger to the optical industry. It includes a computer-ized router-type lens generator that can cut any plastic lens or a surfacing tool to precise curves. These units are not much larger than edgers and eliminate layout as well since the prescription, already in the lab's computer, totally directs the generator operation. Coburn and National Optronics have introduced similar type generators.

The other new development is robotic lab equipment. LOH Optical Machinery is currently delivering robotic lab equipment that may well represent the future for labs. One laboratory in Germany is presently operating a completely robotic laboratory with only a few workers.

Lenses produced today in the average laboratory are

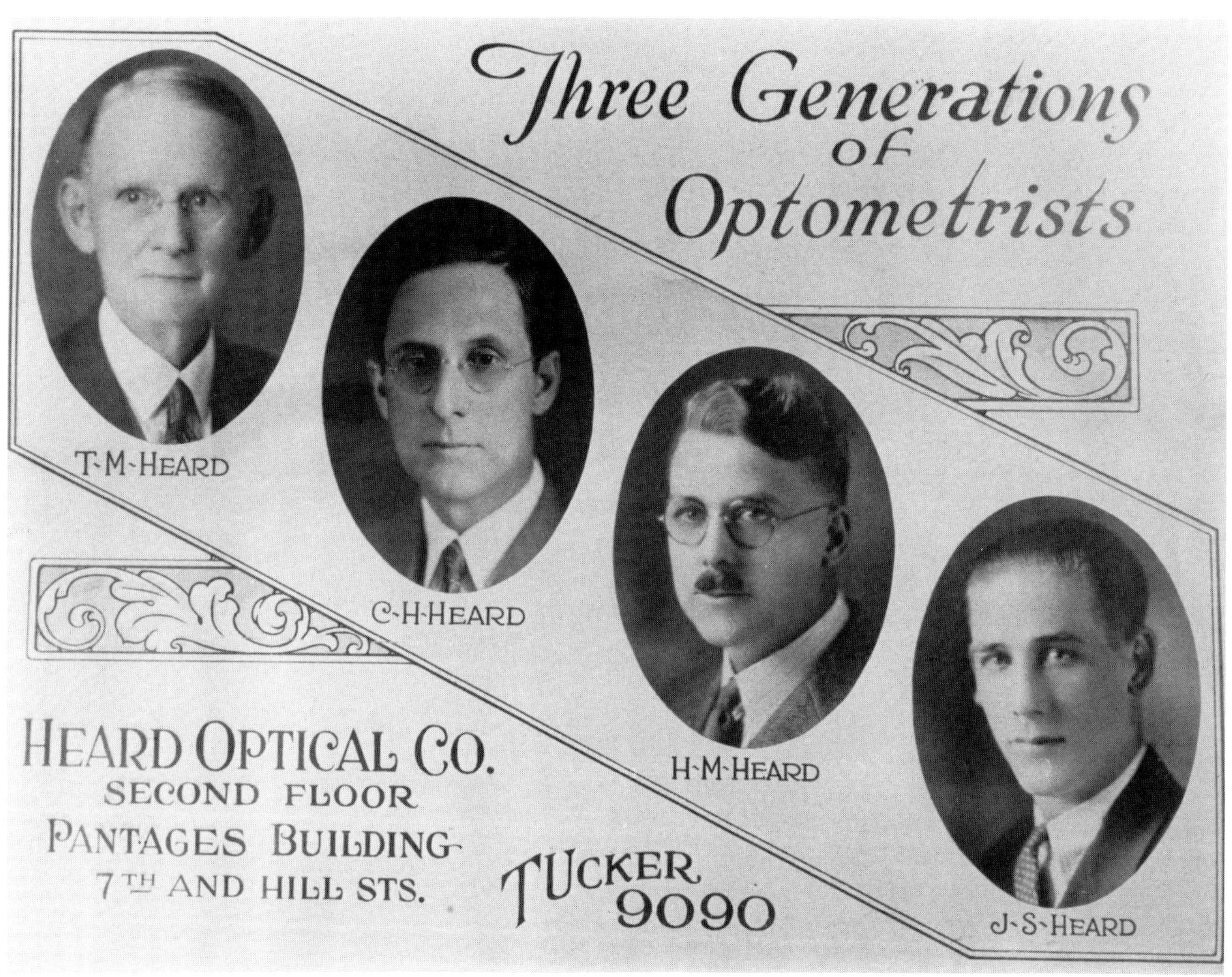

PHOTO – HOWARD HEARD FAMILY

In this chapter, T.M. Heard, an early optician, tells how he became interested in eyeglasses and vision, two subjects that were to become his life's work. He had three sons, one of whom became an oculist and the other two were optometrists. His son C.H. Heard was the first student and first graduate of the Los Angeles School of Optometry (1904-05), known today as the Southern California College of Optometry. C.H. had two sons, H. Marsalen Heard, graduated as an optometrist from Los Angeles Medical School of Ophthalmology and Optometry in 1922 and Joseph S. Heard, an optician who founded Heard Optical Company, today a major wholesale laboratory in California. H. M. Heard's son, Howard Heard is an optician who was a Trustee and staff member of So. California College of Optometry for years. Howard has three sons, each of whom is also in the optical business. T.M. Heard also had a son who practiced as an oculist in Iowa.

Chapter 12
Refracting Opticians

In July, 1928, the following memories were written for his son by pioneer refractionist Thomas M. Heard. Eighty three years old at the time he tells his story, Mr. Heard's personal experiences dramatically illustrate, in a very human way, the state of the fledgling industry and the optical professions during that period when he developed and honed his fascination with the human eye (1860-1900). Here, one man's personal story graphically illustrates how a simple trade that started as not much more than a barter system was gradually transformed into the three eyecare professions we know today. His story begins in 1865 as he is discharged at the age of 20 from the Grand Army of the Republic at the end of the Civil War.

Mr. Heard's Story

"Less than sixty years have passed since the first attempt was made to lengthen the life and usefulness of the human eye. We should stop and recall that eighty years ago, a man or woman having reached the age of fifty whose occupation required good eye sight, they were compelled to give up their work for the lack of proper glasses and were classed as old people. If they did find a pair of glasses they could use, they were the crudest form of frames and the lenses were known as magnifiers.

After being discharged from the army in 1865, I became interested in the study of medicine. In order to obtain an education in this profession, I went to work for a doctor living in the central part of Ohio. I took care of his horse and buggy and did odd chores around the place, for which I received two dollars a week and had the privilege of studying from the doctor's books, helping to mix up pills and accompany him when he was called to the bed side of the sick.

This Doctor was considered one of the most learned men of his time and took quite an interest in me, teaching and imparting to me his knowledge of the human body. I recall many times the great difficulty he had to read, being unable to obtain any glasses that would help him. He tried many different pairs obtained from the drug store, but they always made his eyes smart and burn. I soon formed the habit of reading to him for hours at a time. One cold winter evening as I read to him by candle light, I said, "Doctor, what is the matter with your eyes, they do not look sore, yet you can hardly read any more." He said, "If they were sore, I would soon cure them. They are simply wearing out, they are old eyes." Yet, he was only fifty seven. This noted doctor was able to explain everything about the human body excepting the eyes. I could never find one word in any book in his library that told how the eyes functioned. It was no wonder that this good old Doctor could not answer my questions.

While still with this Doctor, I was quietly inquiring of two other doctors living this same town, asking if they knew how I could obtain a book on the eyes. One said he had never heard of such a book. The other said, "Why there is nothing wonderful about the eyes, there's no need of a book". I replied "Yes, but a lot of people that have well eyes cannot see". "Oh, well", he said, "They can buy a pair of magnifying glasses". When I mentioned that the Doctor I was studying under could not find a pair he could see with, he replied, "Well, don't you know why? He has worn his eyes out by too much reading. A great many persons do the same thing. No help for them."

I told the Doctor I was going to leave him and work in

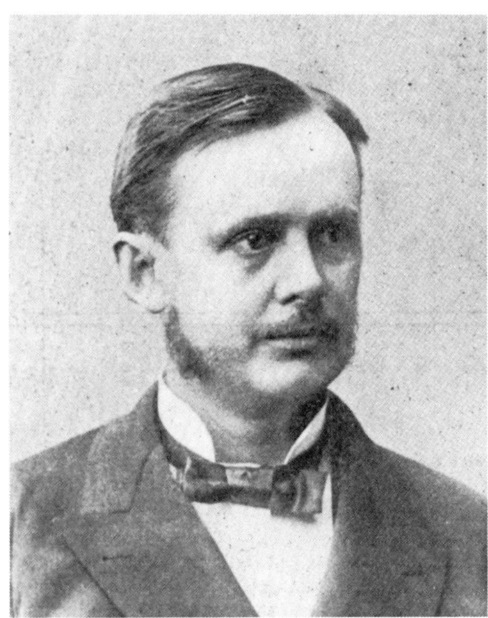

T. M. Heard. This photo appeared on the first page of his famous book "T.M. Heard's Book on the Eye", published in 1885. Thousands of these booklets were sold during lectures presented in various cities around the country.

the drug store and learn what I could about fitting people with spectacles, he said, "Tom, young fool, the less you know about eyes, the more chance you will have to sell spectacles". I had a long talk with the druggist who thought I was crazy, telling me they did not sell enough spectacles in a year to pay me what the doctor paid me in three months.

It seems strange to me after all these years I should be writing this story of the early struggles of my profession, now known as Optometry, for my son, grandson and great grandson, making four generations. When I look back over all these years (I trust you gentle reader, will pardon the musings of an old man for just a minute) and recall my early struggles to obtain some knowledge of the human eye. When I told the Doctor I was leaving to work in the drug store and learn what I could about fitting people with spectacles, he said, "Tom, young fool, the less you know about eyes, the more chance you will have to sell spectacles".

"The first week I had an old farmer come in to buy a pair of spectacles. I rushed back to the druggist and asked how I would know which pair to sell him. The answer came back, "He won't want you to tell him what pair to buy, he will buy the pair he can see with." I rushed back to my customer and sure enough, he was trying on one pair after another. "Can you find a pair you can read with?" I asked. He said, "Oh yes, I guess so, but I want them for my wife. What kind do you usually sell to the women folk?" that was a sticker, so I called the druggist. He agreed to let the farmer take several pairs for his wife to try, promising to return in a few days. That was the beginning of four generations of Optometrists."

When the druggist's stock of spectacles were almost exhausted, young Heard convinced the local jeweler that profits could be made from spectacles. The jeweler ordered a sizable stock but it took six months before the shipment came in from Germany. By that time, the jeweler decided he had made a bad investment. In desperation, he agreed to let young Tom take the inventory and pay for the stock as he sold it.

Young Tom Continues . . .

"I canvassed the town from end to end with mighty poor success. I soon made up my mind if I could work my way thru the country to some larger towns, I miIght be able to find someone that knew about eyes. I made up a pack like I used to carry in the army and, before leaving town, I called on my old friend the doctor. How he did laugh at me standing before him with my pack on my back and carrying an old carpet bag containing all my earthly possessions. When I told him I was going to find someone that knew about eyes, he said, "Tom, better take along a stock of tinware. You won't sell enough specs to pay for your keep. You'll starve to death." Well, I pretty darn near did. I met with some success and kept on traveling thru the country.

I would frequently meet people living in remote parts of the country, far from any towns who did not know what spectacles were for. What do you do with them, they would ask. They're to read with, I would answer. Often they would answer that if I had a pair they could read with, they would buy them. They'd try on pair after pair until they finally told me I didn't have a pair in my whole stock they could read with. When I asked if they could read, the answer would be that if they knew how to read they wouldn't need a pair of my blamed specs! So I went traveling mile after mile, learning something every day.

The first real city I was ever in was Cleveland, Ohio and when I reached this city I was tired and discouraged with very little money and the need to replenish my stock and my clothes. I found several stores that sold spectacles and when I told those dealers I was traveling thru the country selling to farmers, they very kindly told me where I could order new inventory. When I tried to find out what they knew about fitting glasses, it was the same old story. People fitted themselves by picking out the pair they could see with the best.

I always felt sure there was more to be learned about eyes than just trying on glasses. Many times I found people who knew how to read but couldn't see because I didn't have a pair that would magnify the type large enough. I saw many chances to make a handsome profit if I only had the right kind of glasses to sell. It was not unusual to run across persons that wore two pair of spectacles, one pair on top of the other to have them magnify enough.

I kept on traveling and in the early fall of 1869 arrived in the city of Boston, considered at this time to be the very seat of knowledge. Surely I would find someone here who could instruct me in the fitting of glasses. Again, I found it the same as in Philadelphia, New York and other large cities I had visited. To be sure, I found several large jobbing houses that handled spectacles and eyeglasses, but none made any pretense of any knowledge of how to fit the eyes with the glasses they sold. They were simply merchants and dealers in ready-made spectacles, eyeglasses and carried a small stock of telescopes, microscopes, magic lanterns, surgical instruments and other gimcracks or novelties imported from England, Germany, France and Austria. The spectacle part of their business was a side line.

It was in Boston, I was awakened to the fact that no one knew anything about the refraction of the human eye. It came about in this manner. I was browsing in the largest wholesale house in Boston when I overheard a conversation between two of the employees as follows: "Say, where do you think this Heard fellow picked up his knowledge about the eye. We ought to wise up to him and learn all we can." I was surprised to think that any one should think I knew anything about eyes, especially the very people I expected to teach me.

When I was not hustling around Boston selling spectacles, I would visit different doctors. I formed the habit of reading what books and papers that I found lying around their reception rooms. One day I made a real discovery, an article in a medical paper about a doctor named Donders living in Europe who had written a book on fitting the eyes with glasses. His statements in the book were very drastic and were not taken seriously by other noted European doctors. I was very much interested and anxious to obtain a copy.

When I asked others about Donders, no one had ever heard of him and did not think the book would amount to anything. I finally wrote to him, asking about his book and if he would send me a copy. I was almost certain the book was just what I needed and realized that even if the Doctor answered my letter, it would be a long time before I could hope to get a reply. Then began a long tedious wait. I kept close to the town, making a meager living, hoping against hope to get a reply. Can you, my reader, realize my great delight upon at last receiving a letter from the Doctor telling me he was sending me a copy of his book. He hoped I would study the book carefully, thus become able to help many persons prolong their usefulness with the aid of properly fitted lenses.

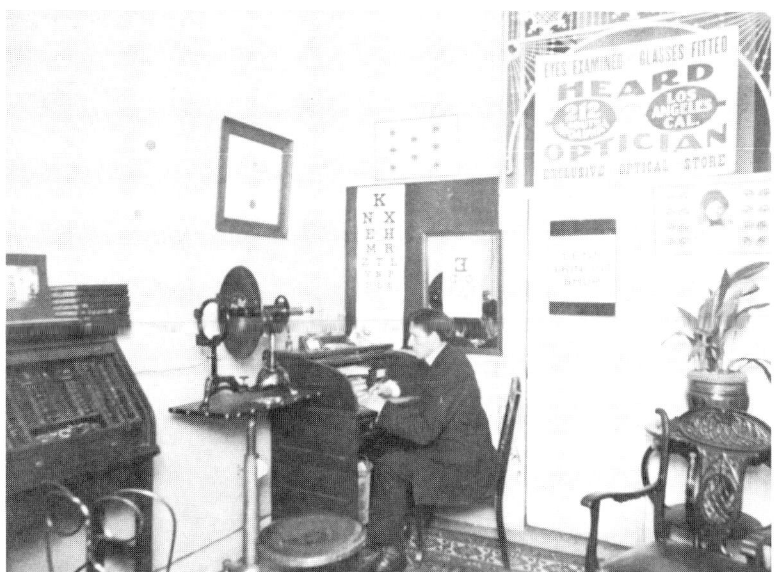

Photo was taken in the early 1900's of C.H. Heard's office in Long Beach.

Donders stated he was presenting to the people of the world a new idea, people reaching the age of fifty need no longer fear they would have to give up their occupation on account of not being able to see. He also stated that after I studied his book carefully, and wanted any further information, to write him and he would do his best to instruct me. I hardly ate or slept for the next six weeks. I kept studying my book night and day for at last I had found what I wanted. The world was mine!

Danders' book was the first book written that really taught the method of prescribing lenses to correct optical defects of the eye, now known as Optometry. The principals laid down in this book are the same now as they were then. Doctor Donders' book is used in every school in the country where ever Optometry is taught. I continued to study this book for the next five years, in fact, was still studying it when I retired from the profession." (See section "The World's Most Influential Optical Book").

"Within five years after this book was published, many changes began to take place and the usefulness of

---

THE WORLD'S MOST INFLUENTIAL OPTICAL BOOK

In 1864, a textbook was published in Holland that would come to influence thousands of individuals in the burgeoning ophthalmic field all over the world. The book's subject was physiological optics and was titled "Accommodation and Refraction of the Eye." It was written by a Dutch eye physician named F.C. Donders. Dr. Donders was proficient in speaking and writing in French, English and German. Reference to his influential book is found several times in this history. The book revolutionized ophthalmology and provided an explanation of the defects of refraction and accommodation. The book had greater influence in the United States than in Europe. Many European physicians claimed to have no interest in Dr. Donders' subject.

In Ohio, however, a young optician named Heard, wanting to learn more about fitting the eyes with glasses, wrote to Dr. Donders and obtained a copy. This book is referred to in several chapters of this history.

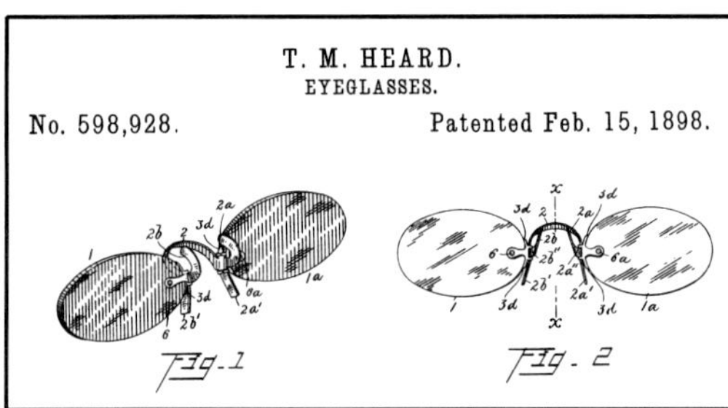

This was another of T.M. Heard's patented mountings.

many persons were prolonged by the aid of properly fitted glasses. I began to meet with great success after studying this book and returned to Ohio as I had acquired knowledge beyond my fondest expectations. On returning to the small town I had left six years previous, I called upon my old friend the Doctor who had told me the less I knew about eyes, the better success I would have selling specs. I had the great pleasure of examining his eyes and fitting him with the first pair of glasses he had ever been able to read with for any length of time. These lenses were strong cylinders and were made in Europe and required four months to get them.

The optical business at this time was in a terrible condition, the spectacle makers of Europe manufactured only one size and shape and were mostly black and blue frames with little bit of lenses. And Europe being the only place they could be obtained, it took several months to get them and, when received, they were more often wrong than right.

I settled in a small town in Ohio and bought a horse and buggy and started out to teach the people the necessity of having their eyes examined for glasses instead of picking out a pair that magnified. Money was scarce and I frequently had to take in exchange, butter, eggs, potatoes or anything they had in exchange for my spectacles. I soon found that people were willing to come to me for glasses, so I quit the road and opened an office in Warren, Ohio."

Dr. Heard later moved to Cleveland and opened the first office in that city for what he called "the scientific examination of the refractive requirements of the human eye". During this period *(mid 1870s)* he still called himself an optician and he tells of jealousy among the competitors.

"The word Doctor was not used or thought of at this time. I decided that it would be well to use the word Scientific Optician and that was the first time the word scientific was used in connection with the optical business, but it was not long before it was adopted by all engaged exclusively in fitting of glasses. It was about this time the first wholesale optical house was opened in Cleveland and many men now became engaged in selling spectacles and would try in numerous ways to find out how I examined eyes. Often they would come in to have me examine their eyes and from their many questions, I would tell them I was on to them. I would ask if the wholesale house sent them to me. They would invariable say "Yes" and try to bargain for me to teach them the business.

In order for the wholesale houses to sell optical goods, they soon found it necessary to give lessons on how to fit eyes and would call on jewelers and offer to teach them how to fit eyes if they would buy a stock of spectacles. From that time on, jewelers added the word optician to their names, such as John Smith, Jeweler and Optician. I think this did more to retard the advance of the science of optics than anything that had occurred until then. The jewelers did not know anything about fitting the eyes and only received enough instructions to sell specs. It soon gave a "black-eye" to the business and brought into the field doctors who treated diseased or sore eyes and who thought they were the logical person to furnish glasses.

So the wholesale houses, in order to obtain a greater out-put for their wares, began to instruct the doctors how to fit eyes. All the wholesalers asked the doctors to do was buy a test-case and set of test-cards and then write down the prescription for what they thought the person needed. The doctor would then send the patient to the wholesale house where they bought the glasses that they thought the doctor had ordered. The wholesale house would charge the person bringing in the order the wholesale price and send back the difference to the doctor. This soon became so great a business that the doctors did not really do any fitting, just made a few figures on a paper and sent them to the wholesale house where some slick clerk who knew something about the business would really do the fitting.

It was not infrequent in the early days to pay the doctors anywhere from five to ten dollars a head for each person sent to the wholesale houses. Not unlike it is done today, only now doctors really do send a prescription with the patient and they receive a rebate of all moneys received above the wholesale prices plus one dollar for dispensing."

> (Editor's note: Rebating profits to the oculist when the laboratory dispensed eyeglasses was a common practice during the 1920's, 30's and 40's, until stopped by the Federal Government.)

"It is a far jump from the old split bifocal lenses invented by Benjamin Franklin to the new invisible bifocal used today (Editor's note: Heard is referring to fused bifocals, considered "invisible" bifocals by 1928 standards). *I had gradually built up a large following in Cleveland by this time and had a great deal of trouble in having lenses properly ground to fill my prescriptions. I decided to take a trip east and buy some machinery and have my own prescription shop. I again visited New York and Boston and then went to Rochester and managed to obtain what machinery and tools needed. After installing them I could not find*

anyone who could do the work for me as I was busy all the time fitting eyes. I did finally employ a man that had some knowledge and at once hired several young men to come in and learn lens grinding and edging under him.

A few years later the cement bifocal came on the market. I was unable to find out how they were made as no one appeared to know about them in Ohio. So I made another trip to Rochester and learned how to make cement bifocals. They are the most simple form of bifocal made and the method was so simple that it is laughable to think of the long trip I made to find out.

We had only flat lenses in those days. No one knew about toric lenses until some years later, while today, no one would think of prescribing a pair of flat lenses any more than a person would think of wearing a pair of split bifocals. Times had changed very rapidly during those last few years and we opticians no longer were jealous of each other for the doctors coming into the field made us get together and improve our methods of eye examination. It looked like the field would soon be invaded by the oculist and we were wise to do so as we now became specialists and were known as Eye Specialists. We were bitter competitors of the doctors who soon found out that the eye-specialists were getting the cream of the business. They were soon trying to have laws passed in different states to force the eye-specialists out of the field altogether. The eye-specialists or opticians formed an organization called the American Optical Association and fought them tooth and nail. They helped to establish schools for the teaching of optics. Also, the opticians had laws passed in many states whereby an optician or eye-specialist was compelled to take a state board examination in order to qualify.

Many scientific instruments began to be manufactured for examining the eyes and greatly helped to cut down the time necessary for an examination. Many new ideas were put forth and we ran thru a period of using colored lenses such as blue lenses. A little later the London-smoke was used. Then a man who made a trip to the North Pole, but is now residing in one of Uncle Sam's boarding houses for some crooked work, came back from the Pole and told how they would all have become snow-blind if it had not been for the yellow glasses they had with them. Almost overnight people began to ask to have their glasses made with a little yellow in them and to this day you will see them on the street.

Then again a school started up in the middle west and began to preach prisms. Everyone must wear prisms. Everyone had muscles unbalanced. The whole country would have been wearing prisms if it had not been for some of the wiser opticians who realized that, no doubt

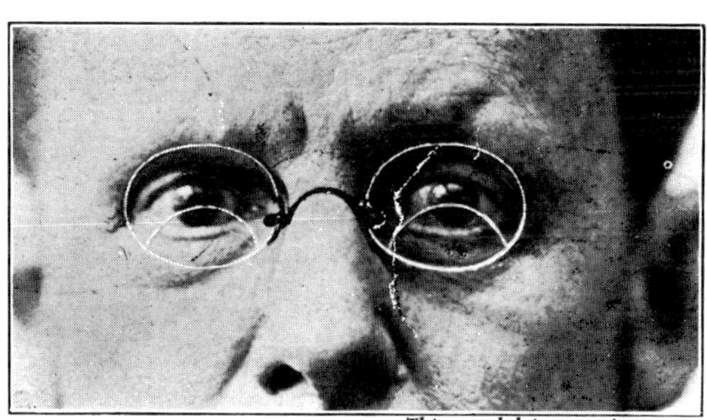

there were cases that required prisms, not one in fifty persons did need them. More prism lenses were ground during the next two years than have ever been made since.

One of the greatest frauds ever perpetuated on the American public was put over by some slick men who styled themselves Eye Doctors. They traveled about the country and inveigled old people into letting them examine their eyes. A great many had cataracts and, while not entirely blind, were nearly so. They would at once pronounce the case one of cataracts and tell the person they would take the cataract off for anywhere from fifty to five hundred dollars. Then they would go through a lot of nonsense and irritate the eye a little and show them the cataract they had removed. The cataract was always a fish scale that they carried about with them. Of course the person could not see any better but were told to keep the eye bandaged for a few days. By that time, the Doctor would be many miles away.

During my early years in the work, I tried to keep my knowledge to myself. What a change came over me. I not only wanted to teach others, I wanted to tell the whole world. I began to write articles for many different publications. I had reached the point now when I had the great pleasure of fitting the eyes of many prominent people. They came to me from far points. I numbered among my patients such names as President Garfield, President McKinley, Mark Hanna, Tom L. Johson and many, many other prominent people who have long since passed away.

I had written a lecture on the eye and delivered it in all the large cities in Ohio, usually engaging the largest house in town and later on, had this lecture printed in book form. More than five hundred thousand copies were printed at different times, but it has long been out of print.

The profession has gone forward with leaps and bounds. It has advanced so much since I retired that should I want to engage in it again, it would be as it was when I first started. I would have to learn it all over again. It has finally become a science which is recognized as vital to our health and happiness and not as it was in 1865 when, if one paid over twenty-five cents for a pair of specs, he was cheated.

Yours for better eyesight was my slogan then and is now and ever shall be.

Thomas Marsden Heard

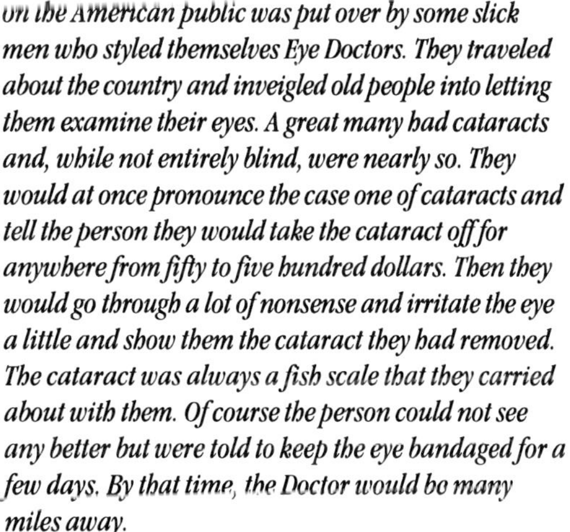

This model is wearing Heard's most popular mounting. Notice the very obvious cement bifocals. It's easy to understand why the much less visible Kryptok bifocal became such an overnight success.

ILLUSTRATION – HOWARD HEARD FAMILY

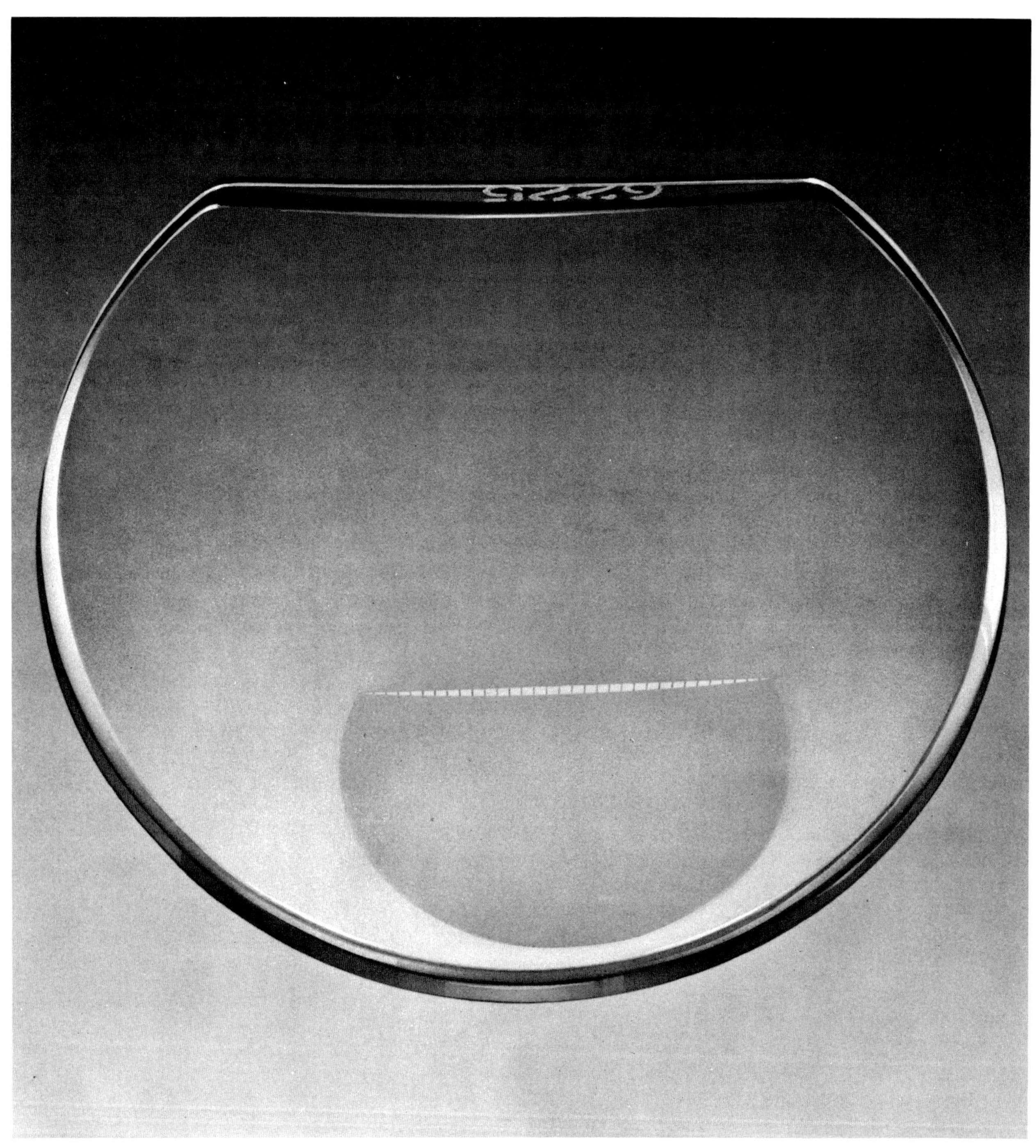

By the time flat top bifocals became the dominant multifocal (mid-1950's), brand identification had become an important issue. It was difficult for practitioners to tell the difference between a top-of-the-line flat top produced by Univis, B&L or AO and less expensive flat tops manufactured by their competitors. Univis dominated the flat top market and the photo above illustrates one method Univis used to identify their products. By 1975, they had adopted the trade name "Sentinel" for their glass line and started applying faint frosted bars to the top edge of the segment, identifying the lenses as genuine Univis (the trade called these marks "railroad tracks"). Sentinel lenses were advertised as "the world's only brand-identified lens". American Optical later applied a gold coating to the top edge of their segments. Patients didn't always appreciate this branding of bifocals because it made the segments more noticeable. In the mid-50's, Univis had tried etching a "U" within a circle on their lenses. Breathing on the glass lens would show the logo. Unfortunately, the next winter practitioners had thousands of patients complaining about blemishes they noticed when they walked indoors during cold weather. Coming into warm air, glass lenses would fog up and show what looked like a flaw to the patient. Univis dropped that idea until they came up with the "railroad track" idea.

Chapter 13
Lens Manufacturers

A list of companies manufacturing ophthalmic lenses during the past 100 years would be a long list and one that continues to grow. The companies chosen to review in this chapter do not include all lens manufacturers but only the more interesting or significant organizations. Some companies no longer exist while others continue to produce innovative new lens products. Any present-day lens manufacturers not included in this review is only because of space limitations.

CONTINENTAL OPTICAL

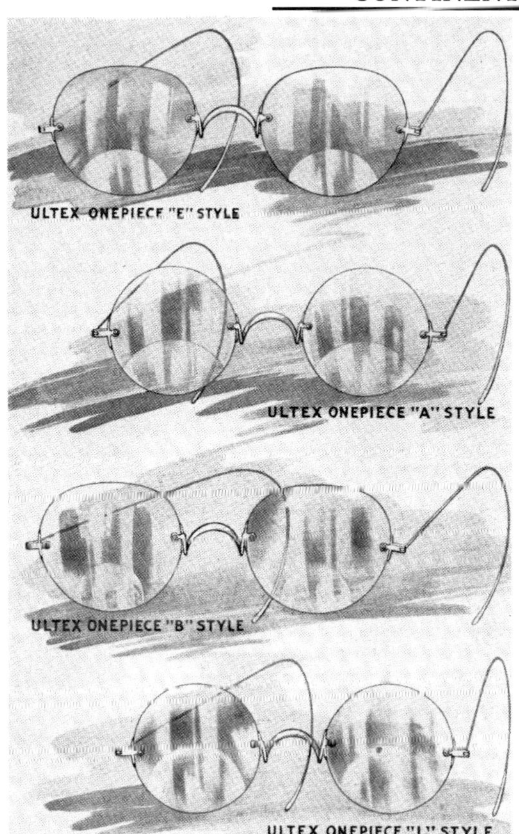

Early Ultex ad. The wide variety of segment styles available in Ultex bifocals offered advantages not supplied by Kryptok which came in one basic segment size (22mm).

On October 23, 1902, a young Indianapolis optician named Charles W. Connor applied for a patent on an improvement of the Franklin bifocal. His bifocal was made from one piece of crown glass. He then set up a company called the Indianapolis Optical Company but changed the name to Onepiece Bifocal Lens Company, a name used until mid-1925.

During the company's early years, the entire industry watched with envy and awe as the Kryptok Company took over the bifocal market with clever marketing and aggressive patent litigation. Taking a page out of their book, Onepiece hired William P. Hall as general manager. Hall had been instrumental in setting up the Kryptok license distribution plan and brought this system to Onepiece. The first thing he did was set up territorial rights, much as Kryptok had done. He induced American Optical, Bausch & Lomb and Wall & Ochs of Philadelphia to take out manufacturing rights in exchange for continuing royalties. Meanwhile, the Connor patent application came into interference with a patent application made by a man named Alexander. During this same period, a patent was granted to a man named Mayer in 1905, the patent office overlooking both the Connor and Alexander patents because they were in the Patent Department of Interferences *(meaning those patents were being contested)*. Connor prevailed and was granted the basic patent on onepiece bifocals. Mayer continued making his onepiece bifocals, resulting in another District Court suit which was decided in favor of the Onepiece Bifocal Company in 1917.

The company's patents covered both product and production method, which meant that even retailers who wanted to merely edge these lenses had to take out a license. Hall coined the name "Ultex" for these onepiece bifocals. He added a prominent scientist and lecturer named L.W. Bugbee, Sr. in 1918 *(Bugbee's son would end up running B&L's Scientific Bureau)*. The company became known as a young man's organization because of Hall's habit of hiring young men of promise who had no other optical experience. The company enjoyed rapid growth during the years 1918 through 1922.

In 1925, the Onepiece Bifocal Lens Company merged with the New Jersey Optical Company *(frames)*, the Simpson-Walther Lens Company *(lenses)*, and the C.G. Aldrich Company *(cases)* to form the Continental Optical

Corporation. That company was later succeeded by the Continental Optical Company. The Onepiece Bifocal Company, because of its size and efficient sales organization, became the dominant factor in the combined organization. William Hall became president of the new company.

Hall, encouraged by the success of their bifocal, induced L.W. Bugbee to develop an ideal single vision lens as a running mate for the Ultex. The company's policy was to produce only quality goods without trying to compete head-to-head with the mass producers *(AO and B&L)*. Bugbee completed his lens design and the company introduced Kurova lenses in 1921. Continental later claimed these were the first corrected curve single vision lenses made in America. The name Kurova came from Latin roots meaning "correct vision."

A new Ultex trifocal was introduced in 1924. This was an improvement over the 1920 trifocal because it could be surfaced by the laboratory, something evidently not possible with the earlier lens. The RedeRite reading lens was introduced in 1929 for "the hitherto neglected emmetropic presbyope." Apparently to answer market demands, the company introduced the Conoptex single vision series, a less expensive toric lens to team up with Kurova, their top of the line. Ultex K, a minus side one-piece lens that looked much like the Panoptik bifocal was introduced in 1941. The company continued to grow during the 30's and 40's, also marketing frames produced by the old New Jersey Optical Division. Much of Continental's strength lies in the fact that they were number four on the totem pole for independent laboratories. Since B&L and AO distributorships were almost impossible for new labs to obtain, independent wholesalers would turn to Shuron, Continental and Titmus, usually in that order.

In 1963, the company was acquired by Shuron Optical and the merged company became Shuron/Continental Optical. Tom Hood, president of Continental took over the reins of the combined company.

Producing glass lantern globes that wouldn't break in rain or snow led to the development of Corning's Pyrex® glass.

PHOTO – BETTMANN ARCHIVES

CORNING, INC.

The first corporate laboratory in the United States glass industry was established in April, 1908 when the Corning Glass Works set up a research laboratory. The first project for Corning's new lab director was to produce a better lantern globe for trainmen. The globe on

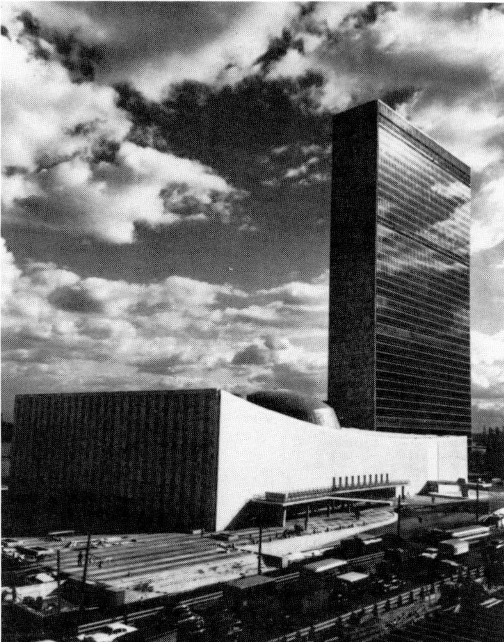

The north side of the United Nations General Assembly building is clad with Corning's photosensitive glass.

PHOTO – CORNING

signal lamps used by railroad workers often became overheated when the oil flame played directly on the glass. When the overheated glass was subjected to rain or snow, it often broke at a time when that lantern signal might be a matter of life or death. This story is particularly interesting because the borosilicate glass developed by Corning's fledgling research laboratory in answer to the railroad's problem led directly to development of a wide range of heat resistant glasses known today as Pyrex®.

Corning traces their inception to 1851 when the Bay State Glass Company in Somerville, Mass. was founded by Amory Houghton, Sr. After absorbing several other glass operations, the company moved to a larger plant in Brooklyn and then to Corning, N. Y. in 1868. The move was accomplished through use of barges on the New York State canal system, at that time the most practical method of inland shipping. The new operation, called Corning Flint Glass Works, was eventually incorporated as the Corning Glass Works in 1875.

The First Optical Glass

The first commercial production of optical glass in the United States was in 1891 in Elwood, Ind. by the Macbeth Glass Company. This company produced optical glass only until 1897, finding it impossible to compete with imported optical glass coming into this country virtually duty-free. That company ultimately became part of the Corning Glass Works.

Eventually this situation changed. The supply of optical

glass from Europe was suddenly cut off by the advent of World War I. Completely losing the source of all optical glass was a crisis for this country and led to a highly successful government-led crash program to establish a domestic source for optical glass. Corning played almost no part in those first efforts, providing only a small amount of crown glass in slab or rod form to customers such as American Optical. The company had an interest for a time in developing a way to produce optical glass but, as a 1934 company memo pointed out, "While optical glass is a most important product, especially in times of war, the volume in total is small."

The worsening international conditions in Europe during the 30's, however, changed many people's minds. Eastman Kodak, at that time, imported 70 percent of their glass from overseas *(all camera lenses were glass)*. Fearful of being cut off from European glass sources, Eastman came to Corning and proposed a cooperative research program. Corning soon developed and patented a unique tilting melter that produced a special "blended" glass by pouring the material back and forth from one sealed container to another. In 1942, the Federal government built a plant in Parkersburg, W.Va. to produce optical glass. This plant was designed and operated by Corning until the end of the war.

Several years later Corning developed a continuous optical melting tank. The first of these new units was lit in January, 1945. This was the first time large volumes of uniform quality glass were continuously melted and formed into finished rough blanks, a major development for the industry. This development, combined with Corning's improved formulas, enabled the company to provide lens manufacturers with ophthalmic lens blanks of uniform quality. Even lens manufacturers who had been making their own optical glass found it expedient to switch to this new source.

Photosensitive Glasses

The development of a light sensitive glass began in 1938 with work by Corning chemist Robert H. Dalton. A physical chemist named S.D. Stookey took Dalton's early work and explored it further. The company wasn't sure what uses this new glass might have. Today, if you examine the north side of the United Nations General Assembly building, you'll find it is clad with Corning photosensitive opal glass in a marbleized pattern.

The family of photosensitive glasses developed by Stookey and his team led to a photochromic glass first described at the New York Physical Society meeting in January 1964. The new form of glass introduced at that meeting is now being used for sun control windows, electronic data processing systems, photographic and holographic recordings and, of course, the familiar spectacle lenses whose sales now represent approximately half of all glass spectacle lenses sold in the United States. In 1994, Corning released a new formulation of this photochromic glass that permits lenses to be made thinner than the conventional 2.2mm center thickness while still passing appropriate drop ball tests.

GENTEX CORPORATION

The story of the Gentex Corporation is, in many ways, the story of polycarbonate ophthalmic lenses. The first involvement of this company into the field of optics came as a result of making flight helmets for the U.S. military. Shortly after World War II, Gentex contracted to make these helmets, each of which incorporated transparent face shields. Rather than source the visors out, the company began making their own visors out of acrylic plastic in the mid-50's.

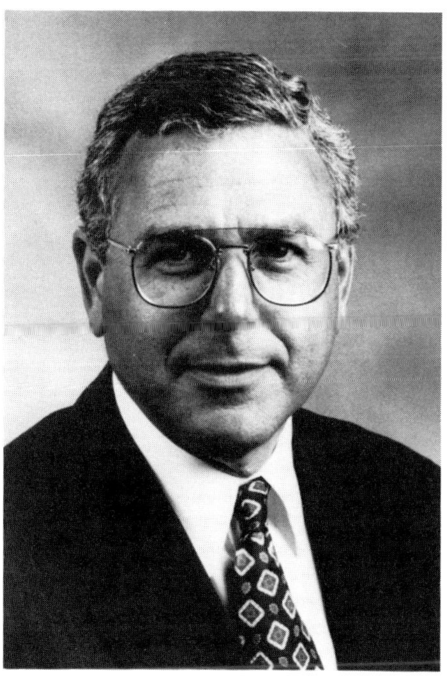

L. Peter Frieder, President of Gentex Corporation. The company's involvement with polycarbonate developed from research involved in the production of flight helmets.

In the 1960's, polycarbonate had been introduced as a tough, impact-resistant material for making burglar-, vandal- and bulletproof windows for banks, schools and other such uses. Gentex soon became a pioneer in developing other uses for this exciting new material.

In 1960, a new company named Omnitech sprung up in Dudley, Mass., formed by a group of former American Optical employees to do research and development with plastic optical products. Among the initial products developed and produced by Omnitech were a nuclear flash-protection system for flight helmets, sunglass lenses and a line of welding filter plates *(which are still successfully marketed by Gentex)*.

An association between Gentex and Omnitech occurred early during the development of the nuclear flash-protection system. During the late 60's, Omnitech continued to develop expertise in optical applications for polycarbonate and L.P. Frieder, Sr. *(father of Gentex's present owner, Peter Frieder)* began to recognize the great potential that existed for polycarbonate, assuming the scratching problem could be resolved. The material, in its natural state, is extremely soft and must be coated for virtually any use.

During this time two things occurred that ultimately resulted in the establishment of an Ophthalmic Products Division for Gentex in Dudley. The first thing that happened was that the DuPont Company developed a hard coating material that seemed ideally suited for polycarbonate. The second was Frieder's purchase of

Omnitech in 1970. Simultaneously with that purchase, he acquired the rights to DuPont's hard coating, taking a considerable gamble that polycarbonate would have commercial optical uses beyond helmet visors.

During this period, Gentex entered the plano *(non-Rx)* safety lens field, drawing heavily on the acquired optical experience they now had in their new optical division. The first Gentex lens coating system was developed and built and is still in use in the company's Carbondale, Penn. plant for safety product applications. The company developed a broad range of industrial safety lenses made in polycarbonate and is a major lens supplier in the industrial field.

Between 1970 and 1980, the safety lens business grew substantially and, during this period, as technology for making, molding and coating polycarbonate improved, Gentex turned their attention to the dress lenses made of polycarbonate. This wasn't as easy as it might seem for several reasons. First, they discovered that quality concerns for dress wear were somewhat more critical than for industrial lenses. Next, it was found that dress lenses were more likely to be dyed. Since only the coating on polycarbonate lenses accepts dye, the coating had to be formulated to permit dying and this sometimes compromised the effectiveness of the scratch protection. Lastly, few labs were proficient in processing polycarbonate and it was a long, slow process to bring labs up to speed on this new process.

It's safe to say that had Peter Frieder and Gentex not persevered licking these problems during those early days, there might not be a polycarbonate lens market today. The new material, however, had enough promise for labs that some of them endured the lengthy learning process and by 1990, 15 percent of wholesale labs were processing polycarbonate. Four years later, most labs in the U.S. are now routinely processing polycarbonate lenses and the quality of polycarbonate lenses rivals that of any other material.

In the spring of 1980, Gentex moved the ophthalmic lens marketing operation from the original Omnitech facilities into a new manufacturing plant and officially changed the company name to Gentex. In 1986, the name was changed again to Gentex Optics. The facilities expanded in 1986, 1992 and again in 1994 in the attempt to keep up with the exceptional growth in demand for polycarbonate ophthalmic lenses.

Today Gentex Optics has expanded their manufacturing, lens design, coating, R&D operations and is reaping the benefits from the lengthy process of establishing polycarbonate as a viable ophthalmic lens material. The Gentex product line covers all ophthalmic lenses, ranging from finished and semifinished single vision, through all multifocals and includes aspherics and progressives. Gentex Optics serves as a primary source for polycarbonate progressives sold by a number of ophthalmic lens suppliers throughout the world.

The company's entire ophthalmic lens line is made of polycarbonate and the recent surge of polycarbonate usage has resulted in considerable expansion of the company's physical facilities. They recently introduced a new line of sun lenses utilizing a unique new synthetic diamond coating that promises to have broad applications for the future.

OPTIMA, INC.

Optima is a relatively new company, having been established in 1984 by Nick Niejelow, initially as an importer of conventional glass lenses. Later plastic lenses were added and, in 1988, the company began selling high index plastic lenses.

Niejelow had been a commodity trader before spending ten years with Welling International where he established a lens division for what had been a frame importer. He left Welling to go into business for himself, setting up Optima to sell glass lenses. Niejelow had developed a very close relationship with Asahi, a Japanese lens manufacturer and, sensing a need for improved lens products, he and Asahi established a research and development department to explore new kinds of lens products. They were looking for an innovative product with benefits that could be effectively demonstrated to consumers as well as labs and eyecare professionals. Working with several chemical manufacturers, they searched for an improved transparent material for lenses. That search produced a number of possibilities and from them, the resin that became Optima's 1.60 high index plastic material was chosen.

Optima's first lenses made of the new 1.60 plastic were first introduced in the United States. If Optima wasn't the first 1.60 index material, the company was certainly one of the first to produce lenses in this index and it was their 1.60 product that made the greatest impact on the American market. One of the difficulties faced initially was cost. The 1.6 high index resin was extremely expensive and when Optima lenses were first introduced, there was serious doubt in the industry whether consumers would pay such high prices for single vision lenses. Once retail offices began showing and demonstrating the new lenses, they quickly discovered that price was no barrier. From that point on, high index plastic lenses gradually became a significant part of the lens market. At the time Optima lenses were introduced, high index lenses represented about 1 percent of the total lens market. Five years later, high index lenses are

Nick Niejelow, President of Optima.

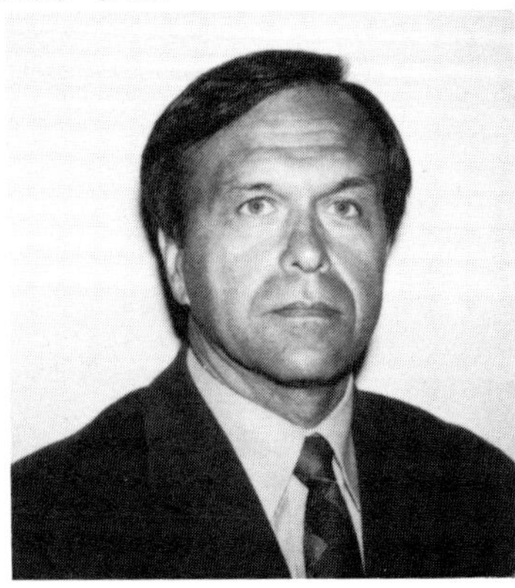

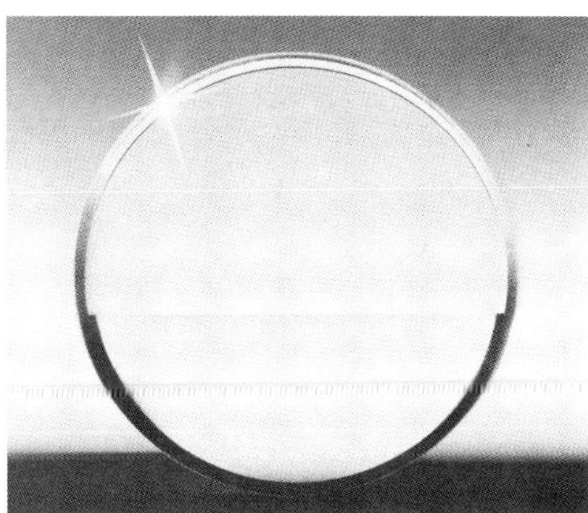

Glass molds used in casting CR-39 executive-type blanks were expensive and difficult to produce. ORC developed a way to create a stainless steel master mold and then replicate it with metal molds, eliminating glass molds. This lead to establishment of the Orcolite Division of Optical Radiation.

estimated to be more than 16 percent.

Optima was the first company to introduce a 1.66 index. They were the first to produce a high index aspheric lens and were also a prime mover in creating a market for AR coated high index stock lenses. Since the introduction of AR stock lenses, the AR market has increased.

Optima lenses are manufactured by Asahi Lite Optical, Ltd. in Fukui, a small city in Japan. Asahi is a postwar major lens manufacturer in Japan, producing only high index lens products. No manufacturing is done in the United States. Niejelow's company, Optima, has since merged with Asahi and Optima serves as the marketing arm for the parent company. Nick Niejelow is President and C.E.O. of Optima and also a director of Asahi. Niejelow believes the future for lenses lies with new lens materials and new lens designs and Asahi is actively working in both those areas. Research and development of new products is currently being done both in Japan and the United States.

OPTICAL RADIATION CORPORATION

Richard D. Wood, an engineer, worked for the Electro Optical Systems division of the Xerox Corporation. He eventually came to the conclusion he would rather be working for himself. The first product of his new company was the by-now familiar police helicopter search light seen so often on the evening news.

Much of the technology of Wood's new company was built around optics, chemistry and radiation, hence the name Optical Radiation Corporation. Radiation referred primarily to the ultraviolet curing involved in many of the company's products and chemistry is involved in how

their coatings do their work. The three elements are a common thread running through many of the company's products.

On the lens side of the business, ORC developed a technology in 1972 in which they were able to take a stainless steel master mold and replicate it over and over. Wood knew how difficult it was to produce the franklin or executive type multifocal because of the fragile glass molds used in manufacturing that type of lens. Using their new mold technology, ORC introduced their first executive-type product to wholesale laboratories and it proved to be an immediate success, so successful that, before long, they were producing their "full seg" multifocals for other lens manufacturers as well. The company goal has always been to produce resin products that commanded decent prices with reasonable profits for them and for the processing labs.

In the meantime, during the early 80's, Wood began to believe there was a need for a lighter, thinner resin and, hopefully, one with greater impact resistance. Polycarbonate was already in the marketplace, primarily as an industrial lens. He believed a polycarbonate dress lens could be produced with a 1.5mm center and better optics than the professions had come to expect from polycarbonate. Orcolite *(the company's optical division)* had watched labs struggle with learning to process polycarbonate lenses. At that time, less than 5 percent of labs were processing polycarbonate. ORC was very aware of how long it took CR-39 to get firmly seated in the market and they decided the only effective way to launch a new polycarbonate lens was to develop their own wholesale distribution. By this time, ORC engineers had developed a proprietary process for producing polycarbonate lenses. The Omega lab was acquired primarily as a means for manufacturing and distributing this new lens *(given the name "LiteStyle"®)*. This polycarbonate lens was further enhanced in 1992 with the introduction of Ultra LiteStyle® with 1.0mm center thickness.

The company is still betting heavily on polycarbonate as the ultimate lens material. ORC continues to manufacture CR-39 lenses, but recently discontinued producing 1.60 high index lenses. Problems in producing quality polycarbonate lenses are all in the past and the company feels confident in concentrating their efforts in proven materials like CR-39 and polycarbonate rather than diverting the company's resources in another new material. ORC also has an Opthalmic Surgical Products Division, producing intraocular lenses, corneal topography equipment and a new procedure for changing the cornea with a non-laser procedure.

Benson Eyewear Corporation and ORC recently announced an agreement for Benson to acquire Optical Radiation, an acquisition expected to be completed by October, 1994. Benson is already actively seeking buyers

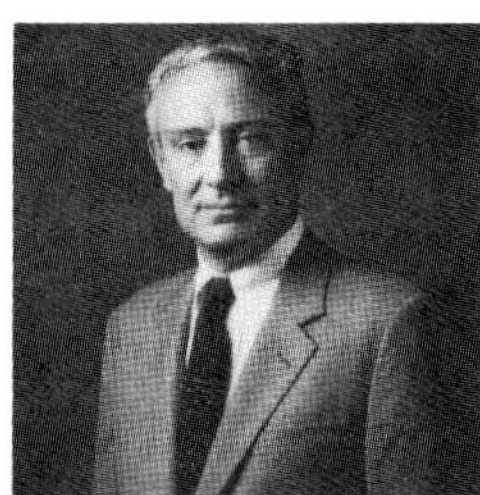

Richard D. Wood, founder of Optical Radiation Corporation.

for their retail operations and expects to be out of retail by year's end. With new ownership and a continuing quest for new products, Orcolite plans to continue doing what they do best — produce superior products that are profitable for labs to process. ORC management remains in place and the company is comfortable with a game plan that's been very successful for them during the past few years.

ROBINSON-HOUCHIN

S.W. Robinson & Company was founded in 1903 by S.W. Robinson, a onetime Dean of the School of Mechanical Engineering at Ohio University. Robinson's son Erdis, a civil engineer working in Mexico for the Mexican Central Railroad joined the company in 1910, two years before his father died. The name was then changed to Robinson Optical.

Meanwhile, a young man named Lowell L. Houchin was working as a shop superintendent for F.A. Hardy in New York. In 1915, he went into business for himself under the name Houchin Optical. He sold the business in 1921 and followed a popular dream of the day to go to California. That didn't work out and he ended up in Okmulgee, Okla., buying a half interest in a retail optical shop. In 1927, he moved to Columbus, Ohio and joined Robinson Optical Company, at that time a manufacturer of machinery. Houchin & Robinson *(note the reversal of names)* was a lens manufacturer. The two firms combined in 1931 and became known as Robinson-Houchin Optical Company, making both machinery and lenses.

Their principle lens product was Ultex bifocals. As the industry gradually changed to fused bifocals and labs grew to prefer grinding minus cylinders instead of the bothersome plus cylinders required for Ultex lenses, Robinson-Houchin developed a one-piece bifocal with the reading portion on the front side. This had limited success but by the 1950's one-piece bifocals had been reduced to a very small part of the multifocal market.

RODENSTOCK

Born in 1846, founder Josef Rodenstock started his career at age 14, traveling the countryside with his father selling barometers and thermometers to farmers and peasants. Prospering, they later added spectacles which they learned to repair and later to make. This success enabled the younger Rodenstock to pursue his heartfelt desire to become an optician. He apprenticed under a local optician and studied that famous book that inspired so many other optical pioneers, Professor Donder's "The Anomalies of the Refraction and Accommodation of the Eye".

The Company is Launched

On December 1, 1877, Josef Rodenstock founded the company known worldwide today as Rodenstock in the town of Würzburg, Germany. It was intended to be a fine-mechanical workshop for producing barometers, precision balances, spectacle lenses and frames. By 1879, Josef had already obtained a patent for an improvement in spectacle lenses. Two years later, he added glass blowing and grinding to his workshop. Another patent was issued for a "spectacle measuring apparatus" much like the trial frames of today. In 1882, he opened a branch in Munich which became the production and company headquarters in 1885. The move enabled him to drive his machinery with water power. By 1891, the company had 120 workers with affiliated branches in Berlin and Cologne.

Regen Works

In 1898, Josef Rodenstock built the Regen Works, a lens grinding factory located deep in the Bavarian Forest. Before long, over 100 workers *(mostly former forest workers)* were at work producing lenses. By 1900, more than 200 workers were producing lenses and by 1905 the figure reached 300 out of a company-wide total of 550 employees. Between the years 1900 and 1914, Rodenstock developed and produced new and improved spectacle lenses. Photography was a growing fad and the company took an active interest in producing precision lenses for this new field. They opened agencies in Milan, Brussels, New York, Bilbao, Moscow, Vienna, London and Chicago.

The outbreak of World War I was a disaster for Rodenstock. Overnight, all export was cut off. While there were many orders from the Army, those demands were difficult to meet. Following the war, galloping inflation became the enemy. The world economic crisis in 1929 collapsed the German export business and the number of Rodenstock employees dropped to 800, nearly half. It was feared that another 400 would have to be cut and the entire company was in peril. Overnight the National Socialists gained power *(1933)* and the German economy took a sudden turn for the better.

World War II

The period from 1933 to 1939 was much like the years from 1924 to 1929 for Rodenstock. By 1938, 30 percent of the company's production was sold to the armed forces. When war broke out on September 1, 1939, Rodenstock's production was taken over by the Ministry of Army Supply. From 1944 on, the owners had no say in the company's affairs. Most company workers were sent to the front and replaced with foreign labor. Oddly enough, even the severe air raids on Munich in 1944/

1945 failed to affect production. The company's optical production had been moved underground in the "Burgerbrau" beer cellar. Alexander's son Rolf was wounded on the Eastern front and returned to Munich in 1943. May 1, 1945 found American tanks standing before the closed gates of Rodenstock's Munich works.

The War Ends

More than 30 years later Professor Dr. Rolf Rodenstock described the events surrounding this dark hour in his personal memories.

"In the night before April 30th we could hear artillery fire from the West. German troops withdrew over the Wittelsbacher bridge. The American Troops entered Munich during the afternoon of April 30th. Early in the morning my Father and I had driven to the works in our old Opel to await there whatever might come. But since nothing happened throughout the afternoon and my Father was not in good health we wanted to return home to Solln. Because of the close approach of the battle activities I chose, on the way back, what I thought was a safe small road running along the Isar. Quite unexpectedly, in Thalkirchen, I met the first American tanks. I got out of the car and explained the purpose of my journey. To my astonishment I was allowed to return to the car and asked to drive back to the factory."

"On the next day I thought it wiser to go to the factory by bicycle and I found there American officers who asked me about the production, number of workers and many other details. Although in their advance they had seen Dachau they were not explicitly hostile. I was only compelled to give up my Swiss wristwatch as "booty". During the next few days however the situation became clearly less comfortable. The troops occupied the works. All the steel cabinets were forced open but they contained nothing special. In our offices and work-shops, foreign workers of both sexes made themselves at home. Understandably, many things that were of any use disappeared. Our typewriters and calculating machines found work in a French service post. A few weeks later we managed to get most of them back."

"The American City Commandant had become the appropriate authority for everything. No German administration existed any longer. There were two requirements I had to settle: first, obtaining a produc-tion permit, and secondly, to get the works cleared of the uninvited guests. At first I did not get much understanding from the captain in charge. At last, however, my argument that it was vitally important to be able to supply the public with glasses prevailed and I received a production permit for Munich. Then I went to the military police who after much exhortation agreed to remove the unwanted guests from the factory."

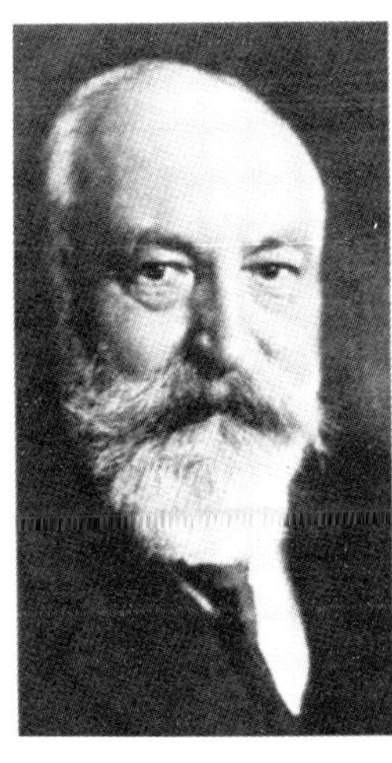

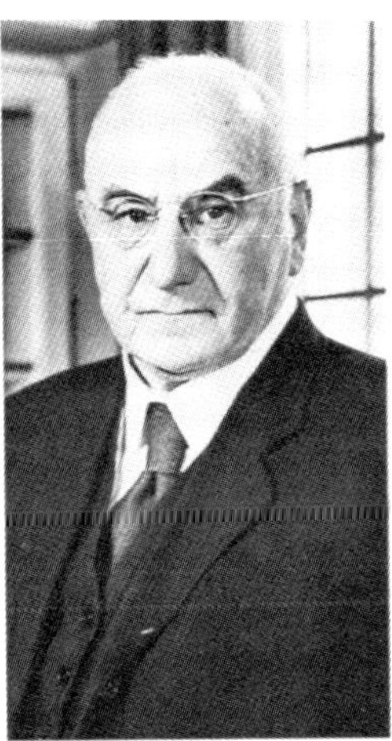

Rodenstock's founder, Josef Rodenstock, left, with his son Alexander on the right.

As some of our old employees gradually returned to us they were given work in clearing up and repairing. Regardless of position, all members of the firm participated in this work. By the beginning of June 1945 we were in a position to begin with the urgent production of spectacle lenses and the preparation of prism-binoculars and theater glasses for the use of the occupying forces."

Management of the company was assumed by 28 year old Dr. Rolf Rodenstock. German industry was some 10 years behind American technology. Rodenstock's Regen Works was again mass producing lenses but using worn out prewar machines. New equipment had to be designed and built. Completely new production lines had to also be built for frames.

In 1972, Rodenstock Precision Optics opened in the United States for the manufacture of precision optics. The following year, the company established a zyl frame production plant in Puerto Rico. In 1975, Rodenstock, USA was established in Danbury, Conn. and an instrument division established in 1977. In 1980, Rodenstock acquired Felix M. Mendelson Company, a company that had been their exclusive frame distributor in the western United States. For a period of time, thereafter, the company sold their frames direct in the western states and through distributors *(mostly labs)* east of the Mississippi.

In 1982, Rodenstock set up an agreement for Coburn Optical to distribute Rodenstock R and Rodenstock Lensometers. In June 1988, the agreement ended and Rodenstock opened up a U.S. Lens Division to distribute Rodenstock lens products to U.S. distributors. In 1991, the company changed their U.S. frame distribution

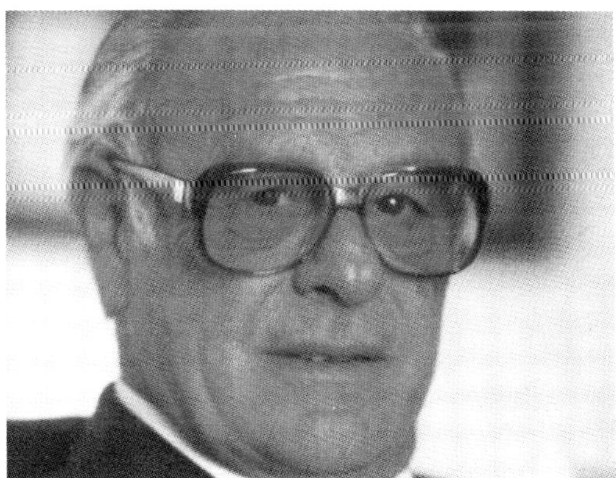

Professor Dr. Rolf Rodenstock was wounded on the Eastern front during World War II and returned to Munich to join his father's firm in 1944. He headed the Rodenstock company from 1953 to 1990, expanding them in many fields of ophthalmic optics. The story of how he and his father awaited the Americans on April 30, 1945, the day American troops entered Munich, is told in his own words.

system and hired a national sales force to sell frame products direct in the east as well as the west. Today, the U.S. Lens Division is solidifying lens distribution through wholesale channels by developing even closer ties with labs that want to be more closely linked to Rodenstock.

SIGNET ARMORLITE, INC.

The company's name comes from a combination of two separate companies: Signet and Armorlite. Armorlite had been the larger of the two and was founded in Burbank, Calif. by Dr. Robert Graham shortly after the end of World War II. Armorlite is generally considered to be the North American pioneer in plastic *(CR-39)* lens casting.

Shortly after receiving his Degree of Optics at Ohio State University, Dr. Graham went to work at Univis Lens Company. One of the things that attracted Graham was that Univis was working on developing plastic lenses. Six years later, Graham was sales manager of the company but his favorite project, plastic lenses, was getting nowhere. Univis spent a third of a million dollars and had achieved little, if anything. A company called Tulca in Beverly Hills was compression molding plexiglas lenses, using metal molds. Univis had bought the company for their technology but then Combined Optical Industries claimed to have conceived this method and sued Univis. Discouraged, Univis dropped the whole project.

Graham decided the company was too easily disheartened and so did some of the top technicians who had been working on the project. They lost their job and Graham resigned. Graham moved from Dayton, Ohio to Pasadena, Calif. with those technicians coming in as stockholders. The first plastic lenses produced by the Armorlite Lens Company were made of polymethyl-methacrylate *(PMMA)*, an ophthalmic quality plastic also known as Lucite or Plexiglas. Injection molded PMMA lenses had been tried but were unsatisfactory. Armorlite developed a method of turning discs made of the polymer on a lathe to the approximate power. The blanks were then finished by being pressed between highly polished glass dies under considerable heat and

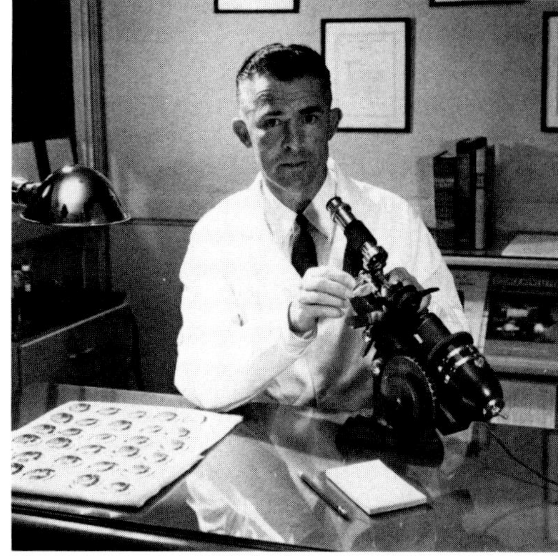

Dr. Robert Graham had worked on plastic lenses while with Univis and when that company abandoned their plastic lens project, he took a few key technicians and moved to Pasadena, California to continue the quest for a lightweight replacement for glass lenses.

pressure. This minimum-flow process produced a product that was very fine optically and free of stain and minute machining grooves. The lenses were only moderately successful. Much like earlier styrene lenses Armorlite had tried, the material was just too susceptible to scratching.

For some time Dr. Graham had known of CR-39, an allyl resin developed by PPG as a bonding solution for combat airplanes. CR-39 had first been used during World War II in bomber planes. Sheets of the material were sandwiched between two thinner pieces of glass, strengthening the glass sheets and reducing their weight. This lowering of gross weight lengthened the flight range of the bombers. It had been classified as a military property and hadn't been available to Univis. With the war at an end, CR-39 became available and Graham and his crew started working with it. It took three more years but they eventually solved the problem of creating plastic lenses.

Like PMMA, CR-39 was optically clear but this new material turned out to be thirty times more abrasion-resistant than PMMA. There was several major problems with casting lenses in this material, however. CR-39 was a bonding agent and separation from the molds was a problem, particularly when using metal molds. Fortunately, Graham's group had always favored glass molds. Another problem was that lenses experienced a 14 percent shrinkage during the curing process. This was not a problem when casting plano lenses but in lenses with power, the differences in thickness between the center and the edge led to differential shrinkage that resulted in optical distortions.

Few labs in the U.S. were capable of surfacing plastic lenses when Armorlite lenses were first introduced. To sell their stock lenses, the company was forced to provide prescription service for corrections beyond the stock range. This price list shows the complete range of plastic lenses available in 1959.

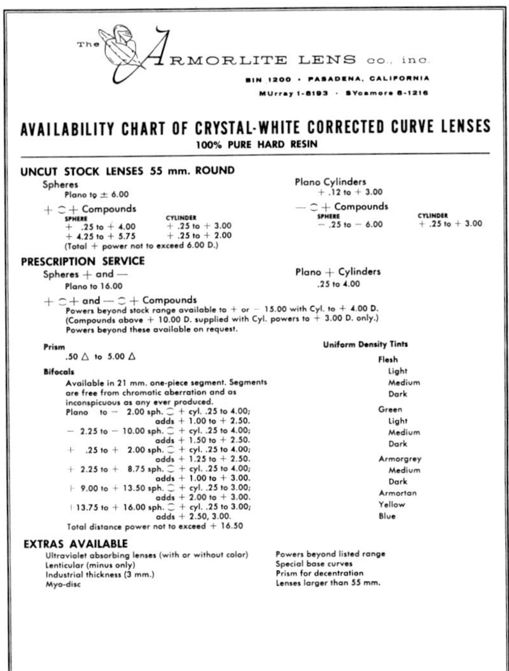

The **ARMORLITE LENS co., inc.**
BIN 1200 · PASADENA, CALIFORNIA
MUrray 1-8193 · SYcamore 8-1216

AVAILABILITY CHART OF CRYSTAL-WHITE CORRECTED CURVE LENSES
100% PURE HARD RESIN

UNCUT STOCK LENSES 55 mm. ROUND

Spheres
 Plano to ± 6.00

Plano Cylinders
 + .12 to + 3.00

+ ○ + Compounds

SPHERE	CYLINDER
+ .25 to + 4.00	+ .25 to + 3.00
+ 4.25 to + 5.75	+ .25 to + 2.00

(Total + power not to exceed 6.00 D.)

− ○ + Compounds

SPHERE	CYLINDER
− .25 to − 6.00	+ .25 to + 3.00

PRESCRIPTION SERVICE

Spheres + and −
 Plano to 16.00

Plano + Cylinders
 .25 to 4.00

+ ○ + and − ○ + Compounds
 Powers beyond stock range available to + or − 15.00 with Cyl. to + 4.00 D.
 (Compounds above + 10.00 D. supplied with Cyl. powers to + 3.00 D. only.)
 Powers beyond these available on request.

Prism
 .50 △ to 5.00 △

Bifocals
 Available in 21 mm. one-piece segment. Segments are free from chromatic aberration and as inconspicuous as any ever produced.
 Plano to − 2.00 sph. ○ + cyl. .25 to 4.00;
  adds + 1.00 to + 2.50.
 − 2.25 to − 10.00 sph. ○ + cyl. .25 to 4.00;
  adds + 1.50 to + 2.50.
 + .25 to + 2.00 sph. ○ + cyl. .25 to 4.00;
  adds + 1.25 to + 2.50.
 + 2.25 to + 8.75 sph. ○ + cyl. .25 to 4.00;
  adds + 1.00 to + 3.00.
 + 9.00 to + 13.50 sph. ○ + cyl. .25 to 3.00;
  adds + 2.00 to + 3.00.
 + 13.75 to + 16.00 sph. ○ + cyl. .25 to 3.00;
  adds + 2.50, 3.00.
 Total distance power not to exceed + 16.50

Uniform Density Tints

Flesh
 Light
 Medium
 Dark

Green
 Light
 Medium
 Dark

Armorgrey
 Medium
 Dark

Armortan
Yellow
Blue

EXTRAS AVAILABLE

Ultraviolet absorbing lenses (with or without color)
Lenticular (minus only)
Industrial thickness (3 mm.)
Myo-disc

Powers beyond listed range
Special base curves
Prism for decentration
Lenses larger than 55 mm.

Graham later wrote of these early days. *"We will never forget those nights, month after month, when we sat by the ovens listening to the sound of cracking glass molds!"* Eventually, however, after a great deal of trial and error, they developed a successful way to cast prescription lenses.

That year, 1947, the Armorlite Company was incorporated and CR-39 lenses were in production. For the next six years they were the sole source for this exciting new type of ophthalmic lens. During this period, Armorlite was both manufacturer and lab processor. There were no labs equipped to process these new lenses and for out-of-range powers, semi-finished lenses were required. With no labs to process them, Armorlite became the only place where lenses were being generated in CR-39. Eventually, they had to decide which they wanted to be - processing lab or manufacturer. They decided they had skills that were of most value in manufacturing and they were confident that processing labs would spring up. They gave up processing.

Even with growing acceptance, however, one factor still held back these new light weight lenses from universal acceptance — scratches. Many other materials were tried but even after 30 years, the original CR-39 is still the most used plastic material worldwide.

Armorlite's inventive scientists tried everything in their quest for better scratch protection, reviewing more than 2,000 patent abstracts for abrasion resistant treatments. Their problem was a difference in the thermal-coefficient of expansion between coatings and substrate. This usually resulted in crazed surfaces after exposure to any variation in temperature.

In the early 1970's, the famous 3M company came to the conclusion they might have the answer. Coatings had always been one of 3M's technological strengths, but finding the right coating for CR-39 eluded even these innovative scientists. One of the things they discovered was that cleanliness requirements for coating lenses exceeded that of any other production situation. The answer, they discovered, was a facility that reduced airborne particles to a minimum.

From 1974 to 1976, 3M refined their process and set up laboratories to evaluate treated lenses. It will surprise no lab person that lenses that looked fine to the 3M chemists working on the project were totally unacceptable to lab technicians, better trained in what to look for. Eventually 3M offered the coating service on a test market basis in five states. More than 25,000 pair of hard resin lenses with the new 3M treatment were sold in the test market from April 1978 to December 1979. At the end of the 20 month test, 3M found that all the test labs wanted to continue selling the coated lenses. The

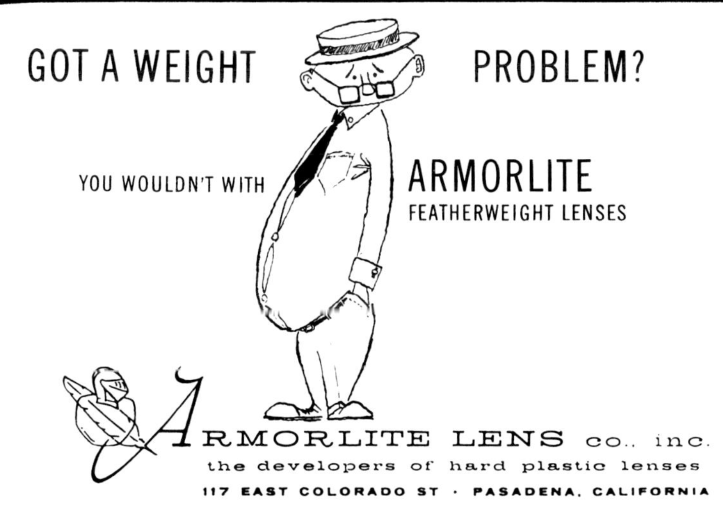

treating technology was then transferred to Armorlite. Just prior to this time *(1978),* 3M, deciding they had a real handle on the optical business, bought the Armorlite Company

The value of 3M stock offered to Armorlite stockholders was $70 million on the day of the agreement and, two days later when the stockholders gave final approval, the stock had increased in value to $72 million. Dr. Graham was to later state, "The quickest $2 million I ever made." Dr. Graham became a consultant to the new company for five years and his son Robin took over as head of the operation. The new coating treatment, called Armorlite RLX, was introduced nationally, putting 3M solidly in the optical business.

Signet

Signet was a younger company than Armorlite. The company was started in San Diego by two entrepreneurs, Doug Campbell, manager of Armorlite's mold department and Don Chatelain, a business-trained executive Named Signet Uptown, it was an all-plastic wholesale laboratory *(a rarity in those days)* that cast their own lens blanks. Signet rapidly became a major lens manufacturer and, by 1971, was producing single vision, bifocal and trifocal lenses as well as an innovative new cataract lens design called HyperAspheric™.

Early Armorlite ad showing how plastic lenses were positioned against glass lenses.

ILLUSTRATION – SIGNET ARMORLITE

Guy Vareilles, shown here with some of the first Silor lenses, had joined a small frame company named La Lunette de Paris in 1964. The next year, this company started importing lenses from the French company Lissac. La Lunette changed its name to Silor in 1969.

PHOTO – ESSILOR OF AMERICA

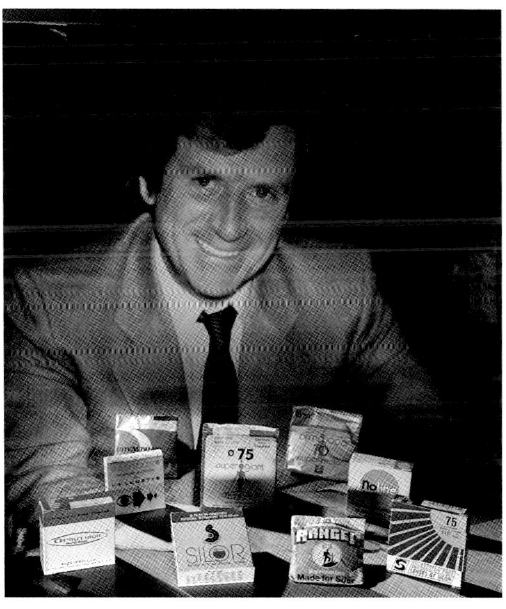

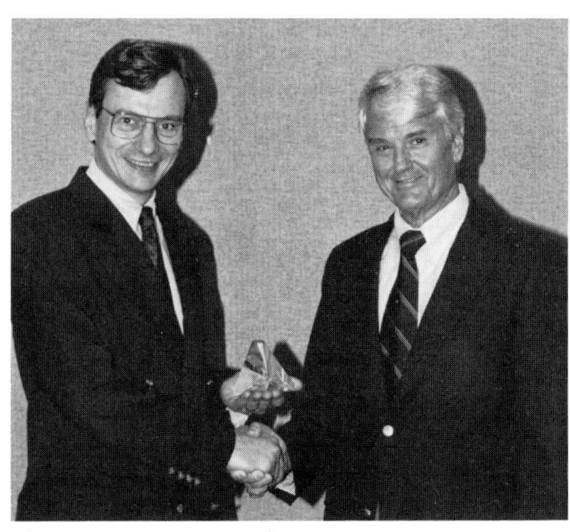

Silor won a 1990 OLA Award of Excellence for their Thin & Lite 1.6 lens. Jacques Stoerr, President of Silor, left, congratulates Hubert Dreckman, President of Essilor of America Manufacturing.

In 1976/77, Campbell and Chatelain sold their company to American Hospital Supply Corporation who sent Richard Ormsby to serve as general manager. In 1981, Ormsby, along with Robert Jepson, purchased Signet from American Hospital Supply Corporation. In 1981, Ormsby and Jepson also purchased Armorlite from the 3M Corporation and merged the two companies to form Signet Armorlite, Inc., the largest semi-finished plastic lens manufacturer in the United States. They expanded into Europe in 1988 by opening in Gloucester, England. From that point on, the company was an affiliate of Jepson Corporation. Signet Armorlite was later purchased from Jepson by the Eagle Corporation. In 1993, Signet Armorlite formed a joint alliance with Industrie Ottiche Europee. Each company continues to operate independently.

Brand Names

In 1993, Signet Armorlite initiated a new marketing plan that may indicate a trend for the future. Consumer-recognized brand names for frames and sunglasses have become an accepted marketing tactic. Patients seem to relate the quality and effectiveness of brand name frames with the highly recognizable names attached to them. Whether this marketing principle will follow through for ophthalmic lenses is still uncertain, but clearly Signet Armorlite believes it will with their newest progressive addition lens carrying the brand name Kodak. It's too early to predict how effective a consumer-recognized brand name will be in the highly competitive progressive market but it's safe to say that other brand names will probably show up in the lens field.

SILOR (ESSILOR OF AMERICA)

The first appearance of an Essilor International affiliate in the United States occurred in 1954 when a company, under the subsidiary name, La Lunette de Paris, was established on Fifth Avenue in New York *(sharing a building with E.B. Meyrowitz)*. At that time, La Lunette was a subsidiary of Freres Lissac of Paris and functioned as a distributor of French frames and plastic lenses. Their most popular frame was the Polymil, a rimless frame with lenses suspended from the brow bar, attached with adhesive.

Lissac had been founded in 1931 by George Lissac, an entrepreneur who, in 1941, introduced marketing to the conservative European optical industry. Lissac created SIL *(Societe Industrielle de Lunetterie)* in 1946 and LOS *(Lentilles Ophtalmiques Speciales)* in 1948. These were frame and lens research and development, manufacturing and distribution operations. SIL launched a whole new trend for the frame industry when they created the revolutionary AMOR rimless frame in 1949. The AMOR name is a condensed version of the French word "Amortisseur" and translates as "shock absorbing" frame

In 1952, LOS developed the ORMA 500 plexiglas lens which marked the beginning of plastic spectacle lenses in France. Plexiglas lenses were only marginally successful, however. After years of continuing research, LOS mastered the difficulties of casting lenses from CR-39 and introduced the CR-39 ORMA 1000 lens in 1956 and patented and introduced the lens worldwide in 1959. In 1960, they changed the lens division name from LOS to LOR *(Lentilles Ophtalmiques Rationnelles)*. By 1961, SIL had introduced the advanced polymil frame. The Lissac group continued on their upward spiral and merged in 1966 with Telegic, a company that specialized in the production of corrective lenses. In 1969, Lor-Telegic joined the other division of the Lissac group, SIL, to form a company in France with the now familiar name of Silor.

Once Orma lenses made of CR-39 were introduced in the United States, La Lunette de Paris began to grow rapidly. In 1965 Guy Vareilles was made president of La Lunette de Paris. In 1970, the two French companies SIL *(Society Industrial de Lunettegy)* and LOR *(Lentilles Ophthalmiques de Rationnelles)* merged under the name SILOR. That same year Silor moved from New York City to Glen Head, N.Y.

Meanwhile, another significant French company, Essel, began to use it's company name for marketing the Nylor frame developed in 1955 and the Varilux progressive lens introduced in 1959. The Nylor frame was an improved version of the AMOR frame that Lissac had created and the Varilux progressive lens was about to revolutionize the presbyopia market.

Essel was an interesting company, formed in 1848 in France during the Spirit of Labor Cooperation *(the revolutionary sociopolitical worker's cooperative)*. They opened their first subsidiary in London in 1881. In 1955, Essel created the NYLOR frame. This frame enjoyed huge success and the cash flow it generated helped finance the Varilux I *(1959)* progressive lens.

ORMA CR-39 lenses were considered revolutionary when introduced. Tested at the National Institute of Scientific Research and the Aerospatial Medicine School in Texas, these lightweight lenses exhibited more shock resistance *(coated or uncoated)* than glass lenses. The lenses were lighter, safer, and allowed uniform tinting. In the late

1950's, the Federal Drug Administration required all ophthalmic lenses to meet safety standards and the ORMA 1000 and its sister, the ORMA Major were the first plastic lenses to meet these requirements. In the meantime, style had hit the eyewear market by 1960 and new plastic lenses met the growing needs of frame fashions. Subsequently, ORMA Major, Major 70 and Major 75 were introduced worldwide.

The "marriage" of these two companies brought recognized ophthalmic brand names - Nylor, AMOR, Varilux I and Orma 1000, research and development teams, and major manufacturing and distribution networks together. A plan to rotate the presidency began at this juncture, with former president of Silor, Rene Granperret, initially serving as president of Essilor, rotating the position with Anatole Temkine, whom initially served as vice president. The two most important French optical companies became ESSILOR INTERNATIONAL.

The following time-line helps in tracking the growth of this company in the United States:

1971   A joint venture between Silor Optical and the Milton-Roy Company is established to manufacture CR-39 lenses in the U.S. Milton-Roy, located in St. Petersburg, was an industrial manufacturer in the healthcare field. During the same year, a merger between Essel and Silor in France creates Essilor International.

1972   The Milroy-Silor joint venture facility is completed in February with 17 employees and the first lens cast in March. The first production is semi-finished single vision lenses but bifocals are quickly added. France is producing a curve top bifocal and working on developing a flat top bifocal. All molds are produced in France.

1974   65, 60 and 55mm FT25 and Aspheric Lenticular SFSV and Round 22 bifocals are added to the line.

1975   Silor expands the U.S. facility again and Milton-Roy is more interested in the contact lens business. Essilor buys out Milton-Roy's share in the Milroy-Silor company and renames plant Silor Optical of Florida.

Optical General Corporation is formed to export lenses from the U.S. Flo-lite *(Florida Lite Optical)* is set up as a subsidiary of OGC.

Marvin Silver, in charge of sales on the West Coast, insists on faster service for western customers. A branch distribution center is set up in Sun Valley, Calif., the start of Silor's branch system.

1976   A second branch distribution center opens in Atlanta, Ga.

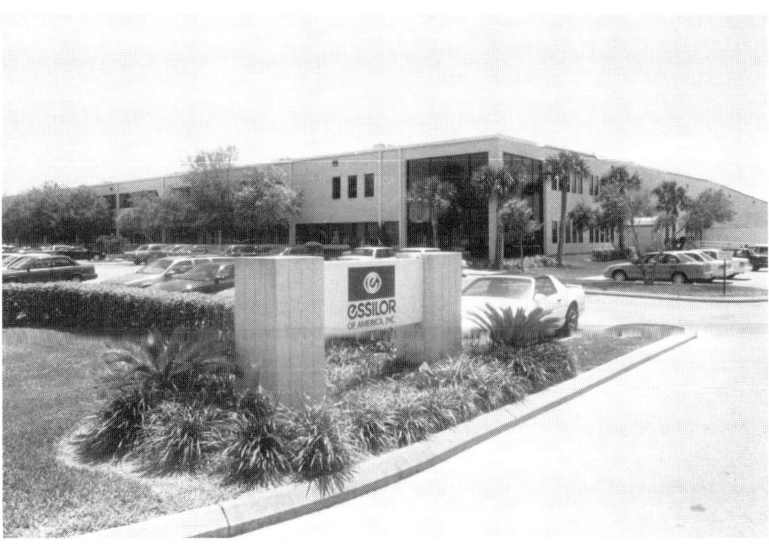

The Essilor of America building in St. Petersburg, Florida was built in 1990 and houses the company's corporate offices.

1977   Florida plant enlarges to 45,000 square feet and 150 employees. The finished 70mm Super Major lens is released.

Due to the rapid expansion of the lens business, Logo Paris is established in Novato, Calif. to handle frames separate from Silor. Silor's machinery business is also turned over to Logo Paris as a subsidiary called Photocentron to sell and service optical equipment, including edgers.

1978   Silor releases 75mm finished lenses. Employment is now 350 in manufacturing.

1979   Florida manufacturing makes fourth expansion to 135,000 square feet and Indianapolis and Dallas distribution centers are opened.

1983   Minneapolis and Miami distribution centers open.

1985   24,000 square foot distribution center is added to lens plant. Reflection Free AR production is established to produce stock AR lenses. SOFI de Chihuahua is established in Mexico to produce finished SV uncoated lenses.

Essilor of America is set up as a holding company for;

        Multi Optics (Varilux)

        Logo Paris

        Silor Optical, Inc.

        Silor Optical subsidiaries;

            Silor Optical of Florida and

            Optical General Corporation

            Optical General subsidiary Flo-Lite

            Photocentron

            Silor Optical of Florida subsidiary

                SOFI de Chihuahua

1986   Essilor Industries opens manufacturing facility in Puerto Rico to produce SF Progressive lenses in coated and uncoated.

1987   Reflection Free opens satellite facility in Sun Valley, Calif.

Lens plant expands in July and adds 14,000 feet in November for additional hardcoating facilities.

1988   Essilor of America purchases minority shares of SunSoft contact lenses.

1989   Photocentron purchases assets of AIT Industries in Schaumburg, Ill. Photocentron changes name to AIT Industries and is based in Schaumburg, Ill.

1990   Essilor of America purchases majority ownership of SunSoft Corporation. EOA and Silor relocate headquarters to St. Petersburg, Fla.

1991   An agreement is signed establishing Transitions Optical as a joint venture between PPG and Essilor International and the first plastic adjustable tint lens is introduced.

Silor Optical, Inc. and Silor Optical of Florida are dissolved. Silor continues to sell and distribute lenses. Essilor of America becomes operating company with Jacques Stoerr as President. EOA acquires direct ownership of Optical General and SOFI de Chihuahua.

Flo-Lite relocates to St. Petersburg.

Flo-Lite Optical, Inc.

In the back corner of Essilor of America's headquarters in St. Petersburg is a seldom heard of international weapon called Flo-Lite Optical. This international arm of the company began in 1976 as a one-man operation to handle selected customers in Canada. After a nine week tour of Latin America, Flo-Lite's current president, George "Papi" Wolf, turned his company's eyes southward. The company opened a warehouse in Miami to serve this new market. Eight years later, the offices were moved to EOA headquarters.

This division has now expanded operations to include Russia, the Baltic States, several countries in the Middle East and South America. Some of these markets are extremely volatile with governments and economies changing overnight. In spite of this and the fact that few understand the company's function, Flo-Lite's sales have increased by at least 10 percent annually.

Today

Essilor International is a large global company, employing just under 13,000 employees worldwide, with annual sales exceeding $1 billion. Seventy-five percent of the company's revenue is generated outside of France, 33 percent of it coming from the United States subsidiaries.

Lens sales are 81 percent of Essilor's total international category of products, with 7 percent accorded to Frames and 6 percent is equally attributed to machinery and contacts. Essilor International is headquartered in France, and it's U.S. subsidiaries and divisions cover all facets of the ophthalmic products industry.

SOFT-LITE LENS COMPANY

It was 1908 when an optometrist in New York City named Morris Singer began importing a pink lens called Soft-Lite, a name suggested by Dr. Cyril Barnert, head of ophthalmology at Mt. Sinai Hospital and a close friend of Singer's. The lens was manufactured by St. Gobain, the French glass-making cartel and sold in Singer's small four store chain in New York City. Morris' son Nathaniel Singer left Columbia Law School in 1920 to join his father's retail business. Nat Singer, deciding the retail business wasn't for him, took his father's Soft-Lite product and offered it to other retailers and laboratories. The product was sold through Lettino Trading Company, Optical Services Corporation, and finally, in 1929, through a new company called Soft-Lite Lens Company.

Having established a growing national market for the product, Singer convinced Bausch & Lomb in 1923 to produce the glass in their eight year old glass plant. B&L was to produce both finished and semi-finished lenses in all lens forms in which B&L made white lenses. This arrangement lasted for the next 30 years and during all that time, there was never a written contract between Soft-Lite and B&L. Those were days when a handshake would seal the deal.

B&L glass makers added a small amount of manganese to their normal pink lens formula to create a lens which would not absorb ultra violet rays from 300 to 360 nm. Because of this, Soft-Lite lenses when exposed to UV light, would not change color as all other pink lenses

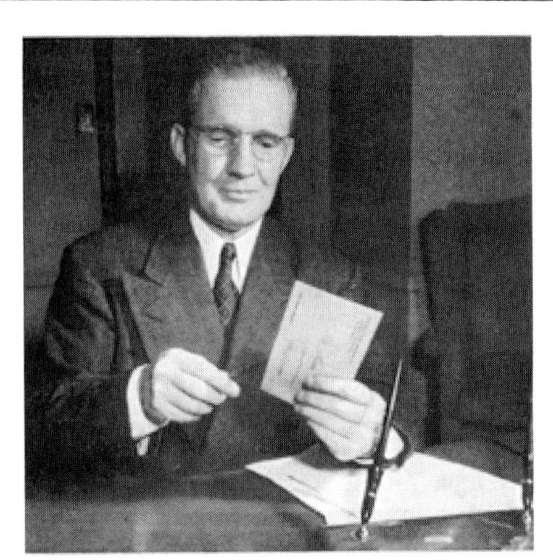

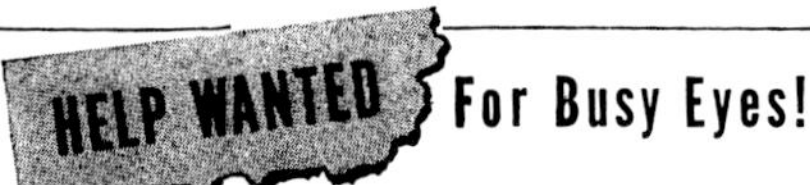

Your patients' eyes work hard all day long. Often they need help when improper lighting of high intensities is reflected at the near point from bright surfaces beneath eye level. *Neutral light absorption*, the 4th prescription component, can help such strained and tired eyes by providing the extra protection from glare that is necessary for complete comfort and increased visual efficiency.

Soft-Lite Lenses provide neutral light absorption. They may be prescribed in a lens form and a degree of absorption for each prescription requirement.

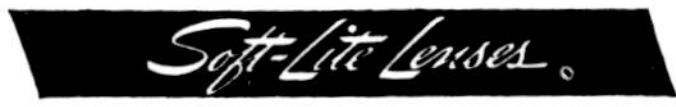

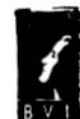

THE 4 PRESCRIPTION COMPONENTS ○ SPHERES ◐ CYLINDERS △ PRISMS ◈ NEUTRAL LIGHT ABSORPTION

did. This provided Soft-Lite with a graphic way to demonstrate that their product was different than any other pink lens. Their marketing strategy was to state "we don't know why the other fellow's lens turns purple but Soft-Lite is the only neutral absorptive lens - the same as white glass."

Pricing

Soft-Lite turned into a cash cow, producing substantial profits for everyone. The Soft-Lite Company paid the B&L factory exactly what a laboratory would pay for a pair of white blanks, plus an extra 6 cents per pair for single vision and 10 cents for bifocals. Because Soft-Lite discounted their bills every month, required no sales effort on B&L's part, placed advance orders each month, and purchased one million pair of lenses per year from 1943 onwards, they soon became B&L's best and most profitable customer. Fifty-five percent of the Soft-Lite lenses produced by Bausch & Lomb were sold to B&L's affiliated labs who paid the same price as independent wholesalers.

Both B&L labs and independent labs loved Soft-Lite because they made more profit on Soft-Lite sales than on any other lens product. Soft-Lite's slogan was: "40 will get you 60" — labs paid 40 cents more than Cruxite *(AO's pink tint and the leading competitor to Soft-Lite)* but could charge 60 cents more at resale. Retailers also made greater profits on Soft-Lite by selling Soft-Lite for $1 more than Cruxite, realizing an extra 40 cents profit on each pair *(a substantial amount often equivalent to half-a-day's wages)*.

As a result of these profit advantages, labs and retailers were anxious to handle the Soft-Lite product but only 200 of the 1200 independent laboratories were permitted to distribute Soft-Lite. It wasn't a coincidence that these happened to be the same 200 labs who were also B&L distributors. Labs had to agree to sell only to retailers selected by Soft-Lite's salesmen and at mandated prices. Selected retailers, or "Licensees" as Soft-Lite called them, were carefully selected by the Soft-Lite salesman for their reputation in the community. They had to agree to abide by Soft-Lite's Fair Trade prices *(until some time after World War II, the federal government enforced price protection for brand name products when sold at retail)*. Retailers had to agree never to substitute a competitive product for Soft-Lite.

Marketing Aids

Retailers received many benefits, including a numbered certificate with each pair of lenses for the patient, guaranteeing they had received a genuine pair of Soft-Lite lenses. Designed to increase the retailers' sales, Soft-Lite produced Practice Builders, including a beautiful Fitting Table Pad, memo books and Soft-Lite samples.

Soft-Lite also published a "Practice Builder" newsletter which gave professional men tips on selling and "Slants" intended to help labs increase profits.

Advertising

Soft-Lite became one of the first national advertisers, advertising in Life, Time, Saturday Evening Post and on the "March of Time" radio show. They also produced cooperative advertising material using top ad agencies. Their advertising program was tempered by the many restraints imposed by the American Optometric Association, the American Academy of Ophthalmologists and Otolaryngologists, and the Guild of Prescription Opticians. These trade associations all insisted the selection of all ophthalmic materials must be left in the hands of the professional. Soft-Lite ads got around this by stating: "See your practitioner and, if glare absorptive lenses are indicated, Soft-Lite Lenses are nice – like cathedral windows, they soften the light." The Soft-Lite trademark featured the famous Rheims Cathedral, a French landmark.

Labs and wholesalers were carefully supervised to make sure there were no infractions of the rules, which would result in delisting and, often, litigation. The Soft-Lite Company had 400 stockholders, mostly optical people who took advantage of the company going public in 1929 to buy stock. Dividends were so substantial that initial investments were quickly returned so that future dividends represented pure profit.

Litigation

In 1943, the U. S. Supreme Court heard the culmination of several years of government investigations and litigations concerning the relationship between Soft-Lite and Bausch & Lomb and Soft-Lite and its customers. The Court abolished the licensee system but permitted the exclusive relationship between B&L as a factory and Soft-Lite as a customer to remain in place. They also permitted Soft Lite to continue selecting and controlling prices of lab and retail customers. This case became landmark litigation, studied by law school students even to this day.

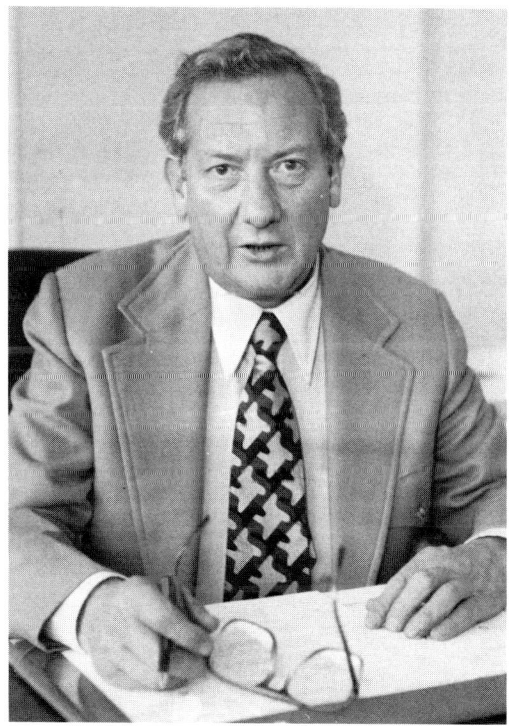

Noel Roscrow, one of the founders of Scientific Optical Laboratories of Australia, the company presently known as Sola Optical.

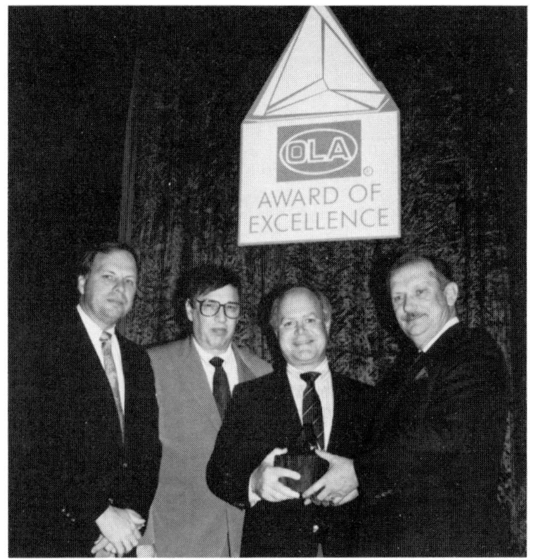

Sola received a 1989 OLA Award of Excellence for Smart Seg. Seen here receiving the Award are, left to right, John Potocny, Bernie Freiwald, Sola USA President Richard Kapash and OLA President Bill West.

Nat Singer remained as president from the company's inception until 1953 when Soft-Lite was sold to Bausch & Lomb for $1.2 million. B&L promptly, despite Singer's vigorous objections, changed the glass formula to match AO's Cruxite, reduced prices to those of other tinted lenses, and never again reached the lowest unit level of 750,000 pairs that Soft-Lite sold in its last year before acquisition.

SOLA OPTICAL, USA

Today's industry knows Sola Optical, USA as one of the world's largest manufacturers of spectacle lenses, but the company evolved from humble beginnings. The first experiments in casting CR-39 lenses in Australia were carried out in 1956 at a time when CR-39 was a new material. It was in that year that the company founders, led by Noel Roscrow, used a gas ring and a saucepan in a garage in a series of experiments to make plastic lenses. Plastic lenses were just beginning to be used in other countries and this small group of Australian optical entrepreneurs were determined to cast lenses in this new material.

In 1960, Roscrow convinced the owners, an Adelaide optometric practice called Laubman & Pank, to let him take his small group and form a small company called Scientific Optical Laboratories of Australia *(now SOLA)*. To produce cash flow during those early years, these nine employees performed binocular repairs for the Australian Army, vacuum coated ophthalmic lenses, made optical instruments and, incidentally, manufactured all rear vision mirrors for cars produced in Australia. Whenever they could steal a little time, they would work on casting CR-39 lenses. A branch was established in Melbourne in 1965 for instrument manufacture and repair but later converted to prescription surfacing and glass mold making.

Noel Roscrow was part of Sola from its very beginning. He had been apprenticed to a Melbourne spectacle maker at the age of 14 and was to spend the rest of his career in the optical industry. On the occasion of Roscrow's retirement, Chairman David L. Pank stated that Roscrow's mixture of knowledge, entrepreneurial drive, energy, persistence, vision and sheer cheek all helped in achieving the company's success.

Plano Lenses

At first, the company concentrated on casting completely finished lenses to prescription. Surfacing and polishing CR-39 was difficult, if not impossible, so casting finished lenses seemed to be the way to go. Gaskets for separating the molds were made by hand and lenses were hand filled individually by syringe. This was slow going and, needing another product, the company began producing plano lenses for sunglasses and industrial uses. Manufacturing CR-39 lenses was new and no one could explain how to do it.

The company decided to concentrate on plano lenses for two reasons. First, planos were easier to manufacture and Sola believed producing planos would provide training to help them solve the greater problems of casting prescription power lenses. Many in the industry believed that manufacturing semi-finished blanks was 10 times more difficult than planos and making finished prescription lenses 10 times more difficult than semi-finished. The second reason was that Sola's broad distribution of plano plastic lenses would help convert the world to the benefits of these new, lightweight lenses.

Marketing CR-39 lenses

To establish plastic lenses, they first had to convince the eyecare professionals. One of the early marketing promotions Sola implemented was to make thousands of clip-on sunglasses and bundle them into groups of five. These were shipped out to hundreds of opticians and optometrists. One pair was free and the other four were billed at a special low price. Seventy percent of the retailers kept the sunglasses and paid for them, 15 percent kept them and never paid and 5 percent wrote to tell how impressed they were with Sola's positive attitude regarding plastic lenses. The rest complained bitterly about such "cheeky" sales tactics. The end result, of course, was a growing acceptance of CR-39 lenses.

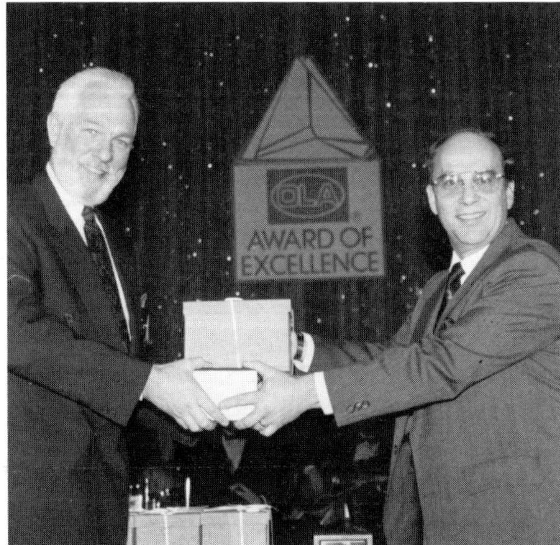

Sola won another OLA Award in 1993 for ASL FT28 in Spectralite. Accepting the Award is Sola USA President James Cox, left, and OLA President Al Willenbring.

World Production

At this time, there were only three companies in the world making any serious attempt to manufacture plastic lenses. These were Orma *(Essilor in France),* Armorlite *(United States)* and Sola. Strangely, for some unknown reason each company selected their own niche for concentrating their production efforts. Essilor worked on producing finished lenses, Armorlite on semi-finished blanks and Sola on plano lenses.

Manufacturing semi-finished CR-39 lenses created another problem. CR-39 material has a 14 percent shrinkage as the material is cast in the mold and this shrinkage changes lens curves. In the early days, calculating what curves to apply to the molds to achieve the desired front curves was an extremely difficult task. Seven-figure logarithms were required for the calculations. One of Laubman & Pank's people was a mathematician who was persuaded to join Roscrow's group where he was to spend the rest of his life calculating curves for the company's growing assortment of lenses.

Sola quickly recognized that, as big as Australia was, that lens market would never support the kind of manufacturing plant they envisioned for themselves so they focused on export sales. In 1968, a foreign operation was opened in Japan, expanding in the early 1970's to the United Kingdom, Italy, Brazil and, finally, the United States in 1975. By this time Sola had evolved into a global network of companies. Their semi-finished range was manufactured in 68mm diameter, at that time the largest available blank in the world.

Coming to the United States

When Sola came to the United States, a 15,000 square foot facility was opened in Sunnyvale, Calif. During this period, the U.S. lens market was still dominated by glass lenses, representing 70 percent of the market at the time Sola's U.S. plant opened. The company's marketing efforts during the 70's were devoted to aggressively converting the market to these lighter, more impact-resistant lenses. Growing rapidly, the company moved their U.S. manufacturing operations to a much larger facility in Petaluma, Calif., and also broadened the product line. An additional production site was set up in Mexico in the mid-1980's.

One of the main limitations in the growth of the SOLA group has been the lead time needed to expand and maintain the wide range of precision molds required for casting. In 1975 a specialist center was established in Singapore to supply glass molds to plants in Italy, Brazil, United States and Australia. The company maintains a special section involved in machinery design and development and most production machinery for their plants throughout the world has been designed, manufactured and tested in-house.

Pilkington Group

In 1979, Sola was acquired by the Pilkington Group of the United Kingdom. One of the world's largest producers of glass and related products, Pilkington has more than 100 subsidiaries in the United Kingdom and over 300 companies in 40 other countries. One of the reasons for Sola's remarkable growth was the U.S. market's shift from glass to plastic lenses. By 1983, the U. S. market was over 50 percent plastic and by 1992, more than 80 percent. Sola took every advantage of this growing market.

In 1987, Sola's parent company, Pilkington, acquired the vision care business owned by Revlon, including Coburn Optical. The previous Revlon operations were, however, operated separately from Sola. The only exception was the Coburn glass lens business which was added to the Sola organization. In 1988, Sola moved their headquarters from Australia to California and created separate United States and international divisions, calling the combined operation "The Sola Group".

Sola developed a plano sun/safety lens for Apollo missions into which Sola mixed carbon black for some

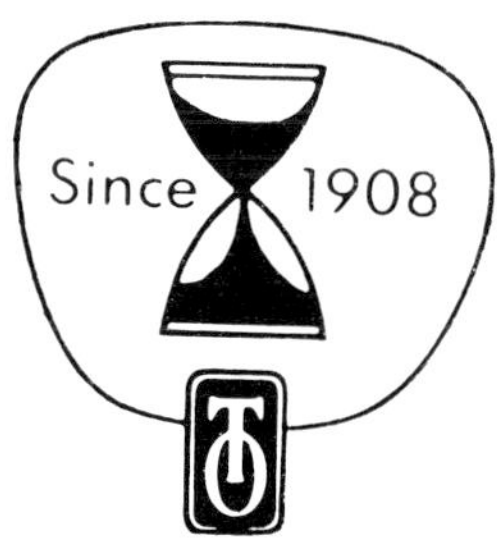

ILLUSTRATION – TITMUS OPTICAL COMPANY

Edward Hutson Titmus founded Titmus Optical as a wholesale and prescription optical business in 1908. Two years later, a fire wiped out much of downtown Petersburg, including the young Titmus Optical.

ILLUSTRATION – TITMUS OPTICAL COMPANY

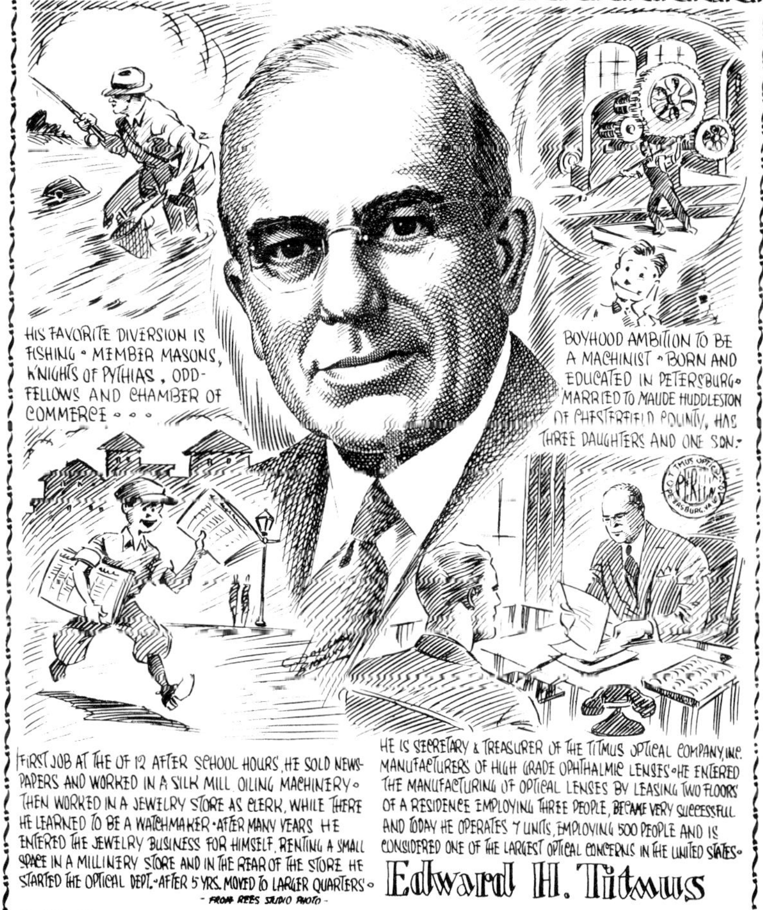

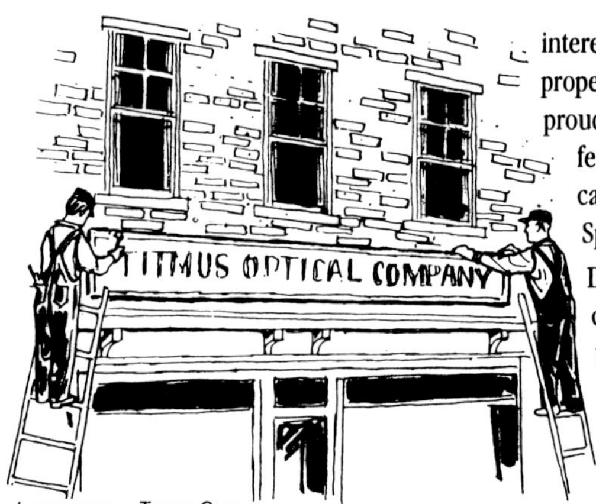

ILLUSTRATION — TITMUS OPTICAL COMPANY

interesting and useful optical properties. One of Noel Roscrow's proudest possessions is a plaque featuring a patch that was carried to the moon aboard the Spaceship America Apollo XVII. During the period Sola was concentrating on building up their export sales, Roscrow traveled all over the world and personally called on many OLA laboratories. On one trip to the United States in 1967, he visited 21 states in four weeks. In one seven year period, he flew around the world 37 times and spent no more than two weeks in any one place. Noel Roscrow retired in December, 1981. His son Ken Roscrow is a company vice president based in the United States.

John Heine took over as chief executive officer in 1981. Under his stewardship, the company's revenues have grown 20 percent per year. Heine was committed to increasing SOLA's presence in Asia and was responsible for SOLA's early entry into Mainland China. As a result, the company has become a major force in that part of the world. He has also been successful in preserving the company's entrepreneurial culture, even after the company became a major optical manufacturer. At the time Heine took over the reins, the company was basically a supplier of commodity plastic lenses. Today, Sola is a major supplier of brand name progressives, high index lenses and coatings.

Company History

A brief outline of Sola's company history would include:

1960   Sola Optical begins selling plastic lenses in Australia with 10 employees.

1961-66   Begins exporting lenses to Japan, England, France, Italy, India and other countries.

1968   Japan operation opens *(This was the first totally foreign-owned operation to open in Japan following the War)*.

1970   UK operation opens.

1972   Hong Kong operation opens.

1973   Started casting lenses in Italy.

1975   USA operation opens. Sola begins casting lenses in Brazil. Sola Singapore opens *(primarily to make molds)*.

1976   Started casting lenses in the United States.

1978   Started casting lenses in Ireland.

1979   Acquired by Pilkington.

1981   John Heine takes over as C.E.O.

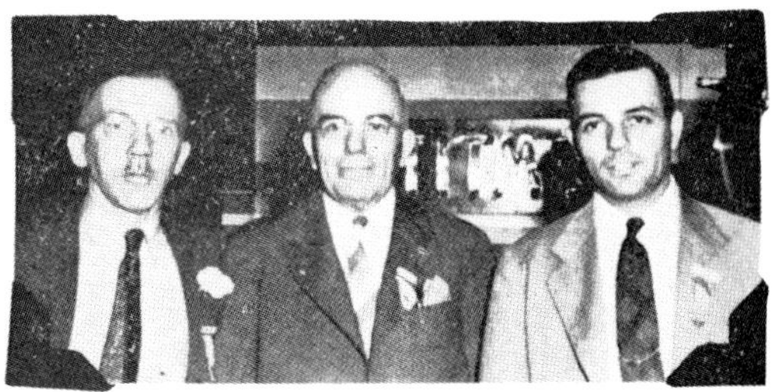

Pictured at the AOA 1940 Convention in Cincinnati are, left to right, Titmus sales manager Gus Berschwinger, E.H. Titmus and son E. Hutson (Hutty) Titmus, Jr. Hutty Titmus took over the company from his father and, following his early death in 1967, the company was headed by Ben Kinsey.

ILLUSTRATION — TITMUS OPTICAL COMPANY

1984   Releases first progressive lens.

1985   Started casting lenses in Mexico.

1986   Sales surpass $100 million *(US)*. Begin casting lenses in Taiwan.

1987   Established coating joint venture in Japan. Acquires Coburn lens business.

1988   Headquarters moved to California.

1991   Jim Cox is made president of Sola, USA.

1992   Sales surpass $150 million *(US)*.

1993   Company sold to AEA Investors.

1994   Introduced Spectralite Transitions, the first photochromic high index lens.

New Owners

In 1993, the Sola Group was purchased by AEA Investors, Inc. This privately-held company, founded in 1968 as American European Associates, Inc., invests in successful, industry-leading companies for long term growth. Fortune magazine once described the group as "The Richest Little Club in the World" in a 1989 story on AEA Investors. The New York City group was founded in 1968 as an investment vehicle for some of the wealthiest families in the world, names like Rockefeller, Mellon, Harriman and du Pont.

As Sola approaches it's 35th birthday, their operations span the globe, operating 12 manufacturing sites on five continents with sales offices in 16 countries. Each week, their customers, located in some 70 nations, order more than one million lenses from Sola. The company believes more than one hundred million people around the world are wearing Sola lenses today.

Even those dreamers in Adelaide couldn't have foreseen all this resulting from their primitive attempts to make plastic lenses in that garage almost 35 years ago.

TITMUS OPTICAL COMPANY

As a lad, Edward Hutson Titmus served an apprenticeship in a jewelry business in his home town of Petersburg, Va., and then attended Philadelphia Horological College where he learned watchmaking, engraving and optical technology *(the only way to achieve academic learning of the optical business at that time)*. Opening his own jewelry retail store in 1902 at the age of 25, he soon expanded his product line to include optical. A wholesale and prescription optical business was chartered in 1908 with an initial capital of $3,000, $2,000 from Titmus and the balance from two other partners. A disastrous fire wiped out much of Petersburg in 1910, destroying the Titmus store. Titmus eventually bought out his partners and in 1916 began producing finished and semi-finished toric lenses, changing the company name to Titmus Optical and Instrument Company. In 1918, the "Instrument" portion of the name was dropped.

At first, only toric lenses were made. These were easy to sell as World War I had created a shortage of optical lenses, with the European supply cut off and larger factories coping with the demand of the armed forces. The postwar era created a buyers market and Titmus Optical Company went through a bad period which ended with a settlement to creditors.

Matters were not helped when AO and B&L, in the early 20's, acquired most of the labs that had been customers of Titmus. In 1923, Titmus added meniscus lenses to their line. Titmus closed his retail store in December, 1927 and devoted full time and effort to optical manufacturing. In 1930, the company initiated multifocal production . Bifocals were successfully produced in 1931 when Carl Haering left B&L bringing his production knowledge to the fledgling bifocal factory. The business continued to develop and additional buildings were added until Titmus became one of the biggest factories in Petersburg.

The business continued to grow through the 1930's, selling lenses at 10 percent less than larger lens factories *(as permitted by AO)*. In addition, Virginia Lens Company was formed and became an outlet for products that Titmus wanted sold below current market prices *(in Virginia Lens packages)*. Titmus stoutly maintained for many years that they had no interest in Virginia Lens which they always claimed just happened to be a lens distributor located in Petersburg.

Frames and Contact Lenses Added

Edward "Hutty" Titmus, Jr. joined the company in 1936 and gradually rose through the management ranks, assuming virtual control after World War II and becoming chief executive in 1953. In 1952, Pete Collier joined the company and set up a frame production facility to enable Titmus Optical to become a fully integrated optical manufacturer. The company's lens and frame sales were, for the most part, to laboratories

not on AO, B&L or Shuron's distributor lists. From 1961 to 1966, the company produced hard contact lenses but abandoned that business because of distribution problems. Titmus, Sr. seldom failed to attend A.O.A. national conventions and the high point of the 1938 convention was a Titmus cruise down the historic James River.

The company maintained a very religious Baptist orientation in deference to the strong convictions of Edward Titmus, Sr. No drinking was permitted in the Petersburg area by any Titmus personnel, endured somewhat unwillingly by salesmen and visitors.

Distribution

Prior to 1955, Titmus had no distribution system and employed only one salesman. The company policy was to price all products at 10 percent below AO's published prices. Suddenly, in 1955, American Optical informed Titmus that a price differential would no longer be tolerated. It must be noted that AO and B&L between them had more than 350 wholesale labs around the country. In addition, they each had a large sales force calling on both independent labs and retailers.

Hutty Titmus came up with a clever plan to set up small "warehouses" in customers' labs. Titmus would maintain a perpetual computerized inventory of each "warehouse" and labs would pay for lenses only as they withdrew them from inventory. In this way, Titmus would finance the customers while controlling their inventories. More than 170 installations were set up around the country, primarily with small and medium sized distributors. While expensive, the program was generally considered a success.

Big Five

Titmus was the smallest of the so-called "Big Five", a term designated to describe the five ophthalmic manufacturers who offered a complete line of products and services — AO, B&L, Shuron, Continental and Titmus. In 1957, Victor Kniss of American Optical informed Hutson Titmus that he planned to lower prices of glass lenses to a point where even the so-called "basement operator" would be driven out of business. At this time, glass represented 95 percent of Titmus' sales. This is an example of the kind of heavy stick American Optical was able to wield over their competition.

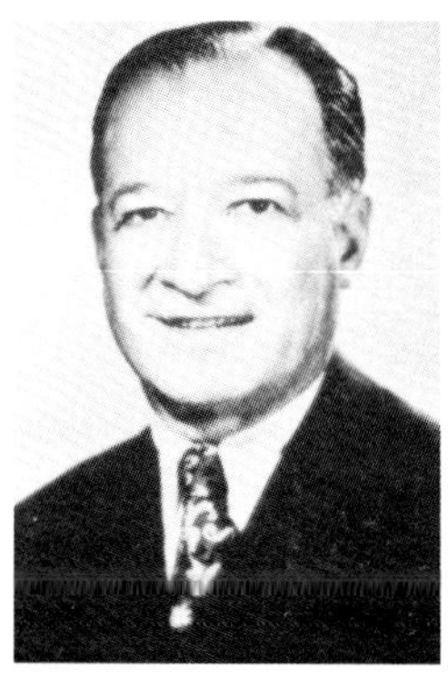

Victor Kniss, a very active American Optical vice president crops up in a number of places in this history. Titmus had traditionally maintained lens prices 10 percent below the majors. In 1957, growing tired of Titmus picking up crumbs from AO's table, Kniss informed Hutty Titmus that AO was lowering lens prices to drive what he called "basement operators" out of business.

Photo – Optical Industry Museum

This early Univis ad shows how Univis promoted the fact that flat tops eliminated the "trouble zone" found in all other bifocals of that day (Kryptok, Ultex and Nokrome bifocals). In truth, the flat top was a better bifocal because it positioned the seg's optical center closer to the top edge, greatly reducing visual "jump" as the eye passed into the reading area.

Illustration – Central States Optical catalog

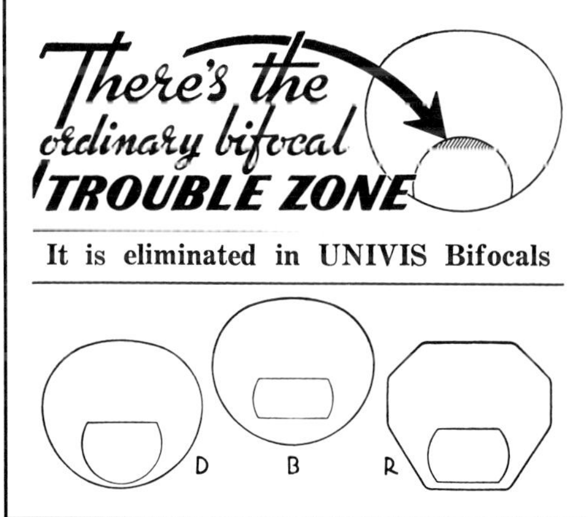

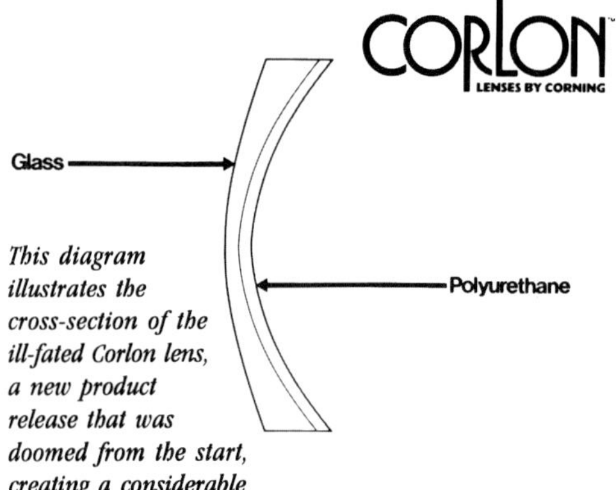

This diagram illustrates the cross-section of the ill-fated Corlon lens, a new product release that was doomed from the start, creating a considerable embarrassment for everyone involved.

OLA OPTICAL INDUSTRY MUSEUM

End of the Family Era

In 1967, when Hutty Titmus died suddenly, the company's lawyer, Benjamin Kinsey, took over as president, operating the company on behalf of the family stockholders until it was sold, in 1969, to a good customer, Dal-Tex Optical. Theodore Shanbaum, the major stockholder of Dal-Tex, owned a very large chain of retail stores, more than 150 in Texas, Arizona, New Mexico, Puerto Rico, and several other states. The Dal-Tex lab, founded by Irving Greenberg was the pioneer in laboratory mass production philosophy. They sold several thousand Rx's per day to their own stores as well as outside accounts. Shanbaum also had interests in radio stations, real estate, and other matters - in fact he was overextended and unable to maintain the conditions of profitability and cash reserves at Titmus as required by his bank loan. His philosophy was to use the frames as bait for lens sales *(or vice versa)* and he was shocked to discover that lenses and frames do not always make good sales partners. He found a buyer in Esterline who, in turn, eventually sold the company to Zeiss of West Germany in 1972.

The business continues today as the American branch of Zeiss. The frame factory is closed and the company distributes the German-made Zeiss frame line. The lens factory produces large quantities of safety lenses, often for their own safety laboratories. The balance of their bifocal production *(single vision lenses were discontinued shortly after the Zeiss takeover)* is shipped to the German parent.

TRANSITIONS OPTICAL

Photochromic glass lenses proved that the public was interested in changeable lenses. As hard resin lenses began to grow in market share, doctors and dispensers began to express interest in a lightweight plastic lens that would also change color in sunlight. Confident that a market existed for such a lens, a joint venture was formed in the early 1980's between Corning and Coburn Optical to produce a glass/laminate lens to answer this need. The new lens was introduced to the trade in late summer of 1982 and called Corlon or C-Lite. It was announced with a blizzard of high-powered promotion and advertising. Every promotional need had been anticipated so that labs could go out and launch this exciting new product. Only one small detail was overlooked — the lens didn't work.

Corlon consisted of a thin photochromic glass wafer fused to a lightweight plastic lens. The problem with laminated lenses is they can delaminate and this is exactly what happened. Another major problem turned out to be the thin glass wafer. Even though it was chem-tempered at the factory, it was almost impossible to mount Corlon lenses in a metal frame without chipping or cracking the lens. It proved to be a major disaster and was immediately withdrawn from the market.

PPG Industries is the world's leading producer of CR-39, a lightweight ophthalmic plastic monomer. The first efforts by PPG to develop a photochromic plastic took place during the period from 1973 to 1980 although nothing significant came out of that work. In 1981, American Optical introduced their Photolite lens which was a commercial failure, primarily because of poor photochromic properties and an unattractive blue activated color. It did, however, demonstrate the interest in an effective photochromic lens. The next several years led to the discovery of an incorporation technique *(imbibition)* that made photochromic lenses possible from CR-39 monomer. In 1983, PPG Industries discovered a new family of photochromics, the blue pyridobenzoxazines.

A joint venture was launched with Intercast - Europe in 1984 to produce the Attiva lens. PPG developed the manufacturing process and transferred the technology to Intercast in Italy. This lens is still manufactured. By 1985, Attiva production reached 3,150 lenses per day. In 1986, an all-PPG venture was started to produce the Visenza lens. In June, 1986, PPG embarked on a one year program to test the technical and marketing feasibility of plastic photochromic lenses. More than $10 million and 55 man-years were invested in the project.

From July 1987 to May 1988, a large consumer use test was launched, along with extensive employee use tests. During this period, budgets were tight and the Transitions people became very adept at finding inexpensive ways to build manufacturing equipment. Bill Adams managed the Tallmadge Facility *(where Transitions manufacturing procedures were developed)* from 1988 to 1991. He explained how some of their problems were handled. They discovered that a Tupperware container with its push button airtight seal was perfect for mixing the photochromic solution. They soon became the local Tupperware saleslady's best customer.

Cleaning the lens was an important step in making Transitions lenses. They spent weeks looking for an effective lens scrubber. One day while Adams was taking a shower, he noticed his wife's facial sponge in the shower caddie. On a whim, he took it to the lab and discovered it worked perfectly. They cleaned out every drug store in town and eventually bought the material by the roll from 3M. The next two years saw continuing process development and the start of test markets for Transitions Comfort lenses. In 1989, Transitions lenses are introduced in test markets - Vermont, New Hampshire, Memphis and Pittsburgh.

In July, 1990, Transitions Optical, Inc. was formed as a joint venture between PPG Industries and Essilor International. The company is based in Pinellas Park, Fla. and the product name changed to Transitions Comfort lenses. By February, 1991, the new lenses were available in 99 percent of North America and limited international marketing of Transitions lenses began.

In October, 1992, Transitions Plus lenses were introduced. These new lenses darken faster and deeper than the original product and have a more appealing warm-gray tint when activated. In 1993, Transitions Plus lenses received the prestigious OLA Award for Best Lens Treatment. By 1994, a new plant in Ireland was opened to serve the European market.

UNIVIS LENS COMPANY

One of the major lens manufacturers during the middle years of the 20th century, Univis Lens Company began its existence as Stanley Optical Company, an optical laboratory in Dayton, Ohio, just before World War I. Just after the War, Mr. and Mrs. M.H. *(Bunt)* Stanley had occasion to visit England where Mrs. Stanley broke her lenses. Visiting a local optician, they learned about a new bifocal then being produced by United Kingdom Optical that had a segment with a flat top rather than the conventional round shape. UKO, formerly Zeiss-England had been taken over by the British government during the first World War and converted to a public company after the war. Stanley secured exclusive rights to their product for the United States, but not for Canada where Imperial Optical was UK's agent. He imported lenses for his lab to distribute as finished lenses or through other labs who would purchase semi-finished bifocals from Stanley Optical. Jack Silverman, the lab foreman, and his brother, Milton, their salesman, established a market for the new bifocal until World War II began. When lenses could no longer be imported from England, Stanley acquired manufacturing rights to the lens.

Controlled Distribution and Pricing

Distribution of the early Univis lenses was very tightly controlled by the Univis Corporation, claiming in a 1936 trade ad in OPTICAL JOURNAL-REVIEW that their *"splendid lens service is protected from the evils of unfair competition by the strictly enforced licensing policy, restricting wholesale and retail distribution to selected establishments."* An ad the following year stated, *"Distribution restricted to selected licensees, with minimum prices established by contract and strict enforcement of sales policy make Univis 'tops' for protected profit."*

Stan Emerson had been running Emerson Optical, the British lens manufacturer bought out by Univis. He was brought to the United States in a returning U.S. bomber in 1945 and proceeded to supply manufacturing know-how to the Univis Lens Company. The bifocals they produced were distributed by selected wholesale labs throughout the USA. To handle sales, the company set up the largest, independent *(i.e. not AO or B&L)* sales force of the day, consisting of 15 men, a first for this industry.

By the end of the war, the company was being operated by the Silverman brothers, Virgil Hancock and Roy Marks, who was in charge of production. Hancock left soon after the war to form Modern Optics, a Texas-based bifocal manufacturer. Hancock was an innovative engineer and introduced a number of "firsts" for bifocal manufacturing. One of these was the introduction of the "arc lamp" as a way of demonstrating surface quality of finished lenses. Hancock's intention was to prove the superior finish of Modern Optics bifocal segments. Unfortunately, the arc lamp also illustrated the poor back sufaces being produced in many laboratories. These were the days when lenses were polished on felt pads and shadows from the felt pad and swirls from antiquated cylinder machines still used in many labs became glaringly apparent. Hancock's arc lamps sold a lot of machinery for Shuron and the emerging Coburn Optical.

Modern Optics was ultimately acquired by Continental. There is an interesting story about how Modern Optics came to be sold. Their plant was on a piece of property that a Texas realtor wanted. In checking out the company, he came to the conclusion the company had greater value than Hancock realized. He ended up buying the company, the building and the land for less than he had been willing to pay for the land alone. The company was then sold to Continental without the land. What he collected for the company was a nice little side profit. Modern Optics ended up as part of Continental and then Shuron when those two companies merged in 1955.

The Strike

In 1948, Univis suffered a major and violent strike that resulted in the company moving to Puerto Rico and Florida to escape the union. Roy Marks, a Univis vice-

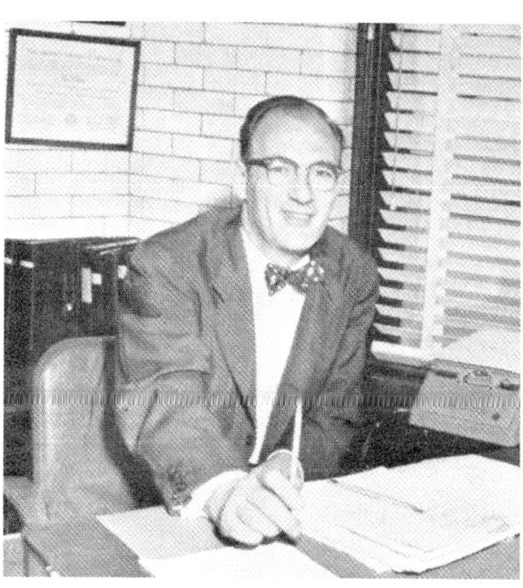

Roy Marks, pictured here during his days as president of Shuron Optical, enjoyed a colorful earlier career with Univis Lens Company, getting his picture on the front page of the Chicago Tribune during a vicious strike in Dayton, Ohio.

Virgil Hancock started his career with Univis and later founded Modern Optical, a flat top manufacturer later acquired by Continental Optical, who had only produced Ultex-type bifocals.

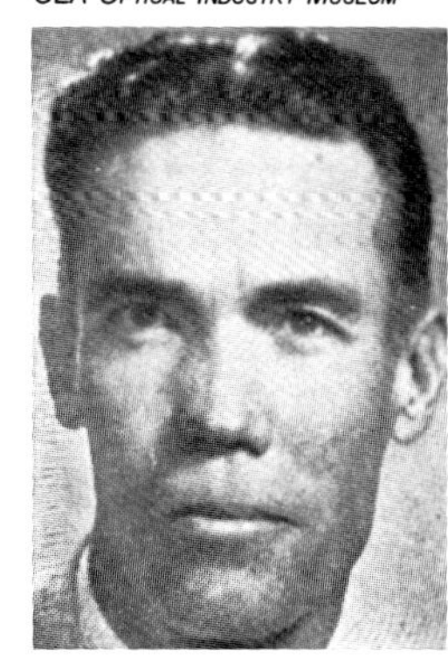

resident was a major figure during the strike. A picture of strikers tossing him out the front gate of the plant appeared in major newspapers across the country. Marks finished his days at Univis as head of sales before leaving for a brief stint with Soft-Lite Lens Company, Bausch & Lomb and then Shuron.

Milt Silverman left the company shortly thereafter, taking lenses for what was owed him for his stock ownership and severance pay, later selling the lenses at reduced prices. His brother Jack retired and Stanley brought in a new team to run what had become one of the largest lens companies in the country. Jerry Weis was brought in from Bendix Aviation as president and head of manufacturing; Bob Barber moved from Bulova Watch Company to take over sales and marketing; Stan Emerson headed research and development; and Art Sowers became treasurer.

In 1954, the four officers banded together to buy the company from Stanley. Since the only one who had any substantial money was Emerson *(he still had the money he received for his British company),* the group sought advice from Soft-Lite's Nat Singer. Together with Soft-Lite's attorney, William Casey *(subsequently to head the CIA),* they put together an early leveraged buy-out in which anticipated future dividends would be used to pay off the purchase price. The quartet then embarked on an ambitious expansion plan, to take advantage of the lessening influence of AO and B&L.

Univis moved to Ft. Lauderdale, Fla., closing the Dayton plant in Ohio to be nearer their major production facility established in the early 1950's in Puerto Rico. Weis died unexpectedly and was replaced as president by Barber. On Barber's retirement, Sowers became president, followed by Jack Cooney who had come up through the sales ranks. A facility was opened in Florida to manufacture CR-39 lenses. They had dabbled with plastic lenses earlier in Dayton, Ohio when Dr. Robert Graham, who subsequently founded Armorlite Lens Company, ran their plastic lens facility. As soon as the tax benefits ran out, they closed the Puerto Rico operation and concentrated all lens manufacturing in the Ft. Lauderdale plant.

Identification

Univis had, by now, developed into the premier bifocal manufacturer. Their bifocal line carried premium prices and, helped by their extensive direct sales force and heavy advertising to the professions, was considered top-of-the-line in bifocal design. Every lens manufacturer had a flat top bifocal by now, and there was fierce competition among the top companies, chiefly AO, B&L, Shuron and Modern Optics. Each company was trying to establish an identity to their flat top so the retailer could know he was getting the genuine product. Univis got the bright idea of etching a small U within a circle in the corner of the lens *(all lenses were still glass)* and introduced it in May. All the doctor *(or wearer)* had to do was breath on the lens and the symbol would show up. What they forgot was what happened to glass lenses in cold weather.

That winter doctors received thousands of complaints from patients who thought there was a blemish on the lens. That idea was quickly dropped. Meanwhile American Optical started gold plating the top edge of the segment. Univis' answer was the famous "railroad tracks" which featured a series of bars across the top of the segment. It identified the product, but actually produced a distracting blur across the middle of the lens.

By this time, doctors and dispensers were beginning to recognize that they had equal fitting success with any first quality flat top bifocal and brand loyalty eventually disappeared. In recent years, a market research organization tried to track brand usage of flat tops by surveying retailers. They discovered that most retail offices do not know, for the most part, whose flat tops they are using. That's how much the lens business has changed since the 50's.

Univis Enters the Frame Business

In 1955, Univis decided to enter the frame business by acquiring Bay State Optical Company, a factory owned by Nat Singer. They had previously experimented with frame distribution, first by designing their own line of frames, made by Bay State, and then by selling Bay State's own line. Their line had been developed by Austin Belgard, a Chicago optician. Belgard and Bernie Spero founded the House of Vision, a major retail

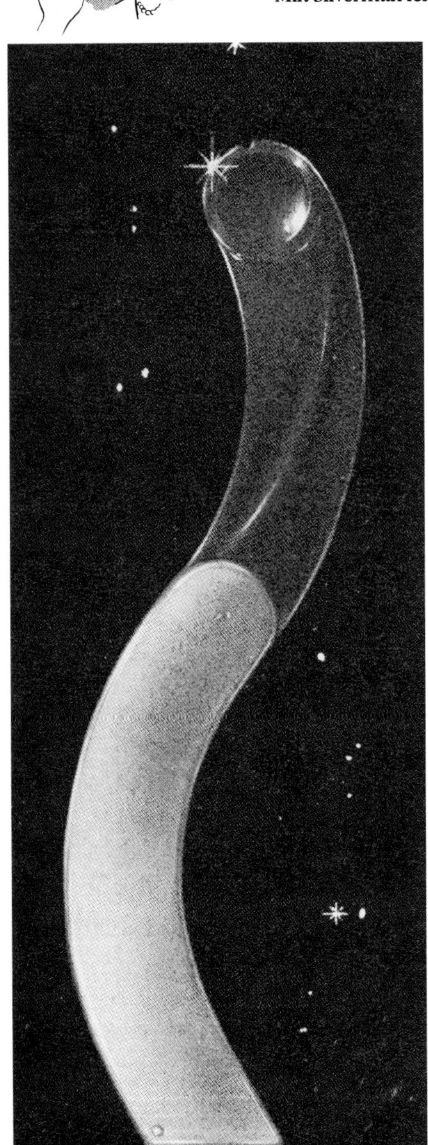

In 1960, corneal contact lenses were coming into their own, but wearers had one problem. There were no effective bifocal contact lenses. Newton K. Wesley (The Plastic Contact Lens Company) came up with an innovative solution. This graceful little tool, called Lorcon, featured a plus lens at one end, permitting contact wearers to discretely read a menu or phone book (reminding one of early fan spyglasses - see right).

dispensing firm in that city. Belgard left to set up his own dispensing business. The Univis frame line included several styles that were ugly and cumbersome and impossible to mass produce. These frames received such poor reception that the entire inventory and tooling were scrapped at a cost of at least a half million dollars. Subsequently, Joe Trahan, a lens manufacturing executive, was put in charge of frame production. The company ultimately shut down frame production in 1957.

Company management was still convinced that selling frames and lenses together would be a natural for their sales force. They had a misconception that laboratories that liked Univis lenses, then the most popular bifocal on the market, would naturally buy frames from their Univis salesman. An unsuccessful effort to utilize Hudson Optical was terminated with Hudson barely surviving the experience. Hudson, on their own again, became a successful frame manufacturer as they had before their experience with Univis.

Next Univis acquired the Bishop Company in North Attleboro, Mass., owned by Jack Baer and including many people who had previously worked for Bay State Optical Company before their move from Attleboro, Mass., to Westbury, Long Island, N.Y., in 1953. Finally, their frame investments began paying off as new styles were introduced and a special marketing group was set up to promote frame sales.

This success was accelerated by the acquisition of Zylite, a leading plastic frame manufacturer in Long Island City, N.Y. Zylite's production was moved to North Attleboro and incorporated with the former Bishop production. Charles Ladew, formerly a sales executive at Soft-Lite Lens Company and then head of sales for Zylite, took over as head of frame sales for Univis. Univis also acquired the services of a Zylite partner, Herman Lieberman, who remained the oldest active salesman in the United States until passing away in 1992 at age 94.

Shortly after the acquisition of Zylite, Alan Glassman purchased the three floor Zylite operation, complete with all machinery, tooling, and raw material inventories. This was the start of Swan Optical Company, today a major manufacturer and importer of inexpensive frame styles.

The Univis frame division became the biggest domestic frame manufacturer by the early 1980's, producing more than $25 million in frames. In 1955, at the same time they acquired Bay State Optical, Univis acquired Vision-Ease, a St. Cloud bifocal manufacturer specializing in special lenses. At a Univis sales meeting in Bear Mountain, N.Y., Eldon Siehl *(Vision-Ease president)* explained the advantages of expanding the Univis line by adding the special lenses his company offered. Three

weeks later, Vision-Ease withdrew from the acquisition, largely because Benson Optical, a major customer of both companies, objected to losing their favorable discount on Vision-Ease prices. Ironically, 30 years later Vision-Ease would end up acquiring Univis.

In 1967 and 1968, Univis, under President Robert O. Barber, attempted to find a suitable partner for the company. A deal was almost finalized with Becton-Dickinson, the pharmaceutical company, but was not consummated. Financial investigations indicated Univis would be a poor purchase for B-D.

On December 31, 1968, Univis acquired White Haines Optical Company, formerly a B&L affiliate, purchased from B&L 10 years before by its employees. Combining the White Haines 1968 financial statements with their own would provide a more favorable financial picture for enticing acquisition of Univis by Itek Corporation, a high-tech manufacturer in Massachusetts. The logic worked and Itek formed an ophthalmic division around Univis and Pennsylvania Optical Company of Reading, Pa., which Itek had acquired in 1967.

Pennsylvania Optical originated almost 100 years before when a medical doctor decided that the public should be able to obtain reading glasses at reduced prices. The doctor prevailed upon a merchant in nearby Lancaster, Pa., who had just opened a mass-marketing store to add his reading glasses. His neighbor happened to be F. W. Woolworth and as Woolworth expanded his "Five and Dime" empire, Pennsylvania Optical reading glasses enjoyed a similar growth. Soon sunglass lenses, safety glasses, and then precision optics were added. Pennsylvania Optical even polished the bottoms of ceramic ware produced by Corning in nearby Corning, N.Y. But the company fell on bad times during and after World War II under the aegis of a "protégé" of the original doctor's son. A committee of local businessmen, employees, and suppliers guaranteed bank loans and hired Charles Baratelli who turned the business around. Baratelli's experience included the start-up of Polaroid and subsequent sunglass designing for American Optical's Polaroid Division when AO took over Polaroid sunglasses after World War II, and manager of AO's case division. Itek paid 200,000 shares of stock for the Pennsylvania Optical acquisition. It was worth $36 per share at the time of the offer, $45 when the directors approved, and $60 when the stockholders approved.

Interestingly, Itek had first turned down this acquisition despite the net earnings of 20 percent Pennsy made on their sales volume, on the basis that Pennsylvania Optical was just emerging from the 19th century while Itek was already entering the 21st. The Rockefeller interests, who owned a controlling interest in Itek, suggested to the Itek board that Itek should return to the 19th century and discover how such profits could be made. The acquisition was then finalized. Itek, after acquiring the combined companies of Univis-White Haines, in 1970 added Kelley and Hueber, the largest and one of the oldest case manufacturers, located in Philadelphia. It was expected that these operations would dovetail nicely with Pennsylvania Optical, which turned out not to be the case. Management for the division was shifted to the frame plant in North Attleboro, Mass., under Alex Torda, a former officer of American Optical Company.

Itek then decided to form a national wholesale division around White Haines as a protection against the onslaught of direct selling of frames, which was already becoming preeminent. They acquired Balester Optical of Wilkes-Barre, Pa., TAT-Fairfield in Connecticut, Northwest-Northern in Seattle, Wash., and Merritt-Peninsula in Florida.

The ophthalmic division was headed by Bob Barber, Univis president, until his retirement. He continued as a consultant while Matt Burns, an Itek corporate manager, took over. He was followed by Jack Cooney, formerly the sales manager of Univis. Rudy Aversano, another Itek executive, became president when Cooney left the company in 1971. Itek had been doing well in the sophisticated instrumentation area, but went through a bad period in the early 1980's and spun off, closed, or sold their ophthalmic division, exiting the ophthalmic industry. The remnants of Univis became known as Camelot Industries under the direction of Sal Macera, a financial executive who dreamed of the possibilities of reestablishing what had once been an industry leader. Camelot struggled along until, after a raider's abortive attempt to acquire the company, it was acquired by a white knight, their previous "almost" subsidiary Vision-Ease. The Univis glass lens line was shut down and the Ft. Lauderdale facility converted exclusively to CR-39. Vision-Ease moved their plastic operations from St. Cloud, Minn. to Florida. The once-dominant Univis sales force was either absorbed or dropped by Vision-Ease and the frame factory continued as a separate division. The laboratory division was sold piecemeal or closed, a dismal end for once proud labs.

The frame division did reasonably well until an abortive attempt during the mid 1980's to bypass their distributors and sell frames directly to retailers in California. This failed miserably, primarily because the frame styles were inappropriate for direct selling and because personnel handling the project was not effective. Selling frames to retailers wasn't the same as selling frames to labs. The failure also hurt Vision-Ease lens sales as laboratories rebelled against this bypassing of their shrinking frame sales. Labs were already experiencing a drastic loss of frame sales from direct sellers and to have

a lens supplier take to the streets against them was a bitter blow. Fortunately, Vision-Ease quickly recognized the error of their ways.

The frame company was sold to Beta Industries, an entrepreneurial company from San Jose, Calif., who had acquired the purchase money from Fleet National, a Providence bank. They had already purchased Universal Optical Company, an East Providence, R.I., frame manufacturer, sold by its original owner, Wally Murray, to I. Stern, a metals manufacturer, and then repurchased by Wally Murray, Jr. Universal had sold off its production facilities and concentrated on imports, reselling them under designer names such as Givenchy. Beta then moved the Universal operation into the Univis facilities, utilizing Univis' factory to augment their imports *(some of which Univis had also been making)* and selling products under both company names, including designers such as Halston, Bill Blass and Evan Piccone.

Beta introduced innovations such as putting wheels under every factory machine to make the production line more versatile even though no machine was ever moved after the wheels had been added. Less than two years after their purchase, Beta's interest was foreclosed by the bank, who had earlier closed out the interests of all trade creditors. Unable to find another buyer, the bank sold the combined company to Charles Huff, a former B&L vice president. Huff had acquired several other companies in this same manner. Huff paid $2 million, all of it leveraged through the bank with only $250,000 personally guaranteed. The loan was paid off within a year by sharply reducing the labor force and streamlining operations.

Universal-Univis is once again operating as a frame manufacturer and importer in its North Attleboro, Mass. facility, the final vestige of the once powerful Univis Lens Company.

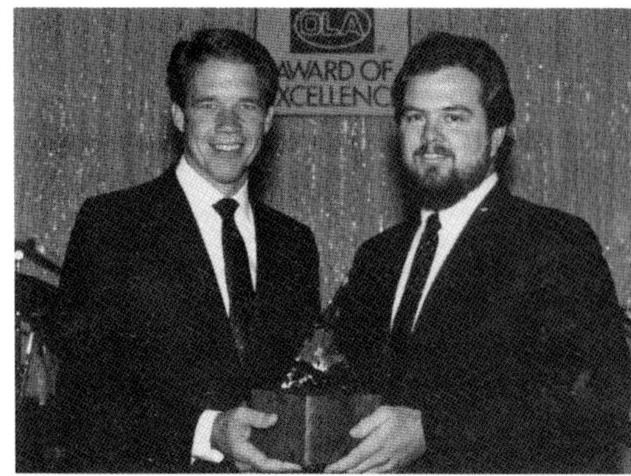

Varilux Infinity design won a 1988 Best In Lenses OLA Award of Excellence. Varilux president Mike Daley, right, accepts the Award from OLA President Gary Duffens.
OLA Optical Industry Museum

VARILUX CORPORATION

The first successful progressive addition lens was introduced in 1959 under the name Varilux I. The actual concept of a progressive lens was patented in 1907 by Owen James but was never produced. The first Varilux lens was designed in France by Bernard Maitenaz as a series of spherical surfaces that would provide a substitute for lost accommodation. Many progressive designs are still based on this principle. Varilux I was introduced in this country in 1969 by Silor.

Maitenaz improved his first design by utilizing aspheric surfaces for both distance and near. The new design, Varilux II was marketed and sold by Multi-Optics Corporation, an Essilor subsidiary company founded in late 1974 by Gerard Cottet and Pierre Le Fahler, its first president. The company was based in Chicago and began processing glass and 6.00 base plastic lenses into uncuts for a dozen or so distributors on the west coast in 1975. The problem was processing aspheric lenses on equipment developed to manufacture spherical lenses.

Multi-Optics provided a Certified Dispenser program as a way of training fitters, one at a time, to insure success of progressive lenses. In February, 1977, the laboratory supplying uncuts to their distributors was closed. The company created a Lab Services division to apply the processing techniques learned about aspheric lens processing to an extensive training program for their distributors.

In the late 70's, distribution was expanded to the midwest and the east. During eight years *(1979-1987)* of leadership under Olivier Mathieux, Multi-Optics experienced dramatic growth in sales and distribution. The company focused on educating independent eye care professionals, one at a time, through a team of sales consultants providing information and dispensing training for optical retailers.

In August, 1987, Jacques Stoerr, presently president of Essilor of America, was named president, following several years as director of professional relations and vice president of marketing. Multi-Optics name was changed to Varilux Corporation in 1988 to more closely associate the company with its product. In this same year, Varilux pioneered the use of consumer advertising for lenses.

As the patents of Varilux II *(presently known as Varilux Plus)* neared expiration, the company launched a new multi-design lens called Varilux Infinity. That design won the OLA Award as "Best Development in Lens Design" for 1988. The company gradually increased lab distribution to Varilux's current level of just over 100 distributors nationwide.

In 1992, the company's headquarters moved from California to Florida to be closer to Essilor of America in St. Petersburg. During and following that move, the company was working on what they considered a breakthrough progressive design. The new lens, called "Comfort", was launched in January of 1994. Feeling they had a real winner in their new lens, the company held up the product release to make sure they had ample inventories for their distributors. Practitioner reaction to the lens even exceeded Varilux's optimistic expectations. There was a period of some three months following release when the company was unable to keep up with incoming orders. That problem didn't last too long and many of their laboratories claimed progressive sales increases of 30 percent or more.

The company's reliance on limited distribution for their product has worked well - for Varilux and for their laboratory distributors.

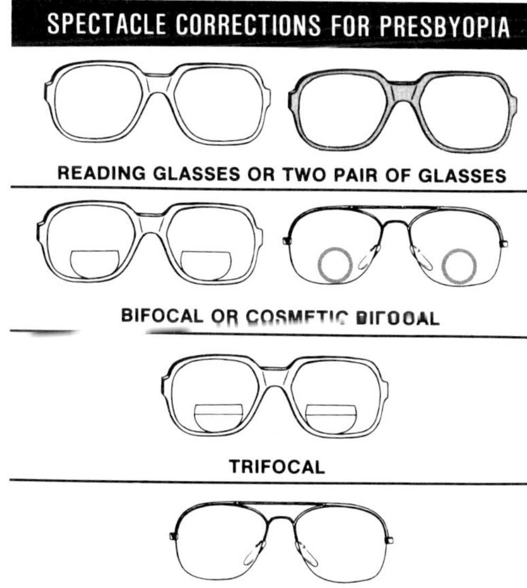

This resourceful ad illustrates how Varilux positioned progressive addition lenses in promotional material aimed at consumers. In one simple diagram, they graphically illustrated the cosmetic advantages and the visual advantages of modern progressive addition lenses.

ILLUSTRATION – COURTESY OF VARILUX CORPORATION

VISION-EASE

In the late 1930's, as the U.S. population continued to expand and visual tasks grew more sophisticated, a greater percentage of the populace required eyecare. This, in turn, meant a greater need for multifocals. Restrictive patents had run out and an opportunity to supply independent laboratories not allied with AO or B&L arose. A new industry sprang up in the area around St. Cloud, Minn. - possibly attracted by the relatively high price levels maintained by Twin City wholesale dispensers such as Benson and Walman. A substantial number of lens factories including Vision-Ease, Lantz Lenses, X-Cel, and Minoco Lens Company all ended up in this area.

It all began when Clair Lantz moved to St. Cloud in 1926 to open a retail optical business. He began making bifocals in his basement at home and, in 1936, opened a factory called Visionez. His operation served as a spring board for most of the other lens manufacturers in that area. In 1948, Lantz sold Visionez to a local businessman named Eldon Siehl. Lantz then formed Lantz Lenses which became a family business including his daughter and son-in-law Val and Audrey Gerads and their

ILLUSTRATION – VISION-EASE CORPORATION

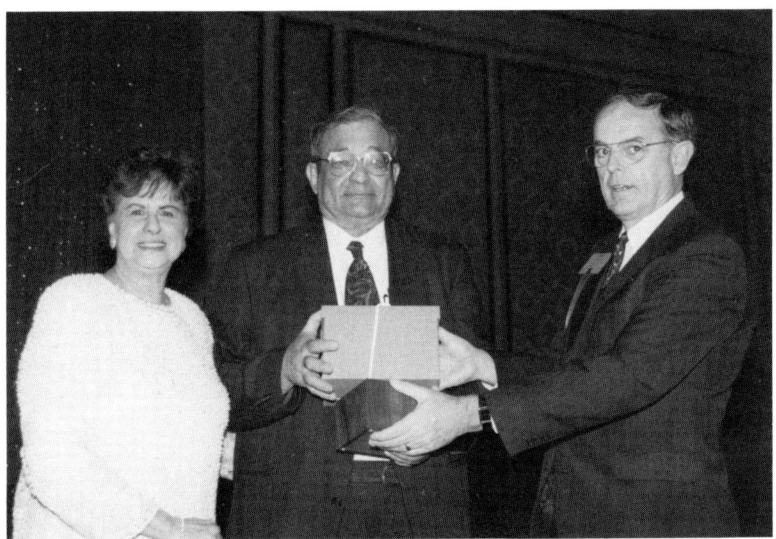

Irving Rips, founder of Younger Lens Company, received the OLA "Directors' Choice" Award in 1992 for his contributions to the ophthalmic industry. In the photo are, left to right, Bebe and Irving Rips receiving the Steuben trophy from OLA President Dave Lea.

sons, Clair and Val, who still run the business.

Siehl expanded his business and, in 1952, changed the spelling of the company name to "Vision-Ease". The company was now manufacturing fused bifocals and trifocals. After the abortive, short-term merger with Univis in 1955, Siehl proceeded to produce increasing quantities of lens products. With the help of Bill Kennedy, a manufacturing executive who had worked with B&L, Shuron, and Univis, he developed new cost-saving techniques and machinery which helped the company stay competitive as the lens market became more and more price oriented. Robert Conn, a local banker, joined the company in an executive capacity and the company continued to grow.

In 1969, Siehl sold the company to a St. Paul conglomerate called Buckbee-Mears, primarily a photographically-oriented organization. Siehl stayed on as president until 1972 when Conn took over. Upon his death in 1975, Carl Bergstrom, a former American Optical executive, was named president.

By 1973 the company had been marketing lenses internationally for four years and growing sales required a move from their cramped, overcrowded plant to a major factory facility in the St. Cloud Industrial Park. In 1981, Vision-Ease *(ironically)* acquired Univis in an effort to save them from an unfriendly takeover. Univis had been spun off from Itek as Camelot Industries. The Univis glass plant in Ft. Lauderdale, Fla. was closed and all of Vision-Ease's plastic lens production moved into that facility. The Univis sales force was either absorbed by Vision-Ease or let go. This was the sad end to the proud Univis name. Their lens products disappeared from the marketplace to be replaced by an expanded Vision-Ease line.

The Univis frame factory in North Attleboro became a separate division under Owen Carroll, another former AO executive, and was eventually sold to Beta Industries.

Buckbee-Mears also sold the Kelley & Hueber case division, obtained through the Camelot acquisition and their contact lens division.

Paul Burke, a former corporate counsel, became president *(replacing Carl Bergman, who headed the optical division for several years),* and moved the corporate headquarters to Ft. Lauderdale, leaving only the glass production plant in St. Cloud. Burke was later elevated to the presidency of BMC Industries *(formerly Buckbee-Mears)* and replaced as president of Vision-Ease by Ray Rogers.

Vision-Ease now produces glass lenses in St. Cloud, plastic lenses in Ft. Lauderdale and polycarbonate lenses in Brooklyn Center, Minn. and has become the largest domestic glass manufacturer. The rapid growth in demand for polycarbonate lenses led the company to double their production capacity in Brooklyn Center. The company estimates their share of the fast-growing polycarbonate market was close to 25 percent by the end of 1993. The most profitable divisions for Vision-Ease are their glass and polycarbonate divisions, both based in the Minnesota area. Recognizing this fact, the company moved their corporate headquarters back to Minnesota in 1993. Vision-Ease today is the largest domestically owned manufacturer of glass and plastic lenses.

In addition to their very significant stake in the optical industry, Buckbee-Mears is also a leader in precision imaged products. They are the only independent non-Asian manufacturer of aperture masks. These masks are critical components used in all color television and computer monitors. They manufacture in both the United States and Europe and are a major supplier to virtually every picture tube manufacturer outside Japan and even to several Japanese companies that manufacture in the United States and Southeast Asia. To maintain this market against the dominant competition from Japan is a tribute to their products.

WEBSTER LENS

Here's another story of a third-generation optician coming to America to pursue his trade and establishing another multigenerational business in this country. Ira Chaffin, born in Russia, had been trained as an optician by his father and grandfather. At the onslaught of the Russian Revolution, young Chaffin set out by himself *(at age 16)* on the Trans Siberian railway, traveling 6,500 miles across Manchuria to Korea, then by steamer to Japan and then across the Pacific to Seattle. From there, he went east to Boston.

16,000 miles later, he settled down in Boston and opened an optician's shop. Several years later, he founded the Chaffin Optical Company in Boston, a wholesale business that survived until 1994 when it

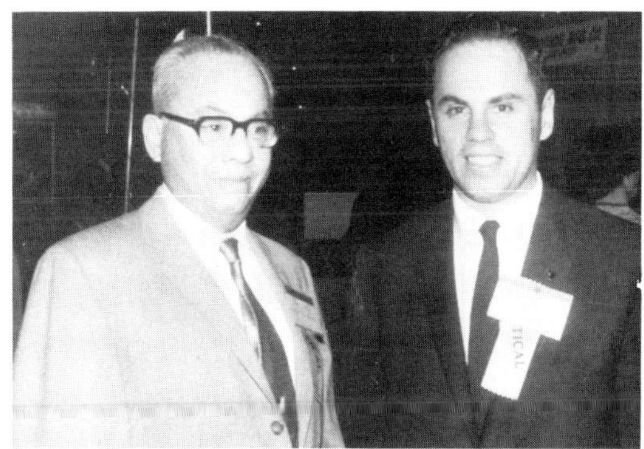

Webster Lens founder Ira Chaffin (left) is seen here with his son Nate Chaffin at the 1966 OWA convention in San Francisco.

ceased operations. In 1934, Ira founded the Webster Lens Company, naming the company after the town in which it was located *(the town was named after Daniel Webster)*. The company grew slowly, suffering several fires and a flood in 1955 that buried the plant under ten feet of water. The company managed to survive these acts of nature and continued producing glass products. Ira suffered a 14 year period of illness before his death in 1978. His two sons, Richard and Nathaniel Chaffin had both joined the company when they got out of college, Dick in 1954 and Nate in 1956. Following Ira's death, the sons took over direction of the company. In 1993, Dick Chaffin sold his interest to Nate who presently runs the company. Nate has six children and his daughter Sara works in Webster's marketing and sales department.

Webster only produces glass single vision lenses but they also produce molds and a variety of other non-ophthalmic lens products. The company was the first to market Schott's 1.70 in semi-finished form and were pioneers in semi-finishing Corning's Photochromic glass and Chance-Pilkington's Reactolite. They are the only company in North America manufacturing a complete line of single vision lenses, a niche market that is primarily Websters. Nate Chaffin sees a secure future for Webster, believing there will always be a market for glass lenses.

Nearly half of the company's sales are outside the U.S. where many countries still use a great deal of glass.

YOUNGER OPTICS

During the 30's and early '40s, during summers and while going to college, Irving Rips supported himself by working for the Cole Bifocal Company, a bifocal manufacturing company owned by his uncle, Paul Rips, in Omaha, Neb. For six years, Irving spent his days studying philosophy and his nights fusing glass blanks. In 1950, he married Grace *(Bebe)* Novick and the newlyweds moved to California to join Irving's brother who was already in the retail optical business.

He worked in the precision optics industry from 1952 to 1954 at Herron Optical in Los Angeles. He was also working long hours after work in his garage trying to perfect a way to make invisible glass bifocals. Whether Irving was aware of the tremendous impact the Kryptok bifocal made when it hit the market in 1899 as an invisible bifocal *(the Kryptok was invisible only when compared to its predecessor, the Franklin bifocal)*, he certainly knew the industry was ready for a truly invisible bifocal. With virtually no funds he was able to develop a crude but effective invisible "blended" bifocal which he began selling to a small but growing list of local area customers.

One day in 1955, he was introduced to Ben Weingart, one of the wealthiest men in California. Weingart visited Rips' home where he was fit with a pair of invisible bifocals. He liked them and decided to assemble a group of investors and turn the new product into a company. The first problem was to find a name for the company. They decided the name "Younger" was the most appropriate name since, without a telltale line, the bifocals made a wearer look "younger".

William Smith was brought into the company in 1956 and for the next six years served as president. Irving's wife Grace *(Bebe)* joined the company to help out in the office in 1965. The company was now producing the invisible bifocal in clear and photochromic glass. In 1967, the company introduced the lens in CR-39 and the following year, Irving's son Ted joined the company. When Dr. Smith died in 1972, Irving Rips became president of Younger.

The company's list of first's is legendary. They include the first oversize plastic blanks, the first high add plastic bifocals, the first extra thick plastic blanks, the first UV or blue blocking lens, the first molded slab-off blanks and the first molded myodisc blanks. The company has carved a special niche for itself by producing specialty lenses no one else has been able to manufacture.

An early Younger ad for their seamless bifocal, the first commercially successful "no lines" bifocal.

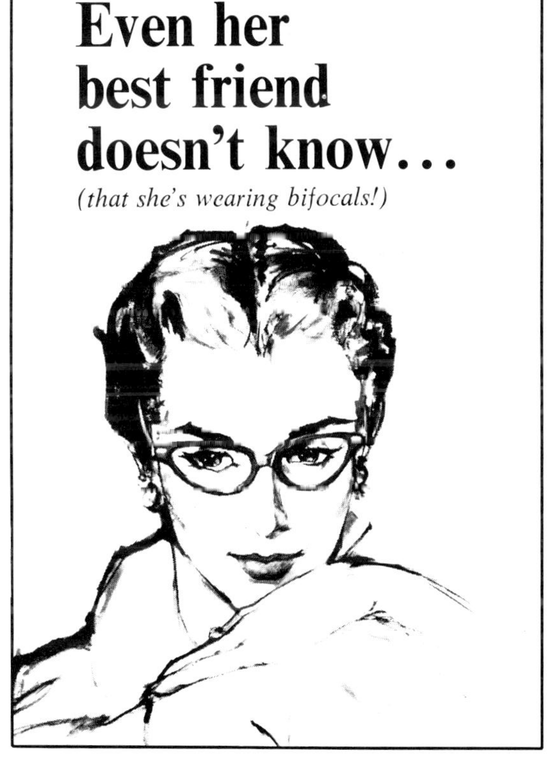

OLA Awards of Excellence

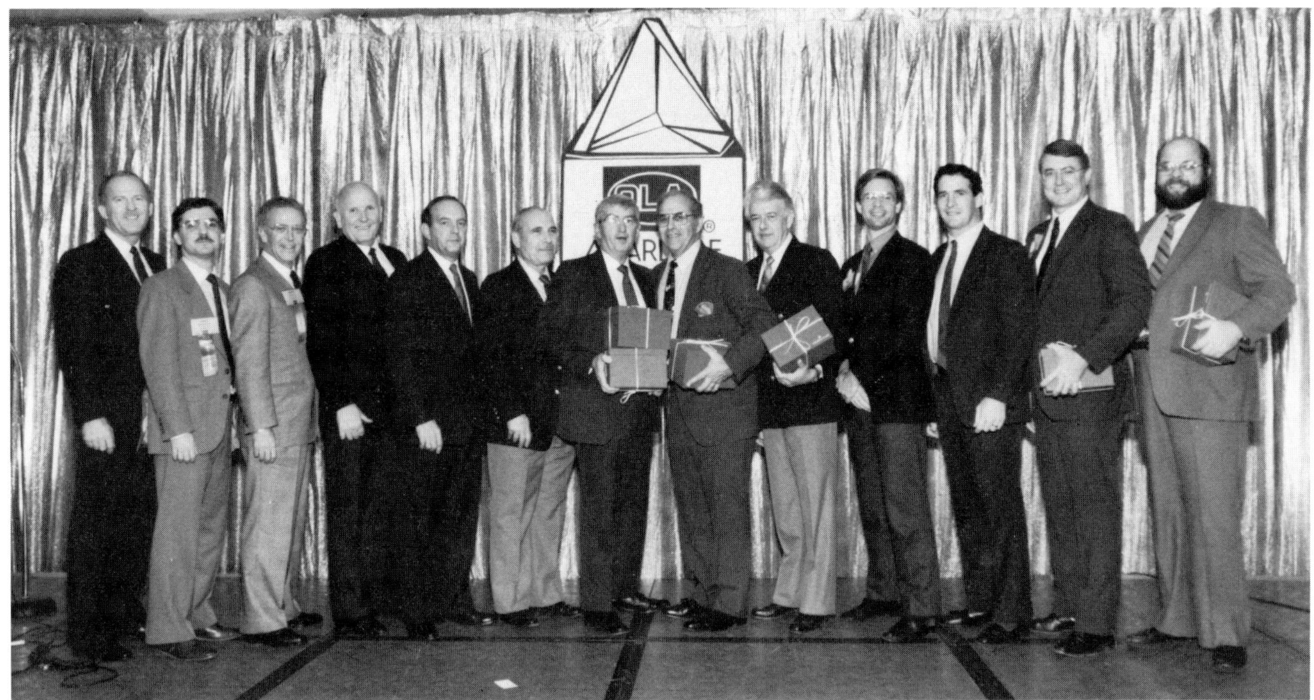

OLA Optical Industry Museum

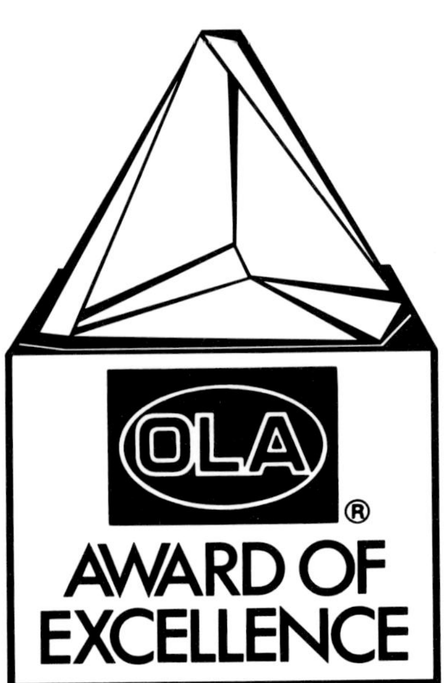

1987 marked the launch of the Internationally-recognized OLA Awards of Excellence program. This annual program was developed as a public way of honoring companies whose products make outstanding contributions to the ophthalmic industry and the optical professions. The OLA believed these Awards would also ultimately interest the consumer press in new eyecare developments.

In addition to the public acknowledgment of receiving this honor, each company winning an OLA Award also receives a custom piece of Steuben crystal, produced by Steuben Glass of Corning, New York. The first OLA Awards were announced at the President's Banquet on November 14, 1987 in San Antonio, Texas. The recipients of that year's Awards are shown in the photo above.

From left to right are; Joe Tardif, FOREMOST OPTICAL, Dan Boucher, YOUNGER LENS, Ron Pincus, FOREMOST OPTICAL, Dieter Beuthien, WECO, John Blocha, COBURN OPTICAL, Fritz Koerting, RODENSTOCK, Phil Eichelberger, LIBERTY OPTICAL, Henry Shyer, ZYLOWARE, William Hernandez, GERBER OPTICAL, David Shute, UNIVERSAL OPTICAL, E.Y. Snoden, UNIVERSAL OPTICAL, Ken White, UNIVERSAL OPTICAL and Ted Rips, YOUNGER LENS.

Products winning an OLA Award of Excellence are permitted to display this logo in their advertising.

Chapter 14
Frame Manufacturers

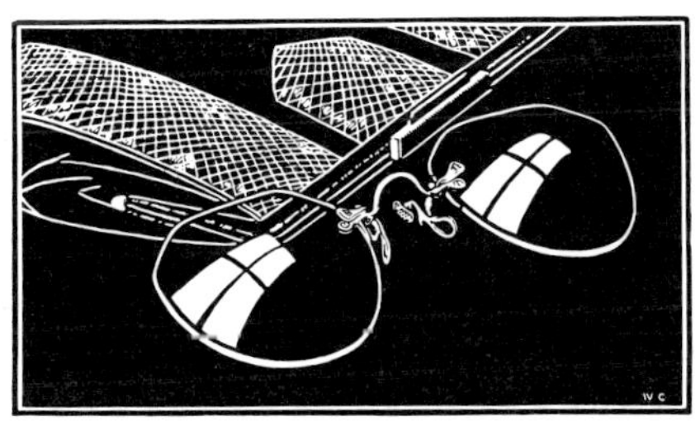

A "Roll Call" of members of the Optical Manufacturers Association appeared in THE OPTICAL AGE *(A trade journal of that day)* published in August, 1923. It was a rather short list of lens and frame manufacturers. The list did not include either AO or B&L who were, by that time, owners of wholesale-retail chains. What is surprising that only one manufacturer member from that era, Martin-Copeland Company, is still in business under the same name. Here is that list, along with the fate of each company where it could be determined:

BAY STATE OPTICAL Attleboro, Mass.	Acquired by Univis in 1953.
THE BISHOP COMPANY North Attleboro, Mass.	Acquired by Univis in 1957.
CENTRAL OPTICAL Southbridge, Mass.	Closed.
DuPAUL YOUNG OPTICAL Southbridge, Mass.	Acquired by Shuron in 1925.
GENERAL OPTICAL Mt. Vernon, N.Y.	Acquired by Shuron in 1930.
MARTIN-COPELAND Providence, R.I.	Still operating in East Providence, RI.
MICHIGAN OPTICAL Detroit, Mich.	Closed.
NEW JERSEY OPTICAL Newark, N.J.	Acquired by Continental Optical, closed when Continental merged with Shuron.
W. P. SHORT, INC. Newark, N.J.	Closed.
SHUR-ON OPTICAL Newark, N.J.	Recently reactivated after bankruptcy.
STANDARD OPTICAL Geneva, N.Y.	Acquired by Shuron in 1925.
UNITED OPTICAL Webster, Mass	Closed.
UNIVERSAL OPTICAL CORP. Providence, R.I.	Sold to I. Stern, now part of Universal-Univis.
WILLSON GOGGLES, INC. Reading, Penn.	No longer in ophthalmic business.

Note that all OMA members were in New England or the New York area *(including Rochester)* except for one in Detroit. Many other manufacturers were in existence at the time but were not OMA members, often because they belonged to what was considered the "black hat" element. These companies were severely frowned upon by the so-called OMA "white hats". This division of the "good guys" and "bad guys" continued for years until a common enemy showed up on the scene - the frame importer.

There have been more than 100 major U.S. factories

producing frames in the 20th century *(along with many more small operations that operated much like a "cottage industry")*. A few of the major players in the U.S. frame industry during the passing years are described here.

ART CRAFT OPTICAL COMPANY, INC.

Two experienced tool and die manufacturers teamed up in 1918 to start a company they called Design Manufacturing Company. The men were Charles J. Eagle and Otto W. Dechau. At the time they started in business, they were making equipment and frame parts for other manufacturers. In 1922, they concentrated on producing spectacle frames and as their sales grew, they changed the name of the company in 1929 to Art Craft, the trade name of their frame products.

A need for increased space forced a move to larger quarters in 1934. Initially, they rented one floor but, in 1945, the seven-story building and the adjoining property were purchased. The company is still located in the same building and occupies the entire building's 70,000 square feet.

Otto Dechau died in 1947 and was succeeded by his son Bert W. Dechau who served as treasurer until his death in 1974. At that time, C. Thomas Eagle became president and Charles Eagle served as C.E.O. until he passed away in 1988.

Frame Style Trends

The company has gone through every fashion trend impacting the frame industry during the past 75 years. 1918 to 1940 was the gold-filled era and the company made a variety of frames in solid gold and gold-filled materials. Styles were three-piece rimless and full-rim frames. Frame eye sizes were small because lens blanks were small but frames were made in a wide range of sizes to fit every patient. Intricate patterns were coined or hand-engraved into the bridges, endpieces and temples.

1941 to 1955 was the "combination era" with frames made of metal/zyl combinations. Metals were yellow or white and aluminum was also combined with gold-filled metal. Art Craft products included the Clubman, Leading Lady and Rimway.

1955 to 1965 was considered the aluminum era and Art Craft produced a number of frames in all-aluminum and aluminum combination styles. 1966 to 1980 was the acetate era and Art Craft began producing pantographed acetate frames. To improve service to distributors, the company opened 9 warehouse locations. 1980 to 1992 was the import era and designer names became important. Art Craft added the Oscar de la Renta line and began supplementing their own production with imported styles from Japan and Italy.

Today, there is a growing demand for US-made frame products. The company presently has more than 250 production workers producing a wide range of frames from a new prescription industrial eyewear line to a variety of designer lines. Five of the company's frames have earned sales of over 1 million units each. They were Clubman, Leading Lady Art Rim, Rimway, Mustang and 100A Ful-Vue, an outstanding record for the volatile frame market.

BAY STATE OPTICAL COMPANY

It was 1862 when a costume jewelry manufacturer was started by two men named Mace Short and Peter Nerney, setting up their business in Attleboro, Mass. Nerney eventually bought out his partner Short. Working with sons Ed and George, Nerney became a pioneer frame manufacturing company when he added eyeglass frames to his product line in 1883. Bay State was located in the heart of the jewelry industry and this turned out to be fortunate because it assured them a ready supply of skilled workers, local availability of jewelry findings *(comprising hinges, screws, etc.)*, well-trained and experienced tool makers, and best of all, a ready source of raw materials.

In 1885, Bay State became the first to introduce gold-filled frames to the young optical industry. Their frames won prestigious prizes at the World's Fair of 1900 in Paris, France, demonstrating the international popularity of their products at a time when few American frames left the U.S. They later pioneered another new concept, combination metal and zyl frames in models such as Princeton Dean, which was a handsome frame with plastic rims and a gold-filled bridge, endpiece, and temples. Another innovation was Zylarc, a Numount rimless combined with plastic rims. These were stylish frames at a time when style was hard to find in frames.

Bay State went on to develop the famous Rimway frame. This was a Numount rimless *(2 screws)* that featured

One of Art Craft's bestselling frames was the Leading Lady, a shape that was copied by dozens of other frame lines. This frame remained a staple of the Art Craft line for years.

OLA OPTICAL INDUSTRY MUSEUM

Banking on a surefire shape, Art Craft produced the Leading Lady shape in their Art-Rim line, their version of the highly popular zyl/metal combination frame.

OLA OPTICAL INDUSTRY MUSEUM

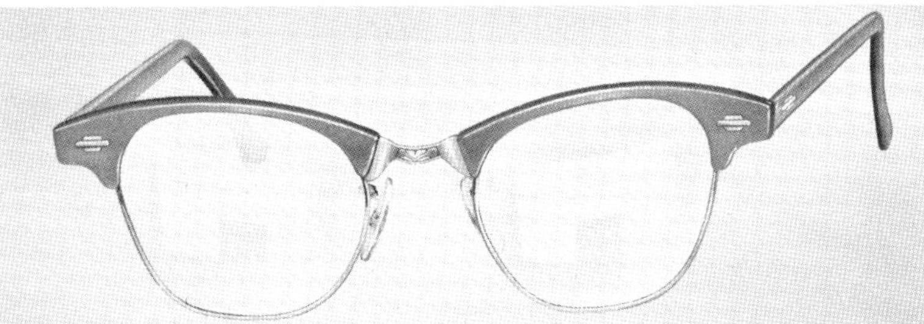

two additional screws at the temporal ends for greater stability. They rather cleverly assigned the patent for this innovative frame to that bully of the industry, American Optical. AO was well organized for policing and administrating licensing and protection of their own patents. Bay State received the net proceeds of some rather substantial royalties after American Optical deducted their expenses. AO's interest in playing this middleman role was primarily because of the control it gave them over their competitors. Ironically, Bay State never manufactured any Rimway mountings.

Bay State also conceived the idea of hydraulically pushing a heated nickel silver core wire into heated plastic blanks to provide wire core plastic temples. This revolutionized what had previously been an extremely difficult process of sandwiching wire cores in plastic sheets and then chopping them out, a system accompanied with more than a few production rejects. This innovative company also introduced the first high quality injection-molded frames which they called Baylok, a clever, rather attractive frame that was extremely unsuccessful because, against the strong advice of Celanese, the material's manufacturer, they used a new plastic material called Forticel for their design. Celanese had warned the material was known to be brittle. Lenses for this frame required precision mounting, exactly as for a metal frame. Once the lenses were carefully fitted by hand, the endpiece had to be secured with a metal clasp called a clevis. This was easy to do if the lab man had three hands. Since most did not, the frame became extremely unpopular with labs and, since most frames were sold by labs, they had the capacity to make or break new frame designs.

Bay State had a spectacular success with their Heiress frame, a gold-filled frame featuring an eyewire suspended behind a gold-filled browbar. This was another patented frame which received the signal honor *(for those days)* of receiving a 20,000 unit advance sale. 10,000 frames were sold to American Optical for $60,000 and another 10,000 units sold to an investment group for another $60,000, all paid in advance. The frames were sold to distributors, mostly labs, for $6.50. The investment group pocketed the fifty cents difference as their profit.

The Bay State company was operated in the first half of the 20th century by Peter Nerney's sons, Ed and George. Ed did the traveling, yet managed to find time to also double as Attleboro's volunteer fire chief. George was responsible for production and administration. A "national sales force" was developed with Arthur Bullock handling the East Coast and L. C. "String" Thurber handling the mid-west. Both men maintained homes in Attleboro. Frank Webster handled the West Coast out of San Francisco. These three men were among the top

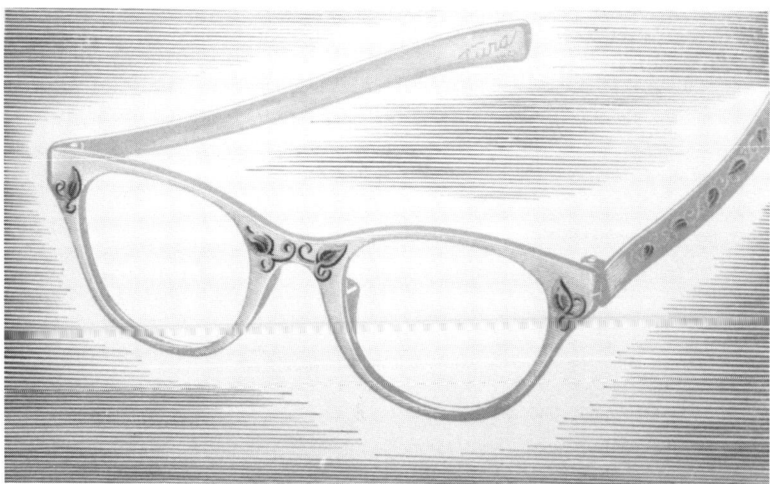

salesmen in the country but, as was the custom with most salesmen in those days, they were poorly paid *(less than $2,500 per year)*. *They* did, however, enjoy unrestricted expense accounts. In those days, it was the custom for sales people to travel almost 40 weeks per year so this worked out well for them. When Ed Nerney died at the end of World War II, Bay State was sold to Soft-Lite Lens Company and a group of debenture holders. George Nerney continued to handle research but a new President, Julius *(Jack)* Hansen took over. He had been a purchasing agent for Bausch & Lomb.

In 1949, after three unprofitable years, the Bay State sales force joined forces with the Soft-Lite sales force. Bay State salespeople were told they now had to abide by the same tight discipline governing Soft-Lite salesmen. Soft-Lite paid their salesmen more than double what Bay State had paid but limited their sales people to $10 per diem expenses. Ten dollars was expected to pay for their hotel room, three meals, and all incidentals. String Thurber, when advised of this at a sales meeting, was heard to say that he was used to spending more than this before arising in the morning *(a bottle of whiskey and a box of cigars, ordered from the bellman, would do this).*

Hansen moved the factory to a large, new building. He had the distinction of introducing the ill-fated Baylok frame. Between these two substantial expenses and the company's philosophy of continuing to sell basic Bay State products at the same price as previous years, created major economic problems for the company. As an example, Bay State's Ful Vue P3 frame, the backbone of their line, sold to distributors for $1.10. Accounting studies proved the frame cost $1.16 to

A revolutionary frame mentioned elsewhere in this history is Tura's original all-aluminum frame, produced in a profusion of anodized colors with a great variety of trims. Monroe Levoy insisted that almost any facial blemish (large nose, pointed chin, etc.) could be offset by properly used trim.

OLA OPTICAL INDUSTRY MUSEUM

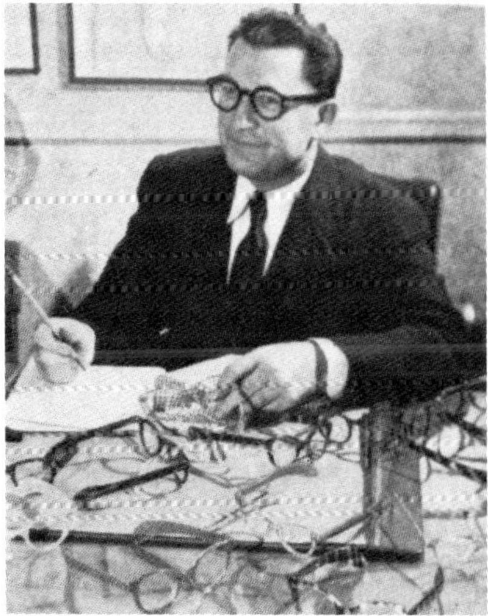

Alexander Kono's frame company was a leading fashion trend setter in the years immediately following World War II. Kono frames were distributed by B&L labs, giving that company their first taste of "fashion" frames.

OLA OPTICAL INDUSTRY MUSEUM

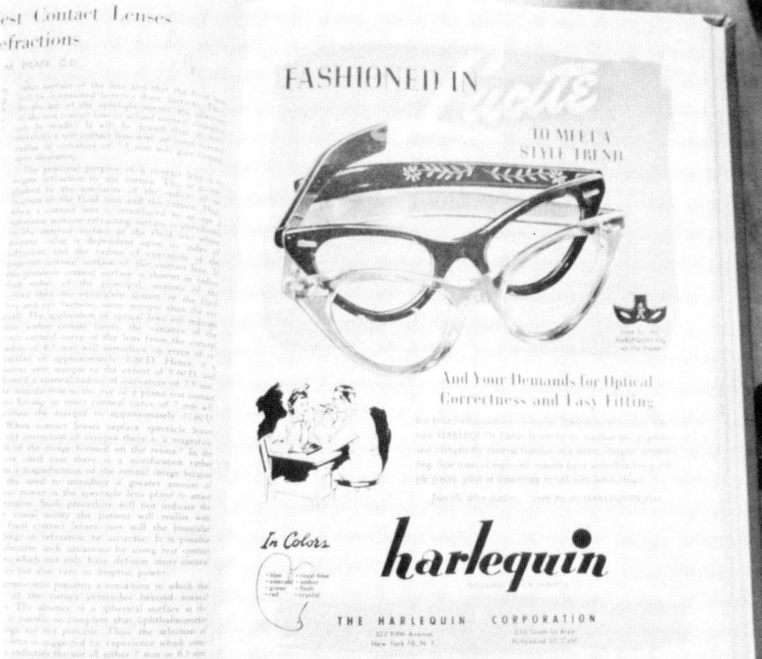

This 1947 ad shows the famous Harlequin frame, these crafted of Lucite (Plexiglas). Lucite produced beautiful frames but were dreadfully brittle and quickly went out of style.

produce. The Bay State sales force strongly resisted price increases on the basis that their customers had supported the company during the war and deserved reciprocity. The company also neglected to upgrade their styling to contemporary standards, other than the disastrous Baylok frame.

The newly combined frame and lens sales force attempted to market Bay State frames exactly as they did Soft-Lite lenses, on a personal basis. In an era of increasing fashion consciousness, this didn't work and frame sales continued to founder. Falling sales kept the company from making any substantial changes in styling because of cost.

Continuing losses saw a procession of managers followed by unionization of the facility. The CIO took over the machine shop, the AF of L took over frame production, and both unions had contracts coming up for negotiation at 6 month intervals. Spiraling costs forced the company to move out of the area in 1953. After an extensive search for a new site, Westbury, Long Island, New York was selected and the company moved there in 1953 along with certain key employees.

Univis Lens Company bought Bay State in July, 1955. They paid no attention to Soft-Lite's mistake of thinking the professions would buy frames from a lens salesperson simply because they liked him or liked the lens product. It failed to work for Soft-Lite and it failed for Univis. Lens people tried to direct the frame operation but with slight success. The factory closed in 1957, ending a 95 year career for the oldest independent frame factory in the USA.

HARLEQUIN CORPORATION

In 1938, the optical professions sold virtually no frames that might be called fashion eyewear. The great majority of plastic frames featured the P3 or PR4 *(perimetric)* shape, rimless frames were either Numont *(2 screws)* or Rimway *(4 screws)* and metal frames were mostly "Fulvue". Almost all frames by this time were Fulvue which simply meant that the hinge was located less than one quarter the distance from the top of the front to the bottom rather than on line endpieces as with all earlier frames *(AO collected a royalty on every frame sold in the U.S. that had above center endpieces. This continued for the life of the patent)*. Frames could be ordered in any color as long as they were pink *(a flesh-tinted color)*, demi-amber, demi-blonde, verdal *(a dark green demi)* or, for the fashion-conscious few, basic black.

The Harlequin frame was introduced into this staid, conservative market, to the utter dismay of most professionals. The new Harlequin company was owned by a woman with the impressive name Altina Schinazi Sanders Barasch Barrett. She was the scion of a wealthy Philadelphia tobacco family, and had been known in her youth as "Bubbles" Schinazi. In concert with a brilliant publicist, Constance Hope, who happened to be married to an eminent New York ophthalmologist *(Dr. Milton Berliner)*, Mrs. Barrett created a "fashion frame", designed by professional designers who came up with the concept of a perfect teardrop propped at a 45 degree angle. This "perfect" design turned out to be less than perfect because it failed to properly fit any nose. The nasal area was then modified to provide a better fit. The two innovative, persistent ladies prevailed upon plastic material companies to provide colors consistent with those currently in vogue and contracted manufacturing of the frames to local New York factories. Ultimately Carl Weitz, a Long Island factory that was to become part of Zylite, took on the project. Initial introduction was accompanied by consumer advertising *(seldom seen in those days)* and a great deal of publicity which was Constance Hope's field.

The new frames got a major boost from Gus Blocker, owner of Lugene Opticians, a fashion-oriented New York optician. The frames were sold through wholesalers and laboratories at unheard-of prices for those days, costing retailers $2 to 3 per frame. Success failed to materialize and the only thing that saved the company from failure was the advent of World War II with its shortages of materials and increased buying power by war workers. Those factors created a modest acceptability for this daring product.

By 1948, Mrs. Barrett had married a Los Angeles doctor and moved to the West Coast. Martin Singer, son of Nat

Singer *(Soft-Lite Lenses)*, purchased the company for $5,000 and continued operations on a limited basis until 1955. At that time, a new marketing plan was introduced together with a high fashion "frame collection". This collection was developed and sold by a triumvirate which included Richard Hirsh *(whose experience in the fashion world and with Tura turned out to be invaluable)* and Sam Haigh, who had been an outstanding salesman for Soft-Lite Lens Company.

Prominent retailers nationwide were solicited to serve as "dealers". They purchased the product directly but on a controlled basis: frames were priced to the wearer with a discount of 50% to the dealer and an additional 20% which the dealer could earn back through volume purchases and through co-operative advertising. The collection was backed by advertising and publicity. Dealers were offered marketing aids that included displays, advertising mats, and consumer literature.

Success in the first half of 1955 was substantial with dealers signed up representing the vast majority of quality dispensing establishments throughout the country. These were mostly opticians with a sprinkling of quality and fashion-conscious optometrists.

In July, 1955, as a condition of the purchase of the Bay State Optical Company, Univis Lens Company was given the right to introduce a lower priced version of Harlequin's first collection. Bay State's factory, owned by Soft-Lite Lens Company stockholders, had produced the frames in the first Harlequin collection, so this was easy to do. Univis sold this new line through lab distributors who made it available to retail customers at lower prices than the original Harlequin line. This created havoc with the concept Harlequin had just introduced to their retailer dealers.

Harlequin overcame the previous year's marketing problem and sales increased significantly during the next five years. In the early 1960s, Harlequin suffered a major setback as dealers became weaker and the influence of AO and B&L waned. Ophthalmologists were dispensing in increasing numbers; and Optometry, with their conservative fashion philosophy, became an increasing factor in frame sales. To cope with this problem, Harlequin's marketing strategy was changed to sell through selected distributors and to forego the dealer plan.

When Univis took over Bay State's factory in 1955, they were unwilling to continue making Harlequin frames. Production was shifted in 1956 to Optical Products Corporation, an old-time manufacturer owned by Bill and Herb Grossman. When OPC closed the following year, production was again switched, the fronts to Zyloware and the temples to Perfect Temple. Harlequin applied the "design details" and assembled and packaged the frames. In 1960, Harlequin acquired a small frame factory in Manhattan from Acousticon, a hearing aid manufacturer.

Unfortunately for Harlequin, unit sales, which had been expanding substantially for the past 9 years, slowed just at the time when economies could be realized because of company-owned production. Finally, by the late 1960s, importers began to sell directly and Harlequin became a victim of the times.

HUDSON OPTICAL

One of the true pioneers of the frame business, still active today, is Irving Hirschman. Starting with OPC as an apprentice in 1924, he advanced to foreman status, and helped settle the first major strike of the Optical Workers Union *(founded in 1926 by Sebastian Ribaldo, another former OPC employee, who remained chief of the union until 1990 when his son succeeded him)*. Hirschman left OPC to help form G&W Optical in 1930. They were a manufacturer of Oxfords and later of metal frames. While still at OPC, with the consent of OPC management, Hirschman worked one day a week for G&W Optical Co., owned by Harry Weissmann and Joe Geller *(Hirschman's brother-in-law)*, and continued to work there until Weissmann left to form Whitney Optical, a metal frame manufacturer.

G&W moved to Hudson Street in Manhattan in 1933 and changed their name to Hudson Optical Company. Hirschmann was most instrumental in helping the Mexican frame industry get started in the early 1950s and still consults with several frame factories in Mexico City.

In 1958, Hudson worked closely with Univis until Univis's method of operation came close to forcing Hirschmann's company out of business. Fortunately, Hirschmann withdrew from the arrangement in time to make his company once again a powerful force in the

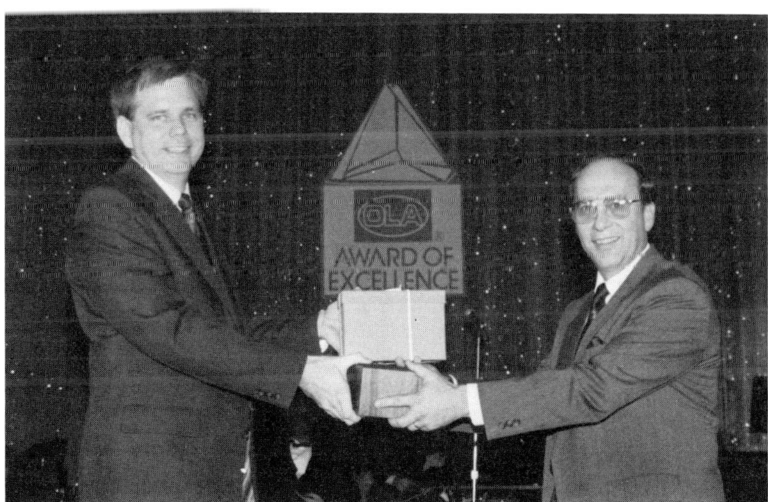

Marine Optical has been a frequent winner of OLA Awards of Excellence. This photo was taken in 1993 when they won two Awards. Marine's John Olson, left, accepts the trophy from OLA President Al Willenbring.

OLA OPTICAL INDUSTRY MUSEUM

industry. He was one of the first importers to utilize Korean production and actually set up his own production facility there in 1980.

Hudson Optical moved to Long Island after World War II and, in 1985, to Bohemia, at the eastern end of Long Island. Much of their product today comes from their Korean factory and the company continues to play a significant role in the optical industry.

MARINE OPTICAL

Another old-time frame factory is Marine Optical in Roslindale, Massachusetts. The Company was founded by Arthur Ditto on July 5th, 1925. Ditto had been Superintendent with the Humboldt Manufacturing Company in Everett, Mass. Starting with three employees, the company had grown to thirty hands by 1929 when they moved to larger quarters. By 1941, they had a staff of 175 and Arthur had been joined by his sons Eugene and Hugo. They produced a well-known line of sunglasses carrying the name Filt-Ray. The Ditto family sold the company in 1974 to Barnes-Hind *(a pharmaceutical company)* who never quite grasped the complexities of the optical frame business.

To illustrate their misunderstanding of the frame business, one of Barnes-Hind's top sales executives visited the author at the time of the acquisition and announced the taking over of Marine. He was very excited about this broadening of their line. He explained that B-H had some eighty contact lens solution detail people calling on every contact lens fitter in the country.

"All we have to do", he claimed, "is have them drop off a Marine frame catalogue in every office. We'll corner the frame market." Sad to say, they did distribute the catalogs in such a way, but it had absolutely no effect on Marine's sales. Harry Hind was an early purchaser of frames from foreign sources and was, perhaps, ahead of his time. Eventually sensing they were out of their depth, Barnes-Hind sold the company to Revlon in 1976. Marine Optical was spun off and sold to Ted Izzi *(a Univis frame executive)* and Bob Kemp. In 1979 the company closed its production facilities to buy product both from domestic factories and by importing.

In 1990, the company was acquired by Michael Ferrara, David duFour, Don Everburg and John Olsen. The company continues to develop and cultivate their distributors *(mostly labs)* and operates very successfully in the Boston area.

MARTIN-COPELAND

Martin-Copeland is the only company still remaining from the 1923 Roll Call of OMA members. Started late in the 1880s by two Providence men, Martin-Copeland produced frames continuously from that point on, but only in a small way until Duncan Martin, a grandson of the founder, initiated a major expansion program in the 1960s Aided by Curt Rogers, who handled sales, and Richard White, a former AO executive who took charge of production, Martin-Copeland initiated the extremely successful Versailles collection which included a number of imported frames, along with frames produced in their new factory built in East Providence in 1975. Rogers and White purchased the company in 1985 but experienced a substantial sales decline, finally selling the company to Lou Schwartz, a New York importer, in 1989.

The company continues in reduced space *(some of the factory having been rented out)* and produces frames domestically as well as importing them. Schwartz died unexpectedly in 1991, leaving his brother to run the operation. In the meantime, the only remaining member from the Roll Call of 1923 continues in business.

UNIVERSAL OPTICAL

Wallace Murray founded Universal Optical after World War I. It became a major frame producer and eventually was sold to one of its gold-filled suppliers, I. Stern of Mt. Vernon, N.Y. who had set up a small conglomerate called Stern-Dent in 1970. In 1980, Stern-Dent decided to withdraw from the optical industry and Wally Murray, Jr. purchased the company back and continued to import and to produce frames in a large new East Providence factory. Several powerful designer names, including Givenchy, were successfully used. But as domestic

The zyl Ful-Vue frame was one of the staples in OPC's all zyl line. This was a uni-sex frame and widely used during the 1940s

OLA OPTICAL INDUSTRY MUSEUM

Joe Shyer, founder of Zyloware, learned his trade working for B.B.W., an early zyl manufacturer. This 1920s ad shows the type of frames sold by B.B.W.

OLA OPTICAL INDUSTRY MUSEUM

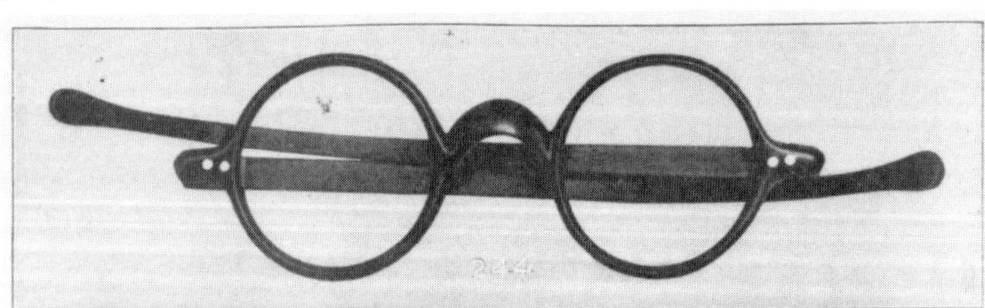

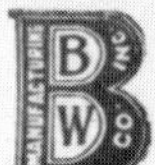

production was replaced by imports, the decision was made to sell off all production machinery at a time when the company was suffering reduced sales.

In 1980, Fleet National Bank, which had financed the leveraged buy-out, facilitated the sale of Universal to Beta Associates, an entrepreneur organization based in San Jose, CA. A year later, Beta also purchased the Univis frame division, using the same bank for leveraging and merging Universal into Univis.

The new company introduced a number of new ideas. For example, they mounted all the machinery on wheels to give the factory more versatility even though the machines were hardly ever moved. They put in an elaborate Cad-Cam manufacturing setup but used it only for two styles of frames. The bank eventually foreclosed and sold the company, less their $9 million debt, to Charles Huff for a leveraged $2 million. Huff, who had purchased seven other companies in the five years since he had left his position as a corporate vice-president of Bausch & Lomb, financed the purchase by reducing the work force from 250 to 100, gradually increasing it as needed. The bank debt was paid off within a year and today the company operates a successful factory and importing business.

STYL-RITE OPTICAL

T&P Optical, a partnership of Tiburon and Pomerantz, manufactured metal frames in Manhattan in the 1920s and, after World War II, changed their name to Styl-Rite Optical, setting up a major factory in Long Island City, N.Y. Jerry Pomerantz, son of the founder, took over control of the company, moving it to Miami, Fla. in 1975, when New York labor costs became too expensive. The move did not solve the company's financial problems and the company was eventually sold to Royal Optical, a Dallas-based retail chain, in 1980. The company continues manufacturing frames in Miami for their parent company (now part of US Vision, a large retail chain) and for other customers.

ZYLOWARE CORPORATION

One of the earliest frame factories in New York was a company named BBW. It was owned by Barney Becker, a local optometrist and Becker had a key employee named Joseph Shyer. By 1923, Shyer decided the time had come to strike out on his own so he left BBW to form a company he called Zyloware Corporation. The name came from DuPont's new plastic material called "Zylonite", used in a variety of items such as combs, pocketbooks and bible covers.

Shyer had been an outstanding salesman for BBW for several years. Believing this would insure the new company's success, two men who had worked in the same Manhattan loft building in which BBW was located, left their jobs to join Shyer. Each of the three invested $2,000 in the new enterprise. This was considered a lot of money in those days and demonstrated their confidence in Shyer and his plans. After a brief interlude in the loft, a factory was located out in the potato fields of Long Island City. They started in the same building from which the factory operates today, although this building has undergone considerable expansion.

Stephen Ray, an engineer, became their toolmaker and Abe Flink served as production manager - both men had experience making plastic buttons, and though the relationship to optical frames may seem remote, it was truly a related industry since buttons were made from the same nitrocellulose used for frames. Each man learned to make frames as they went along, and whatever they were able to produce was sold by Shyer.

Their initial production was aimed primarily at the low priced market. One of their leading products was the Code frame, priced to the trade at 44 cents *(even after World War II)*. Needless to say, producing a frame that could be sold for such a low price meant it had to be produced in the most economical way possible. The least expensive nitrocellulose material was used. Frames were cut out in a single size and shape. They would then be stretched to whatever size and shape was required. Fortunately, this wasn't a major feat since most frames in those days were small and geometrically shaped. The frame was then "polished" by subjecting the parts to an acetone spray, or dip. This gave the frame a rounded, shiny appearance that was quite attractive - at least until worn for the first time. In spite of these shortcomings, this was exactly the kind of product many retail opticians and optometrists of the second quarter of the 20th century wanted. They had to have an inexpensive product for their low-income customers *(this period included the dreary depression years)*.

The company was successful and the management team worked well and remained in place until 1947 when Flink died. His stock was purchased by the remaining

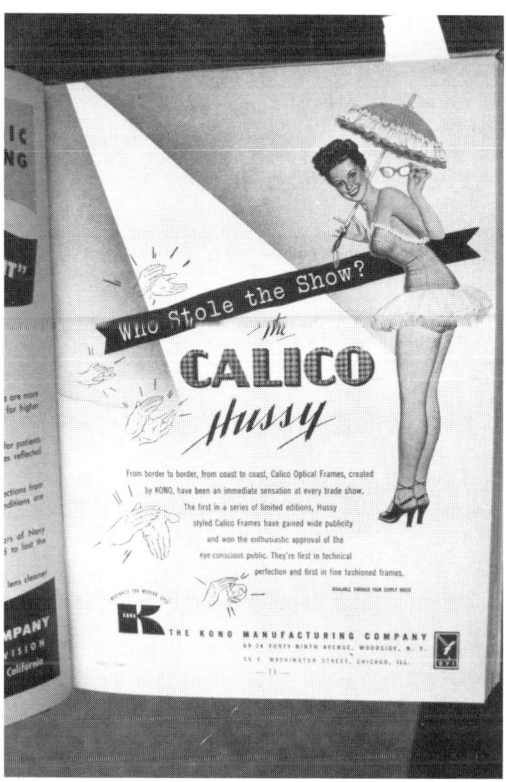

Kono's Hussy was one of the first "fashion" frames, hitting the market about the same time as Victory's Honey. One of the most popular hussy models was made of clear zyl with various colors in calico cloth laminated in the middle.

OLA OPTICAL INDUSTRY MUSEUM

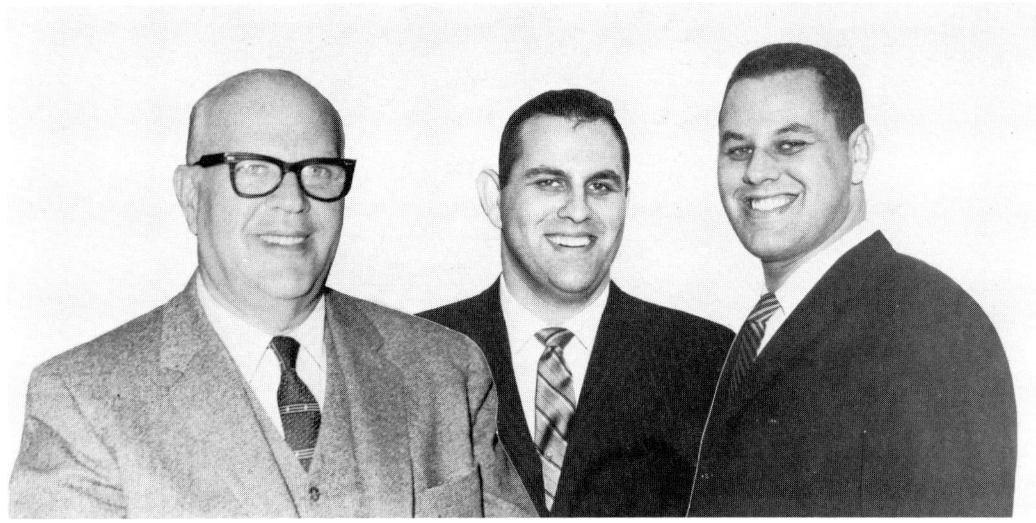

Zyloware has been owned and operated by the same family for more than 70 years. In the photo, founder Joseph Shyer, left, is shown with his sons Henry and Robert. Henry and Robert still manage the company which, by accommodating to industry changes, is stronger and more influential than ever.

PHOTO – ZYLOWARE CORPORATION

partners, and when Ray died in 1957, his stock reverted to the Shyer family which now owned all the stock.

Joe Shyer's two sons, Bob and Henry, joined the business in 1954 and gradually took over from their father during the following years until Joe retired in 1962. The brothers decided it was time to upgrade their line. They improved both styles and quality and set out to distribute their products through the better wholesalers in the country.

In 1962, the company took a major step by importing a nylon frame from France which they named "Invincible". This was a bold move because, at that time, it was considered taboo for a frame factory to import anything and, adding to this unacceptable behavior was the fact that the Invincible was a molded frame, considered taboo by the industry. Adding to all the "no-no's" was the fact that the frame was made from nylon. Nylon frames could only be produced in solid, dark colors and the material tended to be abrasive to the nose. The company overcame these problems in several ways. First, the frame sold for $5, considered at that time to be an extremely high price for a plain frame *(Browline metal/zyl combination frames featuring gold-filled materials sold to retailers for $5.30).* The high price was offset by offering a very respectable profit to their wholesale distributors. These facts, combined with the advantage that the frame was identifiably

different and the superb marketing the Shyers devoted to this new product made the Invincible a remarkable success story. The frame quickly became a top seller with over 20 million Invincibles sold during the last 30 years. Orders for at least 500 of this 30 year old frame still come in every week.

Emboldened by this success, the Shyers embarked on an ambitious program to add other imported, quality products to their line. Some new product would be finished in their own plant. At the same time, the company continued to manufacture quality frames of a more conservative design in their plant. By 1975, they put together a collection under the "Gloria Vanderbilt" name and started a successful national advertising and marketing program for Zyloware and their distributors. The "Sophia Loren" name was added in 1981 and "Stetson" in 1988. The company was substantially aided in their marketing endeavors by Richard Hirsh, an experienced marketing expert whose previous experience included early days at Tura and ten years with Harlequin. Hirsh died in 1986.

Today the Zyloware Corporation is a major frame factory/importer and continues to sell their products through wholesale distributors, many of them laboratories. Thirty percent of the line is produced in their on-premises factory. Ten percent of their sales are represented by export sales. Both Bob and Henry Shyer have served as President of the Optical Industry Association *(OMA)* and Bob has served as President of the Vision Council of America *(VICA)*.

OTHER NEW YORK FACTORIES

In the late 19th century, many factories sprang up in the New York-Newark, N.Y. area, often owned by retail opticians and using production executives from the plastics or jewelry area. One of these, BBW, was owned by Dr. Barney Becker, a New York optometrist, and this

This is the famous Code frame which launched Zyloware on the path to the enviable industry reputation they enjoy today.

PHOTO – ZYLOWARE CORPORATION

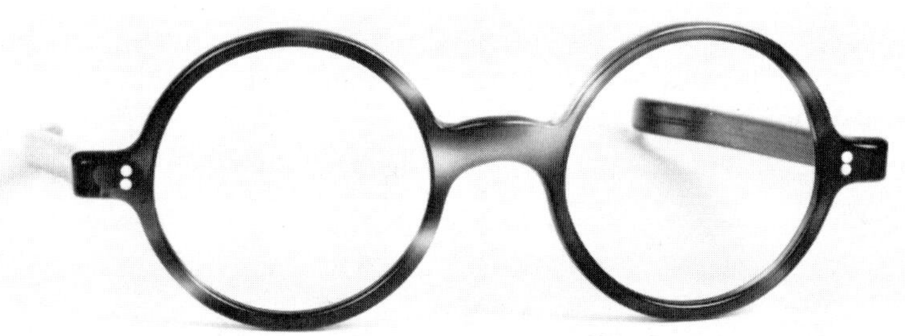

is where Joe Shyer gained his experience. Another was Shellcraft, owned by the father of Sydney Weinrib, a cofounder of Sterling Optical *(a major retail chain)*. The story goes that Weinrib Senior entered his customer's offices with two shoe boxes under his arm: one contained his samples, the other his lunch. When lunch time came, he asked for hot water, made coffee, ate his lunch, and left *(presumably with an order)*. He often slept in his office since he was responsible for frame production as well as sales.

Century Oxford Manufacturing Company, owned by the Levy family, was another early starter, lasting until the 1950s when the glut of manufacturers and obsolescence created by fast-changing fashion frames overcame them. Another grandfather-type factory was Newport Optical, owned by Morris Klein and Dunkelsberg. They were one of the first factories to produce frames from nitro-cellulose material.

Leopold Strauss operated Optical Products Corporation, called OPC, with Dave Ettinger as manager until he left to become head of Riggs Optical, Chicago. His wife, Leila, set up the first union-oriented retail establishment in New York City. The Grossman family operated this business from before World War II until it closed in 1957, another victim of too many factories and too much frame availability.

The End of U.S. Frame Manufacturing

The virtual demise of frame manufacturing in the United Sates, companies both large and small, was the result of several factors: the takeover of the frame market by direct sellers acquiring their frames from abroad *(Hong Kong, Korea, Japan, France, Italy, and Germany being the principal suppliers);* poor designing facilities, failure of domestic manufacturers to invest in new technology as the more progressive foreign factories did; the decline of many laboratories and wholesalers who got out of frame distribution and the policy of accepting for credit any frames the retailer chose to return.

The Pinnacle Group

Laboratories are taking a renewed interest in frame distribution and this interest is being reinforced by changes in the market economy. Eyecare professionals today are inundated with direct selling frame companies. Retailers in Southern California report as many as 60 sales reps a month attempt to call and display their products. Added to this over abundance of product is the need for faster service. Many laboratories are connected to their customers by fax, modem or telephone and the convenience of ordering lenses and frames together is starting to impact frame buying.

In 1992, the Optical Laboratories Association set up a joint venture with a number of U.S. frame companies.

Calling themselves the Pinnacle Group, this is a marketing organization devoted to selling the concept of "one stop shopping" for frames and lenses. While it's too early to tell, the interest and reaction from both laboratories and practitioners seems to indicate that the U.S. frame market is still in a shifting mode and, how frames will be distributed in the future, is difficult to predict.

A New Influence

In the fall of 1993, Vision Service Plan *(VSP)* announced they were going into the frame business. By Spring of 1994 they began distributing their own line of frames *(called Altair)* to VSP panel doctors all over the country. Importing the frames from outside the country, they have priced the frames so they can offer the doctors their accustomed 20% discount, normal for buying groups.

It's interesting to note that their take over of the frame market reflects the expectations of Barnes-Hind back when they purchased Marine Optical. Rather than merely pass out frame catalogs, VSP has established a bank of telemarketing people who spend full time calling VSP doctors and selling frame samples over the phone. They should end up more successful than Barnes-Hind because they do not charge for the frame inventory. Consignment frames provide a powerful incentive to their panel doctors.

At the present time, VSP's contract laboratories are not involved in this frame distribution. Many in the industry believe that frame returns and exchanges will create major problems for VSP, but only time will tell. The basic premise of this new program is improved service for patients and doctors, so laboratories may ultimately be involved in distributing their frames, if only to expedite turnaround time in the lab. In the meantime, every Altair frame sale is taken away from traditional frame importers or distributors.

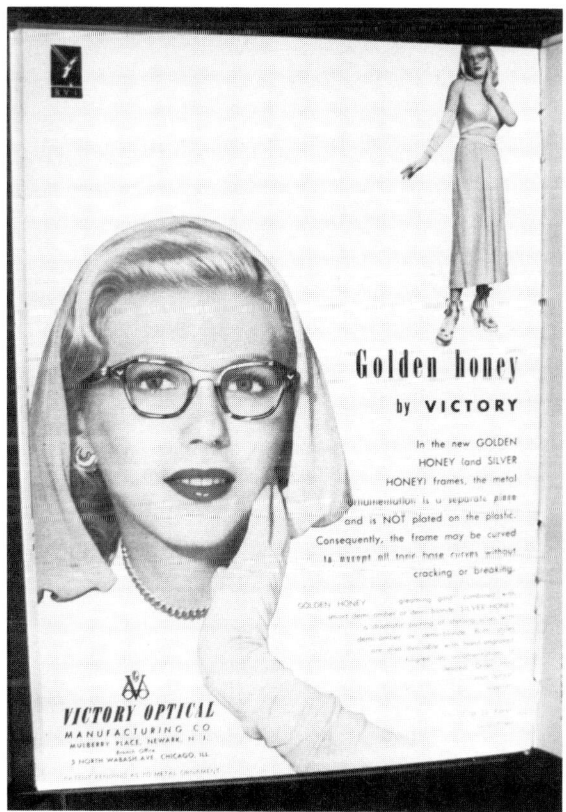

The Honey frame by Victory was undoubtedly the most successful of the early fashion frames. It was produced in great variety and color and continued selling for years.

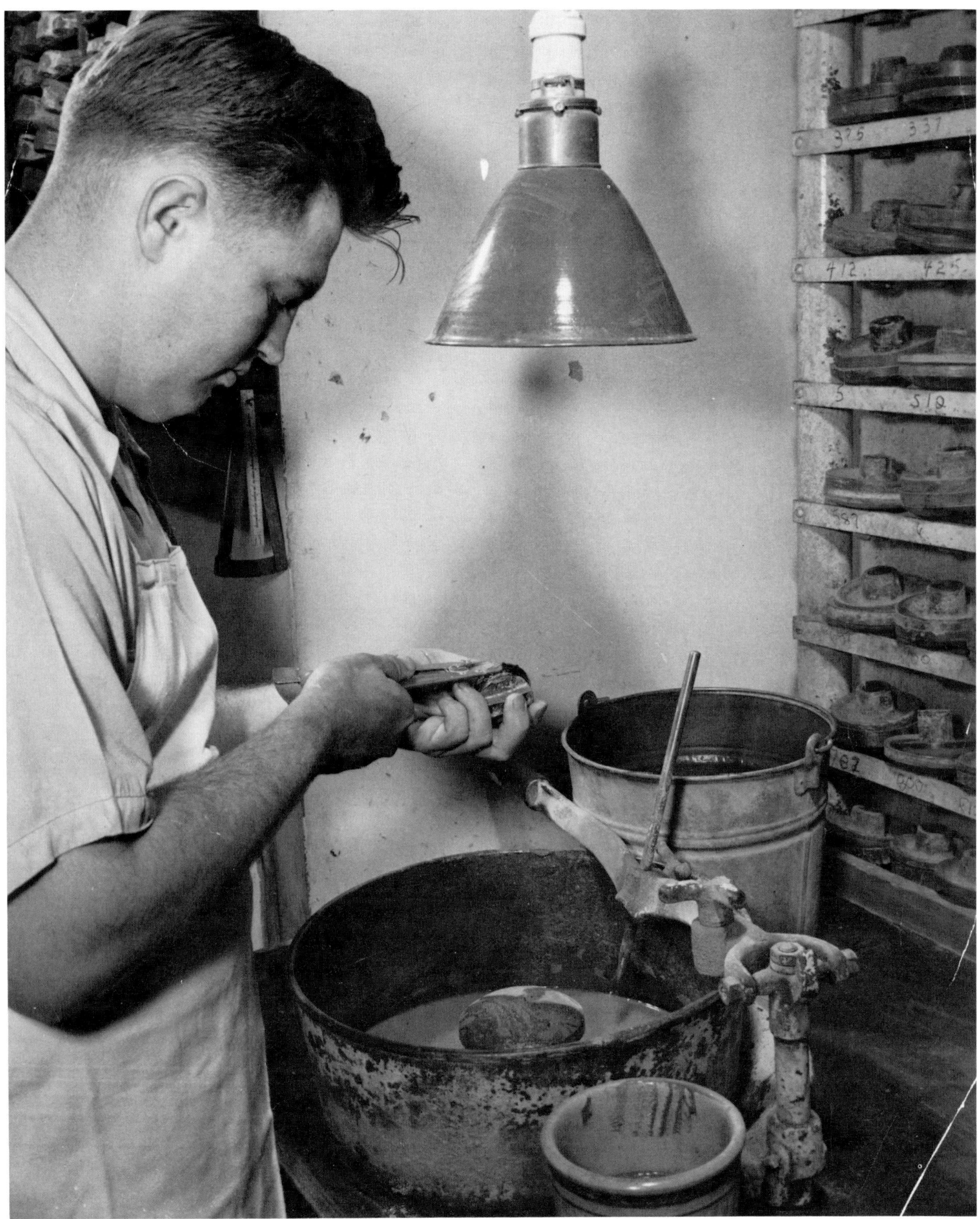

This photograph illustrates, in a most graphic way, the primary difference between producing prescription lenses prior to the emergence of laboratory generators and producing lenses in a modern lab. When laboratories produced lenses by hand roughing in a surface pan, calipers were an essential part of the process. Producing the desired thickness in the finished lens, meant operators had to take the semi-finished blank down to a closely controlled thickness before fining and polishing. Controlling the optical center was also a result of maintaining controlled thicknesses at four sides of the compass around the lens. Anyone who ever worked in or visited a laboratory before the 1950s advent of generators will recall the technicians constantly checking each lens, exactly as seen in this familiar photograph.

Chapter 15
Machinery Manufacturers

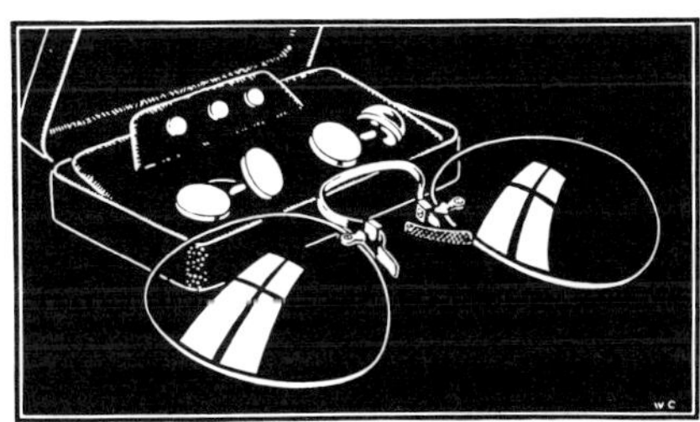

COBURN OPTICAL

Orin W. Coburn's first contact with the optical business was in 1937 when he made a call with his Dad, a water air conditioner dealer, on American Optical's branch in Enid, Oklahoma. The branch was managed by 24 year old Tom Brown *(Fred Reed also worked there and Reed and Brown would later found their own laboratories)*. At age 16, O.W. took a full-time job with AO, learning every job in the lab since it was AO's policy in those days to have each job completed by the same lab person. Once he had the lab work down pat, Coburn showed interest in sales and Tom Brown promptly took advantage of his interest.

In 1942, Coburn, now married, was transferred by AO to Kansas City. Coburn had suffered a back injury that kept him out of the service until 1944 when the Navy finally accepted him. Six weeks later, problems with his back flared up and he was discharged from the Navy. AO promptly hired him back and ultimately sent him to Cheyenne and later to Denver. By now, he was on the road full time selling for AO. Coburn had always wanted a lab of his own and finally, in 1947 he was able to open a new lab in Casper, Wyoming which he called Wyoming Optical. It was during this time he changed his name to "Bill", deciding that Orin was too hard to remember.

Coburn had opened a second branch in Sheridan but was getting tired of the cold weather. In the summer of 1949, Charlie Fehr, who owned Western Optical in Salt Lake City, arranged to purchase Wyoming Optical for $10,000. By this time, Tom Brown had left AO and opened two independent labs in Oklahoma. He talked Bill Coburn into moving to Muskogee to take over that branch.

It was during a 1950 meeting of the A.I.O.W. that Bill met Fred Fritzsche, an uncle of Harold Fluegge. Fritzsche had developed a clever mechanical blocking device for automating blocking, one of the most tedious and disliked jobs in the laboratory. Blocking a lens so it could be worked on during surfacing involved standing over a Bunsen burner, holding a stick of pitch and dripping molten pitch over block and lens blank. At the convention, Coburn ordered two of these new units from Fritzsche and had them shipped to Tom Brown's two labs. Coburn began to see how, if he could somehow get the rights to the blocker, he could make and sell enough to generate profits that would enable him to get back in the lab business.

His first problem was money, but with money borrowed from his brothers and funds advanced by Dr. Lynn Moore, a local optometrist in Muskogee, he came up with enough to purchase the patent rights to the blocker. The Fritzsche process used a heated pot of pitch that pumped pitch up into a cavity formed between the block and the lens blank. The ring holding the block and blank had running water pumped through it to keep the

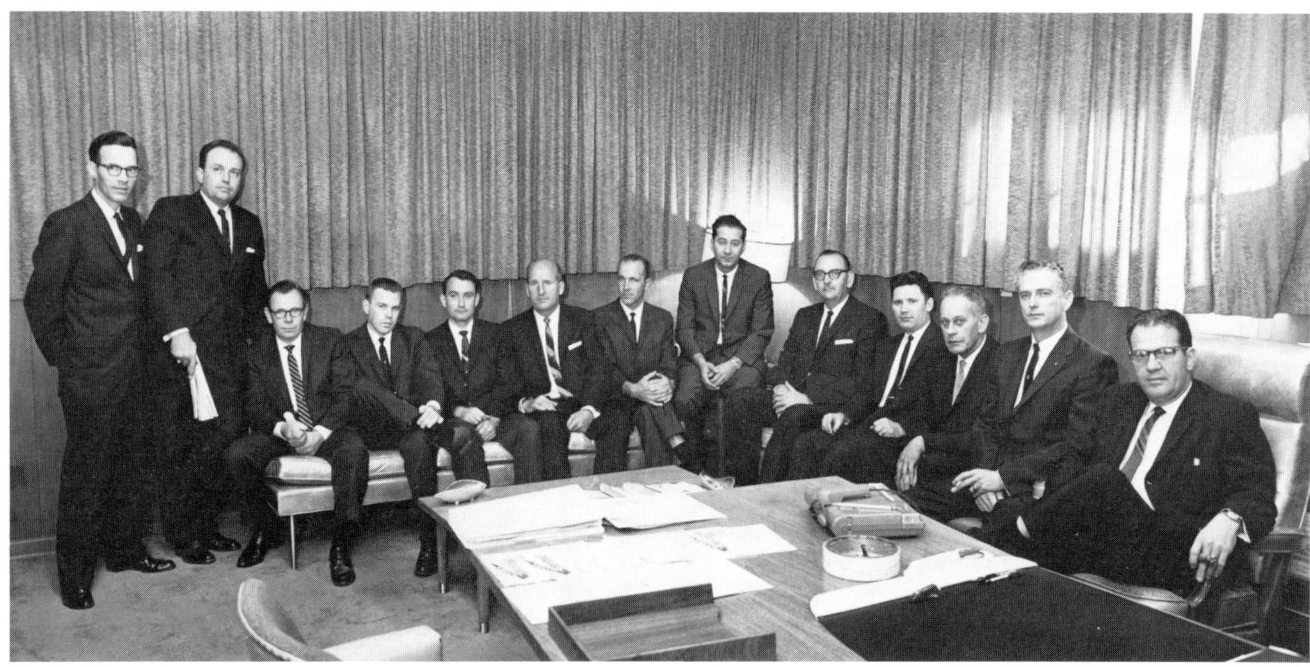

Here is the team that helped established Coburn Optical as a dominant manufacturer of optical equipment sold in every part of the world. Coburn's team consisted of (left to right): John Coburn (O.W.'s brother), Cecil Hornsby, Bill Dunlap (Coburn's first salesman), Brian Barns, Joe Stith, Hank Beute, Hank Gelderman, Herb Cohen, Jack Suddarth (inventor of the original Coburn generator), Greg Szabo, Chuck Douthitt, Bob Roberts (founder of Flo-Bob) and O.W. "Bill" Coburn.

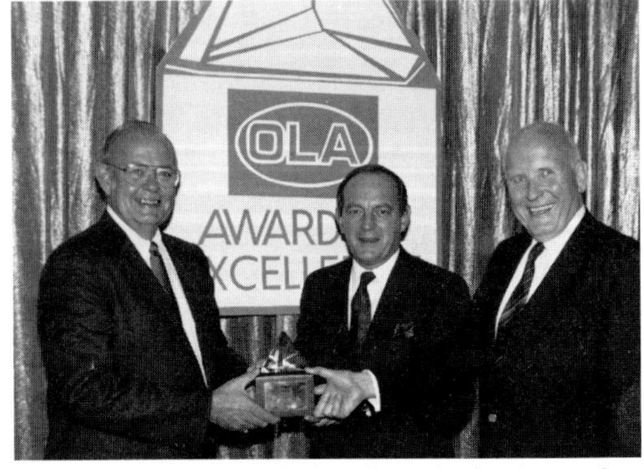

Coburn won an OLA Award of Excellence for their TraceNedge Coburn/Weco edger in 1987. This edger had been developed jointly by Weco and Coburn. Here Coburn President John Blocha (center) accepts the Award from OLA President Keith Caudill. With them is Weco's Dieter Beuthien.

ring cool so pitch wouldn't stick to it. Working out of his garage, Coburn assembled a dozen blockers, placed them in the back of his Oldsmobile Rocket and set out to sell them. As fast as he sold them, he'd head back to Muskogee to assemble some more.

Shuron had also devised a way to partially automate the blocking process by heating the pitch in a pot and dripping it onto the block. Then, if the lab man was swift enough, the lens blank could be blocked in position. Shuron's unit required the use of clear pitch so the axis lines could be aligned with a groove in the bronze block as it was blocked.

Coburn knew a one-product company had a limited life so he looked around to find more products to broaden his line. His most obvious need was a generator, then just starting to be used in laboratories. During the summer of 1953 while in Milwaukee calling on Fluegge Optical, he was introduced to Jack Suddarth. When he heard that Jack Suddarth had patented a generator, he showed immediate interest. That evening they headed out to Jack's home. Jack had been trying to interest someone in manufacturing his generator, which he had conceived one night while sitting in a foxhole on Okinawa with Harvey

Fluegge. Coming back to Milwaukee after the war, Jack refined his original idea and managed to get it patented. He had demonstrated it to Shuron who turned it down since they were already working with Cincinnati Milling Machine Company on converting one of Cincinnati's machines to cut optical lenses.

Jack had stored his prototype machine in his basement. Taking Coburn down there, he removed the motor from his wife Florence's washing machine and demonstrated his machine for Bill. Jack wanted $10,000 for the patent. A deal was struck that night and Coburn left Suddarth's home with the generator in the trunk of his car. By 1958, Suddarth had joined the company as vice president. Acquiring a generator set in motion a long process that ultimately resulted in Coburn Manufacturing Company becoming the largest manufacturer of lens-making equipment in the world.

In 1955, the company introduced the 501 cylinder machine which went on to become a standard for the industry. They also made arrangements with Duffens Optical to build their Quinton-Duffens Modern Polisher on a royalty basis. Suddenly Bill Coburn had a complete line of machinery. The 5000 cylinder machine was introduced in 1987 and received the 1990 OLA Award of Excellence for Best in Surfacing Equipment. Another innovation introduced in 1987 was Coburn's TraceNedge System which eliminated the need to store and retrieve lens patterns. This unit received OLA Awards in 1987 and 1988.

During the lean years, it was Bill Coburn's habit to make a little ceremony every time a generator order came in from a customer. He kept a gold-painted shot gun in his office. Each new generator order meant the company could stay in business a little longer. When an order came in, Coburn would take his shotgun out into the plant and fire off a blank round. Eventually, he had to give up these shotgun announcements. Orders were coming in too fast and his employees were getting too nervous from all the unexpected explosions.

The company continues to develop innovative lab equipment. In 1992, they introduced a radical new type of generator they called IQ. It varied from previous generators by utilizing a single point diamond tool for generating the curves.

There were several reasons why the company grew so fast and became so successful. Instead of spending several years refining and testing new equipment, it was Coburn's policy to immediately start selling each new machine as quickly as possible after it was designed. They would sell the machines on a "satisfaction guaranteed" basis with Coburn promising that any future improvements to the machine would be added to the customers unit at no cost as they evolved. Coburn also knew from personal experience how costly it was to have lab machines out of action for any length of time. He guaranteed free repair, but free service was only of value if it was provided quickly. He required all Coburn salesmen to be able to repair machines as well as sell them and everyone had to be able to fly a plane.

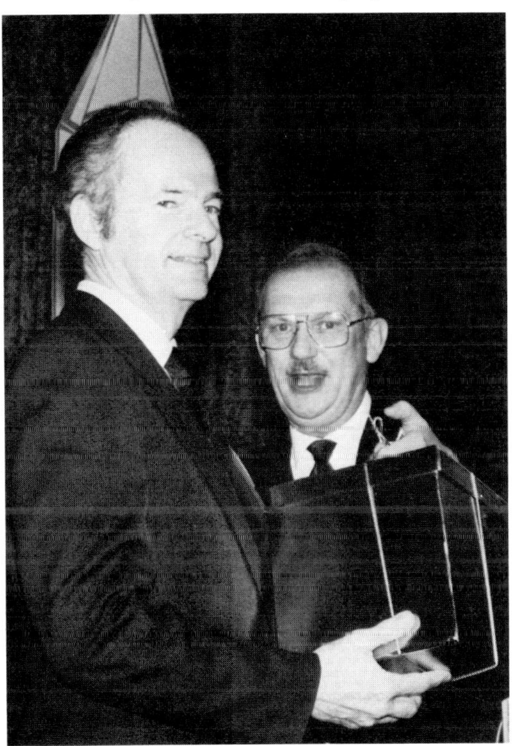

Gerber won an OLA Award in 1989 for their OMS SG-8 Surface Generator, a radically new design concept for generators. Accepting the Award is Gerber Optical President Ken Wood, left, with OLA President Bill West.

The most important order in the company's history came on March 9, 1956 with an order for 50 cylinder machines at $995 each, 22 Rocket generators at $3,995 each and a lap cutter at $2,195 for a total of $139,835 *(fortunately, he was no longer firing off his shotgun by this time)*. The order was from a new lab called Dal-Tex, just being set up to produce 5,000 jobs a day by Irving Greenberg *(see "Texas Labs" in Chapter 18)*. That Dal-Tex order, more than any other single thing, established Coburn Optical as a major contender in the industry.

In 1971, Coburn purchased a small company called Vareco in Colonial Heights, Virginia, anticipating that plastic lenses were about to become an acceptable material for eyeglass lenses. Coburn sent his son Tom to run the plant and the business increased from $100,000 annually to almost $20 million by 1978.

The company went public in 1972. Their sales at the time were over $14 million with profits estimated to be in excess of $2 million. Three years later, in 1975, Coburn Optical Industries was purchased by Revlon. In 1987, Pilkington Visioncare bought the company from Revlon, adding it to their other eyecare properties. In 1992, Pilkington sold Coburn Optical to a Coburn management team along with the Jepson Corporation, an investment group that had once owned Signet Armorlite. The company is completely out of the lens market but still maintains a strong position in optical machinery, a heritage that dates back to Bill Coburn and that pitch blocker.

GERBER OPTICAL, INC.

Gerber Optical is one of four divisions making up Gerber Scientific, Inc. The parent company was founded by H. Joseph Gerber, a refugee from Nazi Germany who came to the United States in 1940 at the age of 15. He worked the 4:00 p.m. to midnight shift in a bakery in East Hartford, Conn. while he was going to high school. Attending Rennselaer Polytechnic Institute on a scholarship, he devised a variable scale, the first of more than 650 domestic and foreign patents that have been issued in his name. Gerber Scientific was incorporated in 1945 when Gerber was 21 years old.

In the late 1960s and early 1970s, Gerber Garment Technology developed the first in a succession of precision, computer-driven cutting systems for the apparel industry. Today, these cutters are the mainstay of Gerber Scientific's business. More than 2,500 cutters, worth approximately $1 billion are presently in use for cutting parachutes, sails, auto interiors, helicopter blades and more than 70 other items.

Gerber Scientific Products produces systems for sign-making and graphic arts industries. Gerber Systems Corp. makes productions systems for the printing industry.

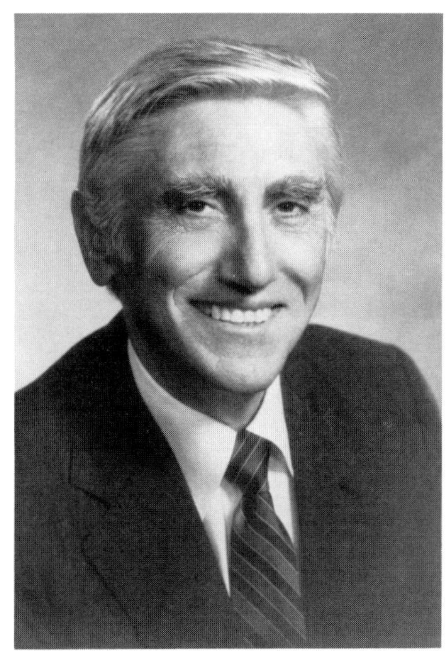

Gerber Scientific was founded in 1945 by Joseph Gerber when he was 21 years old. Gerber holds more than 650 domestic and foreign patents. Gerber Optical is one of four divisions of Gerber Scientific.

Optical Division

The optical division produces lab equipment for the optical industry and represented 4 percent of all sales in 1993. This division was established in 1987 with a single product. Today, the company produces an extensive laboratory system. One of the strongest assets Gerber had when entering what was, for them, a completely new industry, was total inexperience with optical machinery. Ken Wood, a 21 year veteran of Gerber Scientific, was chosen to head up the new optical division.

Wood believes that having no optical experience permitted the company to view lens production from an unbiased view. With no preconceived notions of how lenses should be produced, the company also benefited from having no existing product lines to protect. What they did have was extensive expertise in multi-axis technology. Their first product was a tracing device to produce precise patterns for edging lenses. The second product was a network for linking retail offices to laboratories for transmitting prescriptions and scanning information direct to the lab. The third item was the most revolutionary - their SG8 surface generator, at the time, a completely new method of surfacing lenses. Lab operators who first saw this generator at 1988's OLA Convention couldn't believe that a square metal box not much larger than a vacation cooler could generate lenses. They had never seen a generator like this. This became the first in a new series for multi-axis generation of lenses, a far cry from the industry's old surfacing pans, at one time, the only way to produce curves on lenses.

Gerber Optical's newest innovation for laboratories is a Step One Blocking System. Laboratories have been anxiously awaiting something to replace alloy blocking, the process used in almost every laboratory. The problem with alloy is the hazard of handling the material combined with serious disposal problems. Lead and cadmium present in alloy are extremely dangerous to lab personnel and must be filtered out of waste water before the water can be disposed down the drain. Gerber's new process uses a unique thermoplastic adhesive to fasten lenses to blocks during the surfacing process.

EPA Joint Venture

In June, 1994, Gerber Optical President Ken Wood signed a Cooperative Research Agreement with the Environmental Protection Agency (EPA). This program creates a three-way partnership between the optical industry, the EPA and the Naval lab (NOSTRA) in Yorktown, Virginia and is expected to lead the way toward completely eliminating lead-based and other hazardous materials from laboratory processing.

LOH OPTICAL MACHINERY, INC.

It was on March 17, 1922 that Wilhelm Loh opened a toolmaking shop in his home town of Wetzlar, Germany. He chose a small house on the Liebfrauenberg and hung a modest sign board out in front that read "Mechanical Workshop, Toolmakers and Locksmith of Wilhelm Loh". Hiring one assistant and one apprentice, he set out to earn a living as a toolmaker. During the first few years, the company focused on spindle manufacturing and micro-lens work.

Starting a small business in those days wasn't much different than starting one in today's economy. It's never easy. From the beginning, young Wilhelm's biggest problem was dealing with the fierce inflation raging throughout Germany. The Loh's made their new business a family affair and refused to give up in spite of the difficulties created by the uncertain economy. Wilhelm's wife Käte Loh nee Zörb handled the new company's books and looked after the commercial side of their business.

Within a short time, the Loh workshop began to be recognized for excellent handicraft skills and top workmanship. This growing reputation, aided by shrewd business planning, helped Loh remain profitable even during those prewar years of high inflation and strained economic circumstances. Within three years of the founding of the company, the Loh family began

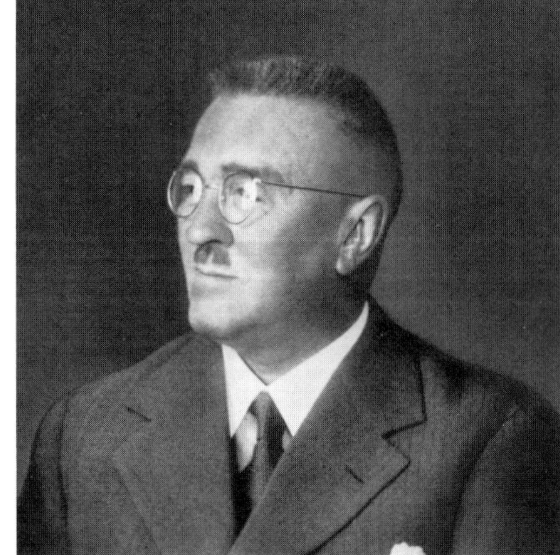

Wilhelm Loh started his company in 1922 as a small toolmaking shop in Wetzlar, Germany. He ran the growing company until his death in 1950.

construction of a larger workshop that became known as the Friedenstrasse Plant.

Integrated Equipment Introduced

Moving to these larger facilities enabled the company to expand its manufacturing capabilities. The company began to produce multi-spindle machines for grinding and polishing lenses and prisms. These became the company's first complete range of machines and represented an important milestone in the history of LOH Optical Machinery.

The company has always considered their employees to be an "extended employee family" and this became a company priority. The Loh family maintained a holiday cottage for their employees and sponsored one of the best employee football teams in that part of Germany. This fellowship has been a vital part of the LOH corporate philosophy ever since. The company prospered for a number of years until World War II began when all nonessential production and growth came to an immediate halt. The war was a serious setback for the company and all developmental work was delayed during those years.

Postwar

In the Post War Reconstruction era, Wilhelm Loh helped make his birthplace Wetzlar, Germany, synonymous with quality and top flight workmanship in the optical industry. A complete range of equipment for processing of precision and ophthalmic lenses was soon developed. The company began to supply equipment and machinery to clients throughout the world. This worldwide recognition led to further expansion of production facilities and equipment lines. Unfortunately, in 1950, just as the company began to rapidly grow, Wilhelm Loh passed away. Wilhelm's son, Ernst Loh became the company's new president. Ernst continued to build on his father's successes and has moved the company into a position of prominence in the optical industry. The company believes one reason they are able to control the quality of their finished products is because they manufacture all machine parts used in their machinery. Avoiding reliance on outside contractors guarantees consistent quality of output.

In the early seventies, LOH launched their North American presence through representation by Universal Photonics, formerly known as Universal Shellac & Supply Company. LOH successfully exhibited for the first time at the 1974 OLA Convention. LOH has exhibited at every OLA convention since. LOH continues to maintain a strong presence at OLA Conventions where they exhibit and often present technical seminars and workshops. More than 50% of the top 25 labs in the United States are LOH customers and 46% of all LOH customers are OLA members. LOH understands and acknowledges the importance of maintaining close ties to an organization like the OLA that is so linked to technology.

In order to strengthen the company's position in the market and enhance after-sales service and technical support, LOH incorporated in 1981 and established U.S. headquarters in the Chicago area. On the 10th anniversary of their incorporation in the U.S., North American LOH broke ground for a new facility in Milwaukee, Wisconsin. The new 15,000 foot facility provides a support system for North American customers and contains a complete customer training facility, live surfacing laboratory and parts inventory.

The company recently developed a computer integration program that provides an advanced manufacturing system. Incorporating a similar program into their own business and manufacturing environment, LOH moved into a new corporate Headquarters and integrated manufacturing facility in 1992. It features sophisticated computer-controlled material handling capabilities, CAD layout and design stations and an advanced customer training area. LOH still calls Wetzlar, Germany its home, but company headquarters are now located on Wilhelm Loh Street, dedicated to its founder. Fifty years ago, there were 3 people in the company's first workshop. Today there are almost 200 engaged in their workshop.

LOH has set up joint ventures with WECO and Balzers to provide a complete system from blocking to AR coating equipment. They are also doing extensive research and product development in robotics and automation to further enhance the work flow process for labs.

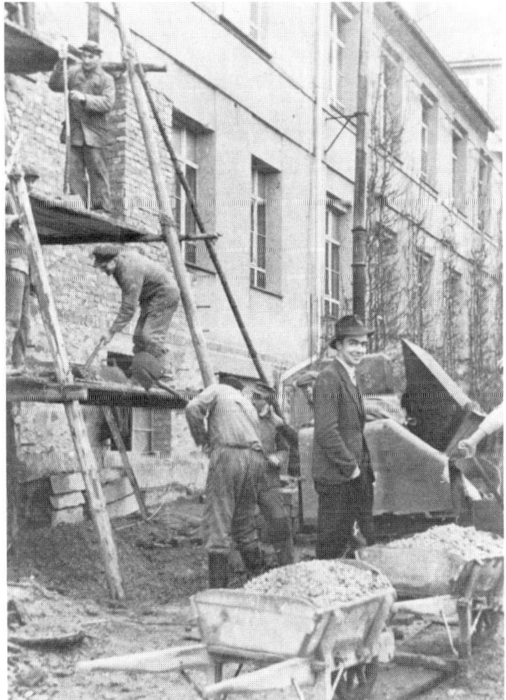

The war very nearly finished off Loh's company and all developmental work ceased during those years. Following Wilhelm Loh's death, his son Ernst Loh succeeded his father as President. In this photo, Ernst is shown overseeing reconstruction work on the company facility following World War II.

Photo – Loh Optical Machinery

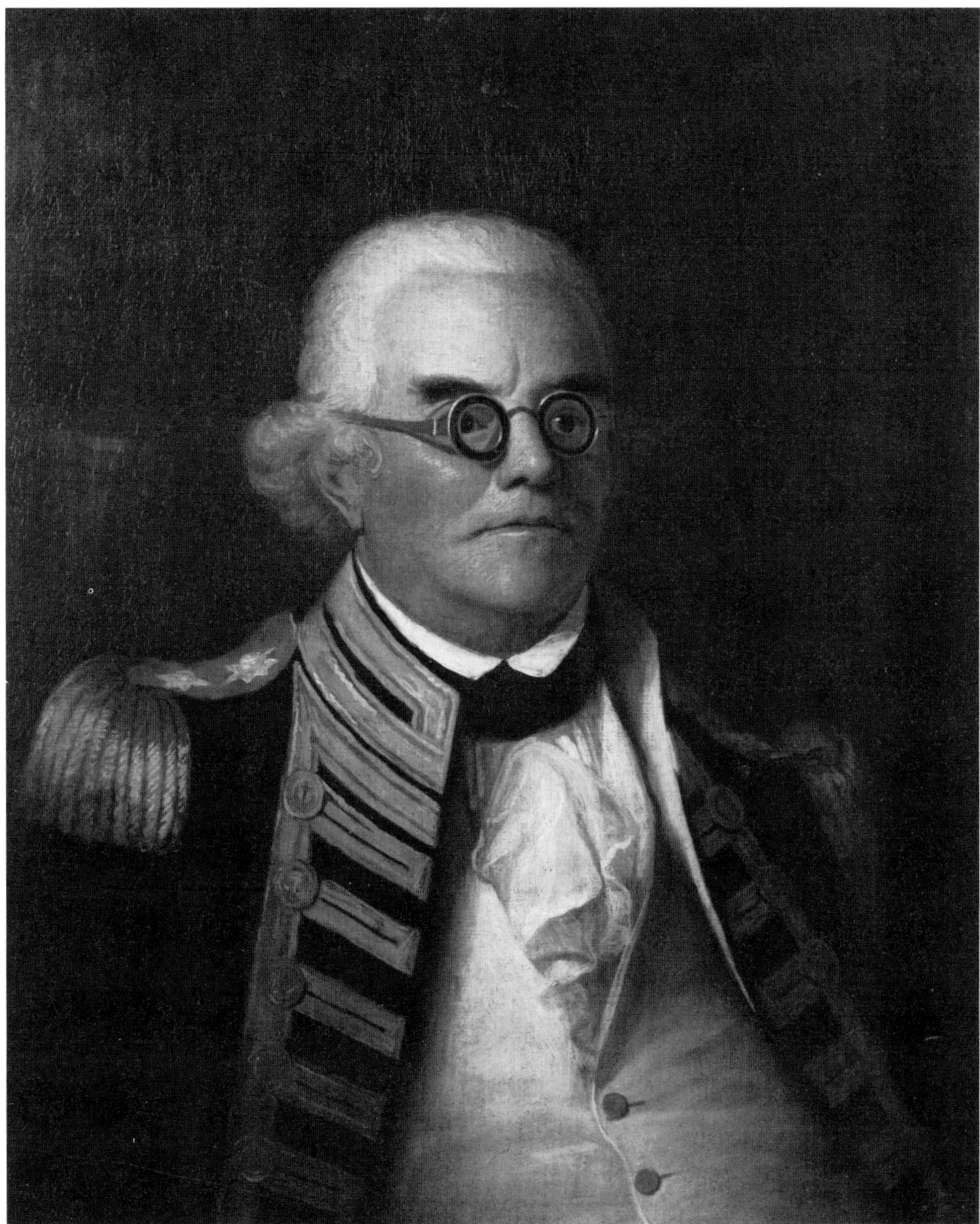

This painting (attributed to Thomas Hickey, 1741-1824) *shows Admiral Peter Rainer* (1741-1808) *who entered the British Navy in 1756. He was badly wounded during the capture of an American privateer in 1778 and was promoted to post rank by the Admiralty for his conduct during that action. He saw action in the East Indies as Commander-in-Chief of a large convoy and remained in that post until 1804. He was made Admiral in 1805 and served as Member of Parliament for Sandwich during his retirement.*

The Admiral's spectacles must have been a regular part of his wardrobe since he chose to have his portrait painted wearing them. His glasses have lenses fitted with "Martin's Margins", made of tortoiseshell or horn. Their inventor, Martin, described his invention as "a safeguard to the eye against all other foreign or extraneous light that may come upon it sideways". What Martin did not mention in his advertising was that use of horn rims such as these enabled opticians to use smaller lenses. Admiral Rainer most likely wore pebble lenses (see Chapter 7) and pebble lenses in small diameters were less expensive. We are indebted to the British College of Optometrists and their Honorary Curator Hugh Orr for this superb portrait.

Chapter 16
Legal Actions that Shaped the Industry

Three legal actions, all undertaken by the U.S. Justice Department, ultimately changed the entire industry — for independent laboratories, for manufacturers and for eyecare professionals. The years between 1920 and 1946 had been tough years for all who tried to compete with the two industry giants, AO and B&L. Suddenly, however, with World War II out of the way, the old ways were no longer tolerated. The world was expecting great things from the exciting postwar years. It was probably inevitable that the house of cards AO and B&L constructed over the years would fall. The first action started just as war clouds began to spread over the world.

#1 - UNITED STATES V. AMERICAN OPTICAL, AN ASSOCIATION, ET AL.

This Federal action was first filed in 1940 under the Sherman Antitrust Act and Clayton Antitrust Act. It charged that 13 manufacturers of eyeglass frames and mountings, a national trade association, 6 wholesalers, 2 patent holding companies and 13 individuals conspired to fix prices and restrain trade in ophthalmic goods. The suit resulted from practices of AO and B&L that are discussed elsewhere in this history. To understand the significance of this case, however, some background is helpful:

For some time, American Optical had controlled three major patents used by almost every frame manufacturer. These included the Ful-Vue patent which applied to any frame where the endpiece was located higher than the center of the lens *(this included virtually every current frame at that time)*. The two basic rimless styles of the day, used worldwide, were the Numont *(2 holes)*, and the Rimway *(4 holes)*. Every manufacturer of rimless mountings produced versions of these two styles. Where they could sell and at what price they charged were all policies dictated by the patent holder. The Numont patent was owned by Uhlemann Optical and the Rimway by Bay State Optical. Both companies, however, had assigned their patents to American Optical, who handled the bookkeeping, policing and collection of royalties *(remitting all royalties to the owners)*. Controlling these patents were a key factor in AO's control of the industry.

Under the Ful-Vue license, for instance, manufacturers were required to distribute their Ful-Vue frames only through licensed distributors. Distributors *(wholesale laboratories)* could only sell the frames to authorized Ful-Vue retailers. All parties were told at what prices they could sell the frames. The wonder is that such a restrictive system lasted as long as it did. The Numont Ful-Vue Corporation printed books each year that listed every "Authorized Dispenser". The title page stated "As required by your License Agreement, sales of Numont Ful Vue products to Dispensers may be made to only authorized Dispensers".

Another aspect that needs to be understood is that there were two wholesaler associations during these years. The more influential of the two was the OWNA *(Optical Wholesalers National Association)* run by Guy Henry. OWNA members included those laboratories owned by manufacturers *(AO and B&L)*. OWNA members could vote for each location they owned. This put association control solidly into AO and B&L's hands. Further, it was AO and B&L's policy only to issue listings *(wholesale distributorships)* to labs who belonged to the OWNA. Adding to the OWNA's influence was the fact that many leading manufacturers would only grant listings to laboratories who had been classified as wholesalers by the OWNA. Obtaining a "wholesaler" classification required laboratories to submit detailed financial information to the OWNA. For years, independent labs believed that confidential information submitted to the OWNA was filtered back to AO and B&L and used competitively in their own marketplace.

In 1939, a new wholesaler association was launched in Chicago specifically to address these important issues. The Association of Independent Optical Wholesalers *(AIOW)* permitted membership only by wholesalers who were neither owned nor controlled by manufacturers.

Independent wholesalers had another major complaint about the giants. They claimed that B&L and AO often favored larger retailers with "big dealer" discounts, bypassing wholesale laboratories and keeping these large retailers as "house accounts" of the two factories. This, then, was the setting for this first antitrust action.

The original complaint had been filed on September 16, 1940. All parties appeared and stoutly denied any violation of the law. Before the case could be heard by Judge John Woolsey, the trial was postponed at the personal request of the Secretary of War and the Secretary of the Navy. War was just over the horizon and war production was the greatest concern *(the War Department needed AO and B&L)*. Antitrust had to take a back seat until the war was won.

On September 17, 1948 the defendants came back to court and indignantly requested a mistrial on the basis that Judge Woolsey had died. Instead of dropping the case, the Justice Department renewed their interest and pursued the issue. The case ended when all parties consented to a final judgment without the facts ever being heard in a trial.

The resulting Consent Decree stipulated the following regarding the patent licenses involved in the suit:

New York World Telegraph
May 27, 1940

Bausch & Lomb Fined $40,000

Nolo C...
Pleade...

N.Y. Times   7-10-40

OPTICAL GOODS TRUST ENDED BY INJUNCTION

Federal Decree Entered Here With Consent of Bausch & Lomb

The final court action to end a monopoly exercised by an American and a German optical company on military optical goods was taken yesterday with the entry of an injunction, by consent of the Bausch & Lomb Optical Company. The decree was signed by Federal Judge William Bondy.

A world monopoly was alleged in an indictment obtained last March by members of the Department of Justice's anti-trust division. It was said to have been organized in 1921 in an agreement between Bausch & Lomb and the German company, Carl Zeiss. Bausch & Lomb, three officials who were named in the indictment, refused to fight the charges, and Judge Goddard exacted fines totaling $40,000 on all the Bausch & Lomb defendants.

The agreement, as charged in the indictment, bound Bausch & Lomb and the complaint, to refrain from selling optical goods to any outside the United States and, in return, agreed, the rest of the world would refuse to order country. ...

D. C. Optometrist Trips Lens Trust'

By MARY SPARGO

Glasses and gasoline! A strange mixture but a District optometrist threw the two together with plenty of fight as a binder and got Justice Department suits against 29 corporations and 68 individuals as the product.

David S. Block, head of the Ideal Optical Service at 802 F-st nw, today told the story behind the filing of four civil suits in the U. S. District Court in New York yesterday which opened a Government attempt to break an alleged monopoly in the optical business.

The first of the suits, directed against substantially all the important companies in the business of making lenses and frames, charges violation of the Sherman Anti-Trust Act.

KNEW IN ADVANCE

"I had known for a long time it was impossible to buy certain types of lenses and frames unless the retailer charged the regulation price," related Mr. Block. "If yo ucut your prices, supplies were refused.

"When the Supreme Court handed down its decision on the Ethyl gasoline case, March 25, this year, I realized I could start my battle against the glasses monopoly.

"The next day I went to New York and purchased 1000 pairs of a patented, price-restricted type of frames. I advertised them in The Washington Daily News at a price greatly below that set by the company which controlled the manufacture."

JUSTICE DEPARTMENT ACTS

Within 24 hours, Mr. Block claimed, a manufacturer's representative was "first cajoling, the nthreatening" him to maintain the price.

The fighting occulist appealed to the Justice Department. The battle was on.

In his book, "The Bottlenecks of Business," Asst. Atty. Gen. Thurman Arnold describes the opening of Mr. Block's drive to smash the alleged monopoly. A cop yof the book he gave to the District optometrist is inscribed, "To David S. Block, a good ally in a good fight. Thurman Arnold."

- Patents involved were cancelled and decreed to be null and void.
- Licenses and agreements between the Ful-Vue Sales Company and AO were cancelled.
- Licenses and agreements between AO and Uhlemann were cancelled.
- Licenses and agreements between AO and B&L were cancelled.
- Licenses issued by B&L were cancelled.
- AO, B&L and Uhlemann were required to license any manufacturer who wanted to produce frames under those patents *(including any improvements they might make to the patents)*.
- Any person whose license had been cancelled in the past would get one upon making application *(Products involved were Ful-Vue, Numont, Arcway, Rimway, Toprim and Zyl-arc)*.
- Patent holders could not collect damages for infringement.
- They could not grant new licenses or enforce these patents for five years.
- They were enjoined from controlling resale prices.
- They could not enter into any Fair Trade resale agreements for two years *(The Fair Trade Act controlled retail prices of branded retail products and was enforced by the Federal Government to assure that Fair Traded goods were not sold at discount prices)*
- For 10 years, AO and B&L were restrained from acquiring any more wholesale companies *(B&L was permitted only to acquire any outstanding stock in affiliate companies where they owned a controlling interest)*.
- The two major manufacturers were forbidden to exchange information, to own optical patents jointly or to grant exclusive patent licenses to one another *(in other words, the good old days of working together were over)*.
- AO and B&L were forbidden to sell to retailers at lower prices than they charged distributors and they could not sell products at different prices in the same trade or competitive area.

All the named manufacturers were enjoined from selling or leasing equipment that could only be used on their products - or from selling products that could only be processed on their equipment. The OWNA was restrained from collecting information relating to businesses or operations, unless it was from an OWNA member. The association was also forbidden to collect, distribute or disclose any data regarding wholesale or retail distribution of optical goods.

AO and B&L were restrained from becoming members of any association that had the purpose of classifying companies or restraining competition in optical goods. They could no longer refuse to sell to companies not listed on the Ful-Vue Distributors List, not members of the OWNA or those not classified as a wholesale distributor by the OWNA.

HOW THE FIRST CONSENT DECREE AFFECTED THE INDUSTRY

These were very tough terms and this judgment finally broke AO and B&L's stranglehold on manufacturing and distribution of optical products. Suddenly, the playing field was a little more level. There was another long-lasting result from this case. The OWNA lost a great deal of that organization's clout and as AO and B&L's involvement in the lab business declined, so did the influence of the OWNA. The AIOW, representing independent laboratories, gained tremendously in membership, stature and clout. Eventually the OWNA was absorbed by the AIOW to become the association known today as the OLA.

#2 - UNITED STATES V. AMERICAN OPTICAL COMPANY, ET AL.

On July 23, 1946 the Justice Department filed a complaint against American Optical and a list of individual medical eye doctors. The author remembers well the impact of this case when it was filed. The Chicago Tribune *(and most other U.S. newspapers)* treated the case as a major news story and even included a list naming all the doctors involved in the suit. Many of these oculists were pillars of their communities and were highly embarrassed to have their friends and patients learn they had been receiving kickbacks on all glasses purchased on their prescriptions *(the Tribune's list even stated the amount of their rebates)*.

As a result of this action, a Consent Decree was eventually issued on May 16, 1951 perpetually enjoining each defendant doctor from accepting payment *(in any form)* from any dispenser connected with dispensing to any patient. American Optical was perpetually enjoined from making any payment to any refractionist *(specifically including any oculist)* arising out of dispensing.

During the course of this action, American Optical raised the court's ire by suddenly discontinuing dispensing in all company branches *(without notifying either the Justice Department or the Court)*. AO transferred the dispensing branches and those assets connected with dispensing to others *(mostly AO ex-branch managers)*. On September 18, 1950, the government filed a supplemental complaint against all those who had taken over AO's retail branches *(designating them as "transferees")*.

The final Consent Decree stated that AO could not enter into any agreement with transferees *(buyers of their previous retail dispensing businesses)* that required the transferees to purchase materials or lab work from American Optical. They could not fix or suggest prices charged by their transferees nor could they control where the transferees sold their goods. The Decree specifically stated that AO could not reduce the debt their ex-managers' incurred in buying the retail dispensing branch in exchange for lab work or merchandise orders. This, in effect, took away every possible benefit AO could have expected to recover from their previous retail branches. AO was also enjoined from dispensing or owning a dispensing business for 10 years. They could not set consumer prices for ophthalmic goods or services or even suggest retail prices.

HOW THE SECOND CONSENT DECREE AFFECTED THE INDUSTRY

Apparently seeing the handwriting on the wall, AO was already out of the dispensing business *(but only after the government suit had been filed)*. If AO had hoped to control or at least capture lab work from the new dispensers they had created, that hope was expressly forbidden in the final Decree. The end result was that AO was solidly out of the retail business - with no hope of benefiting from their previous retail business. This is certainly not what they had in mind.

B&L, who had duplicated virtually every aspect of AO's dispensing business, realized their options were also exhausted and proceeded to sell off their retail branches as well. With this one action, the Justice Department effectively ended AO and B&L's domination of the industry. Without the highly profitable retail business to support AO and B&L branches, it was only a matter of time before both companies began closing or selling off their labs. This was the second blow to AO and B&L's house of cards.

Another effect of the Consent Decree, of course, was that it effectively ended the up-to-then common practice of rebating to oculists who referred patients to dispensers for glasses or contacts. The Decree became binding, not just on the doctors named in the suit but every oculist in the country and had a profound effect on all retail dispensing.

#3 - UNITED STATES V. AMERICAN OPTICAL, BAUSCH & LOMB

The final blow to the giants' domination of the industry came from an almost overlooked complaint made by a Wisconsin voter to his U.S. Senator. Senator Alexander Wiley's constituent owned a small independent laboratory called Madison Optical located in Milwaukee. The lab owner claimed he was unable to get a listing from B&L and AO and the two companies were conspiring to put his lab out of business. Senator Wiley turned the complaint over to the Justice Department and their action came to be called "The Milwaukee Case".

The case was filed on December 29, 1961 under the Act of Congress commonly known as the Sherman Act. It was settled by a Consent Decree in 1966. Under the Consent agreement, AO and B&L were enjoined for 20 years from opening more than five new wholesale laboratories a year. Neither company could engage in the retail business for five years. For a further period of 15 years, neither could acquire a retail dispensing business without consent of the Department of Justice. For 20 years, both defendants were forbidden to fix or attempt to fix factory or wholesale prices of their products and they could not establish prices with the intent to eliminate independent laboratories.

More importantly, for 20 years, starting in 1967, each company had to submit profit and loss statements for each of their branches. They had to bill their branches at the same prices charged to independent distributors. Each branch had to be charged for services rendered by the factory at standard market prices. Any lab branch operating at a loss for three out of any five year period *(two of the three years being consecutive)* would have to be closed or sold and the factory could not open another wholesale lab in the same area for two years. For a period of 20 years, neither defendant could refuse to sell to wholesale labs because of the price at which they sold their goods.

HOW THE THIRD CONSENT DECREE AFFECTED THE INDUSTRY

Forcing the two manufacturers to operate their wholesale laboratories on the same basis as independents was a costly blow to AO and B&L. For too many years, AO and B&L labs leaned on the economic advantages they gained from being owned by the factories. When they lost that financial clout, they could no longer compete effectively. Independent labs, owned mostly by ex-AO or B&L men, had all the advantages and incentives that come from personal ownership as well as the contacts and personal relationships built up during the years they worked for the two manufacturers.

Was the downfall of the two giants inevitable? Of course. Much like the railroads, the oil industry, and many other segments of U.S. industry, American Optical and Bausch & Lomb had taken every advantage of the "laissez-faire" attitude of the Federal Government during the years prior to World War II. None of those practices are permitted today and, to be sure, no one misses them. An interesting aspect to the story of the three Consent Decrees that shaped the industry is that the present generation of one litigant, the OWNA, is today's highly respected Optical Laboratories Association, which only proves that we may not be able to select our parents but we certainly can control our destiny.

U.S. Indictment Accuses 95% of Optical Trade

14 Leading Manufacturers and 21 Individuals Are Named as Price Fixers

Fourteen of the largest manufacturers of spectacle lenses and frames, five wholesalers and three trade associations, said by the government to comprise virtually the entire American optical industry, were indicted yesterday by a Federal grand jury for alleged restraint of trade and price fixing in violation of the Sherman anti-trust act.

The indictments, four in all, charge that the defendant corporations and associations and twenty-one individuals associated with them, who were also named defendants, have conspired for more than a decade to maintain artificially high prices for eye glass frames and lenses.

Although the indictments do not allege to what extent prices have been artificially raised, a spokesman for the anti-trust division of the Department of Justice, which has been investigating the optical industry since last November, said that the government's inquiry has shown that spectacles which could be sold at $7.50 at a profit are sold at a fixed price of $20. Similarly, spectacles which sell at lower prices could be proportionately reduced without doing away with a legitimate profit for all concerned, the government spokesman said.

Predicts Cut in Prices

"If the government prevails in these cases, it is expected that existing high prices for eye-glasses and spectacle frames will be drastically cut," Samuel S. Isseks, Special Assistant Attorney General, in charge of the investigation said.

Mr. Isseks announced also that the government will soon institute civil suits against all important optical goods manufacturers. The suits, also under the anti-trus laws, will be directed at price-fixing agreements which are in the form of patent licensing contracts. One of the suits, Mr. Isseks said, will relate to optical frames and mountings; another will concern itself with bi-focal lenses.

Principal defendants named in the indictments are the American Optical Company, Southbridge, Mass.; Charles O. Cozzens, vice-president of the company in charge of sales; Charles N. Shelden, described as trustee and zone manager of the American Optical Company; Ira Mosher, trustee, vice-president and general manager of the company; Frank N. Kreisel, Chicago zone manager of the company; and Irving W. Wilson, in charge of frame sales for the American Optical Company.

Also the Bausch & Lomb Optical Company of Rochester, N. Y.; Ben A. Ramaker, its sales manager; the Colonial Optical Company, Inc., optical wholesalers of New York and an affiliate of Bausch & Lomb; Thomas J. Byrne, president, and Louis W. Joeger, secretary, of the Colonial company; Riggs Optical Company, Consolidated, of Chicago,

and the White-Haines Company, of Cleveland, ... filiates of Bausch & ...; D. Hubbell, preside... Haines, and Roy ... president of Riggs ... tire, Magee & B... wholesale affiliate ... Lomb, of Philade... Klein, vice-preside... delphia firm.

More Corpor...

Also the Shuro... Inc., of Genev... Chew, its presi... linson, chairma... rectors, and ... company's spe... charge of sal... land Compa... versal Optic... Providence; ... pany, of Ro... Manufactur... Brooklyn; ... facturing ... T & P O... York; Th... Attleboro... cal Comp... mus Opti... Virginia... Petersbu... Other ... Wholes... York; ... dent; ... York, ... mana... the ... Asso... defe... of t... tio... Fr... sa... w... B...

$66,000 Fines Levied by U.S. In Optical Suits

14 Corporations, Seven of Their Officers Plead to Anti-Trust Act Charges

Fourteen corporations and seven of their officers, responsible for almost all the manufacture and distribution in the country of spectacle lenses and unpatented frames, have pleaded nolo contendere (no contest) in United States District Court to Sherman anti-trust charges filed by the government May 28 and were fined yesterday a total of $66,000. The fines were imposed by Judge Edward A. Conger on the recommendation of Samuel S. Isseks, special assistant to the Attorney General.

Six corporations and five corporate officers were fined $45,500 under the indictment charging price-fixing of spectacle lenses, and eight corporations and two corporate officers were fined $20,500 under the unpatented frames indictment. Four indictments were handed up last May affecting 95 per cent of the optical trade. On Nov. 15, eight corporations and eleven individuals named in the indictment concerning second-quality prescription lenses pleaded nolo contendere and were fined $51,000.

Optical ...
Horseheads, N. ...

Not all of the defenda... named in each of the indictments. One indictment charges the manufacturers of 95 per cent of all spectacle lenses in the United States with fixing prices to wholesalers and retailers; another charges the wholesalers and their associations with fixing prices of "second quality prescription lenses sold and distributed in the metropolitan area, as well as in Pennsylvania, Maryland and the District of Columbia; a third indictment charges the three largest manufacturers of spectacle lenses and frames — American Optical, Bausch & Lomb and Shuron—with entering into an agreement to specify which firms could act as wholesalers; the fourth charges frame manufacturers with fixing prices of unpatented frames under a threat by the American Optical Company of a price war.

License Plan Defended

SOUTHBRIDGE, Mass., May 29 (AP).—The American Optical Company said in a statement tonight it believed its patent license plan "in accordance with the law as hitherto interpreted."

"The American Optical Company, instead of seeking to prevent others from manufacturing spectacles under these patents, has granted licenses to its competitors and has thus facilitated the widest possible manufacture and sale of the patented products on reasonable terms," the statement said. "The details of the licensing plan are, I believe, in accordance with the law as hitherto interpreted by the courts."

From
N.Y.Herald-Tribune
5/29/40

Form H 9

FILE	Cataloged
H	Abstracted
	Duplicate

INDEX
Opt. Industry
Publicity
SOURCE
N.Y.Herald Tribune
1/21/41

Together with the fines imposed yesterday and with fines imposed in a fifth indictment relating to military optical instruments, the government has received $157,000. Outcome of the remaining criminal indictment handed up last May, concerning alleged discriminatory selection of optical wholesalers, is pending. Four civil anti-trust suits in the optical industry are also pending.

The following fines were imposed yesterday in the lens case: American Optical Company, $5,000, and Charles O. Cozzens, its vice-president in charge of sales, $5,000; Bausch & Lomb Optical Company, $5,000, and Ben A. Ramaker, its sales manager, $5,000; Shuron Optical Company, Inc., $5,000; George J. Nagle, special vice-president in charge of sales of Shuron, $5,000, and Beverly Chew, the company's president, and John W. G...

Pleas End Part Of Federal Suit In Optic Case

Eight Groups and Officers in Lens Business Fined Under Anti-Trust Law

Eight corporations and associations manufacturing a large percentage of all spectacle lenses in the United States and eleven of their officers and directors named in a Sherman anti-trust action May 28 for alleged restraint of trade and price-fixing have pleaded nolo contendere (no contest) in United States District Court and have been fined a total of $51,000, the anti-trust division of the Department of Justice announced yesterday in dismissing the indictment.

The indictment was one of four handed down by a Federal Grand Jury last May involving twenty-two manufacturing and wholesaling corporations and trade associations and twenty-one individuals associated with them, who were accused of conspiring for more than a decade to maintain artificially high prices for eyeglass frames and lenses.

The specific indictment affecting those who pleaded nolo contendere charged that the defendants had entered into a price-fixing conspiracy on eye-glass lenses. They were accused of having conspired to fix uniform prices for the sale by optical wholesalers of individually ground lenses. In recommending acceptance of the plea, Samuel S. Isseks, special assistant to the Attorney General, told Judge Samuel Mandelbaum that if any of the defendants violated the anti-trust law in the future the government would ask the court for jail sentences.

The government also has pending in the court four civil suits alleging violation of the Sherman act by twenty-seven optical companies and sixty-eight individuals. These suits are directed at price-fixing agreements which are in the form of patent-licensing contracts. Still another action against Bausch & Lomb Optical Company, of Rochester, and three of its principal officers, was terminated May 27 when the defendants agreed to pay a $40,000 fine on a plea of nolo contendere that they entered into a secret agreement with Carl Zeiss, German optical firm, to monopolize the world market in military optical instruments.

The defendants who pleaded yesterday and the amount of fines each paid follow:

The American Optical Company, Southbridge, Mass., a voluntary association, $5,000; the American Optical Company, its subsidiary, of Southbridge, Mass., $3,500; Charles O. Cozzens, vice-president of the latter company in charge of sales, $5,000; Charles N. Shelden, trustee and zone manager of the company's New York branch, $5,000; the Colonial Optical Company, of New York, optical wholesalers and an affiliate of Bausch & Lomb, $5,000; Magee & Brown Company, of Philadelphia, wholesale affiliate of Bausch & Lomb, $5,000; Samuel Klein, vice-president of the Philadelphia firm, $5,000.

Also, Thomas J. Byrne, president of the Colonial Optical Company, $5,000; Louis W. Jaeger, secretary of the same company, $1,000; the Hilbert Optical Company, wholesaler, of Baltimore, $3,000; Simon Edelstein, president of the Optical Wholesalers National Association, Inc., of New York, $2,000; Roy D. Martin, of Horseheads, N. Y., treasurer of the association, $2,000; William B. Jones, of Rochester, a director of the association, $1,500, and Clarence J. Brauch, of New York, chairman and secretary of the Optical Wholesalers of Northern New York, $1,000.

Also, Arthur Frank, president of the Optical Wholesalers Association of New York, Inc., $1,000; the Optical Wholesalers National Association, $1,000; Guy A. Henry, secretary-manager of the Optical Wholesalers National Association of New York, Inc., $1,000, suspended; the Optical Wholesalers Association of New York, $1,000, suspended, and the Philadelphia Association of Wholesale Opticians, $1,000, suspended.

From N.Y. Herald Tribune 11/10/40

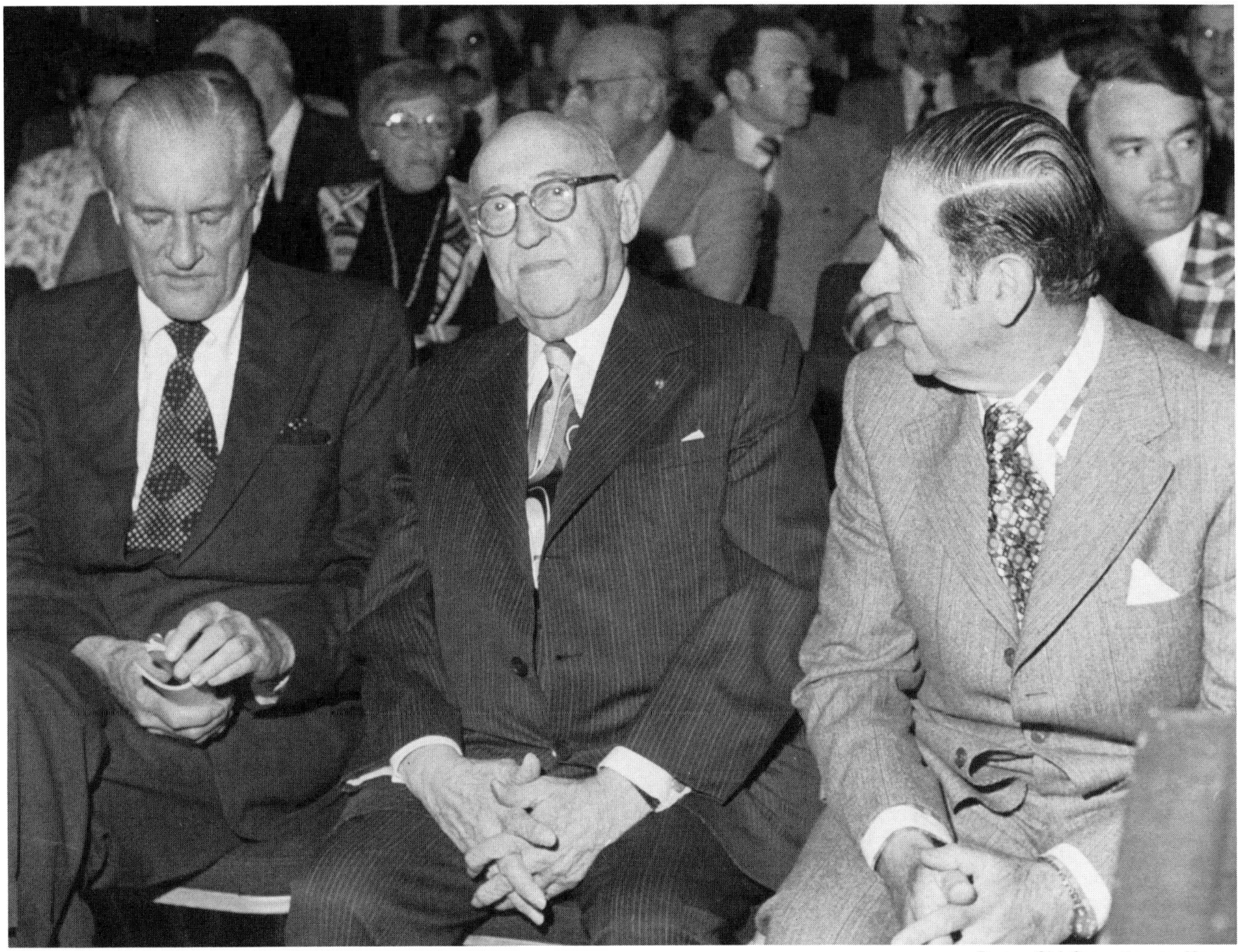

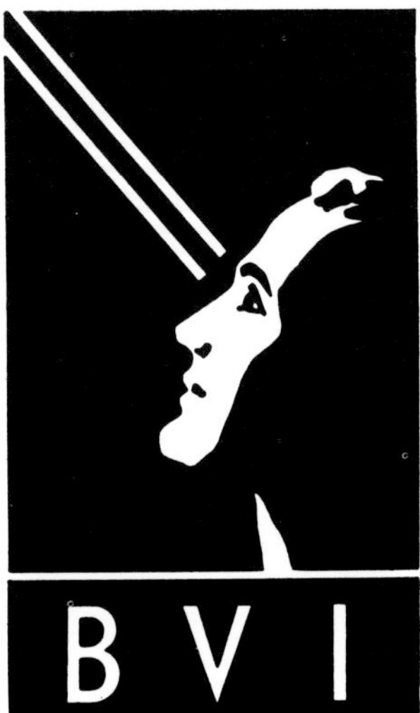

The Better Vision Institute held a Washington Conference on Vision care in April, 1974. The BVI always considered their basic job to be "Keeping the public aware of the importance of vision care". Three prominent speakers at the Conference included TV commentator Eric Sevareid (left), Frank Wiseman (right), a well-known representative of the British optical industry and Dr. Morris Fishbein (center), popular Editor of the Journal of the American Medical Association. Mr. Wiseman reported on England's experience with national health programs and astronaut William Lenoir reported on vision problems in space travel. The conference resulted in extensive national publicity for vision care and the BVI.

Chapter 17
Chowchow

Certain subjects do not fit well into the other chapter headings and have been included in this "catchall" section. One extremely important organization, the Better Vision Institute, has played an important part in the industry for many years and their story is told here. Their role has changed somewhat but the organization is still viable and serves the eyecare professions well.

Trade shows have become a major industry element — for manufacturers, laboratories and the professions. The story of how the first industry-wide trade show came to be is included, although old-timers may remember 1954's famous Optical Fair held in Chicago. That comprehensive show *(with no educational seminars)* combined official meetings of the A.O.A., A.I.O.W. *(labs)* and the Optician's Guild and was very successful. It was tried again later but with less success.

Communications are still a vital part of eyecare and a story of the industry's first involvement with communication technology is told in this chapter. Lastly, how could the history of the ophthalmic industry be told without including the subject of contact lenses? This book has mostly told the story of eyeglasses but we have included a brief review of contact lenses, a vital component in present-day eyecare.

BETTER VISION INSTITUTE (BVI)

With the first World War ending, key figures in the optical industry turned their thoughts from merely surviving, their primary consideration as they built an industry, to more lofty goals such as conserving eyesight. Reflecting these new industry concerns, a group called the Eyesight Conservation Council of America was formed in 1920. The Secretary General was Guy Henry, a familiar name, who later served as the longtime head of the Optical Wholesalers Association (OWNA), the organization that eventually became the OLA. The function of the new Council was to spread the gospel of eyesight conservation. The founders decided to concentrate their efforts on educational and industrial fields. The plan was to gain support for the new organization from the public, the optical professions and the industry in general.

During that same year, another group was created, called the Optical Development Society. This was the brainchild of Henry Kirstein, a former President of Shuron Optical Company. Shuron had sponsored an effective advertising program based on "style in glasses". The purpose of Kirstein's new organization was to take this advertising theme and develop it to benefit the entire industry. The difference between the two organizations was that Kirstein's Society was designed to develop additional business while the Council aimed at the more selfless goal of consumer education. The Society enjoyed a rather short life. It passed out of the picture within three or four years. The Eyesight Conservation Council continued but their activities were limited, mostly because of difficulty in raising funds to accomplish their goals.

A time-line on this subject would show the following actions:

1926: The Association of Optical Jobbers appoints a Plans Committee aimed at devising ways to improve the industry.

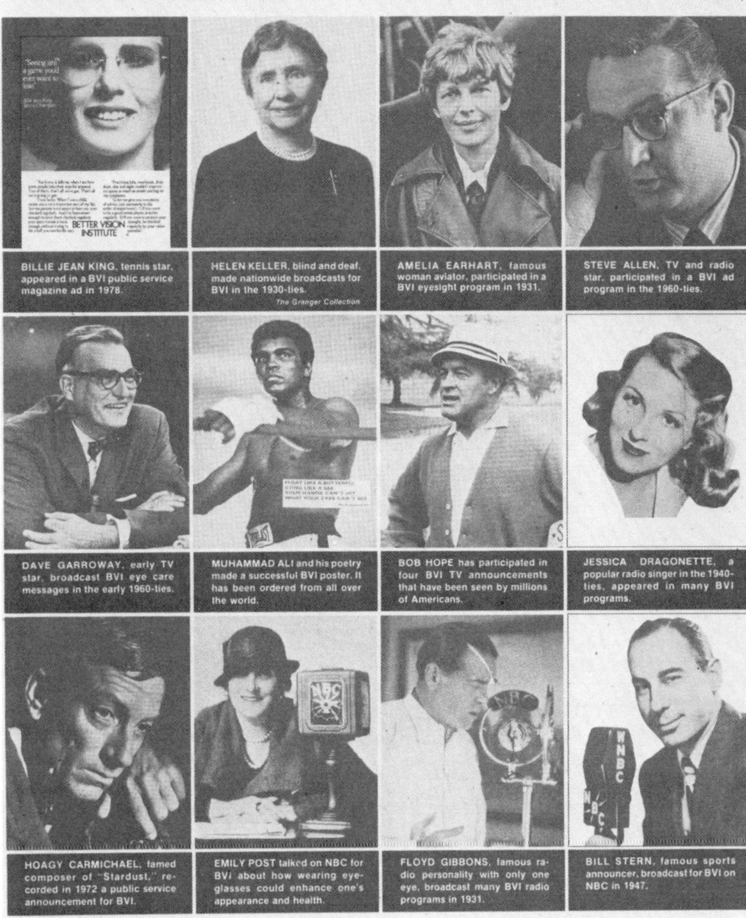

BILLIE JEAN KING, tennis star, appeared in a BVI public service magazine ad in 1978.

HELEN KELLER, blind and deaf, made nationwide broadcasts for BVI in the 1930-ties.
The Granger Collection

AMELIA EARHART, famous woman aviator, participated in a BVI eyesight program in 1931.

STEVE ALLEN, TV and radio star, participated in a BVI ad program in the 1960-ties.

DAVE GARROWAY, early TV star, broadcast BVI eye care messages in the early 1960-ties.

MUHAMMAD ALI and his poetry made a successful BVI poster. It has been ordered from all over the world.

BOB HOPE has participated in four BVI TV announcements that have been seen by millions of Americans.

JESSICA DRAGONETTE, a popular radio singer in the 1940-ties, appeared in many BVI programs.

HOAGY CARMICHAEL, famed composer of "Stardust," recorded in 1972 a public service announcement for BVI.

EMILY POST talked on NBC for BVI about how wearing eyeglasses could enhance one's appearance and health.

FLOYD GIBBONS, famous radio personality with only one eye, broadcast many BVI radio programs in 1931.

BILL STERN, famous sports announcer, broadcast for BVI on NBC in 1947.

The Better Vision Institute used a variety of well-known personalities to carry the eyecare conservation message direct to the public. BVI had as many as 2,000 members during those years and the BVI membership plaque was prominently displayed in their offices.

ILLUSTRATION – LAWRENCE O. AASEN

1927: At their next convention, the Plans Committee proposes conducting an industry-wide survey to determine what should be done. Someone in the group points out that the proposed survey will cost $50,000 to $60,000 and the idea of a survey dies a hasty death.

1928: At the next meeting of the Jobbers Association, a paper is read by E.F. Wildermuth, a member from White Haines Optical of Columbus, Ohio, a prominent laboratory of that day. Wildermuth points out *(in words that sound very familiar today),* "Who is your real competitor? Not your fellow jobber who is soliciting business on a legitimate basis! Your real competitor is the automobile industry, the radio industry, the clothing industry." He went on to point out that eight years earlier when the Optical Development Society was formed, "We had a one-style market — the zylo market. Today we have a one-style market — the white gold frame. The patient buys it because the retailer says it is the latest. He wears it morning, noon and night, not for six months or a year but very likely for many years."

Wildermuth pointed out facts that everyone knew were true. Retailers in those days bought their frames by the dozen *(sometimes by the hundreds)* and tended to fit every patient with the same three or four favorite frames. Most people on the street wore look-alike frames so patients had no compelling reason to come back for an eye exam, certainly not until their vision began to blur. This limitation on frame styles lasted well into the 1960s. Wildermuth's committee suggested rejuvenating the Optical Development Society or perhaps some other organization. His talk was received with great interest by fellow lab owners and the Association decided to give Wildermuth the job of raising funds to underwrite such an organization. Before the lab owners left Pittsburgh, they contribute $8,000. By the following June, a total of $14,000 had been raised.

1929: On April 25, a special organizational meeting is held at New York's Biltmore Hotel. The new public relations organization is formed, taking the name "Better Vision Institute". Three classes of members are set up; manufacturers, distributors *(labs)* and retailers. Retail members would be called "Associate Members" and pay annual dues of $5. On June 29, the new BVI organization published their first booklet called "Occupational Analysis", advising refractionists to prescribe glasses according to the nature of the patient's visual tasks *(a forerunner of the OLA's "Lifestyle Dispensing").*

1930: The new organization now has 3,045 Associate Members, 59 Contributing Members *(labs)* and 15 Sustaining Members *(manufacturers).* On June 30, Mike J. Julian, an experienced advertising man, is appointed to serve as Secretary and Product Manager *(he would serve the BVI for the next 30 years).* It is agreed that officers and directors of the new association would receive no salary and each would pay their own expenses for attending meetings.

In September, "Donor Member" was added as a class of membership. It was decided to refer to the optical professions as "Eyesight Specialists" to avoid professional bickering. Vogue magazine accepted an article on beauty in eyewear. For the next twenty years, much of BVI's efforts was addressed to placing eyecare stories in national magazines. This was a time before TV, when national magazines like Vogue, Saturday Evening Post and others had tremendous influence on consumers.

1931: BVI sponsors nationwide broadcasts and magazine articles by well-known personalities such as Helen Keller, Booth Tarkington, Emily Post and Lowell Thomas. Three more OD's, three more labs and three more manufacturers are added to the BVI board. It was decided that the Presidents of the American Academy of Optometry, the American Optometric Association, the Guild of Dispensing Opticians and the American Association of Wholesale Opticians *(labs)* would serve as directors at large of the BVI. The BVI was incorporated and the new Articles of Incorporation called for seven

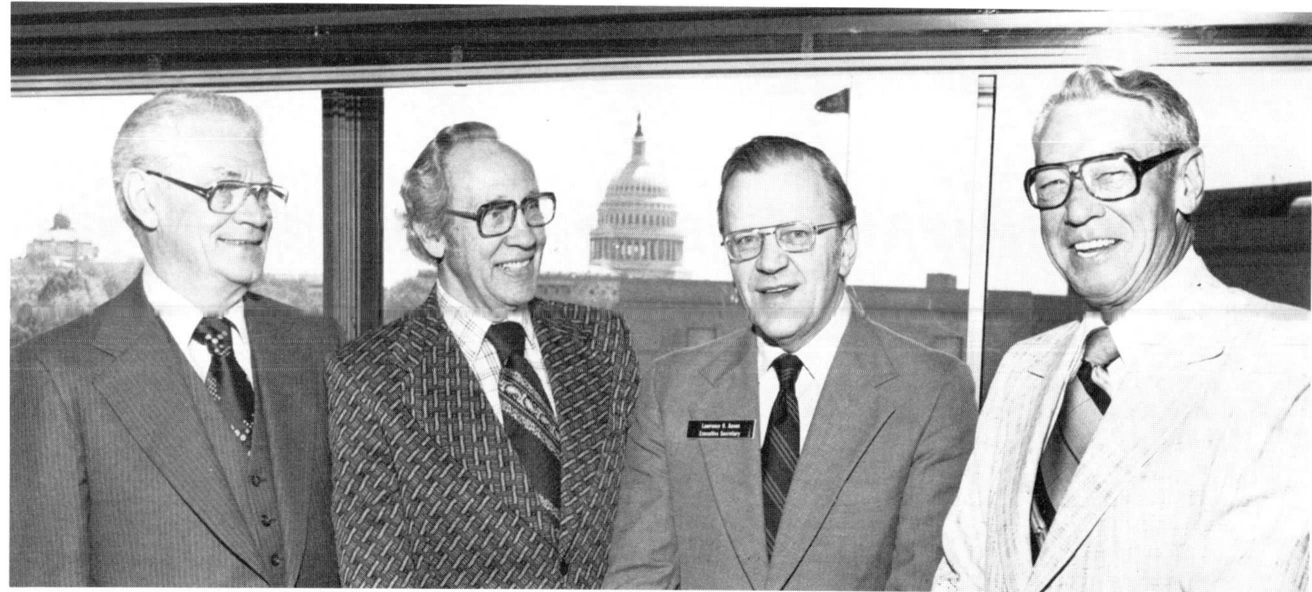

manufacturers, seven labs, seven Opticians, seven Optometrists plus four at-large members to serve as the Board of Directors.

1933: Mike Julian becomes BVI President.

1934: The BVI adopts a new seal and released it for use by manufacturer and laboratory members. It was decided not to make it available to retailers in an effort to keep the BVI seal away from "undesirable elements". BVI membership was 2,000. Over one million booklets were distributed this year. Elizabeth Arden and Amelia Earhart are added as celebrity spokespersons. For the first time, BVI took part in AOA's Save Your Vision Week, due to requests from many OD members as well as a few MD's. BVI sent a model statute to all states not requiring eyesight exams for motorists.

1937: BVI cooperates in preparing a book for young people published by Rand McNally. The organization now has 18 manufacturer members, 39 laboratories and 2,400 retailers as members.

1940: 226 radio stations sponsor BVI programs this year.

1988: VICA *(Vision Council of America)* takes over management and funding of the Better Vision Institute. All VICA health-related public education campaigns from this time on will be done under the BVI name.

1990: Richard L. Hopping, O.D., President of Southern California College of Optometry is appointed BVI national spokesperson.

Present: The BVI Advisory Council is made up of nine vision professionals, representing optometry, ophthalmology and opticianry. The Council guides VICA in creating and implementing its vision education programs. All health-related materials are reviewed and approved by the BVI Advisory Council.

Even though the original concept of a Better Vision Institute was proposed by a laboratory and the BVI's creation was funded by laboratories, labs are not presently represented on the BVI Advisory Council.

OPTICAL TRADE SHOWS

Ophthalmic professional associations *(AOA, OAA, etc.)* have conducted trade shows for their members for many years but it took an unusual event in mid-1977 to launch the first true optical trade show, that is, a combined exhibition and educational conference not sponsored by a trade association.

In 1977, one of the more successful ophthalmic publishers of the day was a company called Advisory Enterprises. Advisory published magazines for optometrists, opticians, vision aides and contact lens specialists and also sponsored a number of successful educational and management seminars in the United States and abroad.

In the spring of 1977, Advisory Enterprises sponsored an all-day marketing seminar aimed at manufacturers and distributors of frames, lenses and equipment. The meeting was held in the Plaza Hotel in New York City and featured a speaker named Gordon Trapnell who had just authored the first definitive study of the optical industry. Dr. Irving Bennett, a partner in Advisory Enterprises, explained what happened that day.

"Mr. Trapnell spoke immediately after the luncheon break. It was either the warm lunch or the temperature of the room or the difficulty to understand and follow statistics - or a combination of all of those - but the audience had difficulty keeping their eyes open.

I served as the master of ceremonies for the event and as soon as Mr. Trapnell finished his formal presentation I literally shocked the audience with a brusque (and

Three BVI Presidents, all members of the Optical Laboratories Association, met during the 1977 annual BVI meeting in Washington, D.C. Left to right, Tom Lynch, Don Gladstone, BVI Executive Director Larry Aasen and Herman Muller. OLA members had always participated in BVI activities but no longer are represented on BVI's Board.

PHOTO – LAWRENCE O. AASEN

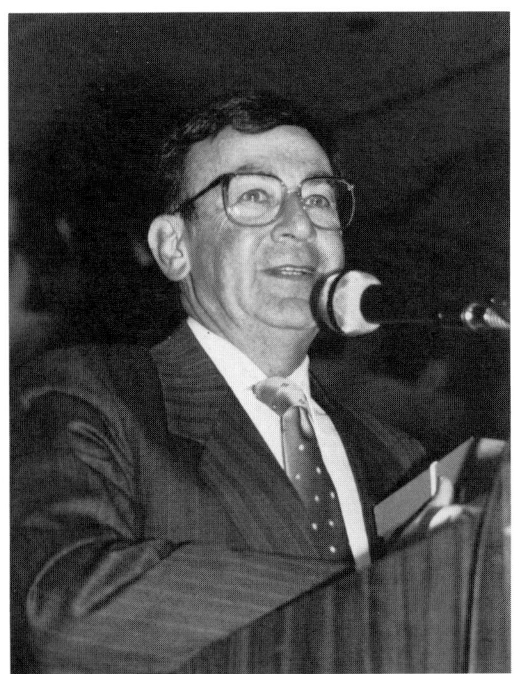

unprepared remark): *"What this industry needs is a show - probably in the Madison Square Garden - that would be open to the optometrists, opticians, and ophthalmologists... and perhaps even the public... to show off all the new innovations in eyewear: frames, lenses and equipment!"*

The declaration was met with spontaneous applause from the audience. And, with a combination of surprise and wonder, from my three partners - Bob Phillips, Jay Gubitz, and Mel Goldberg - who were standing at the back of the hall.

The rest was easy. Advisory spent the next day mapping out when to have the show (Spring 1978) *and where to hold it* (the Hilton Hotel in New York). *Up until that time there had been no national optical meeting in New York for over ten years; the largest "show" was the Annual Congress of the American Optometric Association which had 3,700 persons registered; and the highest charge for booth space had been $500 for a 10 x 10 space.*

Jay Gubitz came up with the name OptiFair and it stuck like glue. Advisory engaged David Cheifetz's firm Conference Management to run the show; Conference Management was a relatively small company with a good track record with trade shows. A booth charge was $750 to demonstrate confidence. And an audience of at least 5,000 members of the optical field was "guaranteed". As a major attraction, Advisory scheduled an ambitious program of educational seminars in one- and two-hour segments. Fourteen seminars were run concurrently but none would be in session when the exhibition was open. There was a total of 160 seminar hours, including a liberal sprinkling of "exhibitor" seminars. No trade show up to that time had scheduled as much variety in any program. And no trade show gave such prominence to exhibitor seminars.

Booth space sold steadily with George Rich of Starline buying the first multiple - three spaces. Large companies like American Optical Company refused to buy any space or participate in the show. A total of 246 booths (a sell out) was achieved. Because of the enthusiasm prior to the show, Advisory and Conference Management reserved space in the Century Plaza Hotel in Los Angeles for "OptiFair West" but told no one about this decision. The second show was to be announced only if the first one was a success.

There was little incentive for early registration of optometrists and opticians. So it was frightening to have only a few over 700 advance registrations before the show opened on March 7, 1978.

I personally came down the elevator to the registration floor at 7:00am on the morning of March 7. What a feeling! The registration area was literally packed with people filling our registration forms, standing in line to be validated, waiting for the seminar rooms to open. The show was "electric". The aisles were chock full of lookers and buyers. The enthusiasm of sellers was great as the buyers. The after-glow in the lobby of the Hilton, that is the time after the show closed, was an extension of an up-beat industry just arising from the doldrums.

The rest is history. Final attendance at the first OptiFair was 6,857. And these were only eyecare professionals. No exhibitor representative, spouses, or friends were included in the totals. Oh, yes, OptiFair West was announced on the last day of the New York show by placing advanced registration forms in each booth with a statement that space for OptiFair West could be reserved at 11 a.m. that morning. The line of space buyers gathered early and within an hour the west show was sold out and a prioritized waiting list was begun.

Those not getting guaranteed space in the west were irate since they had supported our initial effort. The Century Plaza did not have sufficient exhibit space to handle more than 200 booths and agreed to have a tent put on the grounds. Fortunately that was not acceptable. As it turned out the temperature in Los Angeles at the time of the show was over 100 degrees!

Advisory and Conference Management elected to drop the Century Plaza and move the show to Long Beach where it was held on September 26-28, 1978 with 314 booths and an attendance of 5,361 optical persons. OptiFair relocated to Anaheim in 1979 for its permanent home. In 1980 OptiFair Midwest was begun in St. Louis. That show was shifted to Chicago the following year."

In their second year, the New York OptiFair had 7,025 attendees with 368 booths. By 1986, attendance at the New York show had grown to 10,047. OptiFair was eventually phased into Vision Expo, but before that happened, a total of 30 successful OptiFair shows were held. OptiFair and Dr. Irving Bennett are widely acknowledged as originators of the concept of an exhibition and educational trade show that includes all ophthalmic professions.

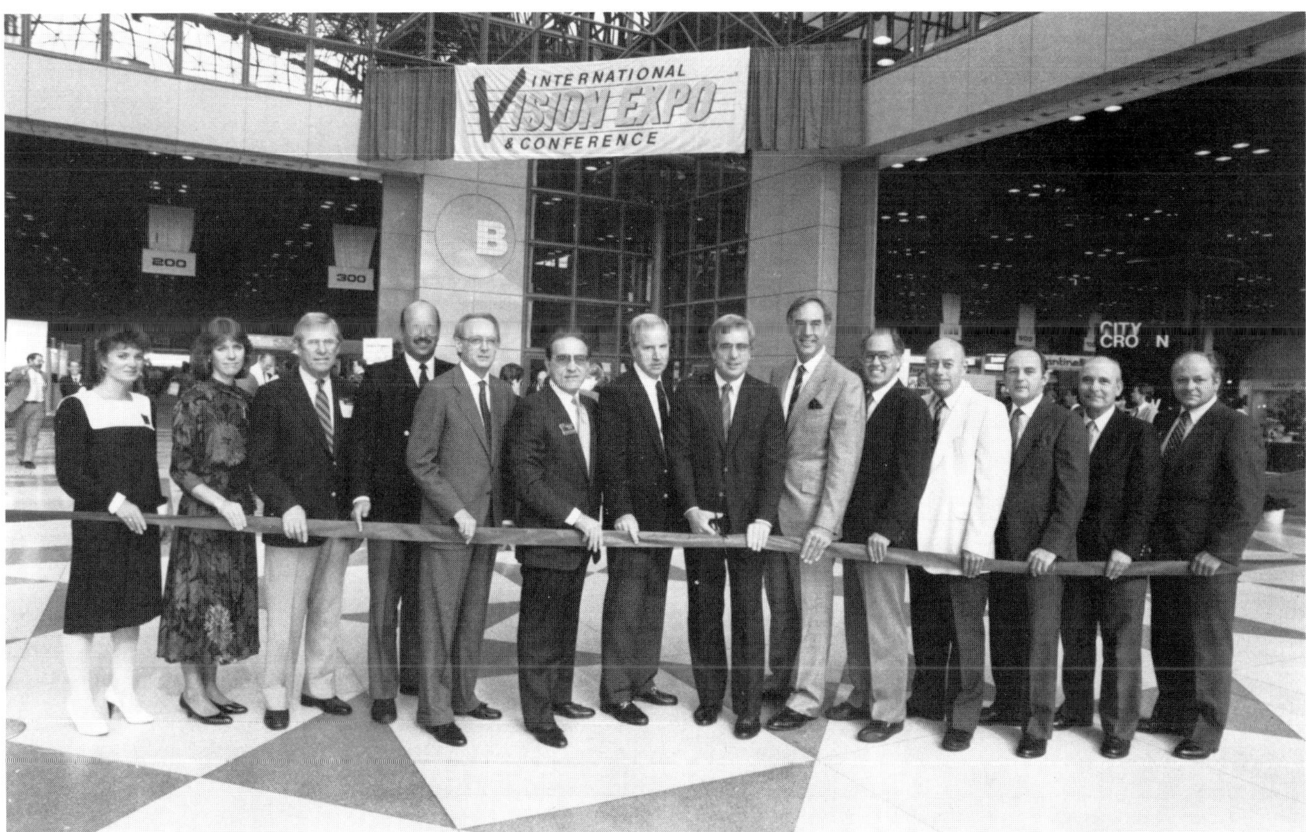

ORDERING EYEGLASSES

Many present-day wholesale lab operators assume that utilization of modern fax machines is the first use technological advancement for faster transmission of lab prescriptions. They remember the introduction of "one hour service" in 1987 and the increased importance of providing faster service for retail customers. They perhaps forget that laboratories during the early part of this century experienced the same pressing need to provide ever faster turnaround service for their customers' prescriptions. Finding faster ways to transmit orders from the refractionist to the lab became increasingly important as the industry grew. The U.S. population was widespread and many small towns were springing up, usually along the routes of expanding railroads. Many traveling spec peddlers put down roots in these small towns. Even though they were far out in the country, they wanted the same rapid prescription service their big city colleagues enjoyed. Not every town was linked by railroad and this left people living in those towns subject to the uncertainty and sometimes lethargic processing of the U.S. mails *(some things never change)*.

Several labs, including Walman Optical in Minnesota, came up with innovative systems that allowed their customers to bypass the mails with rush jobs. These labs devised a special Telegraph Code customers could use for ordering lenses and/or frames. Utilizing this telegraphic code, customers could transmit prescriptions by telegram in an hour or two. Best of all, using a code kept the word count to a minimum *(Telegram cost was based on word count)*. Since there was little brand identity to the frames of that day, the system worked well. The use of clever marketing methods such as this is undoubtedly one of the reasons independent labs like Walman Optical were able to both survive and grow during the past seventy-five years.

Here is an example of a typical laboratory Telegraph order:

"TORIC RIMLESS ABATE CAGE FAN ABET CAD FAT GAY HOW HIP HOME ACME GAME GIVE HAG." (16 WORDS)

Translated this prescription reads:

Toric Rimless Right $+.50 = +.50$ Cyl Axis 90 Left $+1.25 = +.12$ Cyl. Axis 105, 000 eye, 10K gold Riding Bow Cable, 3/4 Basc, 1/8 Above, 1/16 Forward, 6 1/2 inch Temples, 2 1/2 Pupillary Distance, Angle of Crest 45 Degrees. *(Editor's note: a pupillary distance of 2 1/2 was equivalent to a 64mm PD.)*

CONTACT LENSES

Most of the initial work on contact lenses was accomplished in Europe. The original idea developed about 1827 when an English astronomer named Sir John Herschell suggested a device much like a contact lens to

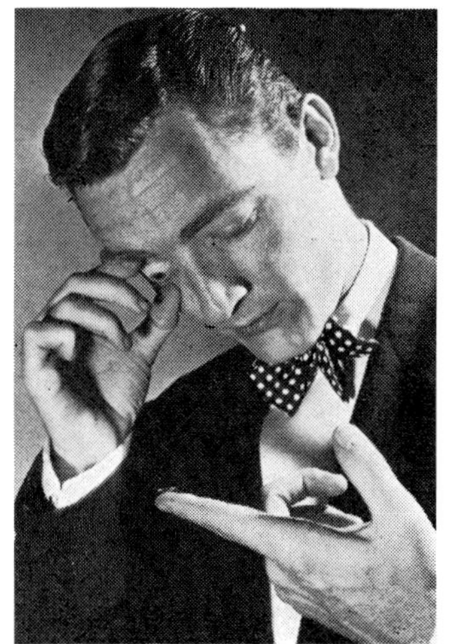

This early photo of the first corneal contact lens appeared in THE OPTOMETRIC WEEKLY in August, 1949. The lens is demonstrated in the photograph by Kevin Tuohy, the man who developed and patented the corneal lens. By the time of this article, 1,300 patients had been fit with this new lens. They were produced by Tuohy's Solex Laboratories in Los Angeles. Solex and Wesley Jessen had conflicting patents and the resulting litigation was ultimately settled by Wesley Jessen buying Solex Laboratories.

protect an eye from a diseased lid. It's not known if he ever made a contact lens. In 1887, the artificial eye-making firm of F.E. Muller in Weisbaden, Germany made a thin blown glass covering to protect the cornea of a patient with a cancerous lid. That patient reportedly wore the lens for years. It wasn't until 1888 that a similar type of glass shell was used to correct vision and subsequently developed into the scleral contact. Zeiss ground the first contact lens for Dr. Salzer to correct malformation of the cornea.

Initially, there were two processes used to make contacts. Muller used blown glass shells while Zeiss made them by grinding glass into the correct curves. From reports, Muller lenses were more comfortable but Zeiss lenses had superior optics. The blown lenses produced by Muller could not be controlled as to size or focal power.

There was a lessening of interest in contact lenses until a German ophthalmologist named Dr. Heine proved their value for correcting sight in 1929. He originated the trial and error system of fitting with a variety of lenses graduated in size. Several years later, the Zeiss Company introduced the first set of trial contact lenses. In 1933, a Hungarian ophthalmologist named J. Dallos developed a way of producing high powers in a contact lens. By 1940, it was estimated that 4,000 people in the United States were wearing scleral contact lenses. In addition to glass scleral lenses, the Obrig lens was developed, made entirely of acrylic plastic. The scleral portion was molded with a ground and polished corneal center.

Between 1963 and 1964, Dr. Otto Wichterle, a polymer chemist with the Czechosovak Academy of Sciences produced a soft compound *(hydroxyethyl-methacrylate or HEMA)* intended for making artificial blood vessels. Eventually his research branched off in a different direction when he produced a spin-casting technique for shaping his material into contact lenses. Meanwhile, Martin M. Pollak, a vice president of New York City's National Patent Development Corporation was in Moscow on business. While there, he heard about a new type of contact lens developed in Czechoslovakia. He met with Dr. Wichterle and arranged to have samples to take to America.

Back home, Pollak needed someone to evaluate these new contact lenses. He approached a well-known contact lens fitter named Dr. Robert Morrison in Harrisburg, Penn. Morrison was intrigued with the possibilities and accompanied Pollak back to Czechoslovakia where they jointly signed an agreement to utilize the Czech technology in the United States. The Czechs were paid $25,000 and were to receive a $1 royalty on every lens sold. On their return to America, Morrison and Pollak had a difference of opinion on how to proceed and National Patent Development agreed to buy back Morrison's rights for $250,000, part now and the rest over a period of time. In addition, Dr. Morrison, who owned a contact lens lab, was to have exclusive marketing rights to the state of Pennsylvania.

Pollak now had the job to convince the country's hard contact lens manufacturers *(mostly small operations)* to use this radically new material. He enlisted the aid of New Yorker Allan Isen, O.D. Typical of the reaction when Pollak and Isen approached the hard lens manufacturers was that of Salvatori of Sarasota, Fla. Pollak and Isen were told that soft lenses would never work. Wesley-Jessen, was the largest contact lens manufacturer in the country. Both Newton Wesley and George Jessen thought the lenses were great but had no interest in marketing them. National Patent Development Corporation had sunk a small fortune in the new material and their investment was rapidly turning into a nightmare. No one had any interest in a soft contact lens.

Then one of NPDC's directors suggested calling on Rochester's Bausch & Lomb. B&L's people, principally vice presidents Jack Harby and Dan Schuman, had the foresight to realize the potential of the new material and on October 6th, 1966, B&L signed a licensing agreement for U.S., Canada, Central and South America and Israel. With B&L's participation assured, NPDC obtained the rights in Western Europe as well. When the agreement with B&L was concluded, Allan Isen went on B&L's payroll. With B&L's product ready for launch,

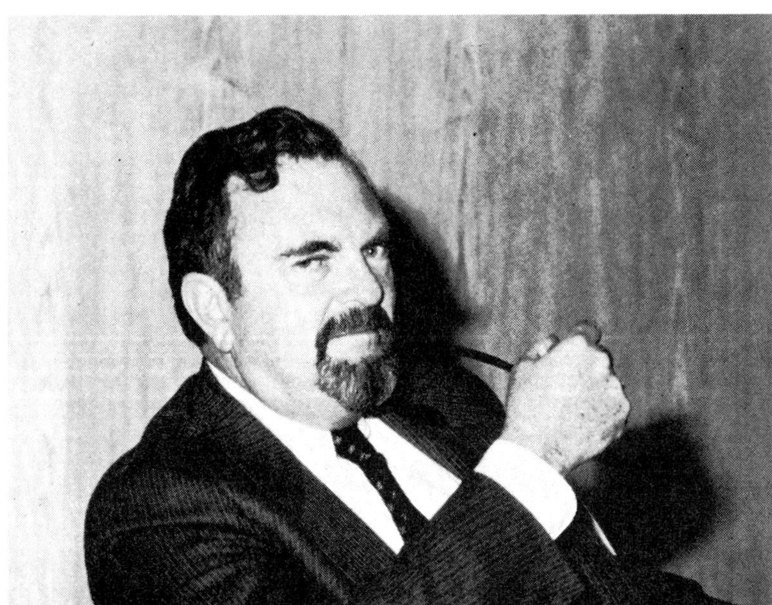

Martin Pollak stumbled across news of a new Czechoslovkian contact lens while on a visit to Moscow. After considerable leg work, his National Patent Development Corporation arranged an agreement to utilize this technology in the United States. This was the lens that ultimately launched Bausch & Lomb into the contact lens field.

B&L asked Pollak to make a cash settlement with Dr. Morrison and the Czech's were asked to change the royalty payment from $1 per lens to 5 percent of sales.

As can be imagined, news of B&L's plan to produce "soft" contacts had a disturbing effect on all the hard lens labs that had turned down the process. Just as B&L was ready to release the product in 1968, the U.S. Food and Drug Administration stepped in and announced that soft lenses were a "drug" that would require FDA clearance. This move on the FDA's part was prompted, it was reported, by the frenzy created by hard lens manufacturers who were cut out of the process. Most of them had written their congressmen and hearings were held before the Senate's Small Business Committee.

This was a whole new can of worms for the optical industry, who had never had to deal with the FDA *(other than tempering glass lenses)* and it took B&L until 1971 to meet the approval of the FDA. This delay undoubtedly pleased the hard lens manufacturers, but with all soft lenses now categorized as a drug, they belatedly realized they had shot themselves in the foot. Now anyone entering the soft lens market had to go through the FDA process and this was prohibitively expensive for small companies. It began to look like the days of small owner-operated contact lens labs was over. The author owned a

contact lens manufacturing company during those years and remembers well the bleak outlook for hard contact lenses. In fact, this led to selling his company and leaving the contact lens field.

In time, NPDC and B&L became snarled in litigation over patent payments. This terminated in 1979 with a $14 million settlement in NPDC's favor. NPDC later introduced their own soft contact lens product.

The Contact Lens Manufacturers Association and others were later able to develop gas permeable materials for use in hard contact lenses, giving a whole new lease on life to hard contact lens manufacturers, many of whom are very successful today, showing the value of not giving up too easily . A number of OLA laboratories are heavily involved in the manufacture and distribution of contact lenses, in addition to eyeglasses.

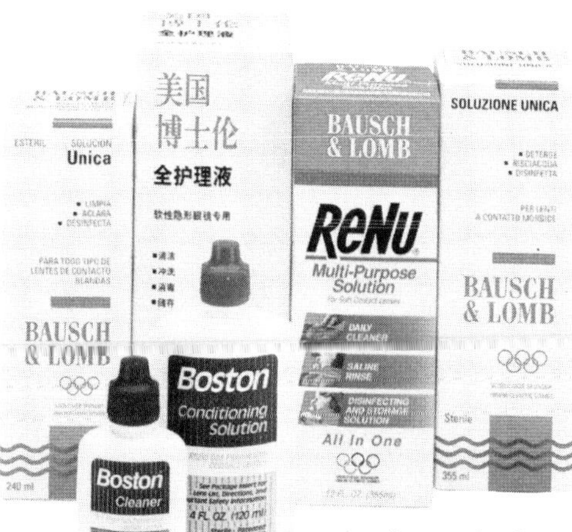

Bausch & Lomb's first contact lens product was released in 1971 and this division grew rapidly. By 1993, B&L had worldwide sales of almost $200 million dollars in their ReNu contact lens solution line alone.

ILLUSTRATION – BAUSCH & LOMB

LINCOLN'S GLASSES

Abraham Lincoln's first pair of glasses were purchased in Bloomington, Ill. Lincoln was in town to take part in a convention to organize a new political party to oppose extending slavery. After dinner that evening (May 28, 1856), Lincoln and a young lawyer named Henry Clay Whitney decided to walk down to the train depot to see who might be coming in from Chicago. On the way, they passed a very small jewelry shop. Lincoln told his friend he wanted to stop in and find a pair of spectacles, remarking that he was 47 years old and "kinder needed them". He tried on a variety of "specs" until he found one he liked that cost him 37 1/2 cents.

Two years later, during the first of the famous debates between Lincoln and Douglas, Lincoln referred to his need for glasses. Douglas had spoken and Lincoln rose to reply. He read a long excerpt from a speech he made in Peoria and evidently had trouble reading the words. "Put on your specs," a man in the crowd shouted. "Yes sir, I am obliged to do so. I am no longer a young man," Lincoln responded.

Later, when he was President, he strode into the optical establishment of Franklin and Company at 244 Pennsylvania Avenue in Washington where he selected and purchased a pair of steel-rimmed spectacles for $2.50, considered a pretty fair price at that time. The owner, Isaac Heilprin, never cashed the check and it still hangs on the wall of the store. It is believed to be Lincoln's only existing uncanceled check. The Riggs National Bank tried to round up Lincoln's checks for "Tad" Lincoln, the president's son, and could only find 14 checks, all canceled.

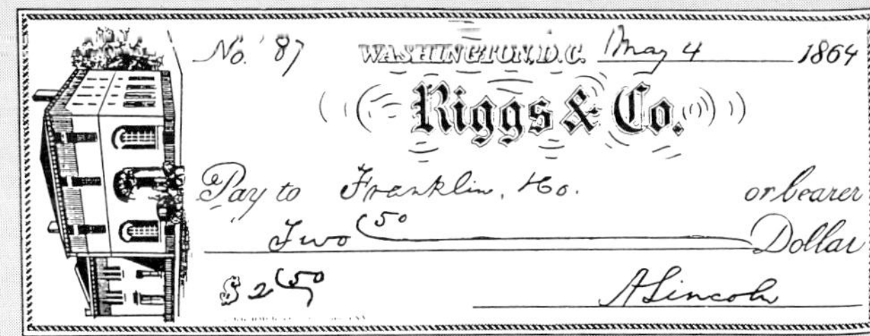

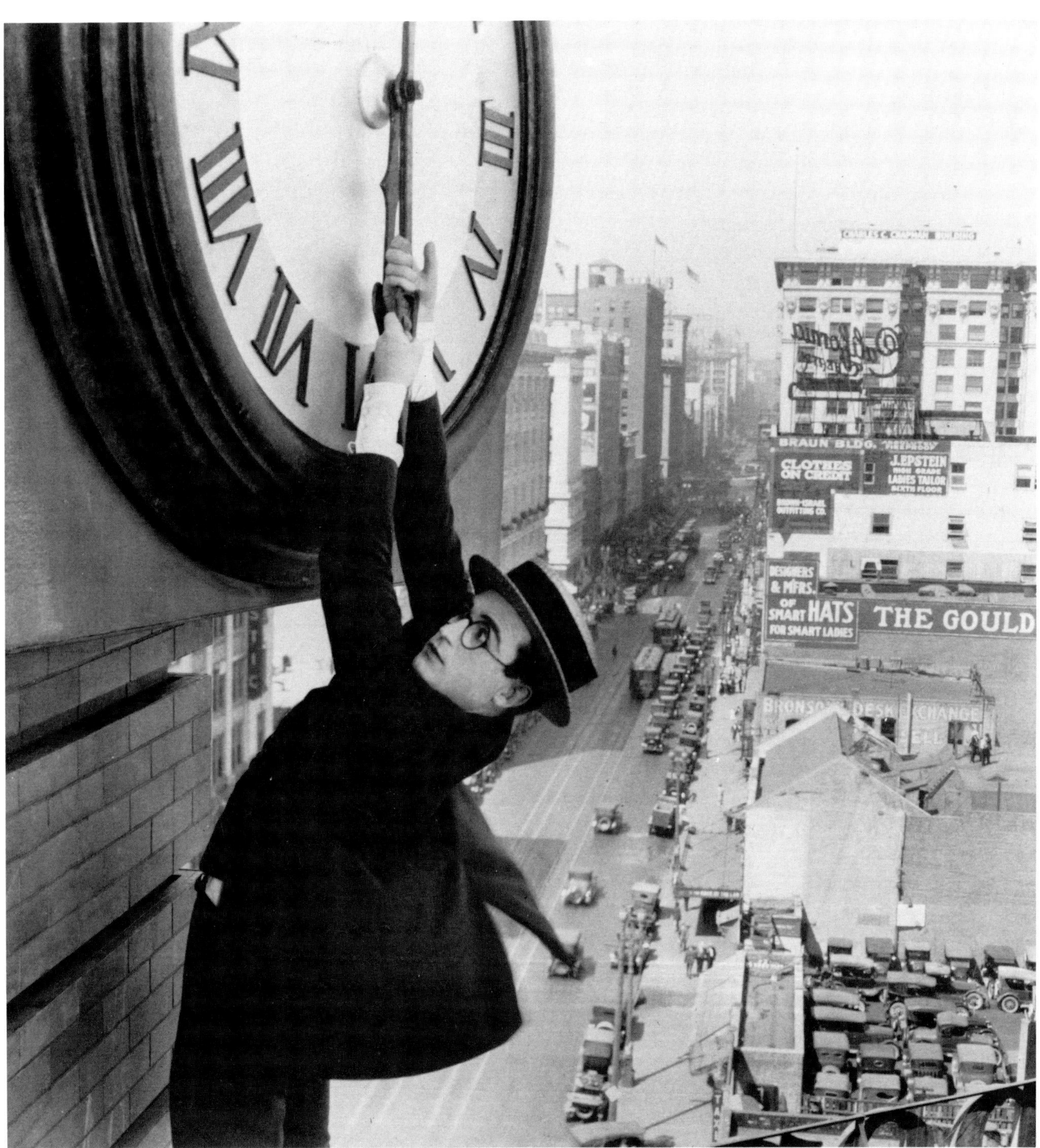

Harold Lloyd was one of the biggest stars in Hollywood during the 1920s. He always played the part of a well-meaning, somewhat nerd-like young man but always managed to get the heroine in the end. He was never seen on the screen without his trademark shell frames, starting a craze that swept the country. Before long, almost every frame manufacturer had added shell frames to their line. The frames Lloyd wore on screen were produced by Optical Products Corporation, a prominent frame producer that no longer exists.

Chapter 18
Pioneer OLA Members

Many members of the Optical Laboratories Association have been in existence for 2 or more generations. This chapter contains thumbnail sketches of a few of these companies. Readers will find common threads linking many of the individuals listed here with earlier wholesale laboratories that no longer exist but are reviewed in Chapter Five. It serves as a graphic illustration of how closely intertwined the ophthalmic community has become. Most of the companies reviewed here are laboratories but several represent OLA stock house members who wholesale frames, lenses and other optical products.

ADVANCE OPTICAL (1922)

Founded in 1922 by Louis Gwirtzman, Advance Optical started as a supply house operating out of a back bedroom. Two years later, Lou's brother Sam joined the company selling frames and stock lenses. Sensing opportunity, sometime during the 1930s, a laboratory was added and a branch laboratory was opened in Buffalo.

During the 1940s, Louis commuted from Rochester and managed the Buffalo branch while Sam ran Rochester. Greyhound Express was the link between the two branches. The brothers worked seven days a week and established a reputation for quality work. Following service in the war, Louis' son-in-law Mort Erenstone became a company sales representative, filling the position for the next 35 years. It was truly a family operation. Morley Gwirtzman *(Sam's son)*, the present head of the company, had worked as errand boy, in the mail room and at a variety of other jobs from the time he was eight. Morley, with no interest in the optical business, graduating from the University of Michigan in Business Administration and immediately left for New York to work in the advertising field. A year later his father called with news that Louis was going in the hospital, asking him to come home to Rochester to help out while Lou was recuperating, promising it would just be for the summer. That was 1961 and Morley never returned to New York City.

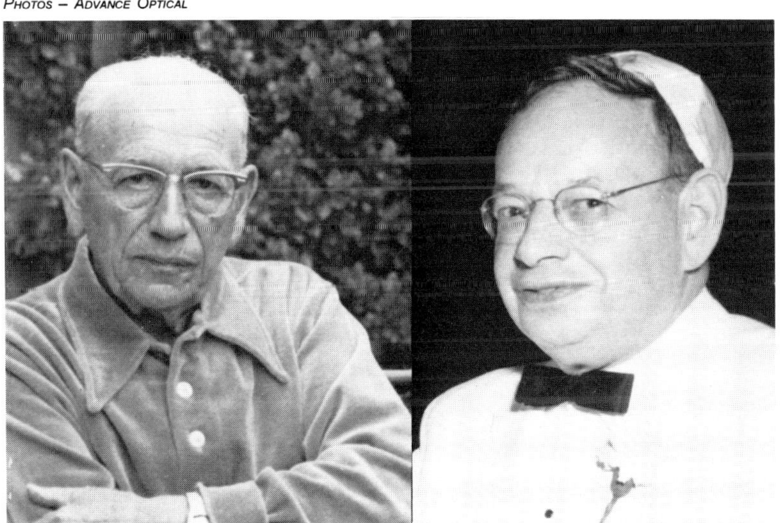

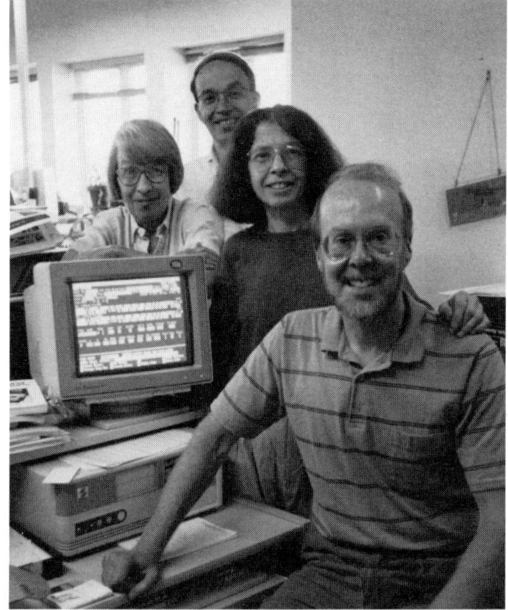

The current management at Advance. Left to right are Honi Lang, Morley Gwirtzman, Ann Kolko, Arthur Kolko.

The family had a tradition of spending Sunday at the office. Morley and his sister would fold mailing boxes or do whatever else was needed while their mother and father opened mail and lined up jobs for Monday. Following that, Sam took them all out to dinner. The company continued selling frames and lenses along with laboratory service and frames continue as an important part of the company's business in the '90s.

During the '40s and '50s, when Kryptoks were the most-used bifocal, Advance maintained a large inventory of blanks. Morley remembers his Dad saying, "One thing you can be sure of, Morley. Kryptoks will never go out of style!"

The Buffalo office was sold to a branch employee named Frank Woodward in the '60s. It became the present Franwall Optical. Shortly after, Louis retired. Late in the 1960s, Sam became ill and Morley took over direction of the company and Morley's sister Ann joined the company.

The company has always been deeply involved in frame sales and Morley remembers the impact of the Cambridge frame. For at least six months, sales were so heavy, factory back orders were a common event. Advance determined not to run out and during the peak years of Cambridge sales, the company kept a year's inventory of that frame on hand. Their first designer line was Sophia Loren and Advance did more business with Zyloware in the month after it came out than they had in years previously. With Art Craft as a neighbor in Rochester, Advance has distributed Art Craft products for years. Art Craft is celebrating their 75th anniversary as Advance celebrates their 72nd year.

Ann's husband, Arthur Kolko, joined the company in the '70s. With a computer background, Arthur had the job of expanding the lab and bringing them into the computer age. The company had occupied four different locations through the years in downtown Rochester. In 1982, the main Rochester post office moved out of the downtown area and Advance Optical followed and built a new facility a mile from the new post office. Morley and Ann's sister Honi Lang also joined the family business. Morley, Ann and Honi each have children who worked at the company as they grew up. None has shown any sign of wanting an optical career but Morley keeps remembering that 33 years ago, he also had no interest in optical.

Today, Advance's lab is completely modernized and still carries a wide range of frames and accessories. They are open 12 hours a day and on Saturdays during the winter months, continuing the tradition of quality and service backed by the family's philosophy. The only difference today is the family no longer spends Sunday's at the office.

BALESTER OPTICAL (1934)

A three-generation family business, Balester Optical was started by Fred Balester, Sr. in 1934 in the basement of his home. Despite cramped quarters, the company did $1,700 business the first year *(considered good in that depression year)*. Balester was no novice to the optical field, having started doing odd jobs and delivery work for an optical retailer in Scranton in 1913 *(he was 13 years old)*. Balester had six people working in that basement before a 1936 flood forced a move to larger quarters. The company continued to grow.

Fred, Jr. *(Fritz)* started running errands in the summer he was 13. Fritz left college to join the Marines in World War II. With the war over, Fritz returned and called his father the Thursday evening he hit town,. His father said, "Great! We'll see you at work in the morning". Fritz talked him into waiting until Monday. Balester Optical now consisted of Fred, Sr., Fritz and his brother Jim. The three formed a partnership and moved into their own downtown building in 1952. An OPTICAL INDEX story

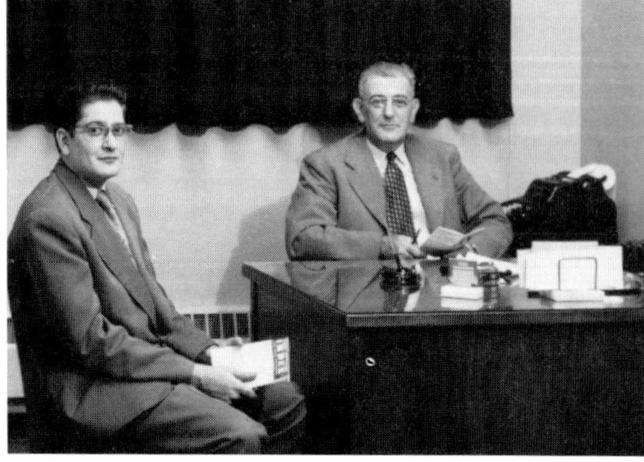

In this 1952 photo, Jim Balester, left, is seen with his father Fred Senior, founder of Balester Optical.

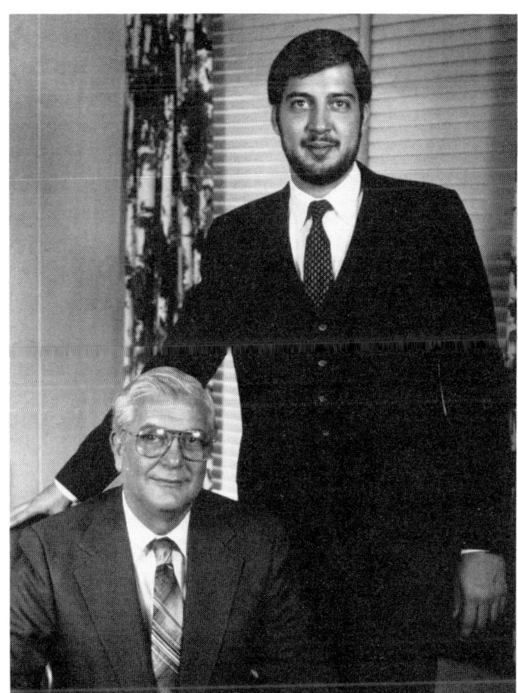

Fred Balester, Jr. (Fritz) with his son Jonathan. Jonathan Balester is currently head of Balester Optical.

claimed this was the first building ever designed specifically for a wholesale lab. The building was later expanded and ultimately sold to the Wilkes-Barre Chamber of Commerce. Balester's had 50 employees at the time they moved in their new building in 1962.

In early 1972, Itek Corporation expressed an interest in buying the company. Fred, Sr. was ready to retire and, to Fritz, this seemed like a good way to insure his father's retirement. Fritz sold the company, expecting to stay with Itek. Alex Torda was his new boss and they had a great deal of respect for one another. However, Torda later left Itek and was replaced by Rudy Alversano. Balester grew disenchanted watching Itek run their laboratories like a factory. He made the mistake of telling Itek headquarters what they were doing wrong and was promptly fired. The laboratory division became a disaster for Itek and eventually Itek approached Fritz to buy back his old company. He refused and Itek countered by saying they would make an offer he couldn't refuse. They did and he purchased Balester Optical in 1979. When Balester returned to take over the company, it was to find a lab that had been doing 1,000 jobs a day when he sold it now doing 300 jobs a day. Today, Balester Optical is the only Itek laboratory that survived into the '90s. All the rest are gone.

Fritz's son Jonathan had started working for a Bausch & Lomb branch in Mansfield, Ohio. B&L sent him to run their Rochester branch when he was 20 years old, making him the youngest-ever B&L lab manager. He left

B&L and was running Waldert Opticians' lab *(Main Optical)* in Rochester when he decided in 1980 to join his father's company.

Since then, the company has grown considerably and the building expanded for the second time, adding another 5,000 sq. feet. Today the company covers a multi-state area around Pennsylvania. The company is very active in frame distribution. Frames are sold by Balester Optical but the company also has a frame outlet called Arcane Optical. Arcane provides less service than Balester and can sell frames at lower prices to meet competitive pressures. The company has never kept their connection with Arcane a secret and the name, in fact, became an in-house joke *(Webster defines "Arcane" as "understood by only a few")*.

Jonathan is now the active head of the company *("hyperactive head", his father claims)*. Fritz has retired to Florida but is often found at Balester. He also consults, working from time to time with other laboratories and manufacturers. Jonathan's sister Heather is vice president and his brother Matthew is in the optical business in the Harrisburg area. Another brother Marc works as a dispensing optician in Austin, Texas. Sister Valerie has a Ph.D. in English rhetoric and teaches at Texas A&M in College Station, Texas. Valerie worked her way through Penn State as an optometric assistant, giving good indication that this truly is an optical family.

BARNETT & RAMEL (1920)

Joe F. Ramel, sole owner at the time of a successful 20 year old independent laboratory organization, sat down to write the history of the Kansas City optical business, as he remembered it. The following material is excerpted from his account, written in 1941.

> *"After working on a farm and then shoveling coal for a coal company, I started in the optical business in 1909, my first job was errand boy for Columbian Optical at $4.00 per week. The company is now Riggs Optical. William Riggs was President and I knew him for some 25 years. I was hired by the Office Manager E.W. Cox who is now the Kansas City Zone Manager for AO.*
>
> *We had no cash register and I never saw any money come in over the counter so it was always a mystery to me just where the money came from that paid us fellows. Nevertheless, we always got our money. That, of course, is where I*

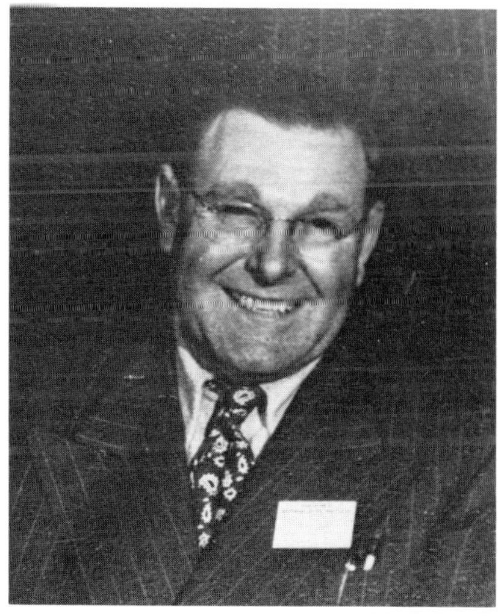

Joe Ramel, founder of Barnett & Ramel. Joe's first job was as messenger for Columbian Optical for four dollars a week.

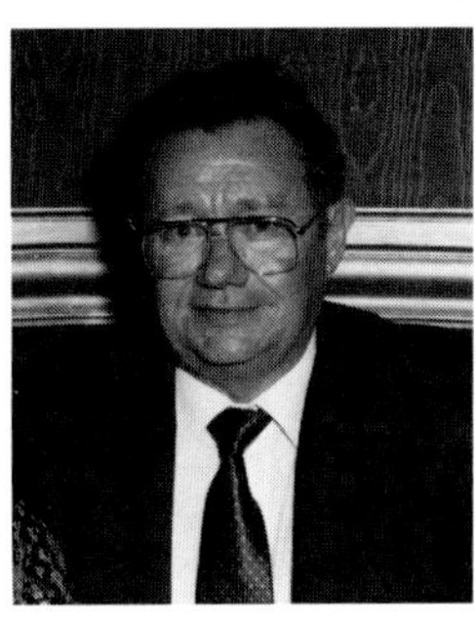

Keith Besch, pictured here, left Rite-Style Optical to buy the Barnett & Ramel Omaha branch in 1957. George Lee told him he'd never make it go and promised to keep his old job open for six months.

learned about credit buying and how things were sold on credit and paid for (at least most of it) through the mail by check.

During this period, Dr. E.A. Lane operated the E.A. Lane School of Optometry in Kansas City with his wife who was also an optometrist. He has since passed away but Mrs. Lane, O.D., is still giving postgraduate courses to M.D.'s in refraction. This school was one of the foremost schools in the country and thousands of students still hold a certificate from it and practice by virtue of its sheepskin. I did not attend their school, but I spent many pleasant hours in the school laboratory, located at 11th and Grand from 1909 until 1920 when they moved to another location.

At this time, the Stead Lens Company was operating a bifocal plant at 7th and Wyandotte. Harold Stead, now of Shuron, was manufacturing Kryptok bifocals and did until 1916 when he decided to close up shop due to patents, law suits and things of that nature. He had one of the most beautiful grinding plants in Kansas City.

In 1909, there were only two wholesale labs in Kansas City, Columbian Optical and Merry Optical. In 1911, O.H. Gerry, Mr. Crosby and Mr. Miller opened up the 3rd lab, Gerry, Crosby & Miller Optical. I went to work for them in 1911 when Mr. Gerry became the sole owner of the company. About 1913, Mr. Murphy, now owner of the O.H. Gerry Optical Company came to work for them as an errand boy.

I left to work for the Merry Optical Company in Des Moines in 1913. In 1915, I helped open up the Gate City Optical in Kansas City with Mr. Fred

Hildebrand, the head of the company."

Working several other jobs and after 11 years of learning the business, Ramel was ready to go into business for himself. He joined forces with F.T. Rupert and W.A. Barnett and opened a lab in Kansas City, Kansas in 1920. The company was called Rupert-Barnett & Ramel Optical Company.

Ramel Continues His Story:

"Our first job happened to be a re-cement job for old "Daddy" Dr. Smith, an M.D. We secured 35 cents cash for this, the first job the Rupert-Barnett Optical Company had ever collected. I picked up the job, re-cemented it, delivered it and collected the money.

In 1920, a yellow dog optical company by the name of Alcoe Optical opened up. They didn't last long but raised plenty of cain in this particular territory with all their cut prices. It was always suspected that this was an undercover yellow dog place operated by people who did not want their names known.

About 1921 or 1922 the Lancaster Optical Company opened in K.C. Then Specialty Optical Company opened a couple more places, one called the Precision Optical Company and one called the Missouri Optical Company. In April, 1934, Ray Optical was opened by C.E. Ray. Caldwell Optical was opened by C.G. Caldwell in 1937 and the Wyandotte Optical opened by W.F. Hunkeler in 1937. These were followed by Star Optical opened in 1939 by Bernard Fenton and Sutherlin Optical Company opened October 18th, 1939 by Ed Sutherlin who was formerly with the

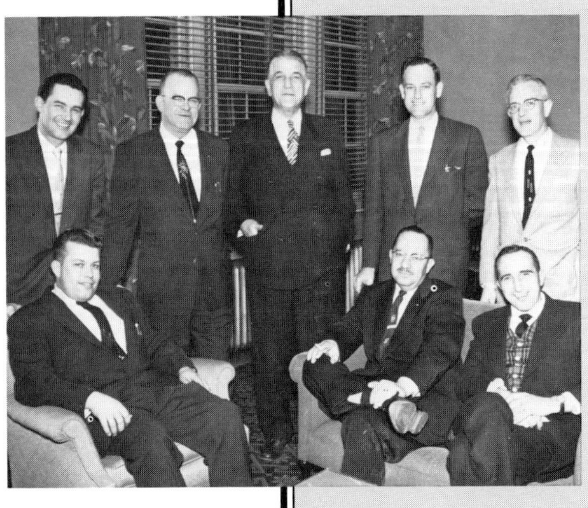

SHURON SALES TRAINING

When Roy Marks joined Shuron Optical, he wanted to capitalize on Shuron's reputation as "the independent's manufacturer". He had a sales trainer hired to go around the country conducting training sessions for laboratory sales people in an effort to help independent lab reps be more effective in competing with AO and B&L's sales people. This photo was taken during one of those Shuron Sales Training meetings held in Kansas City in the mid-1950s. Left to right, standing, Jim Young *(Shuron Sales Trainer)*, Ed. H. Sutherlin *(Sutherlin Optical)*, Chuck Biel *(Shuron Regional Manager)*, Jack Jones *(Shuron Salesman, now with Duffens, Houston)*, Charles Huddleston *(G&H Optical)*. Sitting: Ed. L. Sutherlin *(Sutherlin Optical)*, Ed P. Langley *(Langley Optical)*, Nate Roberts *(Morgan Optical)*.

Lancaster Optical Company.

Along about this time the Owl Lens Company was opened by several shop men who had worked around Kansas City and two other shop men from Merry Optical started the Olsmore Optical Company."

Growing rapidly, Rupert-Barnett & Ramel had to expand in 1924. The city of Memphis was chosen and people were hired to run the new branch. This turned out to be a disaster and Joe Ramel went to Memphis to salvage the branch. Eventually, in 1926, that branch was sold and Ramel returned to Kansas City full of knowledge gained from bitter experience. Sensing greater room for expansion across the river, the company moved to Kansas City, Mo.

That's when the price war Ramel referred to began. The competitive situation made everyone nervous and Rupert decided he wanted out. Barnett and Ramel were "suckers" enough to take a chance and, in 1928, the company became Barnett & Ramel. A branch was opened in Joplin the following year. The partners believed their success was due to their lab system including at least 20 more features than other labs. They coined a new slogan, "20 POINT PRESCRIPTION SERVICE". They added new features to the original 20 points, but the slogan became the banner of the company's success. "Your Friendly Company" was used in place of the customary "Yours very truly" on all company correspondence.

When the depression came, instead of laying off people, they opened a branch in Des Moines. Since they had machinery and men to spare, the investment was minimal. Friends thought opening a branch in the heart of the depression *(1933)* was suicide. The following year they added branches in Omaha and Waterloo. Branches were opened in Oklahoma City, Wichita and, 17 years after they started there, one opened in the "old stomping grounds", Kansas City, Kan. A ninth branch was added in Little Rock in 1941. On May 1 of that same year, just over 21 years after the company's founding, Ramel purchased all the remaining stock and Barnett retired because of ill health.

World War II

George Lee went to work for Barnett & Ramel in January, 1940, joining others already there such as Nate Roberts, Art Appleyard, Ed Ross, Joe Wylie, Cliff Chamberlin, Ed Langley, Earl McClelland, Lyle Schrouf and Harold Thompson. George describes those early years.
"December 7th, 1941 changed everything. The war was on and some of the names mentioned volunteered and others were drafted. By 1943, Barnett & Ramel's Kansas City lab was so busy, mail bags full of incoming orders would sit for a week before they could be opened. With many of our experienced lab people in the service, the sales people were all pulled off the road and were either in the service or put to work in the lab.
The end of the war changed a lot of things. All jobs had been frozen by wartime regulations. With the lifting of the freeze and veterans returning from the service, a lot of people moved around. Nate Roberts left B&R to go with Morgan Optical. Art Appleyard left to join Sutherlin Optical. Joe Wylie opened retail stores. Cliff Chamberlin opened up a wholesale lab in Oklahoma City. Ed Langley opened Langley Optical in K.C., Earl McClelland ran the B&R lab in Joplin. A short time later Lyle Schrouf and Harry Palmer opened a lab in Joplin. Harold Thompson became general manager for B&R in Kansas City. I was made branch manager in Omaha in June, 1946. Two years later, Harold Thompson and I left to start Rite-Style Optical Company in Omaha. Then, over a period of time, the various Barnett & Ramel branches were sold to their managers or closed down."

George Lee remembers one reason he took that first job with B&R in 1940 was that he was told he'd never be without a job in the optical business. Having just come through the depression with some real family financial problems, that was all it took to convince him. He said a real "high" during his B&R days was the year *(1943)* when Joe Ramel, who had started his career working for $4 a week, finally hit the $1 million mark. It was a real triumph.

For at least 50 years the name Barnett & Ramel showed up on résumés of midwest lab people. George Lee explained, *"I remember Joe Ramel telling me I might not make as much money as I would like but I would learn a lot. I will always remember Barnett & Ramel as a great company that created opportunity for many. Some people call it luck, some people call it hard work. Thanks, Barnett and Ramel. You taught many people well!"*

One of the people working for George Lee's lab in Omaha was Keith P. Besch. In 1957, the Barnett & Ramel branch in Omaha came up for sale. Keith and two others decided to take the plunge. Keith went out to George Lee's home to give him personal notice of their plans. George told Keith he wasn't going to make it but his position at Rite-Style would be kept open for him for six months. For years after that, every time Keith saw George he asked if the job was still open and was always told it was.

Eventually Keith bought out his partners. When his son Frank was in his early teens, he spent his summers working in the mail room and coming down on Sundays to help his dad open the mail. Today, Frank is President and CEO and carries on the traditions of this family lab.

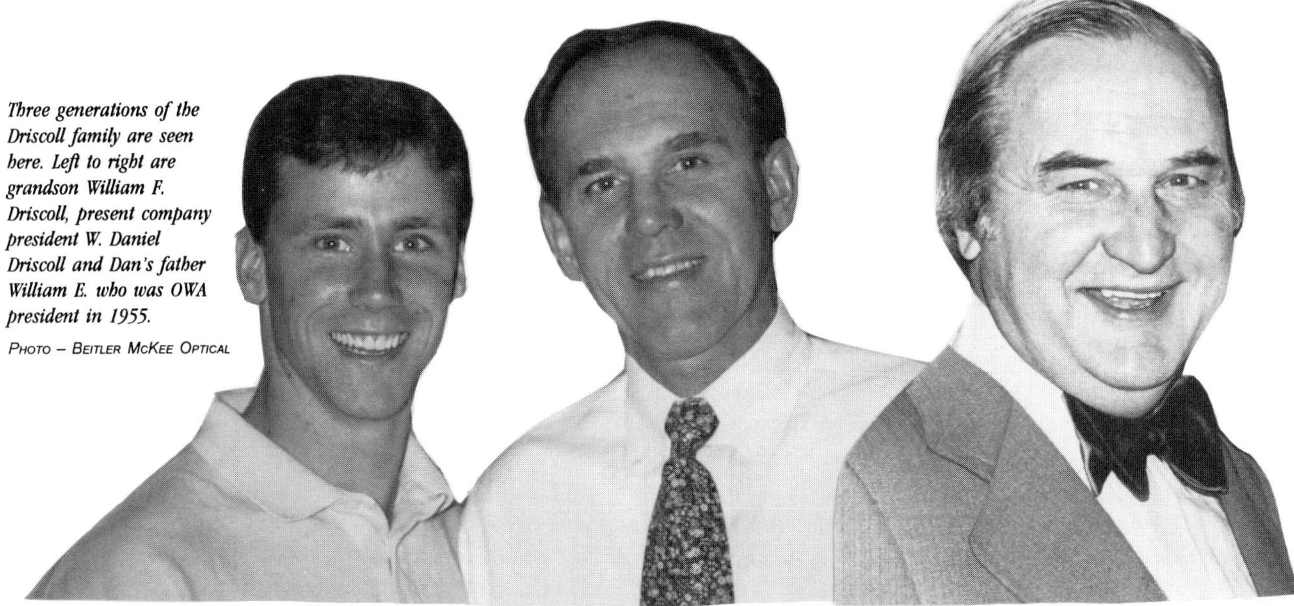

BAUER OPTICAL EXPORT CORPORATION (1939)

Bauer is a stock house member of the OLA and does not operate a laboratory. The company was established in 1939 by Henry H. and Gertrude Bauer. Henry's brother, at that time, worked for a firm in Brazil named Adaga. They were looking for someone in this country to purchase U.S. optical products for their company and Henry was recommended. Handling Adaga's requirements led the Bauers to set up a company to perform similar tasks for other companies. During the war years, Henry went into the service and the company was run by Gertrude Bauer. The war greatly curtailed their activities but the South American market was growing stronger and the company was able to survive until Henry returned. With international trade expanding after the war, Bauer began to handle export sales for a number of major American optical manufacturers.

Today, the company still handles export sales to countries all over the world but they also represent the English firm Pilkington and import their Rapid X photochromic glass and NX-15 glass *(similar to G-15)*.

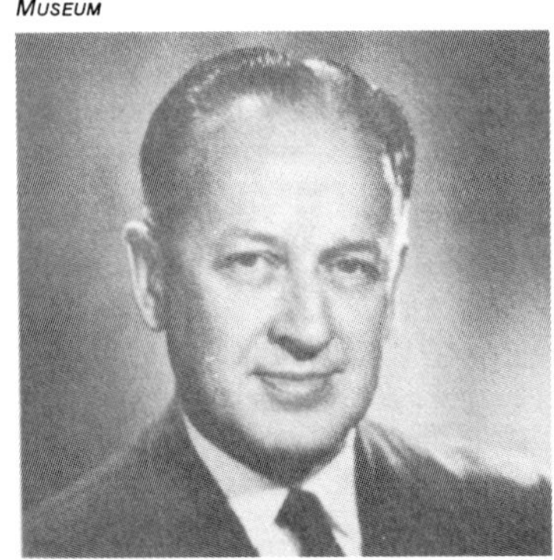

These products are distributed through a number of American laboratories. When Henry fell ill in 1978, the company was sold to Edward J. Klotz who had previously been with Corning Glass and United Lens Company.

Since the company deals with both laboratories and optical manufacturers, their OLA membership is important and the annual OLA conventions give them an opportunity to see all their vendors and customers at one time in one location.

BEITLER MCKEE OPTICAL (1922)

William Beitler and Charles McKee incorporated to form an optical laboratory in 1922 but how they became involved in the optical business is unknown. In 1945, William E. Driscoll, Earl Keller, Stanley Wolfe and Elias S. Wildermuth left White Haines Optical and moved to Pittsburgh to buy Beitler McKee. Wildermuth was the money man and the other three handled sales. Wildermuth died in 1965 and, by that time, Keller and Wolfe had sold their interest, leaving the company in the control of Bill Driscoll. Driscoll got his start handling maintenance at White Haines in Columbus, Ohio when he was 17 years old. Graduating from high school, he progressed from janitorial to stock room to mail room to sales.

Bill Driscoll's son Dan graduated from college in 1963, went in the army for two years and joined his father in 1965. He had worked summers and vacations for his father's company as he grew up. During these years, the company continued to grow and branch offices were opened. In recent years, however, as overnight shipping and fax transmissions developed, the branches were closed, one by one, and the company today is a one-location operation. Bill Driscoll actively ran the company until his death in 1978, when Dan took over the company.

Dan's brother Dave handles sales for the company and a third generation of Driscolls has joined the company. Dan's son Bill and daughter Dana both work for Beitler McKee. Dana runs the company's quality control and Bill Driscoll is in a 10 year training program to take over management of the company from his father. The Driscolls are proud of the fact Beitler McKee is a

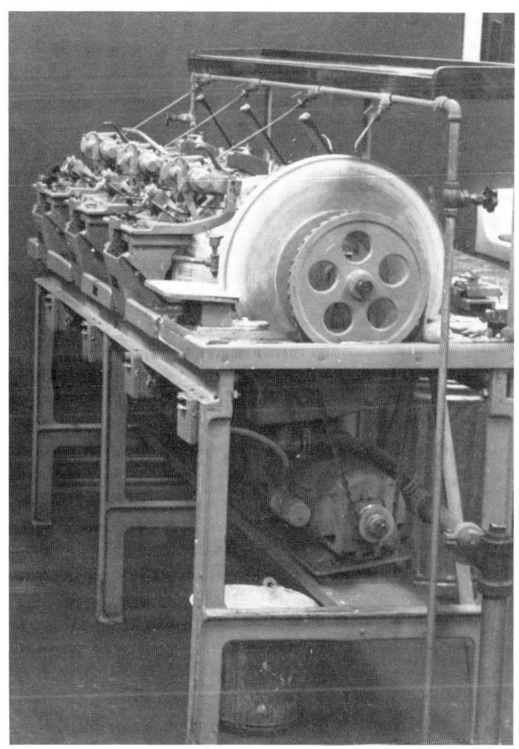

This was part of Bell Optical's edging department in the 1940s. All lenses were edged on these heavy-duty Shuron edgers and then beveled by hand to fit the frames.

Christian company. Simply stated, this means they operate their company on the same Christian principles during the week as they would on Sunday. They view running a business much like a ministry. Their mission statement states, "To help people see a clear vision of God". During the past five years Driscoll has established 12 quality control teams among the company's employees with very positive results.

Dan Driscoll's father Bill served as president of the OWNA in 1955-56 and the company has been a member of the association ever since. Beitler McKee presently maintains a market area extending for a 200 mile radius

of Pittsburgh. The company was a long time member of the "Dirty Dozen" laboratory group.

BELL OPTICAL LAB, INC. (1941)

Bell Optical started as a small two man operation in downtown Dayton, run by Eugene Bell and his wife.

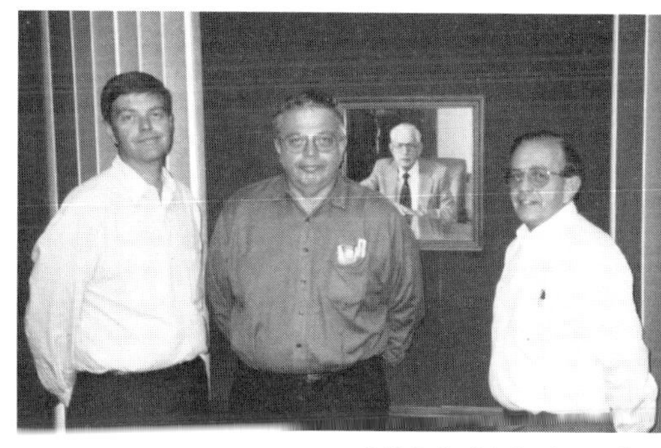

Bell Optical today is run by the second generation Zobrist family, left to right, Doug Zobrist, Hank Zobrist and Tom Zobrist. They are standing in front of a photograph of their father, Joseph Zobrist.

Joseph Zobrist purchased the company from Bell in 1941. Zobrist had spent 15 years with Midwest Optical in Dayton, ending as manager until he left to go into business for himself. Joe Zobrist was conservative by nature and that's the way he built his company, slowly and steadily. The company grew until 1972 when they moved out of downtown Dayton to a 12,000 foot facility in an outlying area. Continued growth made it necessary to add 6,000 feet in 1977 and another 10,000 feet to the building in 1982. Joe's sons Hank and Tom joined their father in the early '60s and a third son Doug came in a little later.

The company began investigating plastic lenses in the early '70s and it was the need for additional room for plastic equipment, as well as the need for a cleaner environment that prompted their move to a new building. Once they were in the new location, plastic processing started in earnest and the company was one of the first in their area to offer these new lightweight lenses. Frames were also added to the services they offered their accounts.

The first Bell branches were in Huntington and Vienna, West Virginia. Both towns had been served by local White Haines branches but as that company began closing down branches, Bell stepped in and hired the people and opened a branch in each town, filling the vacuum left by White Haines. Another branch opened in

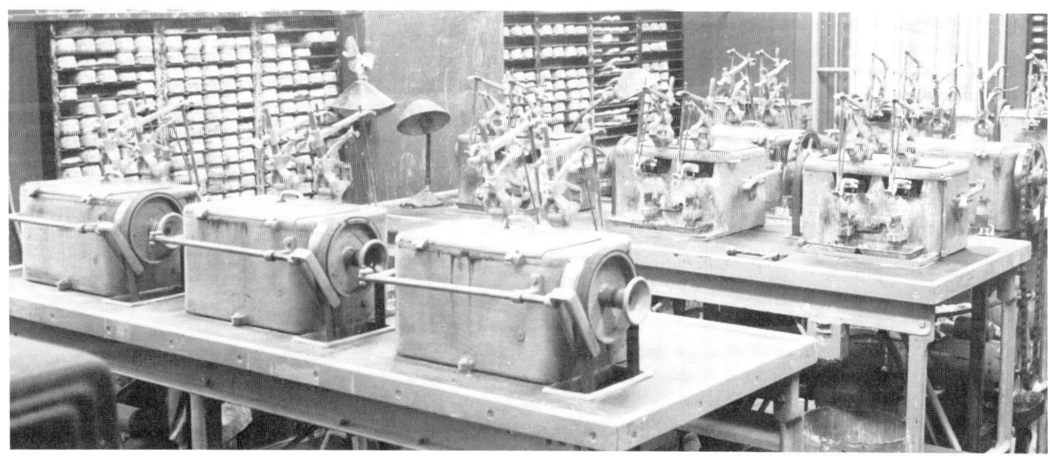

This scene from Bell's cylinder department during the '40s shows the famous Shuron TorCyl cylinder machine referred to many times in this history.

Sandusky, Ohio, but later was moved to Twinsburg, a considerably larger market. In 1989, Bell purchased B&J's lab in Indianapolis and made it a Bell branch. The Indianapolis branch was moved into a brand new facility in August, 1994.

From the sixties on, Joe's sons gradually took over active management of the company until 1988, at age 78, the senior Zobrist retired. The company is presently run by Hank, Tom and Doug. A third Zobrist generation is coming on strong. Tom has two sons, Michael and Steven, both of whom work for Bell and Hank's three sons, Chris, Greg and David are also active in the company. Doug's son, Brian, is still in college but has already had some involvement with Bell's sales department. The company recently brought in David King to serve as sales manager.

In 1987 Bell became involved with Anti Reflective coating, becoming one of the first labs involved in Coburn's Starcote process. AR is a growing segment of Bell's business and the company expects this market to continue expanding. Contrary to the direction taken by some wholesale laboratories, Bell Optical believes frames should be an integral part of products provided by a wholesale laboratory. They presently carry most of the leading frame lines. Their growth continues in a positive direction, due at least in part because of their lab supervisory personnel which includes Chris Wagner in Dayton, Brian Belinger in Indianapolis, Steve Daniels in Twinsburg, Randy Moore in Huntington and Marion West in Vienna.

CENTREX, INC. (1938)

Centrex is a different type of OLA member. Neither a laboratory nor a stock house, Centrex has carved out an exclusive niche as a specialist in ophthalmic international distribution. The company was established in 1938 by Charles K. Austin with a personal goal to become the best independent ophthalmic supplier in the world. During the second World War, Austin established a string of agents throughout Latin America and this became the company's foundation. Following Charles' death in 1947, his wife Susanne Austin ran the company, traveling extensively as she established overseas branches. She also launched a domestic division to serve the American market.

Following Susanne's death in 1982, an Austin cousin, Kenneth Cort, took over the company. He was able to position Centrex to capitalize on business opportunities in Europe, Asia and Africa, making Centrex truly an international corporation.

Thomas Austin Brill, son of the founder, became president and CEO in 1992. Under his leadership, the company continues to grow and gain wider recognition in the ophthalmic community. Today the Centrex organization is recognized and accepted in more than 100 countries. They still strive to fulfill that original goal of the founder - to be the best independent ophthalmic supplier in the world.

H.J. BIRCH OPTICAL COMPANY, INC. (1938)

H.J. Birch Optical was founded by Henry J. Birch. Born in 1901, he started his career in 1917 as a surface man with Uhlemann Optical in Chicago. In 1920, he went to work for Burgess Optical, working for 17 years in the finish department and as a dispenser. While serving in a managerial role with Burgess, he had hired and trained a young man named George Jessen who would later start Wesley Jessen Contact Lens Company with Newton K. Wesley. In 1937, Birch opened a branch office for Burgess on Ashland Avenue in Chicago.

In 1938, Henry took the plunge and opened Birch Optical on the same floor in the same Ashland Avenue building as Burgess. In 1946, Henry's son Dennis returned from the U.S. Navy and joined his dad. Needing more room, they moved a few doors down the street. In 1950, they added a surface room and joined the Optical Wholesalers Association *(at one time, Chicago had 24 wholesale labs in the association)*. Henry served as president of the Illinois Wholesalers group for 6 years and Dennis also was president for 6 years. Henry and Dennis believed that certification and education were

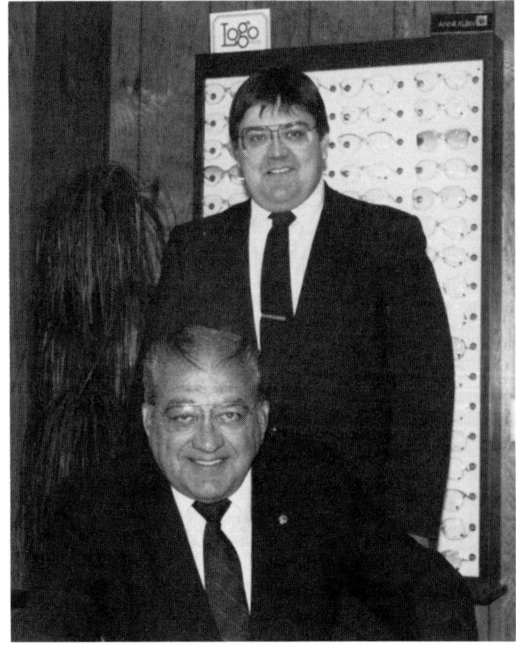

Dennis Birch, seated, is the son of H.J. Birch, company founder. The company is currently headed by his son Paul D. Birch shown standing behind his father.

important and both became certified by the American Board of Opticianry. Dennis was also certified as a contact lens fitter.

Following an auto accident and a long recuperation, Henry retired in 1964 and Dennis became president. In 1967, Birch Optical moved to larger quarters on Milwaukee Avenue, their present location. The lab expanded again in 1975 when the third generation, Paul D. Birch, finished college and joined as vice president. Paul grew up in the business and, following Dennis' semi-retirement in 1988, took over direction of the company. Ken Schmalzer joined Birch in 1974 and is vice president.

Dennis had always wanted a state-wide organization for opticians and in 1977, he and two other Chicago area opticians founded the Illinois Society of Opticianry.

BRENT OPTICAL (1915)

Two brothers, Edgar Brent and William Brent, started this company in Altoona, Pennsylvania. Edgar came out of the watch industry and William from optical. The company started as a jewelry supplier but, due to the influence of William and his wife Elizabeth, gradually gravitated to eyeglasses. Following Edgar and William's death, Elizabeth ran the company until her death in 1978.

The second World War presented the usual problem of losing employees to the Armed Forces but the company survived the war years. The company began offering retail services along with their wholesale work in the '30s but remained mostly wholesale. Today, the company is much more active in retail sales due to shifting market changes but still does some wholesale business.

During the time Elizabeth ran the company, at least 5 opticians had 40 or more years service with the company, making it their life work. When Elizabeth Brent died in 1978, her will specified the company go to 3 employees, James Mattern, Wayne Pheasant and John Hancuff. John learned optical work in the Army, serving in Europe during World War II and joined the company when the war ended. In 1988, Kathy Dempsie purchased Wayne's interest and manages the company today.

With almost 80 years in the Altoona area, it's quite common to have middle-aged patients come in for glasses and remember visiting Brent's when their grandparents came in for glasses.

E.B. BROWN OPTICIANS (1902)

E. B. Brown Opticians was founded in 1902 by Ernest Bradford Brown in downtown Cleveland. At that same time, W.A. Jones was opening a retail store across town. Brown and Jones, though competitors, became good

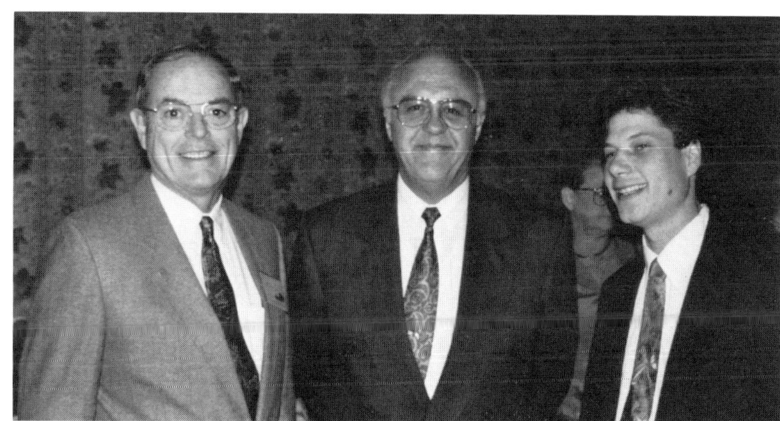

A presidential conference was held during the 1992 Fall California Optical Laboratories Assn. (COLA) meeting. Left to right are, OLA president J. Davis Lea, COLA president Andy Nalbandian and Midwest Optical Laboratories Assn. (MOLA) president Kevin Bargman.

PHOTO – CALIFORNIA OPTICAL LABORATORIES ASSN.

friends and must have been good businessmen as well. 90 years later, both E.B. Brown Opticians and W.A. Jones Optical Company are still going strong.

E.B. Brown was purchased in 1942 by Harry Davis who would later serve as the first President of the Guild Opticians of America. In 1968 the company was sold to Maurice Stonehill and in 1985, sold again to Gordon Safran, the present head of the company. Safran started his career working in the laboratory of Cole National, joining Cole shortly after they entered the optical business in 1961. Following that lab experience, he joined the retail side of Cole as an optician. By the time he left Cole *(1968)* he had risen to administrative assistant to the president of Cole's optical division. Safran had done a lot of traveling for Cole and wanted to settle down. E.B. Brown had just been acquired by Maurice Stonehill and Stonehill was looking for someone to run this latest acquisition. Stonehill hired Gordon Safran to run the company's three stores.

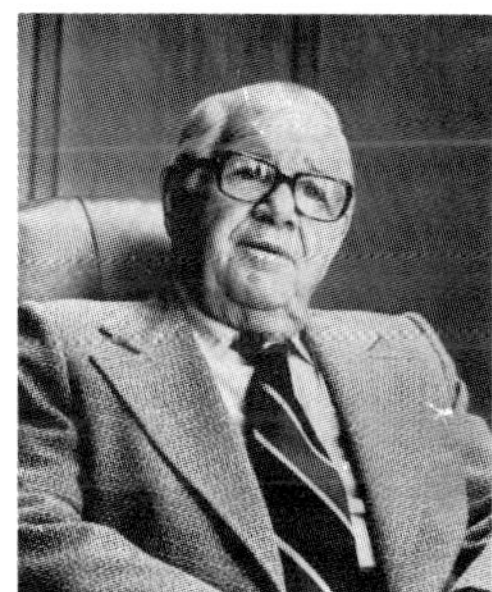

Maurice Stonehill owned E.B. Brown from 1968 until he sold the company to Gordon Safran in 1985.

PHOTO – E.B. BROWN OPTICIANS

In the Cleveland market, E.B. Brown still operates in the traditional medical-referral manner. In other areas where ophthalmologists are scarce or dispense themselves, the company has established optometrists next to their stores. This flexibility may account for why the company has enjoyed substantial growth during the past 25 years. When a branch is in a market that prefers lower priced merchandise, that's what Brown shows and stocks in that office. In more affluent areas, their product mix is high end. Whatever the product mix, their focus is always on producing a quality product and this policy works well for them.

The best indication of how well it works is the fact that, starting with 3 stores, Safran's company now has 41 stores in Ohio, Western Pennsylvania and Maryland with 40 percent of them in malls. Their relationship with ophthalmology remains strong and accounts for much of their strength. They operate three laboratories but most

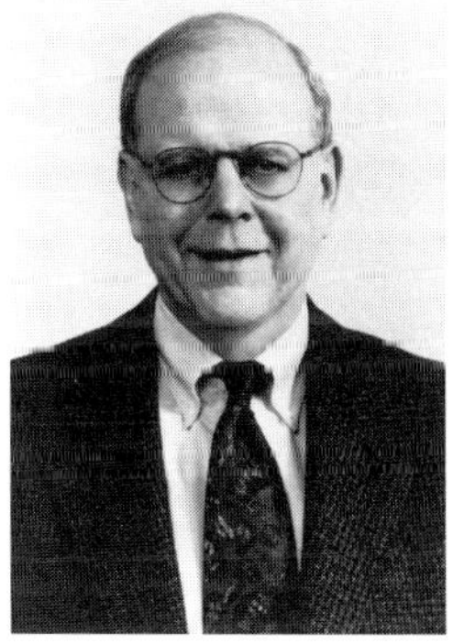

Gordon Safran left Cole National to purchase E.B. Brown Opticians, grown from 3 stores to the present 41 stores.

PHOTO – E.B. BROWN OPTICIANS

work is processed in the Cleveland lab. When branches need fast service they can ask for "Next Delivery" service and get the glasses back the following morning. The company has 230 employees so employee training is important to the company. The low personnel turnover indicates E.B. Brown must be a good place to work.

COLUMBIAN BIFOCAL (1895)

This company has an interesting heritage, having once been part of the famous Columbian Optical Company reviewed in Chapter Five. Tommy Thompson had come to work for Columbian Optical in 1910, 2 years before owner A.I. Agnew died in an auto accident. In 1925, Thompson purchased the Denver branch from Agnew's heirs. By that time, the company name had been changed to Columbian Bifocal, undoubtedly reflecting the important role the company played in the marketing of Kryptok bifocals *(they were one of the few companies authorized to manufacture Kryptoks. See Chapter Eight)*. Tommy Thompson developed many friends in the optical business and was highly regarded by all. Thompson later opened a branch in Los Angeles and, in 1936, another in Portland, Oregon.

Thompson's wife had died and, since he had no heirs, he offered to sell the company to his branch managers following World War II. The Portland branch was offered to the manager, Ben Loman. Loman was interested but wanted a partner if he was to buy it. He approached a returned Army veteran named Joe Seriko, asking if he was interested in joining in the purchase. Seriko had started his optical career in 1930 with Riggs Optical in Portland. He had worked his way through the lab, learning each job and ending in sales, until 1938 when he went with American Optical as a salesman. In 1942, he left AO to join the Army. Seriko returned from the war and rejoined AO until the time of Loman's offer. The two men bought the branch from Tommy Thompson with Loman controlling 51% of the stock. When Loman died in 1972, Seriko purchased the balance of the stock.

Computer Pioneers

One of CB's *(the name most customers use)* most lasting contribution to the industry has been their early involvement with laboratory computers. The story isn't well known and is worth including here. In the early '70s, Joe Seriko had contacted IBM in an attempt to investigate how computers might be used in optical laboratories. Seriko was finding, as did most lab operators at that time, great difficulty in hiring experienced lab technicians, particularly for the crucial surface layout position. There simply weren't enough trained people to go around. He was convinced the only answer for the future was computers. On two different occasions, IBM sent engineers out to Portland to work with CB but the only computers available to handle the job in 1972 required million dollar investments. IBM eventually gave up on the idea, but expressed interest in keeping in touch until the idea became more practical.

Seriko had become friendly with John Chaney, an ex-IBM man who left Big Blue to set up his own company in Portland called Computer Management Service Industry. Chaney had a partner named Art Kazer and both men became fascinated with the long-term prospects of computerizing optical labs. Knowing little about optical, they proposed a joint venture with Columbian Bifocal and one was quickly formed. CMSI hired three or four computer programmers and started work on the long-term project *(turning out to be longer than anyone had figured)*. Columbian Bifocal still had to get work out during the day, so most of the development work was accomplished during long work sessions every night, with CB's Tom Mitchoff and George Weber working every night with the CMSI programmers *(including Gordon Keene who later established his own laboratory*

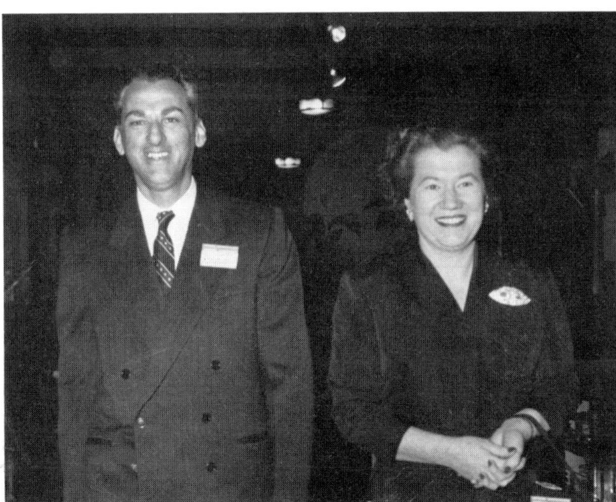

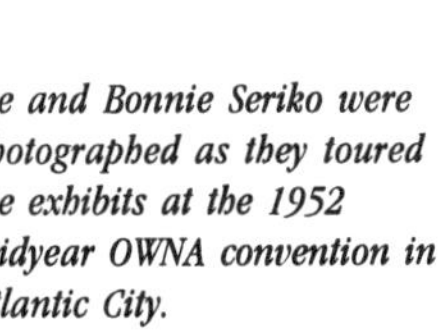

Joe and Bonnie Seriko were photographed as they toured the exhibits at the 1952 midyear OWNA convention in Atlantic City.

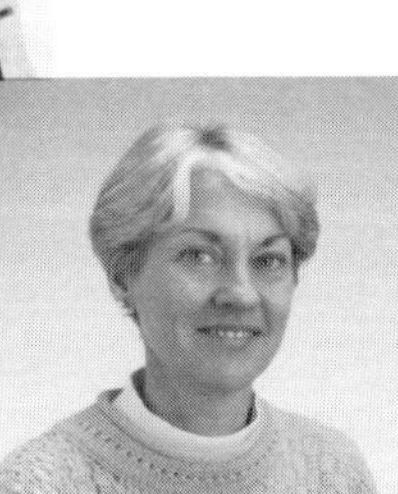

Both Seriko daughters work for the family business. Jo Anne McMahon, left, oversees the company's marketing.

Julie Mitchoff handles accounting and public relations.

computer system). It took 4 long years before CB's computer was able to go on line with the first-ever comprehensive computer program designed specifically for optical laboratories. Hewlett Packard equipment was used and that company also worked closely with the CMSI/CB team. Once the software was developed and on line, it was patented by the joint venture. CMSI presently markets the system which has continued to evolve over the years. In the meantime, CMSI became involved in a variety of important projects in other fields, including water management and hospital systems.

CB has been heavily involved with contact lenses since 1960 when they sent a company employee, Dr. Fred Chinn, to Los Angeles to study manufacturing hard contact lenses with Kevin Touhy. Today they manufacture gas-permeable lenses and distribute many soft lenses as well. At one time, the company had branches in Denver, Honolulu and Seattle. These were not full-service branches, existing primarily to distribute contact lenses and supplies. Today the only CB branch is Salt Lake City but that one is full-service and is newly equipped with LOH equipment in their own building.

Joe Seriko died in 1990 at age 82. His wife, Juanita Sericko, remains active but the company today is headed by C.E.O., George Weber. Weber had worked part-time and summers for Columbian Bifocal while still in high school and joined the company full time in 1956, becoming, in Juanita Seriko's words, the son Joe never had. Juanita's two daughters, Julie Mitchoff and Joan McMahan, are both active in the company with Julie working in accounting and public relations while Joan takes care of marketing. Julie has two children, Joe Mitchoff, named after his grandfather and presently in college, and Michael Mitchoff, about to enter college.

The company travels four sales reps covering the entire Northwestern states. They have always handled frames and still distribute most major frame lines.

DIETZ LAB (1933)

This company started as a retail store, opened in 1933 by Edward Dietz, Sr. during the depths of the depression. Ed came out of American Optical. Borrowing $50 from his boss, he rented a small space in the old Medical Arts Building in Ft. Worth and opened his first store. He had trouble getting lab work that satisfied him so in 1941, he ordered lab equipment and began producing his own. To support his lab, he solicited wholesale work from local practitioners and, before long, the wholesale business was growing faster than the retail.

The one thing people remember most about Ed Senior was that he was an impeccable dresser. His ruby tie tack, his white Stetson hat and his dapper cigarette holder are still remembered by many. He was also acknowledged as a first-rate party man. He could spend all night with the boys, come back to the hotel long enough to shower and show up at an eight o-clock meeting looking like a million dollars.

Ed, Junior worked in the lab while going to high school. Coming in late one day, he was fired, not by his father but by the lab manager. It must have taught him a lesson because there were no more complaints about his work habits. Graduating from high school in 1949, Ed Junior started college and was boxing in Golden Gloves. During his first semester at college, he was clobbered by a boxer from El Paso and ended up in the hospital with a concussion. Going back to school, he was unable to stay awake in class as a result of the concussion. This decided him to go in the service and, in 1950, he enlisted in the Air Force for four years. While stationed in England in 1952 at Bentwaters R.A.F. station, he met his future wife Barbara. Barbara's father was also in the U.S. Air Force, stationed at the same base. Barbara graduated from high school in Washington state in May, went to England in June, met Ed in July and became engaged in September. They married in England in May, 1953 and spent the next year there. Their son Ed, III was born in England in May, 1954. Returning alone with her baby from England to Texas, Barbara was stranded by an airline strike in Chicago. An hour later, she was paged in the terminal and, through the efforts of a U.S. Senator friend of Ed, Senior's, was sent on to Texas on an emergency basis.

Ed Junior was discharged in January, 1955 and immediately joined Dietz Optical. He traveled for the next seven years as a sales rep and, in the early 1960s, Ed and his family moved to Tucson to manage a Dietz branch office *(since closed)*. Several years later, his Dad called and said, "I need you in Ft. Worth." In terms of dress, Ed, Junior was totally unlike his father. Senior was almost never

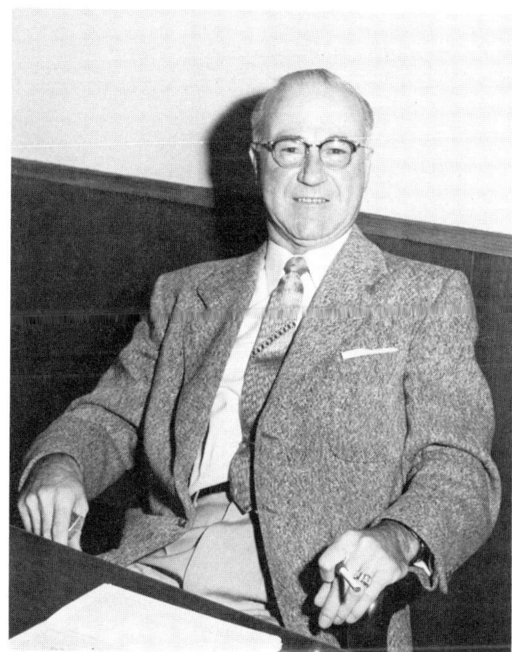

Ed Dietz, Sr. with his ever-present cigarette holder and ruby stick pin. Only his Stetson hat is missing.

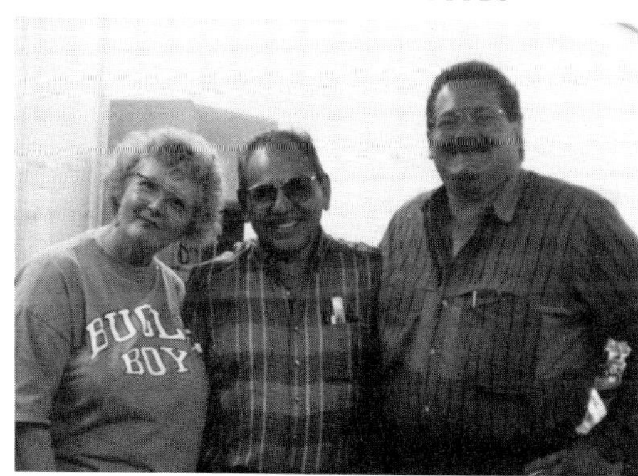

Present head of the company is Barbara Dietz. With her are Pancho Granado, center and son Ed Dietz, III.

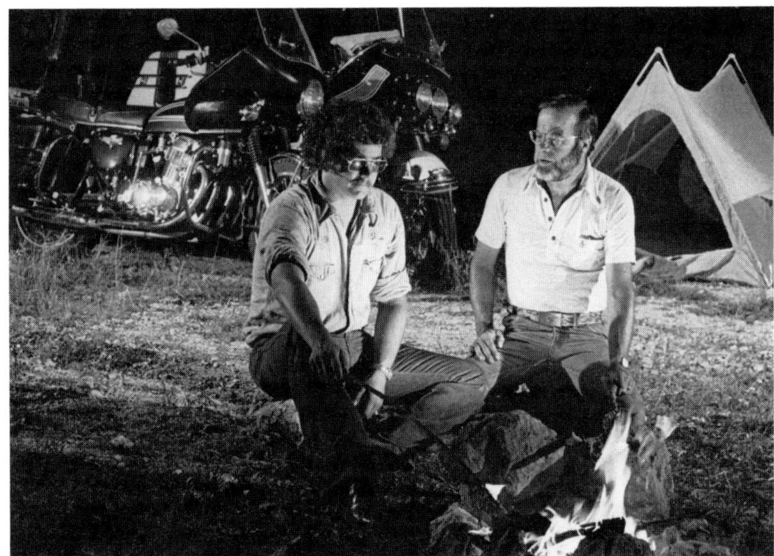

Looking like a scene from the movie "Easy Rider", this photo was taken shortly after Ed Dietz, III graduated from college as he and his father embarked on a 7,000 trip by motorcycle.

seen without a shirt and tie while Ed, Junior seldom ever wore a tie. He preferred more casual attire than his father. Following Ed Senior's death, Ed Junior ran the company until he died in 1990.

The company has been in retail in Ft. Worth for 61 years and had as many as 6 retail locations. The company still operates two stores. One is called Dietz Opticians and the newer one, a boutique type operation, is called "Eyewear by Dietz". The newest store was opened shortly after Ed Junior died. The store was something Ed had discussed doing many times and his wife and son opened it as a tribute to Ed, Junior.

When Ed Dietz, III graduated from college, his parent's gift was a 30 day motorcycle trip with his father. The trip ended up as a 7,000 mile journey. The purpose of the trip was to scout out possible jobs for Ed III who wanted to work at a different level of the optical industry. Their first stop was San Diego. Half way through the trip, they arrived in Brainard, Minn. where the OLA was having a summer Board meeting *(Ed Junior was a Director)*. Returning from the trip, they discussed Ed III's job opportunities and decided Signet offered the greatest potential. Ed, III worked for them for the next fifteen years until his father's death when he returned to help his mother run the family business.

Ed and Barbara's daughter Debbie Dietz traveled and handled sales for the company for 12 years and presently manages the company's retail stores. Dietz Lab, owned by Barbara and Ed III, has 18 employees, two of which have been with the company for 47 years. Paul Rivers runs the surface department and Pancho Granado is bench supervisor. Barbara's father, Jack Smith, retired twenty years ago but soon got tired of that and came to work for Dietz Lab. He's 80 years old and still working in the bench department. The company is heavily involved in stock sales with almost half of their volume coming

from sales of frames, cases, accessories and supplies. They have one sales rep covering Texas and New Mexico.

Ed Dietz, Senior was president of the A.I.O.W. in 1954-55 and his son Ed Dietz, Jr. served as president of the OWA in 1973-74. Barbara Dietz believes the honor of being selected by his peers, next to his own family, was Ed Junior's proudest accomplishment.

DIETZ-MCLAIN OPTICAL (1938)

Raymond G. McLain's optical career began almost by accident while living in Houston with his older brother who worked for Merry Optical Company. One day Ray's brother came home and told him a job as delivery boy was available at Merry. Ray took the job and remained with the company when American Optical bought Merry Optical. Shortly after that, McLain was made salesman. He transferred to San Antonio where he was promoted to AO branch manager and later zone manager.

In 1938, Ed Dietz, Sr. *(Dietz Optical, Ft. Worth)* opened an optical accessory shop in the Medical Arts Building in San Antonio, Texas. The branch suffered the usual problems with unsupervised managers and finally in 1945, Dietz decided he had enough. What he needed was a partner, not a long distance manager. He discussed the problem with Ray McLain who left AO and established a partnership with Dietz, changing the name of the San Antonio office to Dietz-McLain Optical. The company, a wholesale laboratory and a retail dispensing business, started growing. *(Editor's note: During the mid-1900s at least half of all AIOW members were dual operations, wholesale and retail.)*

At this same time, Ed Dietz made similar arrangements with Hobart Dillard in his Temple, Texas branch, changing that name to Dietz Dillard Optical. From that point on, Dietz was, in effect, a silent partner in both companies. This arrangement lasted until Ray McLain

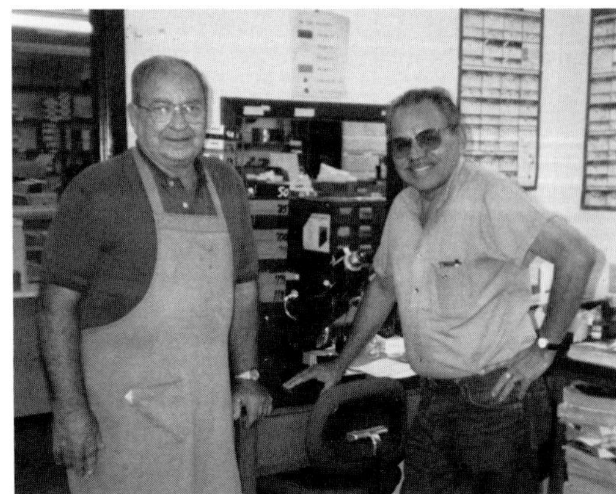

Paul Rivers, left, runs the Dietz surface department and Pancho Granado, right, is bench supervisor.

Photo - Dietz Lab

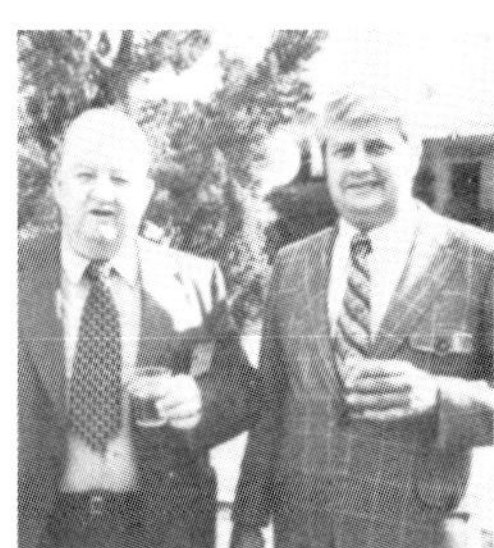

Ray McLain, left, and his son Jim McLain, current head of Dietz-McLain Optical are seen at an early wholesaler convention.

died in 1972. At that time a corporation was formed, owned jointly by Ed Dietz, Sr. and Ray's son Jim. In 1981, McLain bought out the Dietz interests and the company is owned solely by the McLain family. They also own the Temple office, which is operated as Dietz-McLain.

Ray McLain was an active member in the A.I.O.W. *(the early OLA)* and served on the Board of Directors. He served as vice president but during that year, suffered a stroke. Feeling he wouldn't be able to handle the job of president, Ray retired from the board. His son Jim McLain presently sits on the OLA Board and has served as a director for the past three years.

Dietz-McLain Optical is strictly retail today and is run jointly by Jim McLain and his son Drake. The company operates 9 retail branches in the San Antonio area, one in Temple and employs no refractionists. Dietz-McLain Optical has developed a reputation in San Antonio for leading the way in eyeglass technology. Their latest project involves switching patients from conventional CR-39 to polycarbonate. They may be the first retail organization in the country to make polycarbonate the lens of choice for all patients, not just children. Within the first 10 days of their new program, the company had converted over 75% of all new lens orders to polycarbonate.

DUFFENS OPTICAL (1919)

Duffens Optical traces their origin to 1919 when J.T. "Jack" Quinton and R. F. Duffens purchased Morgan Optical in Salina, Kan. and renamed it Quinton-Duffens Optical Company. R. F. Duffens began his career in 1911 at age 14. Due to economic conditions, he had to help support the family and his first job was in Kansas City with the Stead Lens Company *(see Chapter Eight)*. Duffens was an assistant to the man running the automatic countersink polishers which entailed polishing depressions ground into the front surface of blanks that would receive the flint bifocal segments. Duffens' job involved running back and forth with a brush daubing water and rouge on the polishing machine.

Several years later, Stead Lens Company shut down due to patent litigation with the Kryptok Company and young Duffens was hired by Billy Riggs to work for the local Columbian Optical branch *(it was there that he met J.T. Quinton, also working at Columbian)*. Duffens left in July, 1917 and moved to Salina, Kan. to work with

Waitman Morgan who was starting a new lab called Morgan Optical. Duffens purchased a 10 percent interest in the company, investing a small amount of his salary each week. In 1918, Uncle Sam called and Duffens sold his Morgan Optical interest to J.T. Quinton and joined the Navy.

Jack Quinton was an old-timer, starting in the optical business in 1898 with the Grant-Whittlesey Optical Company in Cleveland, Ohio. In 1903, he worked under Jack Brayton at the Julius King Optical in Chicago *(see Chapter Five)*. He later worked for the Eckley Optical company in Memphis but a dangerous yellow fever epidemic chased him back to Chicago where he worked for Almer Coe *(see Chapter Eight)* making the famous three-piece cemented Kryptok. When the yellow fever epidemic abated in 1906, he returned to Eckley which was purchased shortly thereafter by the Merry Optical Company. In 1907, Merry transferred Jack to their Kansas City office and in 1913, he joined Billy Riggs at Columbian Optical Company.

After the war, Duffens returned to Morgan Optical in January, 1919. By April, he and his friend Jack Quinton purchased Morgan Optical and renamed it Quinton-Duffens Optical Company. The new company sold Kryptoks for $8.50 to $11. Kryptoks and onepiece

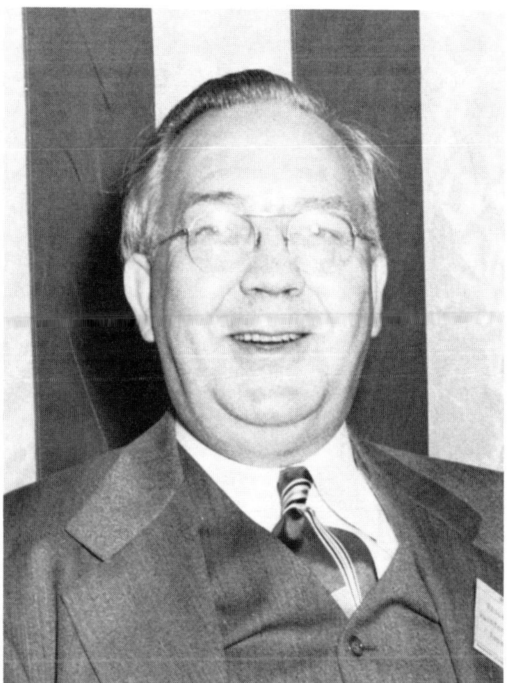

R.F. Duffens, founder of Duffens Optical, a four-generation family company.

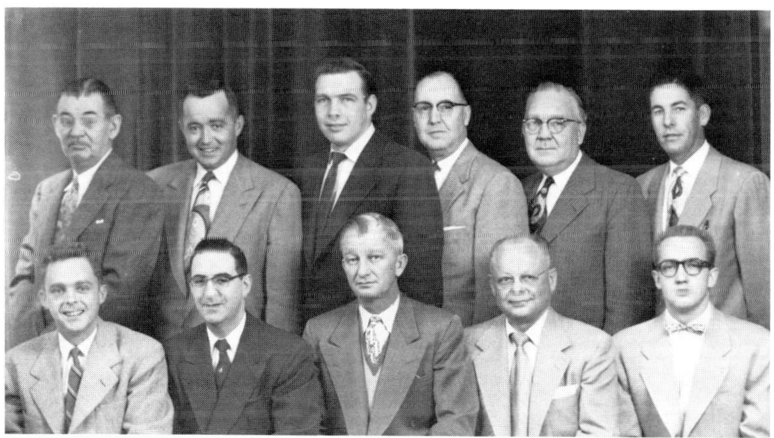

This photo of Duffens Optical's management team in 1952 includes some unidentified persons. In the back row, starting third from the left are Bob Duffens, Art Busche and R.F. Duffens. In the center of the front row is Marshal Becker and Roy Duffens is at the right end.

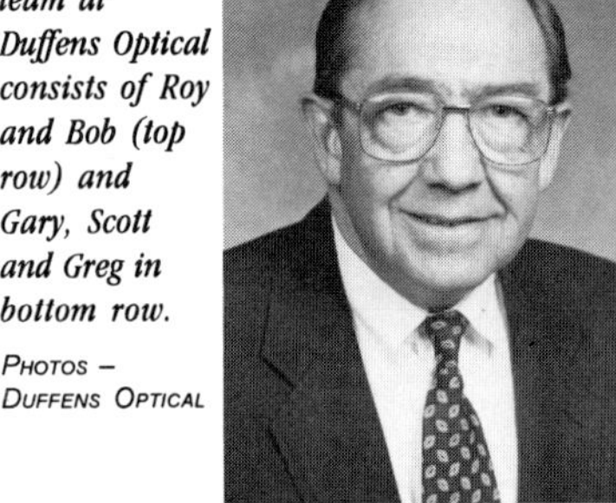
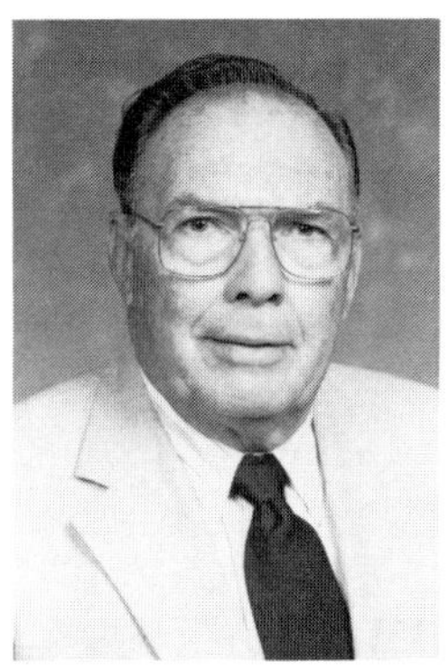

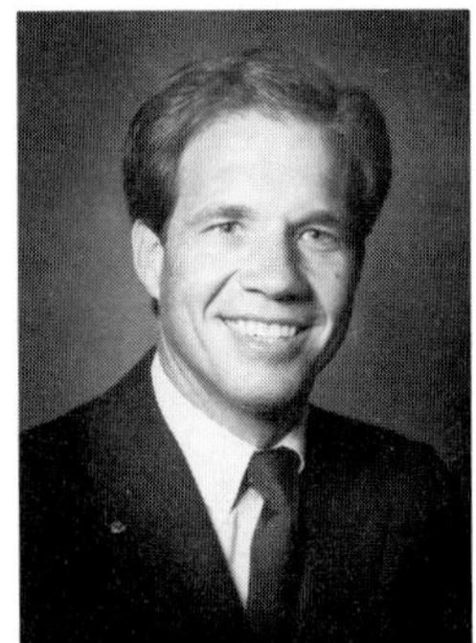
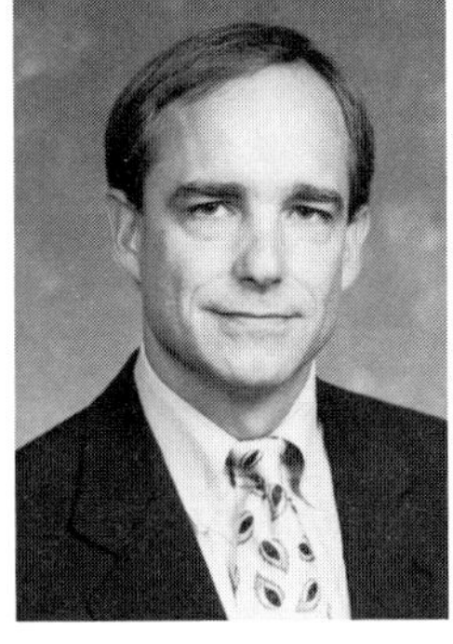
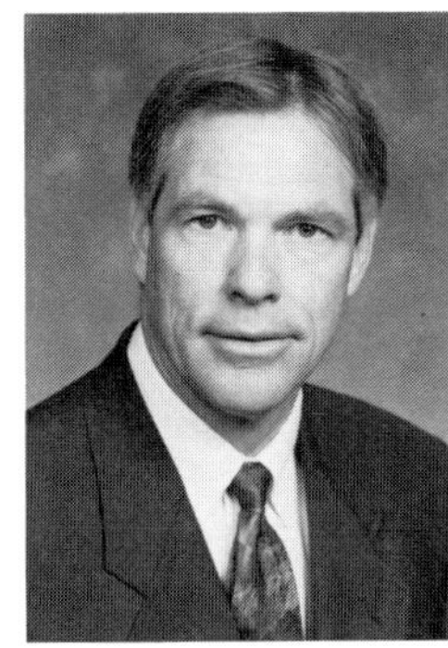

bifocals *(Ultex)* were the top-selling bifocals at the time but licenses to sell both bifocals were tightly controlled. Without a license, labs were limited to producing split or cement seg bifocals. Quinton and Duffens had friends who provided them with Kryptok blanks, but only at a premium price. R.F. would later tell how they were forced to keep the blanks hidden in a closet so inspectors from the Kryptok Company wouldn't find them.

In 1921, they opened an office in Pittsburg, Kan. Riggs Optical, one of the fastest-growing lab chains in the country, was extremely protective of their market area. Deciding they couldn't beat Quinton-Duffens, Riggs offered to purchase their company in 1922 and acquired both branches *(Riggs would later be acquired*

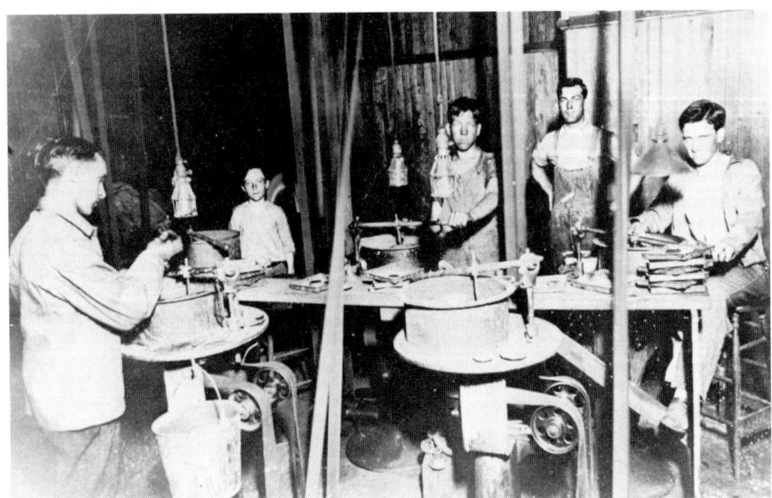

by Bausch & Lomb). Quinton became manager of the Lincoln branch and Duffens remained in Salina as manager.

Onward and Upward

Tiring of working for someone else in 1927, both men submitted their resignations to Roy Wahlgren, then president of Riggs Optical. They opened a Quinton-Duffens lab in Topeka with first year sales of $10,833. R.F. was twenty-nine and Quinton forty-six. Two years later, they opened a branch in Hutchinson, Kan. and in 1934 were able to repurchase their old lab in Salina. During the '30s, R.F. called on customers across the state of Kansas until, in 1938, they added a second sales representative named Marshall Becker. Becker had been a professional golfer and had an engaging personality that quickly earned the trust of new customers. In the late '30s, R.F.'s son Bob started working summers in the lab at age 14.

Quinton-Duffens Polisher

Lens production had changed little from the time in 1911 when R.F. Duffens daubed polish on spinning lenses with a paint brush. Polishing was still accomplished the same way in 1940. Perhaps because of his first job, R.F. was convinced polishing could be accomplished automatically. With the help of a local machinist, he designed a self-contained polishing machine that fed the polish on the lens automatically and could be used for both fining and polishing. Unfortunately, an undeveloped patent had been filed on this automatic feed principal so no royalties could be collected for the idea and it was soon being used by everyone, especially lens factories.

The first Quinton-Duffens polisher was demonstrated at an AIOW convention in Minneapolis in 1941 and was the hit of the show. Lab operators had never seen lenses polished in a hotel room. Thousands of these automatic polishers would be sold to wholesalers in the coming years. In the '50s, Coburn Optical purchased the 501B 4-head cylinder machine developed by R.F. and his son Bob.

Jack Quinton retired in 1943 because of ill health with R.F. Duffens purchasing his interest. The company was renamed Duffens Optical Company. During the '40s, Roy Duffens, R.F.'s second son began working summers to learn optical production. The war years were tough for it was hard to find technicians and even harder to obtain lens blanks. It was quite common to surface both sides of lens blanks, even for single vision *(this was before generators)*. Bob Duffens, had served in the Naval Air Force and returned in 1946 to begin full-time work with the company. Roy Duffens came to work full time in 1952, following a tour in the Air Force.

The company continued to grow, partly through acquisitions of other labs in Indianapolis, Wichita, Shawnee Mission, Denver, Hannibal, New Orleans, Tulsa, Houston, Beaumont, San Antonio and, in 1988, Oklahoma City. During the late '50s, Bob's sons Gary and Greg often spent Sundays at the lab with their father. Their job was to open Saturday's mail and get it trayed up ready for production on Monday.

R.F. Duffens died at age 67 in 1965. By the early '70s, his grandsons Gary and Greg had joined the company full time. Charles Merry, a former AO manager became sales manager. In 1973, Gary moved to Denver, appointed manager of that branch. Kuhns Optical was purchased and merged with the Denver branch. In 1979, Roy's son Scott Duffens joined the company and was assigned to manage the computerization of production and accounting throughout the company.

In 1959, corneal contact lenses started coming into their own. Duffens Optical quickly responded to this new opportunity, establishing a new company, Duffens Contact Lens Company which was headed by Jim Albrecht. The time was right and this new organization quickly expanded to 11 locations. They were producing hard lenses *(PMMA)*, along with related supplies in every state as well as overseas. B&L introduced the first soft contact lens and the entire contact lens market began to change. Duffens Optical sold their contact lens division to Buckbee-Mears in 1981. Also sold was Aquarius Soft Lens Company, jointly owned by Duffens and other distributors trying to market their own soft lens.

In 1985, Buckbee-Mears decided to cut back on their contact lens distribution. Then a gas permeable hard contact lens was developed and, sensing new opportunities in the contact lens market, Duffens reacquired four of their former contact lens branches and reentered the contact field. With contact branches in Indianapolis, Shawnee Mission, Wichita and Denver, they later added new contact laboratories in Tulsa and Houston.

Association Work

R. F. Duffens was president of the AIOW in 1952 and, in 1959 his son Bob also became president of the association. Bob's brother, Roy Duffens, became president of the OWA in 1969 and Bob's son, Gary Duffens, was president of the renamed OLA in 1988. No other family has had as many members serve as association president. Gary's brother Greg Duffens presently serves on the OLA Board of Directors.

Today there are six family members representing three generations active in the company. Roy's son Blair has responsibility for AR coating in the Denver branch. Brian is assistant manager of Indianapolis. Bob and Roy are chairman of the board and president respectively. Gary, in addition to managing Denver, shares with Greg and Scott the managerial responsibilities of the entire company. The company has 12 laboratories employing 500 people and serving more than 5,000 accounts throughout the country.

GULF STATES OPTICAL (1945)

This company was founded in 1945 by Adolph C. and Ladove Huber. Huber had worked for American Optical in New Orleans. The war was just ending and Huber, who had been in the Navy during World War I, would only hire returning veterans as employees, training most of them himself. The new company couldn't afford lab coats for the shop people so they wore their old uniforms in the lab. The uniforms were later cut up and used for polishing pads.

Huber handled sales, traveling the Gulf states of Louisiana, Mississippi, Alabama and Florida while Ladove Huber ran the office. They sold frames along with lab work and the company still sells frames, carrying a private label line called Crescent City Collection. In 1965, New Orleans was threatened by Hurricane Betsy. Mr. Huber came in and told the employees he had just heard the storm had changed paths going up the East Coast. What they didn't realize was the storm would turn again. Returning to work in the morning, they found every window shattered *(they were on the sixth floor)* with trays and jobs scattered all over the lab. Some of the employee's homes in St. Bernard Parish were under water for two weeks.

Huber was a gregarious, well-liked individual who, along with his wife, built a thriving business. In 1949, a young lady named Mary Finnorn was hired *(she is still with the company)*. Huber was in his late sixties and began to tire of traveling. He mentioned this in a meeting with the

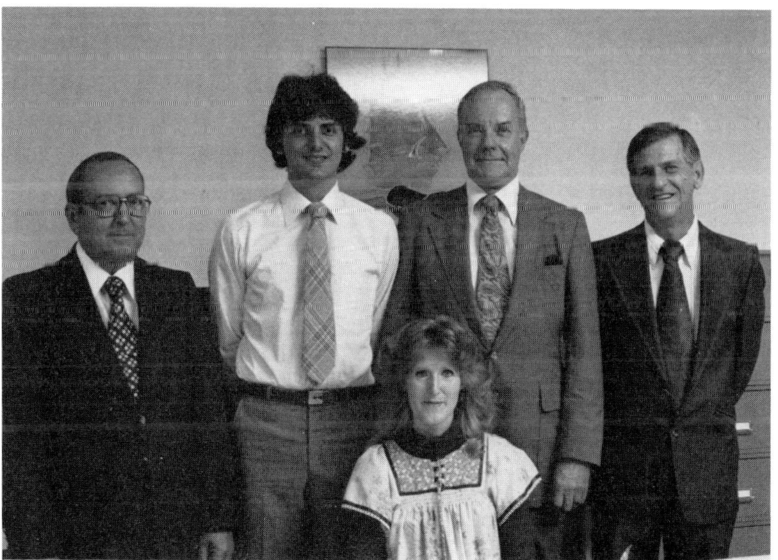

This Gulf States photo, taken in 1979, shows (standing) Stanley Rehage, salesman who retired in 1988, Pierre Bezou, then salesman and now President/Owner, Carl T. Smith, Jr., company president from 1967 to 1993 and Al Durr, general manager and short-term president. Seated is Peggy Young, stock room manager.

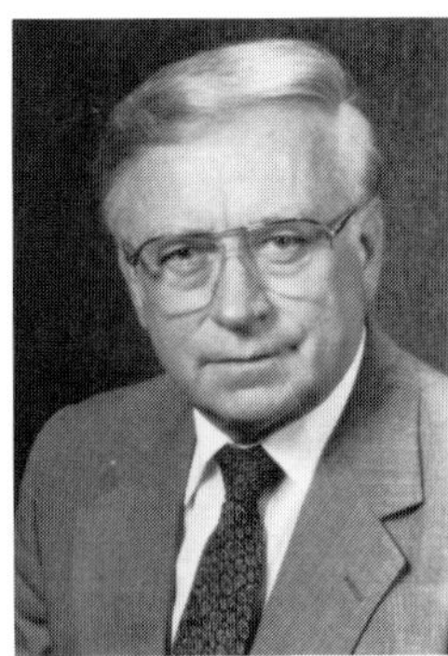
When Robert Dunn purchased Homer Optical from Kay Jewelers in 1973, he ended up with a full-service laboratory but no customers.

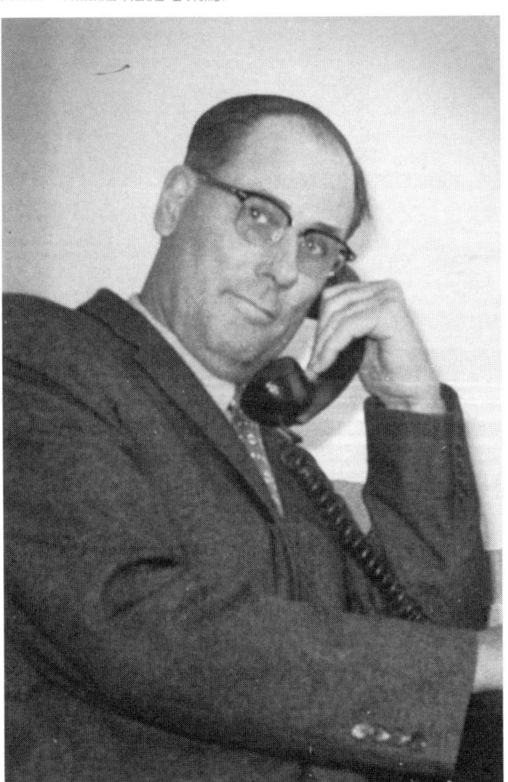
Joe Heard, founder of Heard Optical. Photo was taken in 1957.

company auditor, Felix Hrapmann, Jr. As a result of that conversation, in January, 1967, the Hubers sold the company to Carl T. Smith, Jr., Hrapmann and two other partners in the company's accounting firm. Smith, an experienced sales and marketing person, became president.

The company, located in the Maison Blanche Building on Canal Street, continued to grow, prompting a move to a New Orleans suburb called Metairie in 1982. Eventually the company bought back the accountants' stock, leaving Smith owning the company. In 1977, Smith hired a young man named Pierre Bezou to handle sales for the company. Later promoted to general manager, Bezou became company president in 1982 and is currently the principal stockholder.

Gulf States was always low key and somewhat modest in their sales programs but Pierre Bezou has taken a more assertive approach to marketing, setting up an effective marketing department for Gulf States Optical. The company today covers basically the same territory as that Huber traveled years ago.

HEARD OPTICAL COMPANY (1942)

The history of the Heard family is covered in greater detail in Chapter 12. Joe Heard came from an optical family. His father and uncle were optometrists and he was a grandson of the pioneer optician, T.M. Heard, profiled in Chapter 12. He started this new laboratory in the Times Building in Long Beach in 1942. The company grew steadily until 1958 when increased business made it necessary to move to a larger building. In 1970, they moved again into their present 14,000 square foot facility.

Joe Heard died in 1958, leaving his wife, Dorothy, to run the company with the help of her nephew, Howard Heard. In 1969, Heard Optical was purchased by Dave Current and Dick Cummings, two CPA's who were investors in a number of various companies and also managed the Beach Boys. Current and Cummings bought Heard Optical as an investment. They hired Ron Freese from Spratt Optical

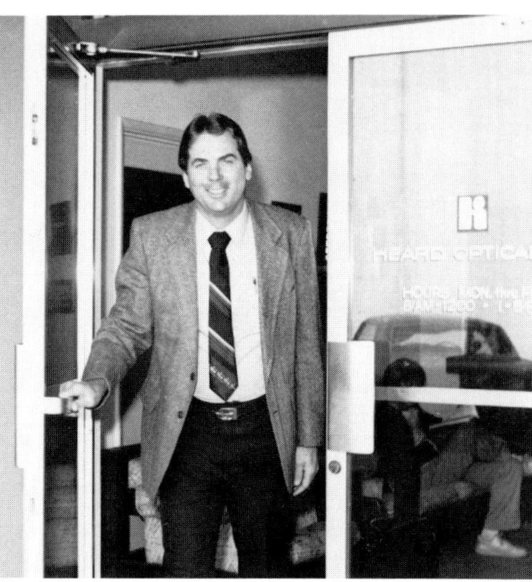
Ron Freese, current president of the Heard Optical Group.

to manage the company. He ran it until 1978 when he purchased the company from Current and Cummings.

Since Freese assumed control, Heard Optical has acquired Bristow Optical, a major lab in Phoenix, Arizona, and Lens Craftsmen located in Tucson. In 1994, Heard acquired Bahnsen Optical and Optical Micro Coating (an AR coating lab) in Salinas, California. The company also operates a 3 branch network of labs in California that offer limited prescription service. The combined companies in the Heard Group cover a four state market area, comprising California, Arizona, Nevada and New Mexico.

HOMER OPTICAL (1940)

The optical industry's roots spring as much from the jewelry trade as any other. Many early optometrists came out of the jewelry trade. With this common heritage, it seemed only natural for jewelry stores to establish optical departments. Thousands of jewelry stores during the mid-1900s had optometrists in their stores, either as employees or leasing the department. Kay Jewelers was a major jewelry chain with optical departments based in Washington, D.C. In the early '40s, a family named Kaufmann set up a laboratory to service the extensive Kay optical departments. By the 1970s, Kay's optical business had shrunk to almost nothing and the laboratory was put up for sale. When Bob Dunn bought the company (1973), Kay Jewelers had just a few optical departments left so that, in effect, Dunn bought a laboratory with virtually no customers. Building from that zero base, the company today has branches in Silver Springs, Maryland and Virginia Beach, Virginia and does business with all three professions in a multi-state area.

The company has set up an in-lab AR coating facility and

was an early supporter of anti-reflective coatings for eyewear. The company enjoys another unique distinction of providing all prescription lenses for the Polaris frame line, specializing in the elaborate faceted edges required for those rimless mountings.

KATZ & KLEIN (1937)

Harry Katz began his optical career in 1914 as an errand boy for R. Mohr & Company in San Francisco. Mohr sent Katz to Sacramento in 1922 to open a branch and kept him there as branch manager. Russell J. Klein got his start in his native Hamilton, Ontario Canada in 1916. Klein eventually moved to the states and joined Riggs Optical in San Francisco, later transferring to manage the Riggs branch in Sacramento.

In 1937, the two men decided fate had thrown them together to do more than just run branch offices for major manufacturers *(Riggs was owned by B&L and the R. Mohr branch was now part of AO)*. The two men were good friends and were well-known locally. Customers had urged them for years to get together and start a laboratory. Once they started making plans, the word quickly leaked. Harry Katz was called to San Francisco where AO's zone manager George Johnston mentioned, "Harry, we hear there's a new lab opening in Sacramento." Harry answered, "Yeah, it's me." Johnston fired him on the spot. Several months later Katz and Klein opened their wholesale laboratory in an inexpensive upstairs location. By the time the lab opened, bags of mail were stacked in the hall filled with incoming jobs. Starting with three employees *(including themselves)*, by the second business day, they added a fourth employee. Continuing growth forced them to move the lab several years later. The year they started in business, the two men created a "building kitty" and, good year or bad, they set aside funds toward their dream. Finally in 1948, that dream came true when they moved into a brand new building, built to the lab's exact needs in downtown Sacramento.

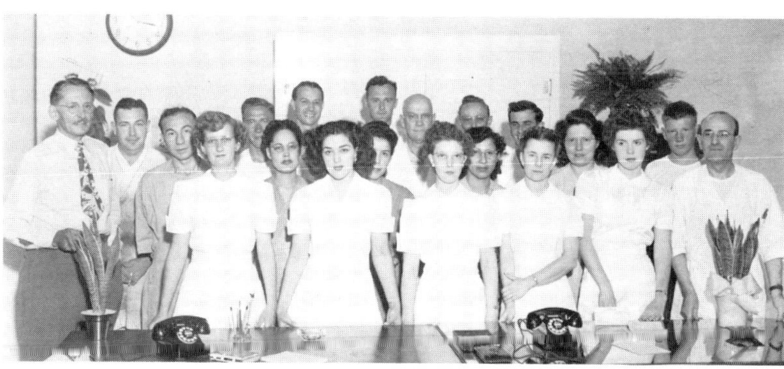

Here is the Katz & Klein crew during a morning break in 1948. The men at either end are Russell Klein, left, and Harry Katz, right. The curly headed young man barely seen to the left of the plant in the background is Ellis Katz, present Chairman of the Board.

Harry Katz had a son named Ellis. Young Katz was running errands for American Optical in 1936 while his father still managed AO's Sacramento branch. From 1937 to 1943, Ellis spent summers and vacations working for Katz & Klein. Service in the Navy followed plus two years of college. While attending college in Sacramento, Ellis tried a number of times to find a part time job to supplement his recreation funds. His father knew everyone and, following each interview, the owner would call Harry Katz to ask if it was all right to hire Ellis. Harry's answer was always, "Tell him if he wants a job, he can come to Katz & Klein." Ellis finally gave up and came to work full time for his father's company in 1948.

Russell Klein retired in 1959 and Harry Katz in 1960. Ellis, Ronald Knight and Art Kirkpatrick bought the company from Harry Katz with Ellis having the controlling interest. When the company suffered a labor strike in 1969, Kirkpatrick came to Ellis and said, "I've been through too many strikes. I don't need another." Katz bought him out and a few years later Knight left to open a dispensing business.

In 1966, the company needed an assistant bookkeeper and Ellis hired a young lady named Corrine Hood for $4.25 an hour. She was placed in charge of the first computer purchased by the company. Ellis, active in the Shrine, knew he was in line to become Potentate of the Shriners in 1979 and realized he had to be grooming someone to run the company while he was involved with the Shrine. In 1972, he asked the company's top 10 employees to select the person who would serve as the company's general manager. Corrine Hood was their choice.

Ellis Katz soon recognized they made the right choice. By 1990, most of the daily decisions were being made by Corrine and Ellis moved up to C.E.O., making Corrine president and Mike Francesconi vice president.

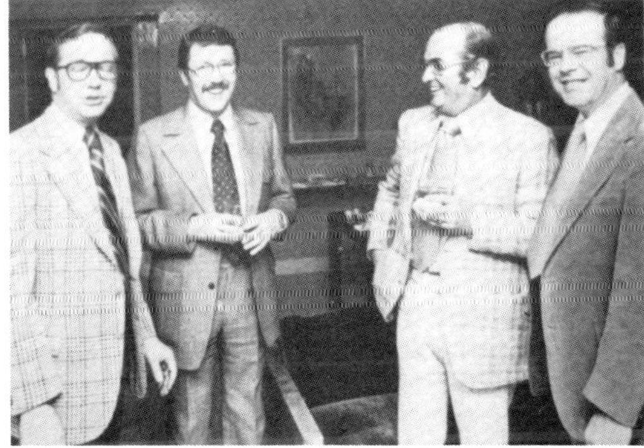

OWA directors are seen in this 1972 photo. Left to right are Roy Duffens, then president Gerald J. Dougher, Ellis Katz and then president-elect Ed Dietz, Jr.

Katz & Klein current management is represented by President Corrine Hood, V.P. Mike Francesconi and Chairman of the Board Ellis Katz, shown during a recent OLA Convention. Francesconi started as a salesman and currently runs the company's sales department.

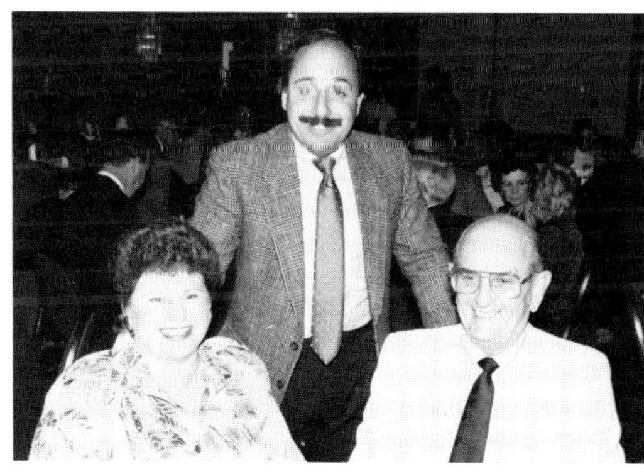

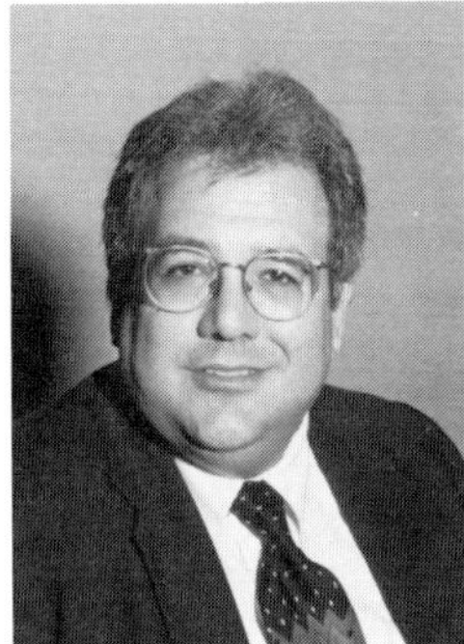

Jeffrey Kosh (pictured here) and his brother Stuart presently run Kosh Ophthalmic.

Ellis remains active and still calls on key accounts but the company's activities are directed by Hood and Francesconi.

OLA Service

Always active in association affairs, Ellis Katz was president of the Optical Wholesalers Association in 1971-72. Carrying on the company tradition of association service, Corrine Hood is currently serving as vice president of the Optical Laboratories Association and is program chairperson for the 1994 Centennial Convention in Kansas City. She is past president of the California Optical Laboratories Association *(COLA)* and has been actively involved with the California legislative process on behalf of COLA and the California optical community for many years.

Katz & Klein also has a long tradition of enhancing the education of students and professionals. Every year since 1970, the company has sponsored an informal gathering of graduating students and doctors from California and Nevada. These affairs are held at the Katz home as a forum for discussing the realities of establishing private practices. The company has contributed significantly to the University of California at Berkeley, School of Optometry, helping to build a wing which now bears the Katz & Klein name. The company also conducts a number of other educational seminars and meetings to teach eyecare professionals how to build a solid patient/doctor relationship and how to market their practice.

KOSH OPHTHALMIC, INC. (1925)

The company was founded in New York City at 106 Fulton Street by Louis Herman Kosh and his brother Abe. Fulton Street was the optical center of New York. Max Zadek had a wholesale shop on the same street. The Kosh lab grew and later moved uptown. A young lady named Rose came to work that first year and within a year had married the boss (Louis). Louis and Rose had a son they named Allan. Abe Kosh left in the thirties and moved to California to start his own optical lab out there.

This photo, taken in 1940, shows the Lehigh shop crew with, left to right, Adam Hamm, John Niedermeyer, Robert Young, E.J. Faust and William Ziegensuss. Dr. Faust was the first optometrist in Allentown, Penn and had his office in the back of a jewelry store.

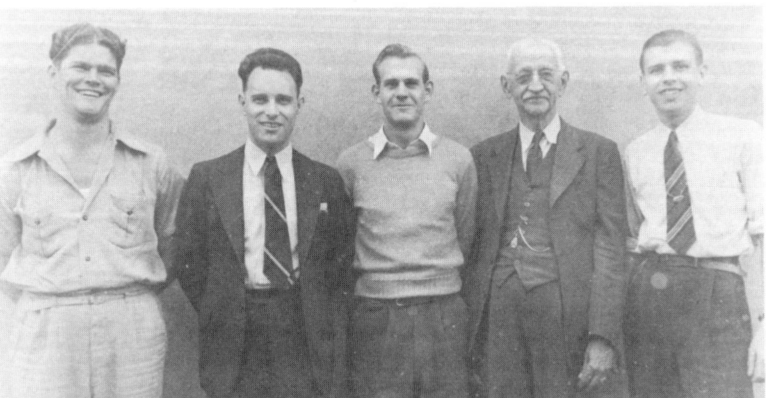

Allan worked for his father as he grew up and eventually came into the company full time.

Allan Kosh married and had two sons, Jeffrey and Stuart. Allan was most proud of his work with the American National Standards Institute (ANSI) during the 1970s. He served as Director and Chairman of ANSI and, until his death, was chairman of Accredited Standards Committee Z80.1 which presides over standards for prescription lenses. He represented the OLA's interest in international standardization and contributed to the U.S. Technical Advisory Group to ISO Technical Committee 172. He was elected vice chairman of ANSI/ASC Z80 in January, 1986. His committee was responsible for developing and maintaining national standards for lenses, frames, contact lenses and low vision aids, among others. Allan passed away unexpectedly on January 7, 1986.

The company is run today by Allan's sons Jeffrey and Stuart.

LEHIGH OPTICAL

Elmer Joseph Faust was born in 1863 and, as a young man, borrowed money from an aunt to travel to Philadelphia to study watchmaking. Once he learned the trade, he and a variety of partners operated a jewelry and watch repair store in Allentown, Penn. Like many other watchmakers, he became interested in eyeglasses and, in 1899, graduated from the Chicago School of Optometry. He became the first optometrist in Allentown, examining eyes and fitting glasses at the rear of his jewelry store.

In 1912, Faust installed a shop in the back of the jewelry store to fabricate the glasses he sold. Several men trained with him in examining eyes and later opened their own offices. Faust began supplying frames and lenses to these optometrists. His became the first optical laboratory in Allentown. In 1918, he received a Pennsylvania license to practice optometry. His son Paul graduated from Philadelphia School of Optometry and opened an office on the second floor of his father's building. Seeing by now where his future was, Elmer moved his office and the lab upstairs and sold his interest in the jewelry store.

By this time, the Philadelphia School of Optometry was turning out many graduates and Lehigh Optical's salesman began traveling the state calling on them. The company also sold linen testers (a type of magnifier) which were used in the many textile mills in the area. Elmer was an accomplished musician and the family remembers many evenings spent listening to their Dad and his friends play chamber music in the family living room.

Elmer's son Henry graduated from Lehigh University in 1931 with a degree in Industrial Engineering. He joined his father at Lehigh Optical and when Elmer retired in

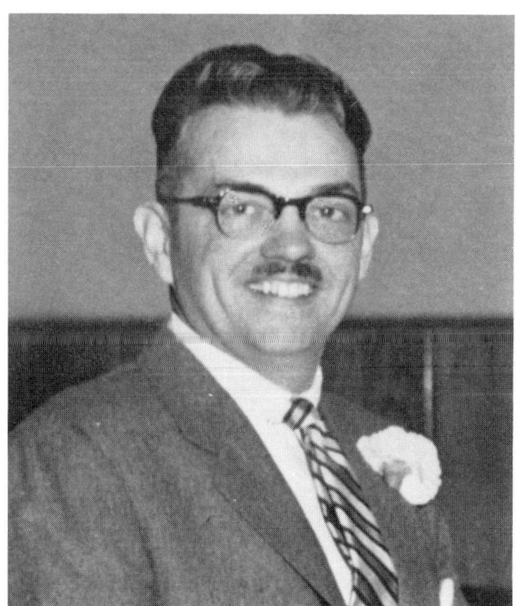

Henry J. Faust, son of the founder, headed the company from 1935 until his death in 1994.

1935, Henry took over the company. His father continued coming to the office every day for years. Henry's sister Louise joined the company in 1934, taking over the bookkeeping and making deliveries by trolley. Henry took over responsibility for sales as he was learning optics and the optical business. Lehigh was approached by Bausch & Lomb to buy the company but Henry turned them down.

Lehigh Optical was a member of the OWNA and Henry Faust served as an officer. Louise (Faust) Haddad retired in 1982 but Henry continued working until age 82 when he became ill. Henry's son Phillip, an MBA, came back to help run the office during his illness and Henry passed away in September, 1994. Fortunately, Henry had built a good team to back him up and the company continues serving Lehigh accounts in Pennsylvania, distributing frames as well as lab work. None of the third generation is interested in coming into the business and the family plans to sell the company.

MCLEOD OPTICAL (1922)

The company opened in downtown Providence in 1922 and operated in that location until they moved to Warwick in 1970. The original family at the time the company started consisted of Norman MacLeod, Sr., his sister Marina McLeod McKeil and brother Ed McLeod. Each learned the optical business at Dechau Optical, a wholesale laboratory in Providence until, pooling their resources, they came up with $1,000 to start a new business. Shuron extended them credit for a two-spindle surfacing machine, a torcyl cylinder machine, an edger and a handstone. The McLeods made a good team with Norm handling the surfacing, Ed doing finishing and Marina handling the paperwork. Whenever Norm got caught up in the surface room, he went out and made calls.

Their fiercest competitors were B&L and American Optical labs. Norm, Senior told of a time early in their operation when they were buying stock lenses for 60 cents and selling them for 90 cents. AO suddenly started selling the same lenses to retailers for 57 cents. Somehow, they were able to weather that kind of brutal competition.

Norm MacLeod and McLeod Optical played a pivotal role in the development of plastic lenses in this country. An English company, Combined Optical Industries Limited *(COIL)*, had developed an acrylic plastic lens in the 1930s called I-Gard. Following the second World War, COIL decided there were opportunities in this country for their plastic lens and established an I-Gard marketing operation in the U.S. They didn't have much luck getting labs to try this new material until, in 1949, an arrangement was made in which McLeod Optical became exclusive distributor for I-Gard in the U.S. Norm MacLeod knew most lab owners personally and COIL believed McLeod Optical's success with the lens would impress other labs. As a result of Norm MacLeod's efforts, a number of major independent labs took on the I-Gard lens. When Armorlite introduced the first CR-39 lens, it doomed the more easily scratched I-Gard lens, although McLeod continued to sell the cataract series *(it was the only plastic lens available for post-cataract use)* for another ten years. McLeod Optical also distributed COIL magnifiers for years and still carry the line.

Norm MacLeod made a major contribution to the development of plastic lenses in this country. Almost single-handedly, his company established that there was

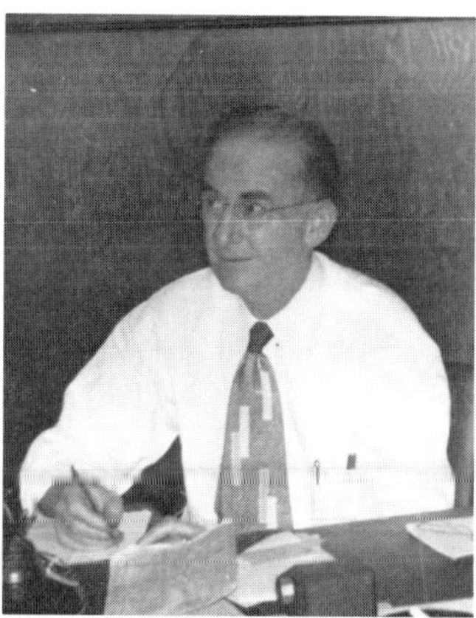

Ed McLeod, Senior, was Norm MacLeod's brother and one of the company founders. Photo was taken in 1949.

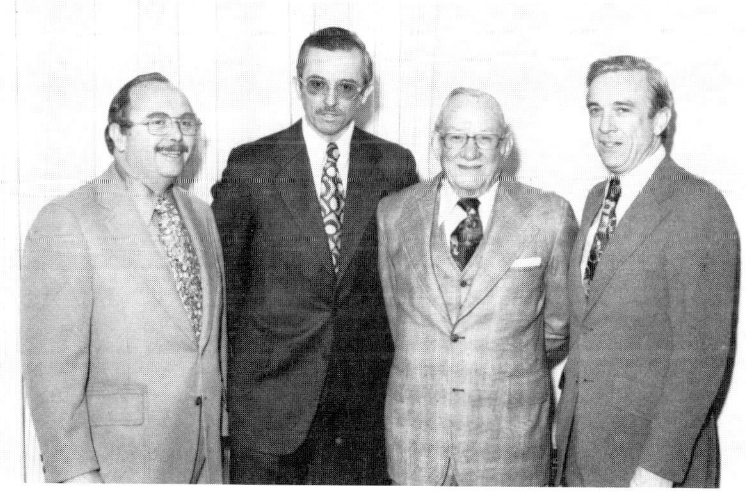

This photo, taken in 1980, shows, left to right, Ed McLeod, Wally MacLeod, Norm MacLeod and Norm MacLeod, Jr.

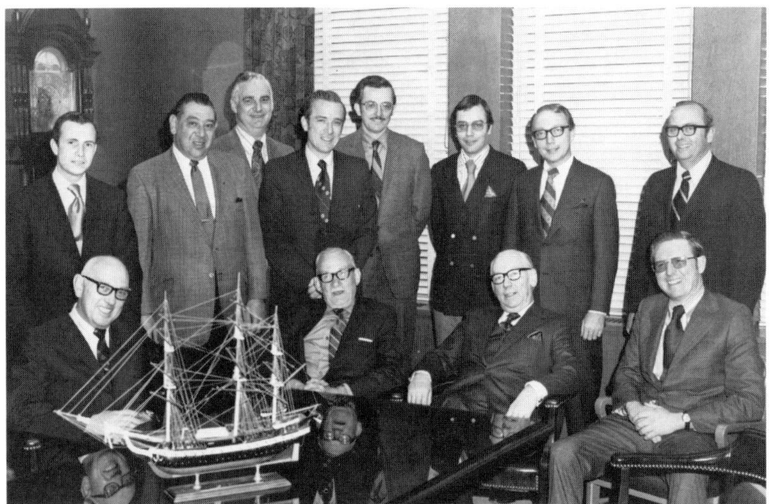

This photo was taken during a presentation from Universal Optical to McLeod Optical on their 50th anniversary in 1972. Seated are, left to right Perry Roberts, Norm MacLeod, Sr., Wally Murray, Sr. and Frank Kelleher (last two with Universal). Standing: Rod McLeod, Mel Beder, Don Wilber (Univ.), Norm MacLeod, Jr., Wally MacLeod, Steve Jobbins (Univ.), Wally Murray, Jr. (Univ.) and Ed McLeod.

PHOTO – McLEOD OPTICAL

a viable market for plastic lenses and McLeod Optical's efforts paved the way for the later success of Armorlite and other plastic lens manufacturers who followed.

Ed's son Edwin joined the company in 1950 after graduating from MIT and Norm's sons Norm, Jr. and Wally, each with degrees from the University of Rhode Island, came to work in 1952 and 1959 respectively. In 1960 the company purchased Belair, Taylor and Merritt Optical, giving McLeod branches in Springfield and Northampton, Mass. A new branch was opened in Waterbury, Conn. and an AO branch purchased in Augusta, Maine. A new branch was opened in Bangor in 1985 and, in 1986, they purchased Wooles Optical in Kittery, Maine. The Northampton and Springfield branches were eventually closed and McLeod Optical presently has 5 offices.

Norm Sr. served as president of the AIOW in 1947-49 and was actively involved in association affairs for many years, passing away in 1982. Current company officers are Edwin A. McLeod, Norman A. MacLeod and Wallace N. MacLeod. A third generation is now active with Ed's son Donald J. McLeod serving as manager of Augusta and Wally's sons Scott W. MacLeod as manager of Warwick and Roderick N. MacLeod serving as sales representative.

MIDWEST OPTICAL (1928)

Midwest Optical is an amalgamation of two optical families and illustrates the part that chance plays in destiny. The original company was founded in 1928, almost by accident. An optometrist named Joe Cline, having a four-man practice in downtown Dayton, received an offer in the mail to become an eyeglass case distributor . . . if he would place an initial order of 10,000 cases. Cline thought this to be a pretty good deal and approached his colleagues in Dayton, offering to share the order *(and the low prices)* if they split-up the initial order. Everyone agreed until the day the cases arrived in Dayton when Cline discovered all his buddies had changed their mind.

Dr. Cline was determined not to "eat" 10,000 cases and had the cases photographed, printed a flyer and bought a national list of optometrists. His first mailing *(nation-wide, excluding Dayton)*, sold out all 10,000 cases and was so successful, he immediately ordered another 10,000 cases. To speed up this story, Cline added frames, parts, accessories and eventually a laboratory to his growing mail-order business. He opened a branch in Cleveland and Trenton, N.J. and eventually left his optometry practice to devote full-time to the company he named Midwest Optical Supply. Then along came World War II.

Even though Dr. Joe Cline was in his late forties, he was determined to serve his country. He sold the Trenton branch to the government *(where G.I. glasses were produced)* and the Cleveland branch was sold to the manager *(it became State Optical but is no longer in business)*. Midwest's key people were brought back to Dayton to run that operation while Cline went off to war.

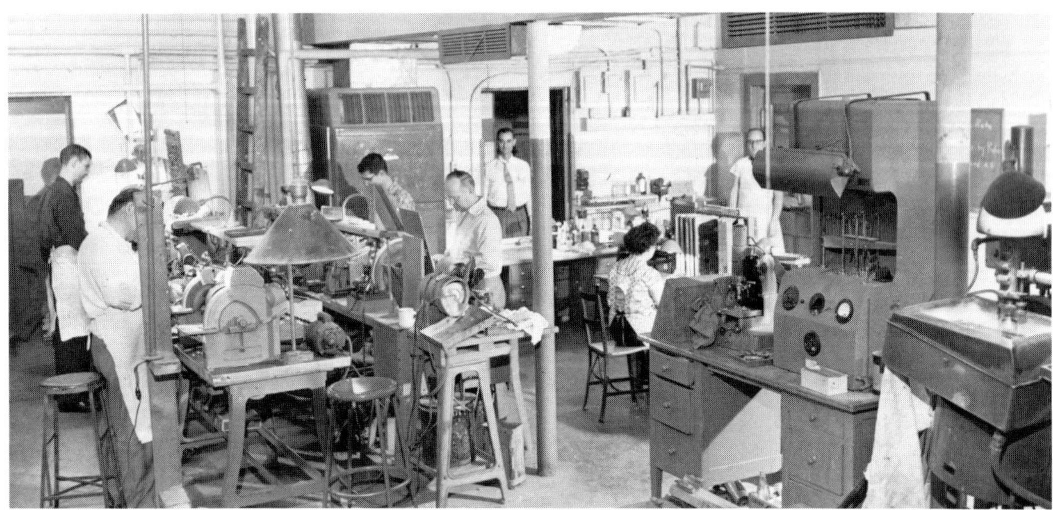

This late 1960s photo of Midwest Optical's lab includes the then-owner Robert Cline standing in the door at the back center.

PHOTO – MIDWEST OPTICAL

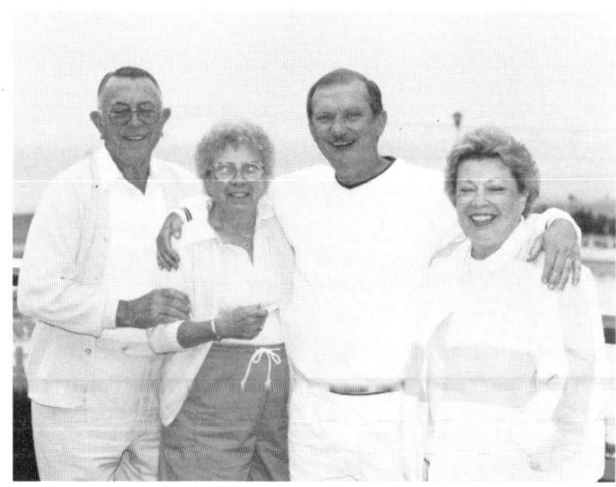

Photographed during a 1989 OLA Board Meeting in Newport, R.I. are Ed Ross and wife with then-OLA president Bill West and Barbara West.

Returning after the war, he was joined by his son Robert and the two ran Midwest as a mail order laboratory/supply house until 1978.

Now we turn our attention to the other family involved in this story. In 1946, R. F. Duffens sent a young man named Edward E. Ross to Ohio. Duffens knew of three Ohio labs for sale and he wanted Ross to determine which would be the best acquisition. Ross looked at all three, called Duffens and reported that the one in Dayton *(owned by the White family of Columbus, Ohio)* was the one to buy. Ross stayed in Dayton to manage this new Duffens lab until sometime in 1948 when Mr. Duffens called and told Ross the branch was going to be sold. Ross asked to have first chance at it and Duffens agreed. Shortly after that the branch name was changed to E.E. Ross Laboratories. The first thing Ross did was arrange for frame and lens distributorships, which he had little trouble doing. It was not until years later that Ross discovered R.F. Duffens had called every manufacturer and personally guaranteed Ross's bills for one year, backing Ed Ross without his knowledge. The story illustrates how personal the lab business was 50 years ago.

Ed Ross hired Bill West in 1949, making him a lab apprentice. Ross and West built a healthy business until 1965 when Ross Laboratories merged with Reese Optical. Three years later, in 1968, Bausch & Lomb concluded a deal to purchase Reese Optical. In 1971, Bill West was transferred to the west coast and in 1974, Steve Ross *(Ed's son)* became a sales representative for B&L following graduation from college.

When Bill West left B&L in 1977, he was San Francisco operations manager. He left to take a position with Uhlemann Optical in Chicago. During that time, he began negotiations with Robert Cline to purchase Midwest Optical in Dayton, his old home town. Steve Ross left B&L in early 1978 and by March, Bill and Steve

were working together under the Midwest banner.

Midwest had the distinction of being one of the first mail order labs in the country, pulling in Rx work and eyeglass case orders nationwide . . . yet, almost none of the work came from the Dayton area. Ross and West simply applied what they knew about regional marketing and began to expand the business locally which is now the strongest market for Midwest Optical. West and Ross never claimed to understand the mail order business, but strangely enough, they still service a few far flung mail accounts that have stuck with Midwest through the years —indicating they must be doing something right.

As a final twist, today Midwest Optical competes against the original E.E. Ross Laboratory — the one that ended up as a Reese Optical/B&L branch. When B&L exited the laboratory business, their Dayton branch was sold to Soderberg Optical.

NEW CITY OPTICAL (1931)

During the depths of the depression in 1931, Simon Gresser, an experienced surface man, got together with his friend Samuel Libowitz, a finishing lab man, to start a new lab they called New City Optical. Gresser got his start working in the Baltimore lab of Bowen & King, later moving to Richmond, Va. to work for Galeskie Optical. Arnold's mother hated Richmond and kept pestering her husband to move to a new city. She finally got her way because they eventually moved back to Baltimore and when Gresser and Libowitz set up their new company, they decided to name it "New City".

The new lab occupied 350 square feet. The initial equipment consisted of a Robinson-Houchins sphere pan, a STOCO Torcyl cylinder machine, a Shuron simplex edger, an Oldfield lap cutter and a set of trial lenses for final inspection.

Business was slow that first year but the founders were able to drum up a little business from local jewelers by grinding, shaping and fitting watch crystals. They had two optical accounts - an oculist named Dr. J.W. Barenburg and an optometrist named Jacob Staimen. Three labs were based in Baltimore; American Optical, Baltimore Optical *(eventually became Hilbert Optical and later Walman Optical)* and McIntyre, Magee and Brown *(later part of B&L)*.

New City Optical founder Simon Gresser with wife Sara. Sara didn't take to Richmond, Virginia when they lived there and kept asking Simon to move to a "new city". Thus the name of their new lab.

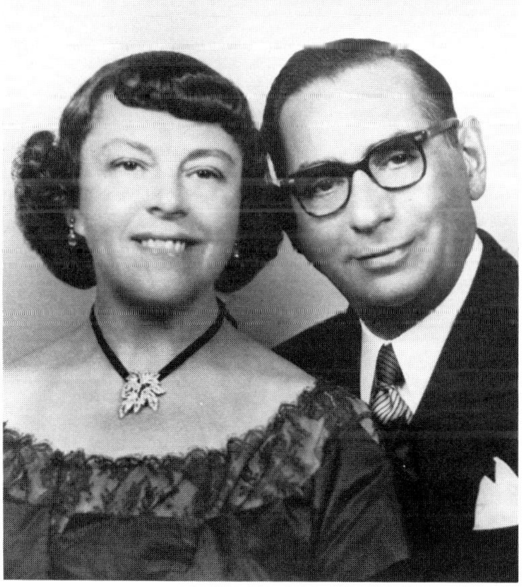

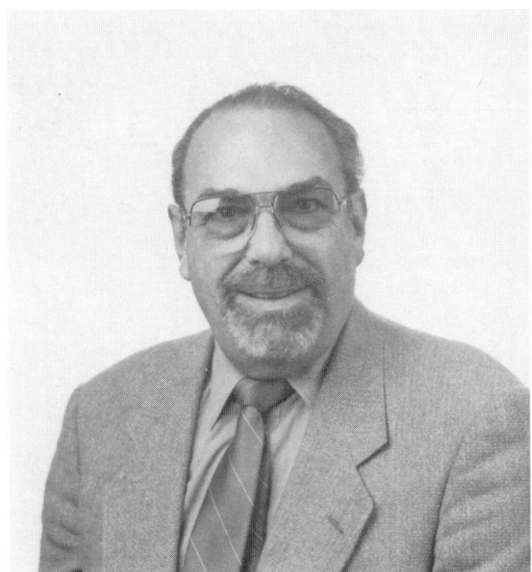

Arnold Gresser, son of the founder, is currently President/CEO of New City Optical.

Arnold Gresser's daughter Jodie Lynn currently works in Rx production for New City.

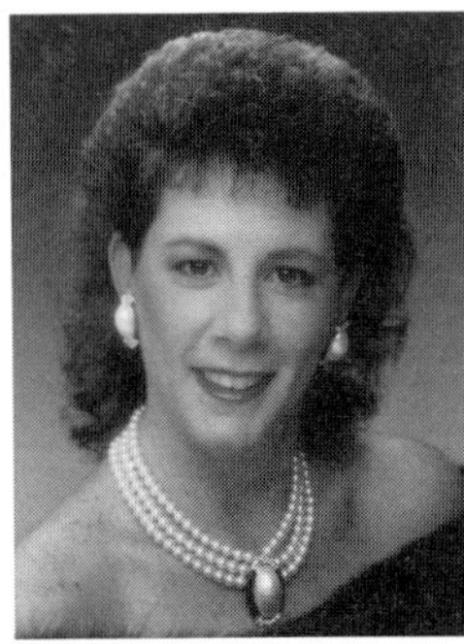

Once New City began soliciting wholesale accounts, they discovered two things. First, Baltimore accounts only wanted to deal with AO or B&L and, second, AO would no longer loan them tools *(loaning tools was a frequent courtesy extended between competitive labs).* That convinced New City needed more accounts. They sent out a mailing on one cent postcards to optometrists and oculists from Providence to Richmond and the business generated by that mailing got them started. The company grew steadily during the 1930s. Glasses were shipped by U.S. Mail in those days when the postal service delivered everything within 500 miles the following day, beyond 500 miles in 2 days.

The company soon added frames to their product line. They became an Art Craft distributor in 1936 and sold frames from Florida to Texas to Tennessee and into New England. Despite the depression, the company's Rx business continued to grow and the company soon employed seven people in the shop. The war years slowed the company's growth because most shop people were in the service and obtaining lenses was almost impossible. The lab had an edging line of 10 Simplex edgers all cranking out lenses. They ran their Simplex edgers until they wore out. The partners would then replace bearings and stone, slap a coat of paint on it and sell the edger to a retailer.

Simon Gresser's son Arnold remembers traveling as a child with his father to Petersburg, Virginia during the war. Simon would take the back seat out of the car and go down to Titmus Optical, take lenses directly off the production line, wrap them in toilet tissue and load them in the back seat. Arnold remembers helping sort the blanks out into stacks of white, Velvetlite A and Velvetlite B when they got back to Baltimore. Producing a simple pair of spheres during the war often meant surfacing both sides of the lenses.

After the war, the company opened their first branch in the Edmonds Building in Washington, D.C. but this office eventually moved back to Baltimore during the early '70s. A second branch was opened in Richmond in 1960 and another in Norfolk at the end of that same year. New City Optical joined the OWNA in 1956 and the Gressers attended their first convention in Cincinnati.

Arnold remembers visiting Oscar Heilman's lab during the convention. Simon Gresser died in 1959. Samuel Libowitz had died earlier when he was only 50.

Arnold worked in the lab during school vacations but was determined to make his career in a different field. He learned shorthand and wanted to work for the Baltimore & Ohio Railroad as a male stenographer. It was unheard of in those days for women to travel with their boss so male stenographers answered the problem. The night he graduated from school, Arnold told his father he was going to work for the railroad for $80 a week. His father offered him $30 a week, a $5 raise over what he had been making part time. His father's argument was that he would learn a trade in the family business and who knew what the B&O might do a year down the line? It was a tough decision to make but, 42 years later, Arnold is still learning his trade.

Gresser spent the first 21 years traveling for the company, 30 weeks out of the year. The first year he was married, he was only home between Thanksgiving and Christmas. Today, New City is a family business that serves the mid and south Atlantic region and employs more than 100 people. The company is still active in the frame business. Arnold Gresser, son of the founder is president and CEO, having purchased the company in 1967. His daughter Jodie also works for the company as a technician in Rx production. One of the company's latest projects has been making lenses for "virtual reality" helmets for the aerospace industry.

ROONEY OPTICAL (1928)

29 year old Frank D. "Pat" Rooney was wholesale sales manager of W.A. Jones Optical at the time American Optical purchased the Jones wholesale division. Rooney took this as a sign it was time for him to go into business for himself. He set up offices in the C.A.C. Building in downtown Cleveland. One of the first employees he hired was Fred E. Blauman who became general manager and minority stockholder. Blauman had come from King Optical where he was general manager. With the

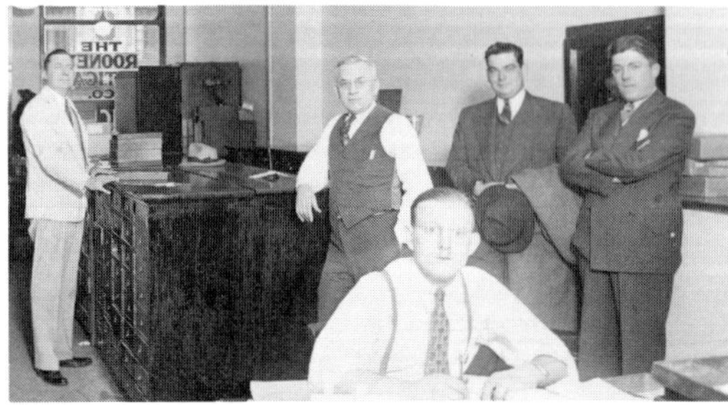

This late 1930s photograph includes, standing at left, Clayton Woodall, to his right is Fred Blauman and at far right is Paul Dougher.

company growing, Rooney found a young man named Paul Dougher selling pianos in Warren, Ohio and hired him as salesman in the fall of 1929.

Cleveland was a tough market for optical wholesalers but in spite of this, Rooney Optical soon made it's presence known. In 1939, Pat Rooney died and Fred Blauman, James Barnes, Paul Dougher, Clayton Woodall and Blanche FitzGerald purchased the company from Rooney's widow. Fred Blauman became president and the others became company directors who would effectively manage the company for the next 15 years. Like most other wholesalers at that time, Rooney Optical also did some retail business but discontinued it in 1950.

Two more Doughers joined the company, Paul's sons Gerald J. Dougher in 1956 and James P. Dougher in 1957. They came in with the understanding that the Dougher family would purchase controlling interest. When Fred Blauman retired in 1963, all remaining original stockholders retired as well, except for Paul Dougher. Paul Dougher was elected chairman of the board and Gerald J. Dougher became president.

When Paul Dougher passed away in 1965, Gerald's brother James became executive vice president. The remaining stockholders, Jack Mastellar, Sr. and John Stang filled the remaining corporate offices. Following John Stang's death in 1978, Stang's stock was purchased by the Dougher family along with Jack Marstellar's shares when he retired from handling sales. The company by now was wholly owned by the Dougher family. After 23 years in the C.A.C. Building and another 15 years at the corner of East 9th Street and Prospect Avenue, the company moved to their present location on 164th Street.

Branch Operations

Service was the name of the laboratory game and Rooney established branches to serve their growing customer base. Youngstown was established in 1937, Canton in 1960, Sandusky in 1970, Latrobe, Pa. in 1979 and Evansville, Ind. in 1982. Rapid delivery systems became more readily available, eliminating the need for regional branches and most branches were closed. Only Rooney Optical of Pennsylvania in Latrobe remains active. The company's commitment to customer service is still paramount as demonstrated by their establishment of a new division in 1993. Called 3-D Optical Coatings Laboratories, Inc., the new division is equipped with the large Satis unit and provides state-of-the-art AR coatings in a timely fashion.

Not long after the company started business they joined both wholesaler associations. Blauman served as director of the AIOW and Paul Dougher was vice president of the

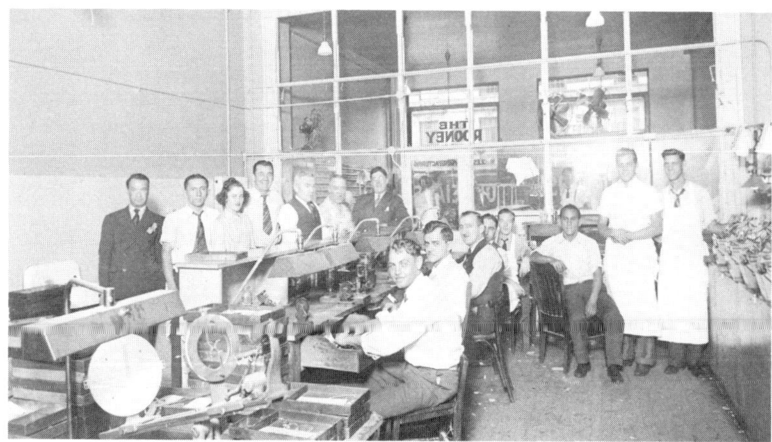

Photographed in the late 1930s, the finishing room crew is ready for the Monday morning rush.

PHOTO – ROONEY OPTICAL

OWNA. After the two associations merged to form the OWA, Paul's son Gerry became President in 1972-73. The Doughers have always been active in association work and expect the third generation to continue this family tradition.

Today, Rooney Optical is truly a full-service company, manufacturing glass, plastic, polycarbonate and high index lenses as well as RGP contact lenses. They distribute frames, stock lenses, soft contact lenses, solutions and ophthalmic equipment. The third generation of the Dougher family is firmly in place and continues the Dougher heritage of top service and quality. Jim has two sons, Mike, in charge of production and Barney, serving as Sales Manager. Gerry's son Kevin has a law degree and serves as company counsel.

When Ellis Katz was OWA president *(1972),* he and Gerry Dougher had the responsibility of finding a new executive director for the OWA. After interviewing a number of applicants, the two selected Irby Hollans, the man who still fills that position today.

SODERBERG OPTICAL (1945)

It was 1913 when the first Soderberg became involved in the optical business through an investment made in a new Minneapolis dispensing firm started by two men named Benson and Walman. Less than two years later, Benson and Walman decided to split up. Walman left the firm to go downstairs and set up his own company which he called Walman Optical. Fred Soderberg remained on the Benson Optical Board of Directors until just before the stock market collapse in 1929, when he astutely sold his Benson stock to Les Meyers and several others. Soderberg, from

The 1994 Rooney team - left to right, Gerry Dougher, Kevin Dougher, Barney Dougher, Jim Dougher and Mike Dougher.

PHOTO – ROONEY OPTICAL

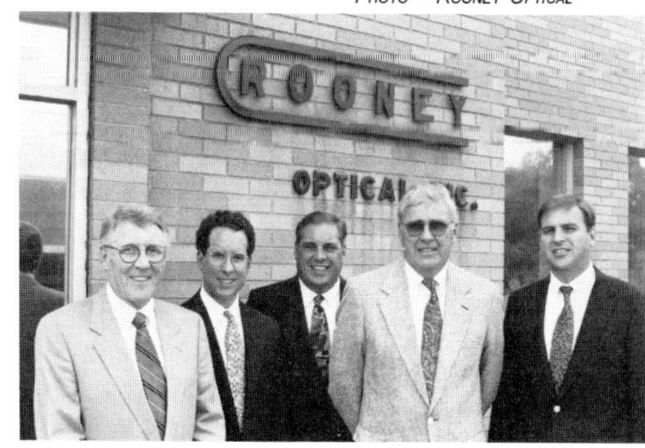

Sweden, came to Minnesota in 1890 earing the name Jonsson. He discovered that every other man in Minnesota was named Johnson. Since he had come from the south of Sweden in the hill country, he took the name Soderberg which translates as "Southern Hill".

Fred had a son named Frederick A. Soderberg. Young Fred graduated from the University of Minnesota in 1938 to find the country in the midst of another business slump. He went to Benson Optical looking for a job but was told they couldn't pay him what a college man would want. Taking an elevator downstairs, he applied at Walman and got a job working in the surface room for $12 a week *(aided by his university degree)*. They gave him the dirtiest job in the shop, polishing spheres with red rouge.

In 1945, Soderberg decided he was ready to set up his own business. Joining forces with Clarence North, they bought a dispensing business from four oculists and then raised the money to set up a lab by selling stock to the doctors *(the same process used when Benson Optical started)*. Their first major decision was to decide who should be president. Fred said, "Let's flip a coin. Heads, you're president, tails I am." The coin turned up tails. Following Bernie Spero's *(House of Vision)* example, they had all their new machinery painted white and installed windows between the lab and the dispensing area so the public could see it in action.

A year and a half later, Soderberg bought out Clarence North. In 1950, Soderberg Optical opened their first branch office in Mankato, Minn. The company continued to grow, primarily because Soderberg had been well trained in every phase of business. While he was with Walman, he had worked in both surfacing and finishing departments and gained valuable experience running Walman's St. Paul branch. This experience turned out to be perfect training for running the company he was building.

Rebating to referring oculists was a common practice at this time, but Soderberg had begun attending A.I.O.W. meetings and learned that rebating would eventually become illegal. Soderberg Optical ceased all rebates in 1947 so when the government stepped in and sued everyone, Soderberg Optical was not involved. In 1950, the company installed the 47th generator Shuron ever produced. Their surface foreman took one look at it and said, "It ain't going to work!"

By 1955, Soderberg realized the company had to be either wholesale or retail, not both. The company got out of dispensing by selling the St. Paul dispensing business *(the only branch where they dispensed)* to the man who still runs it today as Northwest Opticians.

Early on, Soderberg recognized the value of a lab association and started attending A.I.O.W. meetings two years after his company was founded. Fred was close friends with Bill Coburn and became one of Coburn's earliest customers. Shuron Optical and Univis Lens Company were also good friends to the company. Soderberg was selling in the same market as Walman and Benson and obtaining Shuron and Univis listings was crucial to the young company. Roy Marks, written about elsewhere in this history, was a close friend of Soderberg's. Fred and Roy spent a great deal of time together and became close friends.

In 1957, Fred Soderberg was elected president of the A.I.O.W. During his term of office, the A.I.O.W. was involved in a federal lawsuit. Fred remembers a day when he was questioned under oath from 9:00 a.m. until past 3:30 p.m. The action was primarily against American Optical and Bausch & Lomb with the A.I.O.W. only marginally involved. Al Marsters, representing Bausch & Lomb and Victor Kniss, representing American Optical also gave depositions that day. AO had four attorneys at the meeting, B&L had two and several more were there representing the U.S. Government. As it turned out later, the Justice Department was particularly incensed with Victor Kniss because of some of his overt actions at AO. Both B&L and AO had serious concerns over possible damage from the government suit. Fred remembers sitting on Otto Batzli's back porch with Otto, Marsters, Kniss and several others. Kniss, who may have been more worried than he admitted, leaned over to Fred and said, "If I go to jail, there's one other person going with me!" Fred, A.I.O.W. president at the time, asked him who that would be. Kniss' answer was, "You!" For some weird reason, AO blamed the independent labs for all their legal problems, perhaps with some justice since it was usually complaints from long-suffering independent labs that launched the government investigations.

Today, Soderberg Optical has 15 offices, each complete with laboratories and located, for the most part, in company-owned buildings. The company has five contact lens labs and is estimated to be the 5th largest laboratory in the country. Ten of the company's branches were acquisitions of branches of other companies such as Bausch & Lomb, Barnett and Ramel, Fluegge Optical and other independent labs. Fred's son Tom Soderberg

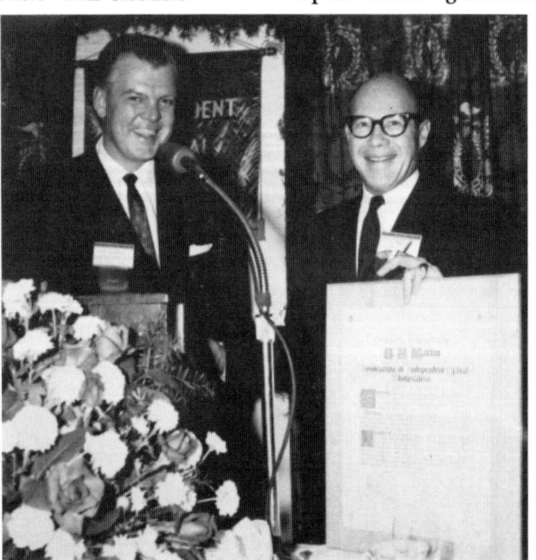

When J.A. "Al" Martin (Uhlemann Optical) left office as AIOW President in 1959, Past President Fred Soderberg (left) presented him with a testimonial plaque.

PHOTO – FRED SODERBERG

runs the company's Milwaukee branch. The company has established a long tradition of service to the industry. Three Soderberg people have served as association presidents - Fred Soderberg in 1958, Robert Honsa in 1980 and Soderberg Optical's current president Al Willenbring served as OLA president in 1993. The company will be celebrating their 50th anniversary in 1995 and Fred Soderberg expects to collect his 50 year service pin that year.

SOUTHERN OPTICAL (1938)

The Sloan family's optical involvement really dates back to 1808 when Tom Sloan's great-great-grandfather, Isaac Salomon, began selling eyeglasses in Dusseldorf, Germany. The family has an 1813 newspaper clipping showing an ad for that company's glasses. The same paper includes a news story of Napoleon's latest campaign, two years before the Battle of Waterloo. Isaac taught the trade to his son Jacob. Jacob passed it on to his son Richard and Richard to his son Harry.

It was Hitler's campaign, however, that drove the 4th generation of Sloan opticians out of Germany. Harry Sloan landed in New York in 1938 with $50 in his pocket, possessing little English and knowing nothing of American business customs. To gain experience, he worked for several months at no pay in what he later described as "sweatshop conditions". Discovering an ad for an optician placed by a High Point optometrist, Harry boarded a train for North Carolina where he worked for the optometrist before opening up a wholesale optical business with his cousin Arthur S. Sloan in 1938. Shortly after that, he married an Austrian woman he met in North Carolina and they later had two sons, Frank and Thomas.

The company grew slowly because the North Carolina market was dominated by American Optical. During the '40s, they were located in several rented rooms in an office building. Their break came as World War II ended. Most labs on the European continent had been wiped out and Harry Sloan was able to renew old friendships and start exporting lenses to Europe. For a period of time, Southern was a major international trader, sending lenses to Switzerland, France, Norway, Sweden and even South America. By 1950 most of the European labs had reestablished themselves and Southern turned their attention to the local market.

Harry's son Frank, in the meantime, having no interest in the family business, earned a Ph.D. in economics at Harvard University and holds a chair in health economics at Duke University. Frank's brother Tom was determined he should follow his ancestors and join the family business. After working summer jobs in the lab, he attended the University of Rochester, the only college at the time offering degrees in optics. After earning both

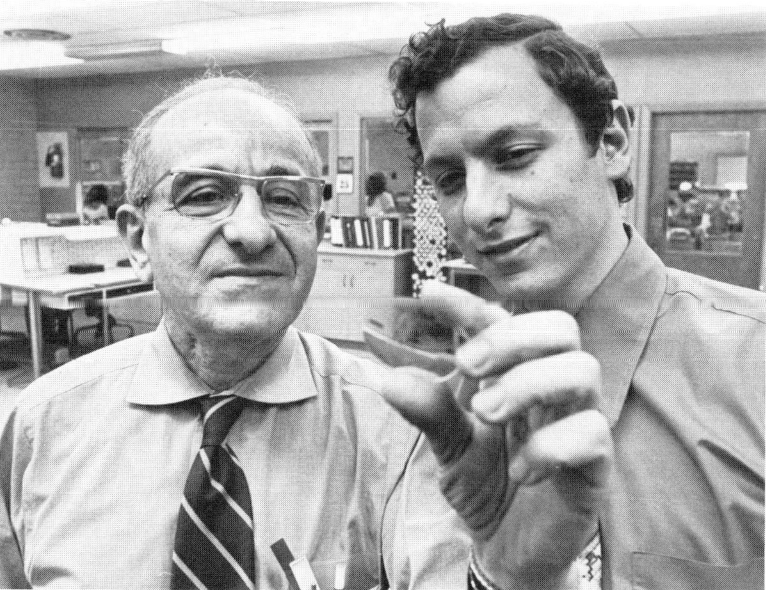

In this early 1970s. photo, Southern Optical founder Harry Sloan shows his son Tom the finer points in checking out a lens.

PHOTO – SOUTHERN OPTICAL

bachelor's and master's degrees in optics, he worked for the Itek Corporation in lens engineering and design while completing an MBA program at Northeastern University in Boston. In 1970, having proven himself in the outside world, he was ready to return to Greensboro and join his father's company as vice president.

Tom Sloan took over as president in 1975 with his father becoming Chairman of the Board. In 1986, Southern Optical merged with the R.P. Scherer Corporation of Troy, Michigan with Tom continuing to run the company as president. Shortly after that merger, Southern Optical acquired Williams Optical Laboratory in Nashville, and subsequently several other locations. Southern operated as a wholly-owned subsidiary of R.P. Scherer Corp. until late 1989 when Scherer became involved in a leveraged buy-out and desired to sell off all its non-core business units. At that time, Tom Sloan led a management group in purchasing the company so that it once again became an independently-owned enterprise.

Today the company operates 12 manufacturing locations in eight states throughout the Southeast. It operates two separate divisions: one geared to manufacturing spectacles and the second involved in selling and servicing diagnostic ophthalmic instruments. Their operations include:

> Southern Optical in Greensboro, N.C., Richmond, VA and Greenville, S.C.
>
> Southern-Piedmont Optical in Goldsboro, N.C, Southern-Pioneer Optical in Bristol, Tenn.
>
> Southern-Williams Optical in Nashville, Tenn., Leeds, Ala., Jackson, Miss., Scott, La.
>
> Southern-Reid Optical, Stone Mountain, Ga., Dothan, Ala.
>
> Southern-Monroe Optical, Monroe, N.C.

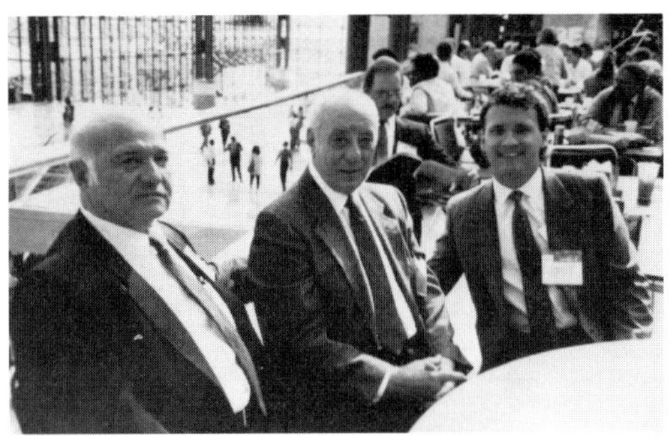

Pictured during the 1986 Vision Expo show in New York's Jacob Javits Center are, left to right, Bill Benedict, Irving Greenberg and Charlie Pendrell. After Benedict sold Omega, Pendrell was brought in to set up the company's new LiteStyle production line, working closely with Benedict who remained as a consultant with Omega.

Southern has traditionally been a leader in introducing new technologies and new products to the industry. Southern was the first Varilux distributor east of the Rockies when they made a major commitment to distribute this new lens in 1977. Today it is one of the leading suppliers of this product in the nation. The company was also one of the first to install their own in-house AR coating facility eight years ago and has since expanded it.

SUTHERLIN OPTICAL (1939)

About the same time Hitler's army crashed into Poland, Edward H. Sutherlin was quitting his job with Lancaster Optical in Kansas City to launch a new laboratory with two partners. The year was 1939 and the company name was Burow-Sutherlin Optical. Within a year, Sutherlin bought out his partners and changed the company name to Sutherlin Optical, a name that's been part of the Kansas optical scene for more than 50 years.

Sutherlin was determined to set up a first class lab. Their first price list reveals that customers could order any bifocal they wanted as long as it was a Kryptok or an Ultex. First division compound bifocals were supplied, cut and edged for $2.25. If you wanted them mounted in a frame, you paid 25 cents more. Polished edges could be ordered for 15 cents extra. First quality single vision lenses were 80 cents edged to a zyl or metal frame. For rimless, the price jumped to $1.15 a pair.

The Sutherlin family has always been responsive to changing technology and the evolving marketplace. Their laboratory today is state-of-the-art and the Sutherlin

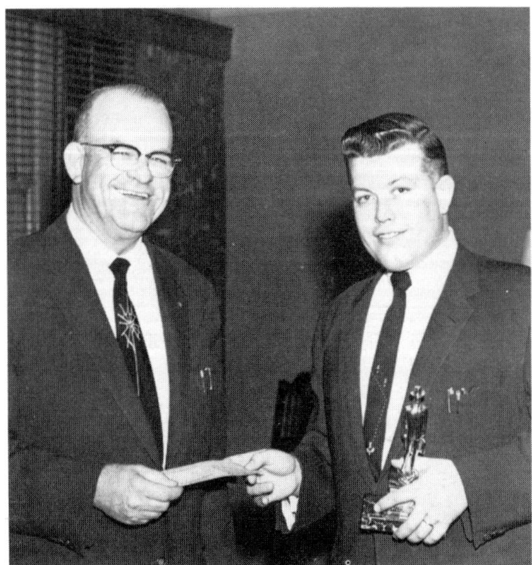

Edward H. Sutherlin presented his son, Ed L. Sutherlin, present-day head of Sutherlin Optical, with a "Salesman of the Year" award (and a check) during the 1950s.

family still runs the company. Edward H.'s son Ed L. Sutherlin heads the company with the assistance of his sons Steven, Michael and John. Ed L. Sutherlin served as president of the OLA in 1978.

TEXAS LABS

For nearly 40 years, there has been a certain mystique about "big volume Texas" labs. Labs producing eyeglasses in large volume are certainly not restricted to the state of Texas, but the concept of high volume production did begin in that state and it all came from the efforts of a man named Irving Greenberg.

Southwestern Optical

The first high volume, mail order laboratory, the kind of laboratory the industry has come to think of as a "Texas" lab, was Southwestern Optical, established during the '30s by Al Bogart. Bogart had come out of the clothing business in New York. As a result of some union trouble he was having, some gentlemen Bogart later described as "Mafia" called on him and told him to get out of town. He wasn't inclined to argue with them.

Landing in Texas, Bogart ended up working in an optical lab. One day in 1942, a young man named Bill Benedict walked in his door looking for a job. Bogart offered him a job as janitor. Benedict agreed to take the job on the condition that he also would be taught the optical business. In those days before generators, everything was hand surfaced. Bogart's company was turning out 50 jobs per day. During this period, three remarkable lab men were employed at Southwestern - Irv Greenberg, Sylvan Ray and Bill Benedict. When World War II began, Greenberg left to join the Army and help set up their mobile optical units. Benedict left to serve in the Navy. Following the war, both men came back to Southwestern. That was when the job flow began to increase from work coming in from the growing chain of Lee Optical retail stores. Southwestern production rose to 400 jobs per day. Greenberg was beginning to develop his mass production theories and these were all passed on to Benedict. Eventually, Greenberg left Southwestern and Bogart made Benedict general manager.

Dal-Tex Optical

Irv Greenberg was convinced that eyeglasses could be produced on a mass-production basis and he started Dal-Tex to prove his theories. Greenberg was a remarkable man. Benedict calls him the "Big Daddy" of the mass-production lab concept. He was an innovator and a teacher and Benedict credits much of his optical knowledge to what he learned from Greenberg while they were both at Southwestern. Dal-Tex soon became the largest lab in the country and everyone assumed there could only be one "giant" lab.

Associated Optical

Meanwhile Sylvan Ray had started Associated Optical in 1950. Associated went national in the late 1950s when Sylvan Ray made a trip to California. Before long, the company was pulling most of its business from California and Texas, with 95 percent coming from outside the Dallas market.

International Optical

Benedict, still at Southwestern, wanted to share in what he was producing and offered to buy 20 percent of the company in 1959. Bogart turned him down cold. Benedict left Southwestern and started a company called International Optical. Six months later, Bogart called Benedict and offered him the 20 percent free if he would return but it was too late. International Optical, established in 1959, was active for 15 years.

Among the lab people who developed "big lab" production techniques working with Bill Benedict at International Optical were John Payne *(Icare Industries)*, Charles Pendrell *(Sierra Optical)*, Bill Sullivan and Buddy Lucas *(Omega)*, Bill Copeland *(Laser Optics)* and Drs. Shannon and Damron *(Apache Optical)*. By 1960, there were now three "Texas" mass-production labs in operation — Dal-Tex, Associated and International.

Pearle Vision

The first time Bill Benedict met Stanley Pearle was as he delivered a pair of glasses for Southwestern to Dr. Pearle's office in downtown Dallas *(by bicycle)*. At that time, Dr. Pearle was running an optometric department in a Zales Jewelry store. Some years later, Dr. Pearle had 14 retail stores of his own, which he had taken in trade for his interest in Lee Optical. Dr. Pearle and Bill Benedict decided to merge Pearle's 14 stores with Benedict's International Optical to form a new company they called Opticks, Inc. based in Georgia. Their first store opened in Savannah. This partnership lasted 14 years and their joint efforts made Opticks so successful it was ultimately acquired by a conglomerate, the Will Ross Company, who operated it as Pearle Vision *(Will Ross was later acquired by G.D. Searle)*. Before long, Benedict found working with the conglomerate mentality too much and retired.

Omega Lab

Retirement lasted for two years and ended for Benedict when he came roaring out of retirement to set up a new lab called Omega. He built the building, installed all new equipment and on the day the doors opened, hired 50 new employees. At the time Omega opened in 1972, the company had one salesman *(in California)*. Benedict got on the phone and personally called all his previous customers. Within three weeks, Omega was processing more than 500 jobs a day and in four months Benedict reached his original goal of 1,000 jobs per day.

Omega then purchased Hensel Optical and, in 1974, added Champion Optical. Some time later, Omega purchased the wholesale operation of International Optical as well as the company that gave Benedict his first optical job, Southwestern Optical. Precision Optical lab in Minnesota was then acquired along with Milroy's two labs *(Chicago and Florida)* and Optimum Optics *(later closed)*. Three years after opening, Omega became the first wholesale laboratory to go public. By the time Benedict sold Omega Optical to Optical Radiation Corporation, the company was processing 10,000 jobs a day, 4,000 in the branches and the balance in the Dallas lab.

Optical Radiation had developed LiteStyle polycarbonate lenses and needed a company to distribute what they felt would be the lens of the future. They ended up buying Omega as a vehicle to distribute LiteStyle. Benedict remained with Omega for one year following the sale before heading out, once again, to retirement.

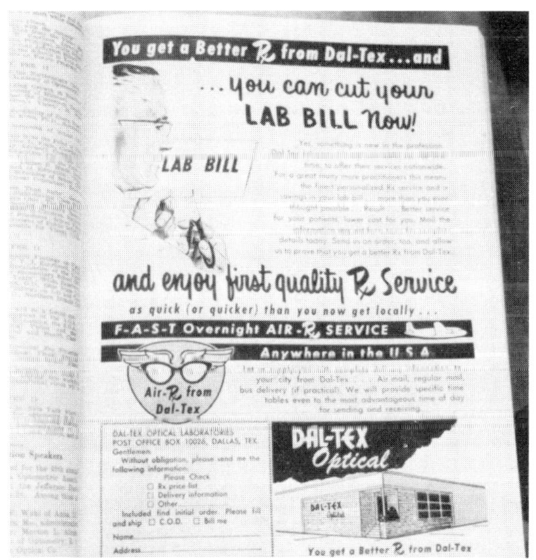

Dal-Tex was the first high volume, mass-production mail order Texas lab and their early ads antagonized local area labs all over the country.

Family Tree of the "Texas" Labs

SOUTHWESTERN OPTICAL — Al Bogart, Sylvan Ray, Bill Benedict, Irving Greenberg

ASSOCIATED OPT. — 1958 — Sylvan Ray

INTERNATIONAL — 1959 — Bill Benedict

DALTEX — 1956 — Irving Greenberg

PEARLE OPT. — Dr. Stanley Pearle

OPTICS

ROYAL OPTICAL — Irving Greenberg, Benton Markey

LASER OPTICAL — Bill Copeland

OMEGA — 1972 — Bill Benedict

APACHE OPTICAL — Dr. Shannon, Dr. Damron

BENEDICT OPTICAL — 1990 — Bill Benedict

This diagram illustrates how the mass-production fever spread out from the original concepts of Irv Greenberg.

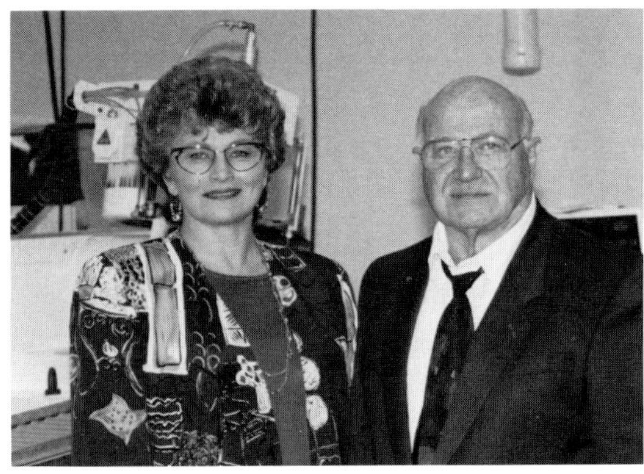

Benedict Optical's founders Donna and Bill Benedict photographed in 1994 in their polycarbonate facility.

Benedict Optical

Benedict's non-compete clause expired in 1990 and, once again, he came out of retirement, this time to set up Benedict Optical with his daughter Donna. By 1994, the company has outgrown their facilities. Their polycarbonate laboratory is in a different location and a much larger plant is already in the planning stage. The Texas "big lab mystique" is still alive.

WALMAN OPTICAL (1915)

Today's Walman Optical chain grew from a single lab founded in 1915 in downtown Minneapolis by optician John A. L. Walman. Leaving Sweden to come to the new country, young Walman attended optometric school in Chicago and continued his training in St. Paul before finally settling down in Minneapolis. In 1913, he and fellow Swede, N.P. Benson, opened an optical firm. The partnership only lasted a year before Walman left to form his own *company (N.P. Benson went on to found Benson Optical).* Walman's company grew slowly with branch offices opened in Grand Forks, N.D. (1922), St. Paul (1928) and Fargo (1932). By 1937, the company employed 45 people in four offices.

In 1939, Mr. Walman began what turned out to be eight years of declining health, followed by his death. Company management during this period was turned over to son-in-law Clarence Welling. Meanwhile, a young man named Otto Batzli had been hired during the mid-1930s to work in the stockroom. Otto Batzli became

This early photograph was taken in Walman's lab in 1917. Founder J.A.L. Walman can be seen in the doorway at the right rear of photo.

majority stockholder and president of the company in 1946, shortly after John Walman died. Batzli acquired 52 percent of the company stock from Walman's widow.

By this time, the company had five labs. Through the 1950s, a new branch was opened every other year. Bob Morrow began working in the Fargo branch surface room for $6 a week in 1937. He was brought into Minneapolis as vice-president in the 1950s after stops in Austin, Minnesota and St. Paul. Shortly before Batzli's death in 1967, his controlling interest was sold to a group of stockholders, all company employees. Morrow was named president in 1968 following Batzli's retirement and held the position for 10 years before creating a new position of chairman. At the time Morrow became president the company was doing $3 million annually. Within a year, sales nearly doubled and by the time of Morrow's transition to chairman of the board, sales had increased 13-fold and employees had grown from 100 to 700.

In the early 1960s, a young man named Ed Reindl started a new job in the lab at Treasure State Optical in Butte, Mont. Within months of his starting, the company was purchased by Walman Optical. Reindl was later made manager of the company's Rock Island, Ill. branch. By 1983, Reindl became president, taking over from Bob Morrow's brother Jack. In 1981, the company expanded to the east coast, buying the former Hilbert Optical Company which added 5 more labs in Virginia, Pennsylvania and Maryland.

In 1986, the company set up Ultra Optics, a company-owned division that markets coated lenses and coating

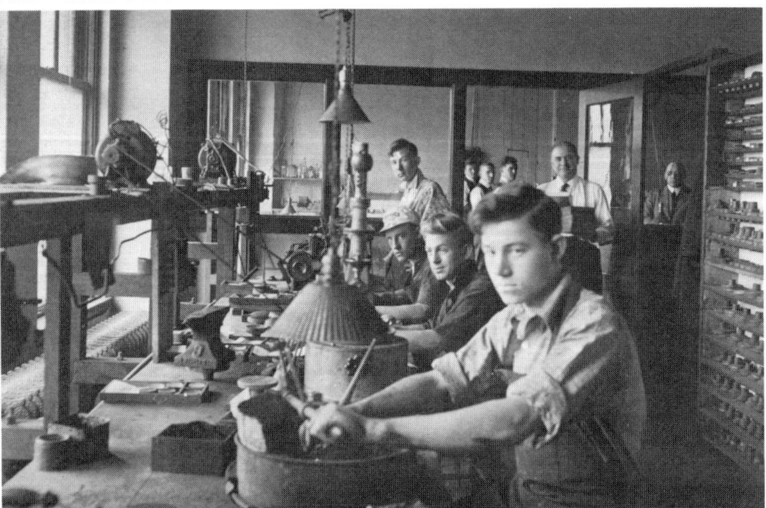

Otto Batzli, shown here, became Walman president in 1946, running the company until his death in 1967.

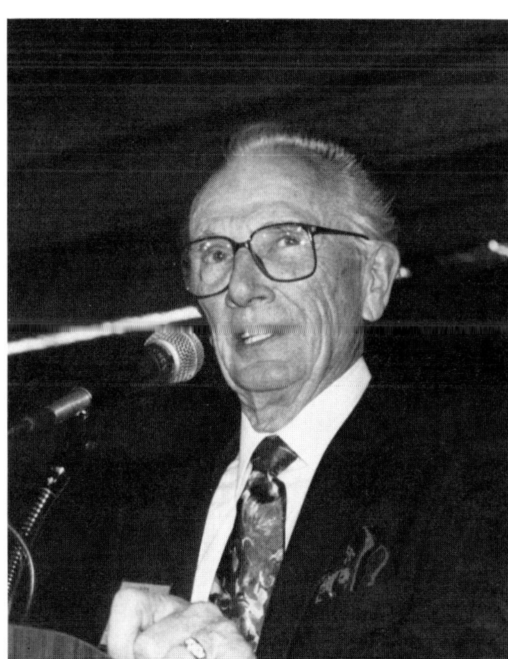

Robert Morrow shown accepting the 1993 OLA Directors' Choice Award of Excellence. Morrow took over as president when Walman Optical was doing $3 million annually and increased sales 13-fold.

equipment. Poly Optics was founded jointly with Vision-Ease to manufacture polycarbonate lenses. Today, the company has 30 branch offices and is wholly owned by its 700 employees.

VICTORY OPTICIANS (1945)

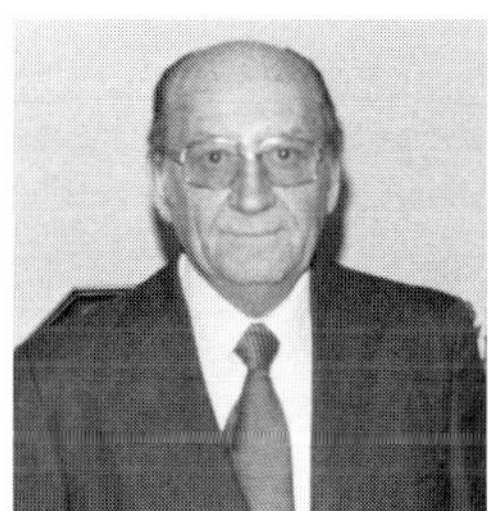

Victory Opticians was founded by Harry Rack photographed here on New Year's Eve, 1975.

Harry Rack had been a bookkeeper with Fluegge Optical in Milwaukee, Wis. when World War II ended. Rack and a Fluegge salesmen named Roz Williams formed a partnership called Rack & Williams. The partnership didn't last long and Harry left to form Victory Opticians while Roz joined Benson Optical, where he served with their sales department for years. Victory Opticians operated as a wholesale-only laboratory until 1978 when the company moved to a new larger building and changed directions by putting greater emphasis on retail operations. They continued to do wholesale and industrial safety work, however.

In 1957, Harry's son Derek joined the company, working through every department in the lab as he learned the optical trade. Derek's brother David also worked in Victory's lab production until his early death at age 29.

When Derek married, the company purchased Rockford Optical, a laboratory in Rockford, Illinois and the young Racks spent their first married years in Rockford. Derek remembers calling on the author's father, Dr. Louis Bruneni, in practice with Dr. Wallace Duncan in Rockford. Victory still operates Rockford Optical and has opened a second store on the East side of Rockford. They also have a branch in Delavan, Wisconsin. All branches are retail operations.

Harry Rack passed away in 1976 and Derek took over direction of the company. His daughter Debbie Rack does the buying and handles all advertising for the company. Her brother Robert, who is much like his grandfather, Harry Rack, is the one they call when anything breaks down on the production line. Robert also oversees the computer department. Derek's wife Bernadette is in charge of the company's financial department.

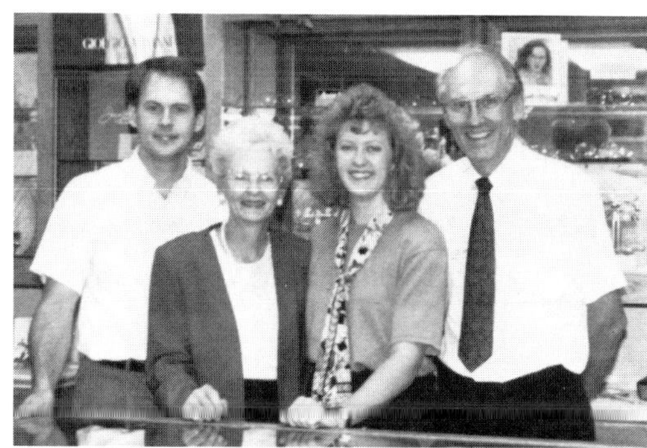

Derek Rack (at right) heads up Victory Opticians. Shown with him here are, left to right, son Robert Rack, wife Bernadette Rack and daughter Debbie Rack.

WAKEFIELD OPTICAL COMPANY, INC. (1939)

This company dates back to June 24, 1939 when Arch Wakefield and his wife Alicia Seawright Wakefield opened a lab in Gastonia, N.C. Wakefield learned his trade as a branch manager with American Optical. The new company gradually grew to 5 offices in North Carolina: Gastonia, Charlotte, High Point, Winston Salem and Hickory. Mr. Wakefield died in 1948 and the branches were eventually closed or sold to their resident managers. Paul Owensby bought Gastonia but later closed it. High Point was purchased by D.K. Miller and had a name change to Miller Optical *(since closed)*.

Mrs. Wakefield, Charles Lookabill, Sr. and Earl Miller remained with the Charlotte location. Lookabill left the company in 1959 to open his own company in Charlotte, Lookabill Optical, still in existence today. Earl Miller took over as President and served until his retirement in 1982. Earl's young sister-in-law, Glenda Heavner, came to work for Wakefield in 1961. Two years following Miller's retirement, she took over as president in 1984. She recently found journal entries in the company's 1945 books showing monthly dues paid to the O.W.N.A. of $24.75. Glenda also has a Diploma from the OWA's 1974 San Francisco convention carrying the somewhat sexist inscription "Know All Men By These Presents" and testifies to her completion of the OWA "College of Optical Knowledge" course.

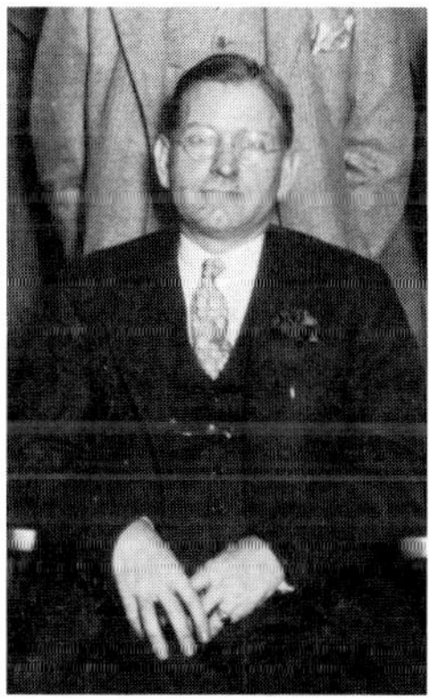

Arch Wakefield attended a Zone 3 American Optical sales meeting in Atlanta on March 11th, 1930 where this photo was taken. Nine years later he started his own company in Gastonia, N.C.

To illustrate how simple the frame business was in the '40s, a Wakefield inventory for that period lists 1,465 pairs of one style, Arcway fronts *(a metal/zyl combination style),* valued at $2.05 each. Today, few labs would carry this many units in one frame, but Arcway was a highly popular frame style that was probably used on 1 out of every 4 jobs. Wakefield also carried 765 rimway fronts *(a 4 screw rimless mounting).* Styles changed slowly in those days and wholesalers like Wakefield weren't afraid to carry in-depth frame inventories on their bestselling frames.

Mrs. Wakefield remained active until the late 70's when she retired, passing away in 1988. John Wakefield, a grandson of the founder joined the company in 1968 and presently serves as secretary of the corporation. The company operates two locations, Charlotte and a branch operation in Spartanburg, S.C., opened in 1984.

WINCHESTER OPTICAL (1902)

John A. Perkins began working in 1894 for a small frame manufacturing company in Winsted, Conn. owned by Franklin Clark *(Winsted Optical).* The spectacles they sold were considered "focus" spectacles, only made with spheres, mounted in frames of solid gold, solid silver or nickel silver since gold-filled metal had not been developed. Clark died in 1898, leaving a tangled estate. Four of the employees bought the machinery and stock, taking the name Winchester Optical Company, from the town of Winchester in which the village of Winsted was located. At this point, fate intervened.

A local Baptist minister named Gates accepted a call from a church in Horseheads, N.Y. He told the Horseheads Board of Trade he knew of a small optical manufacturing concern that was looking for a new location and additional capital. A new factory was built in the village of Horseheads and on January 1, 1902, the Winchester Optical Company machinery was moved into the new facility. The company incorporated with John Perkins as president. The company had six employees and an annual payroll of $5,000. Their only products were frames and rimless mountings which they sold to wholesalers who were, for the most part, optical departments of wholesale jewelry houses.

The company purchased finished lenses to put in their frames. These were mostly spheres, as cylinders were just starting to appear. In August of 1907, a young man named Roy Martin joined the company. The first of many frame improvements came along about that time. Prior to then, most spectacle temples had a small metal ball finishing off the end of the temple. Someone came up with the idea of a "pear tipped" temple. Producing it meant hammering the end of the temple until it assumed a paddle-like pear shape. It was a revolutionary

development and Winchester immediately added it to their frame line. Operators with tufts of cotton in their ears worked all day in a tremendous din, hammering away at temple tips.

From this point on, the story of Winchester Optical parallels the evolution of laboratories and is particularly interesting for that reason. Opticians and about-to-be optometrists were learning how to refract and prescribe cylinders. Orders for factory-made eyeglasses fell off. Retailers were beginning to order custom-made glasses that couldn't be mass-produced in a factory. This is the way the need for laboratories began. That same year *(1907),* Winchester recognized this change and set up their prescription department. In 1906, Winchester had opened a branch in Elmira under the name Elmira Optical to wholesale the eyewear they produced. The company then transferred that wholesale business to Horseheads, combining it with their manufacturing business. Initially, the lab consisted of two men edging lenses. Surfacing was not considered a laboratory function. All lenses were flat and the only bifocals they produced were cement segs.

In 1912, Edward Clark of Dunkirk, N.Y. developed an automatic rimless edger. Excited because he felt his edger made it possible for every optometrist, optician or oculist to edge lenses in their office, he brought the plans to Winchester Optical. With the help of Winchester's toolmaking machinists, they developed what they called the Monarch line of optical machines. A partnership was arranged between the inventor and Winchester. Two years later, Winchester Optical purchased the patents, continuing to manufacture and market the Monarch line.

In the meantime, the lab business was increasing and additional men were added to the Rx department. Frames, however, were getting more complicated as new styles such as fingerpiece mountings became popular. Producing these new styles required considerable expansion of the frame manufacturing facility. By the start of World War I, the company came to the conclusion their future was in optical machinery and wholesale prescription work and frame manufacturing was discontinued. In 1924, a branch was opened in Williamsport and another in Elmira in 1928. Looking westward, the company established a branch in Olean in 1930.

Tom Lynch had come to work at Winchester when he was 14 years old. His mother was trying to support the family by baking bread so young Lynch needed a part-time job. The only opening was as delivery boy, using a company motorcycle to deliver glasses. Asked if he had a driver's license, Lynch, who was not licensed, assured them he did and got the job. He worked all through school, later attending the University of Illinois.

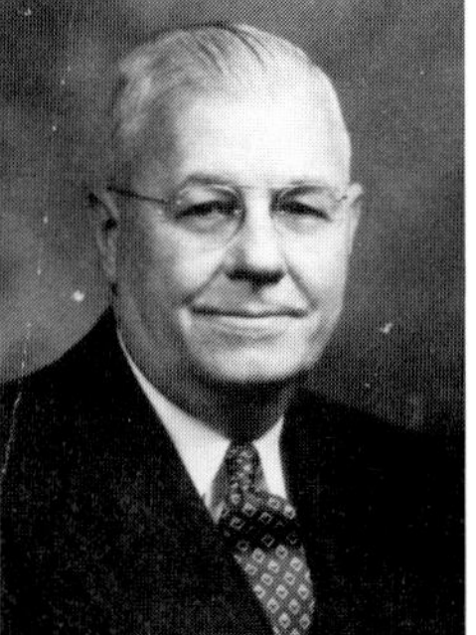

Roy Martin was unusual in association affairs in that he is the only person to ever serve 5 terms as president, with four of them consecutive (1932-35).

Graduating from college, he discovered there were no jobs and the young college graduate ended up back at Winchester working in the stock room. By 1939, however, Perkins put Lynch on the road as a salesman. When the war started, all business travel came to a halt and Lynch was brought back inside. Lab prices were frozen by the OPA during the war and, between that and limited lens allotments, the war almost wiped out the company.

By this time, Tom Lynch was running the company as general manager, with Roy Martin as president. John Perkins died in 1947, leaving his stock to his widow, who died in 1955. While Roy Martin was company president, he owned no stock in the company. Following Mrs. Perkins death, a Perkins son-in-law took over but was immediately contacted by Tom Lynch who made a fair offer for the company, announcing that if it wasn't accepted he was leaving to set up his own company. The offer was accepted and the company sold to Lynch, who then made it possible for Martin to buy in as a partner. Winchester continued as before with Lynch basically running the company. The company moved to Elmira when they built their present headquarters building in 1961. Roy Martin died in August, 1967 and was succeeded as president of Winchester by Tom Lynch.

Winchester Branches

Kirstein Optical had been founded in 1864 in Rochester. The company had a wholesale operation in addition to manufacturing. When Shuron was acquired by Standard Optical in 1925, the wholesale lab division was spun off and sold to some ex-Kirstein employees. That laboratory was acquired by Winchester Optical in 1965 and is presently operated as Winchester/Rochester.

Tom's son Ben Lynch joined the company in 1963. Ben had been a nuclear physicist, coming out of Cornell and graduating from CalTech with a master's degree in Nuclear Physics. He spent his summers working for

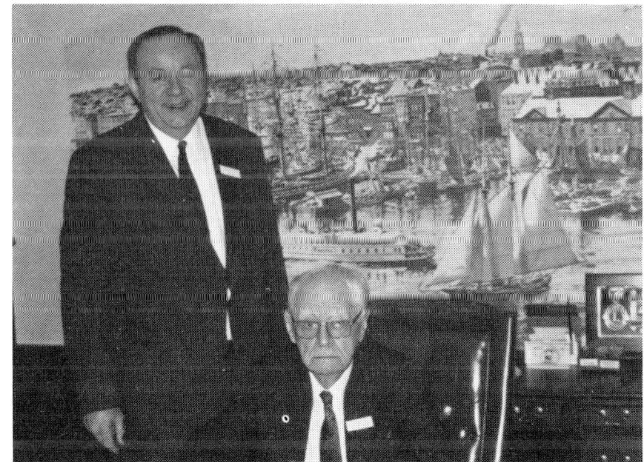

Ben Lynch currently heads Winchester Optical but his father Tom is still active and can be found most days in the lab he ran for so many years.

Winchester as he grew up and, the more he learned about the nuclear world, the better the optical business looked. He spent his first year with Winchester in Geneva where the company was putting up a new building. He's been in Elmira ever since, primarily in company administration.

Association Involvement

Winchester has produced its share of leaders for the laboratory association. Roy Martin served four consecutive terms as president of AAWO (1932,33,34,35) and one term when the group was known as OWNA (1950). In 1965, Thomas P. Lynch became president of the then OWA and Ben Lynch served as president in 1974. Art Waite, the company's sales manager, presently sits on the OLA Board of Directors. Ben was president of the OWA during the period when the association conducted a management study to determine what the association should be doing for the members and the industry. This study led to a number of major bylaw changes as well as the name change to Optical Laboratories Association. This period of association history is described in Chapter Six.

A third Lynch generation presently works for the company. Ben's sons Brian and Mike are both industrial engineers by training. Son-in-law Ken Bassler has a chemical engineering background. Mike and Brian both work in production, Mike supervising Elmira's finishing department and Brian supervising Elmira's surfacing. Bassler primarily focuses on the instruments and contact lens departments. All three are closely involved with the lab and office computer system. The company presently has four branches in addition to the Elmira headquarters - Geneva, Rochester, Greensburg, Pa. and Williamsport, Pa. The Geneva branch has an interesting history. This was the original Geneva Optical, referred to elsewhere in this history. Shortly before Roy Martin died, Geneva Optical went out of business. The Lynches believed this was an opportunity for Winchester but Martin preferred not to expand. To solve the dispute, the Lynch family formed a separate company in Geneva and operated it as Finger Lakes Optical. Following Martin's death, Finger Lakes was absorbed into Winchester Optical.

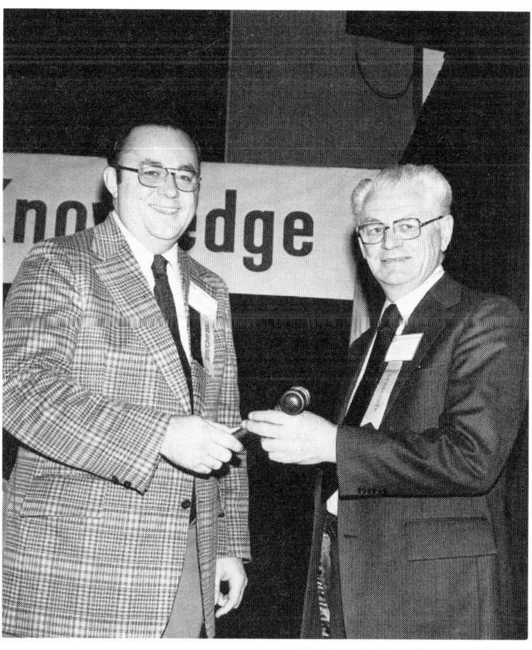

The Lynch family is another in the OLA's history of father/son presidents. Ben Lynch is seen here receiving his OWA presidential gavel from his father in 1974. Thomas Lynch had served as OWA president in 1965.

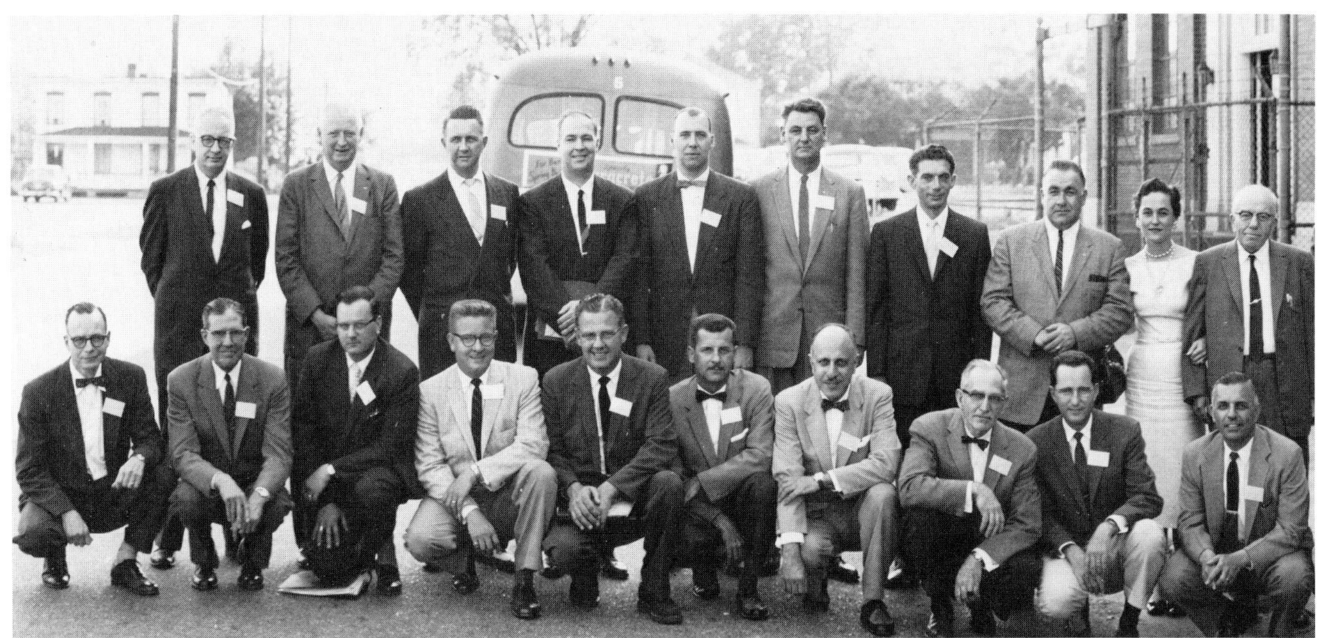

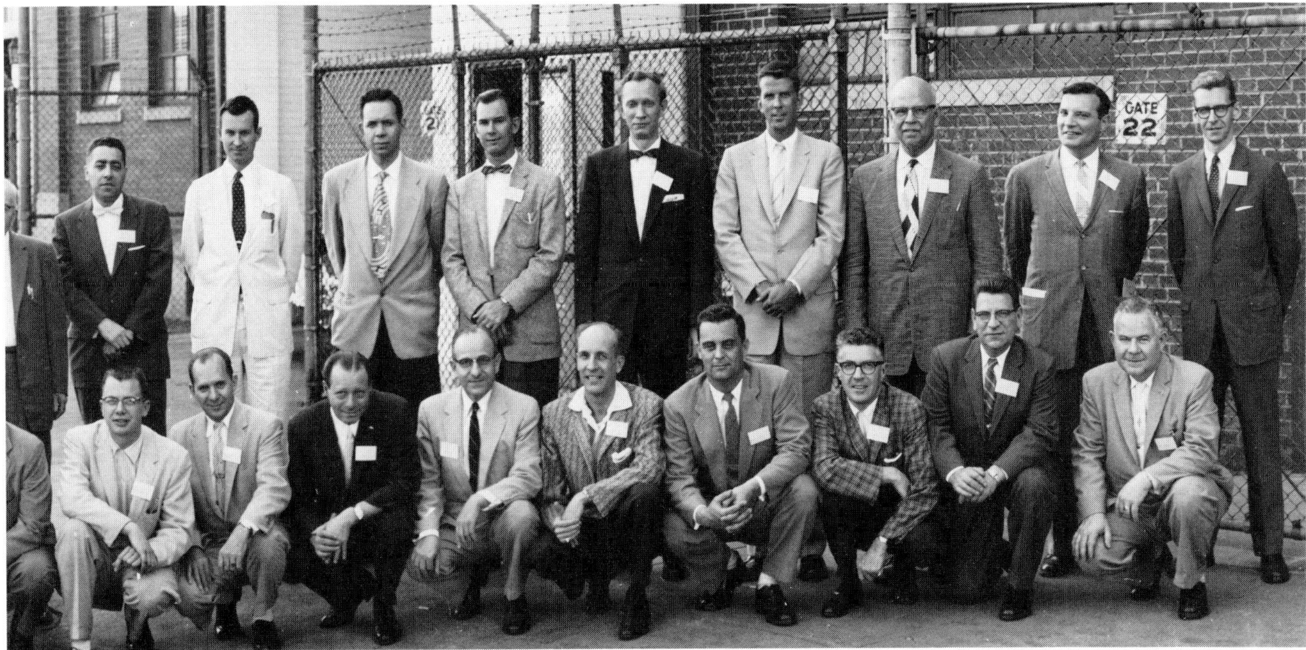

PHOTO – WAKEFIELD OPTICAL

For three days in late May of 1958, Titmus Optical conducted an Occupational Vision Seminar in Petersburg, Virginia. Attending were a number of prominent laboratory representatives who are seen in this photograph (split in two halves to fit the page). Companies represented in this group photo included Titmus, City Optical, C.A. Reilly Company, New City Optical, Littlepage Optical, Mancine Optical, Southern Optical, Geo. Smith Company, Supreme Optical, Blue Ridge Optical, Sperry Company, Northampton Optical, Wakefield Optical, Supreme Optical, Universal Laboratories, Gregory Optical, Alvin Optical, Cleveland Optical, Fairfield Optical, Rooney Optical, Liberty Optical and South Jersey Optical.

<u>Top photo</u>*: third from the right is Titmus popular sales manager Pete Collier with Titmus founder E.H. Titmus at the right end. Between them is Nita Littlepage. Kneeling, 4th and 5th from the left are Wakefield Optical's Earl Miller and D.K. Miller. Fourth from the right is a well-known Optometrist, Dr. Richard Feinberg with Hudson Titmus at the right end.*

<u>Bottom photo</u>*: Standing at the left end is OLA member Clifford Mancine (M&S Optics). Kneeling, at the left end is Martin Suchocki (Parmount Optical) and third from the left is a well-known St. Louis wholesaler at that time, Al Segelbohm (Alvin Optical). To his right is Southern Optical founder Harry Sloan. Third from the right end is Rooney Optical's Paul Dougher.*

Chapter 19
Chronology of U.S. Optical Industry

424BC Aristophanes writes of "burning glasses".

350BC Aristotle mentions eye defects of myopia and presbyopia but suggests no cures.

250BC Ptolemy, Egyptian astronomer draws up tables of refraction and reflection.

60 AD Pliny, Roman historian tells of Nero's use of concave emerald.

80 Plutarch, Roman writer mentions myopia as ocular defect.

450 Actius, Greek physician states myopia is incurable.

1025 Alhazen, Arabian astronomer writes famous scientific treatise on optics, first ever written.

1252 Earliest painting of historical figure wearing glasses.

1266 Roger Bacon describes means of obtaining enlarged objects and correcting weak eyes or those of aged people.

Giordano di Rivalto writes in 1305 that spectacles were invented in 1285.

A manuscript from St. Catherine's Monastery of Pisa says "Brother Alexander della Spina, made spectacles which had previously been made by no one".

1313 Portrait of Pope Leo X by Raphael shows him holding a reading glass.

1450 Nicolaus of Cusa describes concave lenses as being known at that time.

1456 Gutenberg invents movable type, a milestone for the optical industry.

1611 Kepler, famous astronomer, introduces meniscus lenses and publishes first rules for finding focal lengths of lenses.

1618 Sirturus of Milan advocates grading of lenses according to their radii of curvature instead of by age of persons fitted.

1629 Worshipful Company of Spectacle Makers incorporated in England.

1690 "Oxford" type spring glasses introduced at Regensburg. Chinese are using shell-framed glasses with temples.

1727 Benjamin Franklin's store, connected with his printing shop, sold spectacles.

U.S. Post Office established in this same store this year.

1737 First mention of spectacles in America in Pennsylvania Gazette.

1758 Dollond, English optician invents achromatic lens.

1783 John McAllister, Sr. establishes whip and cane business in Philadelphia.

1784 This is believed to be the year Franklin created his bifocals.

1785 Franklin describes his bifocals in letter to Philadelphia optician George Whately.

1799 McAllister adds spectacles to his whip and cane business.

1801 Thomas Young discovers the use of cylinder lenses.

1804 Wollaston issued English patent on meniscus lenses, the first wide angle ophthalmic lenses.

1806 Thomas Jefferson purchases glasses from McAllister

1810 McAllister opens factory to make whips and canes at Mt. Airy and later makes spectacles in this new plant.

Sir David Brewster suggests trifocals.

1811 John McAllister, Jr. enters father's business and firm becomes John McAllister & Son.

1816 McAllister & Son begin to make hand-made gold and silver spectacles

1817 North establishes ophthalmic infirmary in New London, Conn.

1820 New York Eye & Ear Infirmary opens.

1823 George Frick publishes "A Treatise on the Diseases of the Eye".

1827 Airy, the astronomer applies cylindrical lenses to correct astigmatism.

1828 McAllister, Jr. fits first concave cylindrical lens to correct astigmatism.

Henry Clay purchases glasses from McAllister.

1833 Wm. Beecher starts to manufacture spectacles in Southbridge, a town of 1600 persons, the start of American Optical.

1836 Isaac Schnaitmann of Philadelphia invents solid up-curve bifocal.

1838 Charles A. Spencer constructs first achromatic lenses made in U.S.

1840 First steel spectacles made in Southbridge by Beecher firm *(later American Optical Company)*.

1841 President Andrew Jackson orders glasses from McAllister.

1846 Carl Zeiss opens retail optical shop in Germany.

1847 Charles Spencer makes first American microscope and founds firm of Chas. A. Spencer and Sons.

1848 John J. Bausch takes first optical job in Swiss optical shop.

1849 John Jacob Bausch and Henry Lomb, separately, come to America.

1850 The first clinical course in ophthalmology is given at Harvard Medical School.

1851 Von Helmholtz discovers ophthalmoscope and establishes the beginnings of Ophthalmology.

Pierre Gougelman makes 1st artificial eyes in America and establishes his own business.

Bay State Glass opens *(ultimately becoming Corning)*.

1853 Bausch opens optical shop in Rochester.

Queen & Company established in Philadelphia by James W. Queen.

1854 Henry Lomb turns savings over to Bausch.

1855 Lomb becomes active partner with Bausch.

Fritz & Hawley starts in New Haven, Conn.

1858 Spencer Optical Company established in Mt. Kisco, New York.

1860 Albert S. Aloe establishes A.S. Aloe Company retail opticians in St. Louis.

Charles Vickers builds 2 lens grinding machines for Wm. White of New York City.

Donders devises case of trial lenses containing cylinders.

Zentmayer grinds spherocylinder lenses.

1861 Civil war begins.

Henry Lomb goes to war and sends his army pay back to keep Bausch's company going.

Bausch begins manufacture of hard rubber spectacle frames.

Snellen starts experiments with test letters.

1862 Dyer prints test card, in Philadelphia using Snellen principles a few months before Snellen does it abroad.

Bay State Optical starts up.

R. H. Cole & Company formed.

1864 George Washington Wells enters employ of R.H. Cole & Company.

B&L moves into first factory at Andrews and Water streets.

E. Kirstein establishes optical business in Rochester, NY *(later to become Shuron)*.

American Ophthalmological Society founded.

Dr. Donders publishes his famous "Accommodation and Refraction of the Eye" book.

1866 B&L, a retailer, begins manufacturing rubber frames and changes name to Vulcanite Optical Instrument Company.

B&L opens New York office.

Samuel Gregg perfects a cement bifocal.

Nagel advocates the metric system for designating lens powers to replace the old inch system. The term "diopter" proposed by France's Monoyer.

Kirstein Optical opens.

1868 American Hard Rubber & Cement Company agree to allow B&L to be sole manufacturers of hard rubber spectacle frames and other optical instruments.

First rimless eyeglasses manufactured in U.S.

Wm. Y. McAllister receives order from Dr. Dyer which is the first Rx for spectacles in the U.S. taken from a doctor.

Julius King, jeweler of Warren, Ohio, acquires agency for "The Perfection Spectacles" manufactured by Lazarus & Morris.

Celluloid Company is formed.

1869 Cole and Wells form the American Optical Company from their former companies.

A.L. Smith starts to make metal frames in Geneva, NY and starts what becomes Geneva Optical, a forerunner of Standard Optical.

1870 Gile and Thomas Willson issued patent on process of modifying color and transmission qualities of optical glass by adding certain chemicals to glass mixture creating "Arundel Tinted" lenses.

T.A. Willson & Company is founded *(eventually becoming Willson Products, Inc.)*.

Julius King sells jewelry business, keeps optical division and establishes Julius King Optical Company.

B&L starts power lens grinding on small scale.

1871 Cuignet invents retinoscope.

1872 AO constructs new factory.

James W. Queen establishes his own business in Philadelphia.

Bausch renames company "Bausch & Lomb"

1873 T.A. Willson starts lens grinding plant in Reading, PA.

A.L. Smith's optical business in Geneva, NY becomes Geneva Optical Company.

Retinoscope introduced.

1874 B&L makes first microscope.

Edward Bausch joins the company.

AO produces first rimless goods.

1875 William Bausch joins B&L.

Julius King moves business from Warren to Cleveland.

1876 George, John M. and Aaron C. Johnston start optical business in Detroit.

Willson company receives award for exhibit at Philadelphia Exposition. Company also receives silver medal from Franklin Institute for contribution to science of eye protection through their use of specially compounded glass.

Spencer Optical introduces Celluloid frames.

1877 Henry Bausch joins B&L at age 18.

Josef Rodenstock founds Rodenstock company.

1878 B&L enters the general lens market, manufacturing spherical lenses.

1879 American Ophthalmological Society adopts Javal's notation in prescribing cylindrical and prismatic glasses.

First patent issued for frame made from Celluloid.

1880 B&L manufactures first telescope lens.

Wm. Wilson founds American Lens Company of Katonah, NY.

Southbridge Optical opens.

1881 John L. Borsch Company established in Philadelphia.

First Trial Case introduced.

1883 Martin-Copeland Company established in Providence from a gold jewelry manufacturing firm.

B&L begins manufacturing camera lenses for Kodak.

1884 American Optical begins manufacture of its own spectacle lenses.

F.A. Hardy established wholesale optical business in Chicago.

Almer Coe opens retail optical business in Chicago.

Reed McIntire enters industry with Queen and Company.

Cement bifocal perfected by August Morck.

1885 Anton Wagner of Philadelphia patents toric lens.

Bay State introduces first gold-filled frames.

Eye Echo, the first optical magazine is published by J.M. Johnston.

Julius King opens New York office.

THE JOURNAL is published by Frederick Boger for jewelers and opticians.

1886 Perfection bifocal invented by August Morck.

Prentice announces prism dioptry measurements.

Natchet of Paris devises metric system of lens notation.

Julius King graduates from Western Reserve Medical College in Cleveland, source of his title.

Charles Prentice writes book "Ophthalmic Lenses" and builds astigmatic eye model.

The first department store optical shop opens in Wanamakers, Philadelphia.

1887 Ottumwa Optical Company established by Dave Chambers and Charles Inskeep, later to become Chambers-Inskeep & Company.

Wall & Ochs established in Philadelphia.

Eye Echo re-christened Eye-Light.

Adolf Mueller successfully blows first contact lenses.

1888 Morck patents the cement bifocal.

Julius King gives practical course "Instructions on Refraction", and becomes first teacher of optics.

First glass contact to correct vision is produced.

1889 Ottumwa Optical, now in Chicago, changes name to Chambers-Inskeep & Company.

Perfection bifocal patented.

B&L starts large scale production of spectacle lenses and discontinues importing lenses.

1890 John Hardin enters employ of F.A. Hardy.

C.L. Merry persuades Julius King to open Kansas City branch.

Snellen Reform Eye introduced by Germans.

D.V. Brown Company established.

Geneva Optical of Chicago opens.

1891 Channing and Albert Wells start work with American Optical.

Frederick Boger changes THE JOURNAL to THE OPTICIAN *(now Review of Optometry)*, the first optometric journal in the U.S.

B&L installs electric lighting.

George Washington Wells becomes president of AO.

King Optical opens branch in Mexico City.

1892 Geneva Lens Measure, invented by Brayton, is patented.

Globe Optical established in Boston.

Merry Optical opens in Kansas City as branch of Julius King.

George Johnston buys out brothers John M. and Aaron C. and continues to operate in Detroit as Johnston Optical Co.

Keystone View Company established in Meadville, PA.

Philadelphia Optical College started by Dr. Brown.

South Bend College of Optics started by Mr. Thomson.

1893 A.I. Agnew, representing Geneva Optical has a booth at Columbian Exposition.

AO commences manufacture of cylinder and compound lenses and adapts the dioptric system of designating lens powers.

American Optical brings out standardized case of trial lenses.

Geneva Optical separates wholesale and manufacturing. Manufacturing becomes Standard Optical.

Preliminary meeting for forming a wholesalers association is held in Niagara Falls.

Muller, artificial eye maker, comes to America from Germany.

1894 American Association of Wholesale Opticians organized in NYC.

McIntire, Magee and Brown opens in Philadelphia.

Limeburner opens in Philadelphia.

Bay State Optical patents method of making seamless gold plate wire.

Klein School of Optics founded in Boston.

Merry purchases Kansas City branch from Julius King.

Northern Ill. College of Ophthalmology and Otology founded by Drs. J.B. and George McFatrick.

1895 A.I. Agnew opens Columbian Optical in Denver from profits made at Columbian Exposition in Chicago.

Spencer Lens incorporated.

Merry Optical purchases Julius King Kansas City branch.

1896 B&L manufactures first meniscus lenses.

B&L starts manufacturing optical machinery.

Julius King and Rodney Pierce establish Rodney Pierce Optical.

American Academy of Ophthalmology & Otolaryngology formed.

Columbian Optical opens branch in Omaha.

1897 B&L manufactures first toric lenses.

Julius King opens Chicago office.

Will Uhlemann starts work in shop of Julius King in Chicago.

Columbian Optical opens branch in Kansas City.

1898 The first American Optical Association convention is held.

1899 Early cemented Kryptok produced by John L. Borsch, Sr. in Philadelphia.

Borsch issued two patents on Kryptok bifocal.

STOCO introduces Standard Lens Drill, first Rx machine sold to optical trade.

1900 AO begins manufacture of toric lenses.

Dr. Haux Mail Order Spectacle Company started.

1901 STOCO releases Toric Lens Grinder for grinding cylinders.

1902 B&L introduces 6 day/54 hour work week.

Winchester Optical founded by John Perkins.

Connor patents the onepiece (*Ultex*) bifocal.

1903 F.A. Hardy purchases Chambers-Inskeep & Company.

Wall & Ochs incorporated.

S.W. Robinson Optical (*forerunner of Robinson-Houchin*) established in Columbus, Ohio.

Fred Stevens starts Stevens & Company.

1904 Borsch, Jr. applies for patent on new Kryptok design and separate patent for making them.

F.B. Saegmuller joins B&L.

Pollak & Michaels opens in New York City.

Percy Hermant opens branch office in Toronto for Imperial Optical.

1905 Opifex bifocal patented by Albert Bowers.

Jules Cottet invents fingerpiece mounting. Rights are sold to Julius King who turns them over to AO for manufacturing.

Harold Stead joins Merry Optical in Kansas City.

B&L acquires Saegmuller Company, an instrument manufacturer.

Benjamin Mayer patents Bi-Sight bifocal.

1906 R. Mohr & Sons opens in San Francisco.

Merry Optical purchases Eckley Optical of Memphis.

Needles Institute starts in Chicago.

1907 Elwood Riggs opens under name of Omaha Optical in Omaha.

Paul Johnston opens lab in Davenport, Iowa.

Kryptok Sales Company organized.

Harold Stead applies for patent for "Kryptok-type bifocal". Leaves Merry Optical and starts own firm to make this bifocal.

Standard Optical of Geneva starts making lenses.

Morris Singer starts selling first Soft-Lite lenses in his retail optical establishment in New York City.

Uhlemann Optical opens in Chicago.

Roy Martin employed by Winchester Optical.

The OPTICAL REVIEW starts publication.

Sioux Optical Co. founded.

McIntire, Magee & Brown incorporated.

Progressive power concept patented by Owen Aves.

1908 Morris Singer takes out trademark on Soft-Lite Lenses.

Word "Balopticon" chosen as B&L trademark for projection equipment.

Moritz von Rohr in Germany begins experiments on Punktal lens.

Name "Shur-on" adapted for eyeglass mountings.

F.A. Hardy becomes interested in American Rubber and turns management of F.A. Hardy over to John Hardin.

Julius King begins producing safety goggles, develops King's Saniglas.

Kryptok begins selling blanks to designated wholesalers.

Borsch patents issued for Kryptok lens.

Optical Wholesalers Association of New York organized.

Titmus Optical opens in Petersburg, Virginia.

Meyrowitz copyrights name Kryptok in Canada and England.

Henry Lomb dies.

1909 Muller firm of Wiesbaden produces a blown type of contact lens with scleral portion opaque and corneal portion also blown.

Stead is sued by Kryptok for patent infringement.

J.F. Ramel enters optical business.

Geo. S. Johnston opens in Chicago.

1910 F.A. Hardy retires and John Hardin becomes President of F.A. Hardy.

Queen and Company go out of business.

Onepiece Bifocal Company incorporated to acquire C.W. Connor patents.

AO and B&L granted manufacturing licenses by Kryptok.

United Optical Company established in Webster, MA.

Electric soldering developed by Standard Optical of Geneva.

THE WEEKLY started in March by L. Topaz

OPTICAL JOURNAL and OPTICAL REVIEW consolidate and are renamed OPTICAL JOURNAL & REVIEW OF OPTOMETRY.

B&L introduces 6 day/53 hour work week.

Harold Stead develops Steadfast bifocal.

1911 Seymour experiments on bifocal similar to Kryptok called Unito.

Universal Optical Corporation is started in Providence, RI by E. Beatty, Jos. Rosenblatt & Frank Silva, a local OD and his dispensers.

Meyrowitz moves Kryptok Sales Company to Mt. Vernon, NY and changes name of company to General Optical Co.

O.H. Gerry Optical opens in Kansas City.

1912 George Washington Wells dies.

Wm. R. Uhlemann incorporates as Uhlemann Optical in Chicago

Omaha Optical changes name to Riggs Optical.

First Blue Book of Optometry issued.

Clinton Optical established.

Charlie Wilson starts United States Lens Company.

Elmer Faust starts Lehigh Optical lab in Allentown, Penn.

1913 Sir Wm. Crookes produces glass with green color for infra-red cut-out and a glass for ordinary use which cuts out ultra-violet called Crookes lens.

Punktal lens introduced in U.S.

Merry Optical buys Crown Optical in Des Moines, Iowa.

1914 World War I begins.

Kryptok litigation with Stead ends with finding against Stead.

Kryptok Sales Company incorporates.

1915 Charles Cozzens joins AO.

First practical optical glass produced by Bausch & Lomb in new glass plant.

First Red Book of Ophthalmology appears.

Gate City Optical opens in Kansas City.

Harold Stead is employed by Standard Optical of Geneva to promote sales of Kryptok.

Guild of Prescription Opticians founded in Philadelphia.

Walman Optical opens.

Brent Optical opens in Altoona, Penn.

1916 First commercial production of optical glass in this country started by B&L.

AAWO and wholesalers of country indicted and charged with monopoly and conspiracy to fix prices.

Elwood Riggs purchases wholesale department of Woodward-Clark in Portland, Spokane Optical and Standard Optical in Spokane and E. Lalonde in Helena, Montana.

Shuron introduces 66A rimless edger.

Geo. W. Spratt Optical opens in L.A.

B&L establishes 5-1/2 day/49-1/2 hour work week.

1917 U.S. enters World War I.

US Government approves B&L-made optical glass.

Morgan Optical opens in Salina, Kansas. Name changed to Quinton-Duffens Optical when Quinton and Duffens take over in 1919.

General Optical moves to Mt. Vernon, NY.

1918 General Optical buys Tilton Optical and Toledo One-Piece.

Amer. Association of Wholesale Opticians hold first annual meeting in New York with manufacturers attending.

B&L establishes 5-1/2 day/48 hour work week.

American Optical Association changes name to American Optometric Association.

1919 1916 monopoly suit concluded with AAWO and other defendants enjoined from former practices.

Professional Press incorporated and changes "OPTOMETRIST AND OPTICIAN" to "OPTOMETRIC WEEKLY"

Riggs, Portland buys Northwest Optical in Seattle and Globe Optical in Tacoma.

Shuron introduces first bevel edger.

Duffens Optical founded as Quinton Duffens.

AO patents Tillyer corrected curve lenses.

1920 Bay State produces first Princeton frame.

Zeiss produces contact lens made of chemically resistant glass that is ground and polished.

Ultex trifocal announced by Onepiece Optical.

J.I. Morris Company established in Southbridge by J. Irwin Morris.

F.A. Hardy and Julius King sign agreement whereby Hardy sells NY office to King and agrees to stay out of NYC. King sells his branches in Chicago and Davenport to Hardy and agrees to stay out of those areas.

E. Kirstein becomes Kirstein Optical Co. and buys Rochester Spectacle Co. as manufacturing division of company.

Kirstein Optical changes name to Shur-on Optical.

Grodstein and associates open Triangle Optical in Pittsburgh.

Barnett & Ramel opens in Kansas City.

George S. Johnston Optical, Chicago buys Federal Optical in Davenport.

Eyesight Conservation Council formed.

Optical Development Society formed.

1921 Kurova corrected curve single vision lenses announced by Onepiece Lens.

Riggs Optical buys National Optical in Salt Lake City.

Ohio Optical in Columbus merges with George S. Johnston of Chicago.

AO acquires F.A. Hardy, the first in their lab network.

Nokrome seg color-free bifocal announced.

1922 Monaxial Bifocal designed by Tillyer introduced by AO

First issue of Archives of Optometry appears.

Eye, Ear, Nose & Throat Monthly appears.

Morris and Nat Singer start Optical Service Corporation to distribute Soft-Lite lenses.

Riggs Optical buys first Quinton-Duffens branch in Salina and Pittsburg Kansas.

Riggs Optical opens buys Co-operative Optical in San Francisco (*wholesale department of W.R. Johnston Co.*).

Rodney Pierce becomes AO division.

B&L acquires White Haines Optical labs.

Merry Optical acquired by American Optical.

B&L acquires Stevens & Company frame company.

Advance Optical starts in Baltimore.

McLeod Optical opens in Providence, R.I.

Beitler McKee Opens in Pittsburgh.

Wilhelm Loh opens toolmaking shop in Wetzlar, Germany.

1923 American Optical sets up national distribution organization.

B&L produces first pocket microscope.

B&L buys Stevens & Company, a frame manufacturer and adds frames and cases to B&L line.

AO buys out Geo. S. Johnston Optical of Chicago.

AO buys Globe Optical and Federal Optical

Through exchange of stock, AO absorbs Globe Optical, F.A. Hardy, Julius King, Merry Optical, D.V. Brown and Boston Optical to form AO distribution organization. Harden and Fred Merry become Trustees and Vice Presidents of AO.

Dave Ettinger *(OPC)* designs and introduces Silhouette, the beginning of style and color combinations in the zylonite field.

Riggs buys Northern Optical Company

Zyloware Corporation opens

1924 Onepiece Bifocal announces improved Ultex trifocal.

Riggs Optical buys Irving-Beard of St. Paul.

President Collidge signs last state optometric law *(District of Columbia)*.

U.S. Lens Company is absorbed by Standard Optical

B&L arranges to manufacture and grind Soft-Lites for Optical Service Corporation.

AO takes over Consolidated Optical Company of Canada.

Superior Optical opens in L.A.

1925 Continental Optical is formed from Onepiece Bifocal, New Jersey Optical, Simpson-Walther Lens and C.G. Aldrich Company.

AO acquires DeZeng Instrument Co.

Kryptok patent expires.

Marine Optical Manufacturing Company opens in Roslindale, MA.

Riggs Optical buys Fond du Lac Optical. Elwood Riggs consolidates western and eastern companies but maintains separate headquarters.

Riggs sells Riggs Optical to Bausch & Lomb.

Shur-on Standard is formed from a merger of Kirstein, Standard, DuPaul Young and 80% of General Optical common stock.

Louis and Abe Kosh open Kosh Ophthalmic lab.

Tommy Thompson buys Columbian Bifocal in Denver.

1926 B&L introduces Nokrome bifocal.

Geneva Optical consolidates with Riggs Optical.

Riggs buys Central Optical of Chicago.

National Guild of Prescription Opticians is organized.

OPTICAL INDEX magazine appears.

Continental introduces See-Step Bifocal, BiSight Channel Bifocal.

Univis Lens Company is formed in Dayton, Ohio.

Univis B *(bar)* bifocal, invented by Watson & Culver of London, is marketed by Univis.

John J. Bausch dies.

1927 Riggs Optical buys Davies Optical, Portland, Oregon.

Quinton-Duffens opens second branch in Topeka, Kansas.

L.L. Houchin joins Robinson Optical of Columbus, Ohio which has lens making subsidiary, Houchin & Robinson.

OPTICAL JOURNAL & REVIEW OF OPTOMETRY sold to Chilton & Company.

1928 B&L introduces Orthogon Bifocal.

Riggs buys Scott Optical of Chicago.

Stead returns to Standard, Geneva which is now Shur-on Standard.

Diederich Optical starts up in Los Angeles.

Simpson-Walther Lens buys Buffalo Lens of Buffalo.

Midwest Optical opens in Dayton, Ohio.

Rooney Optical opens in Cleveland, Ohio.

White Haines lab proposes organization to promote eyecare.

1929 Better Vision Institute *(BVI)* formed.

M.M. Stanley and Univis introduce the Univis D bifocal on license from United Kingdom Optical.

Panoptik bifocal patented by Hammon Company.

Riggs buys Fergus Falls Optical *(Minn.)* and Davis Optical in Tulsa.

Optical Service Corporation changes name to Soft-Lite Lens Company. Controlling interest remains with Singer family.

RedeRite bifocal introduced.

Southeastern Optical established as a B&L affiliate in Richmond, acquiring wholesale department of S. Galeski, Richmond, Norfolk, Roanoke, Raleigh, Winston-Salem, Greenville, Miami, the C.B. Smith Optical of Petersburg and White Haines branches at Roanoke, Atlanta, Tampa, Birmingham, Chattanooga and Knoxville and starting a new office in Augusta.

Charlie Cozzens becomes General Sales Manager of American Optical.

Better Vision Institute *(BVI)* formed under Mike Julian.

Riggs Optical acquires Geneva Optical of Chicago.

Germany's Dr. Heine originates trial and error fitting for contacts.

1930 Albert Aloe leaves A.S. Aloe Company and opens own firm in St. Louis under name of Albert Aloe, Opticians.

Fused prism-seg bifocal produced by Culver & Emerson of London is marketed by Univis Lens.

First Panoptiks are sold by Perfected Bifocal but made by Bausch & Lomb.

B&L takes over McIntire, Magee and Brown, also Bohling & Gibbs in Philadelphia.

Shuron Optical buys General Optical.

Michaels Optical is sold to B&L.

Riggs buys Mitchell-Harper, Little Rock.

1931 AO introduces Ful-vue bifocal.

B&L introduces Orthogon D bifocal.

Robinson Optical and Houchin & Robinson merge into Robinson & Houchin Optical.

Shur-on Optical becomes Shuron Optical.

New City Optical opens in Baltimore.

BVI begins sponsoring national radio and magazine stories.

1932 First Panoptik patent re-issued.

Fused trifocal issued by Univis.

B&L issues Soft-Lite Nokrome D bifocal.

Colonial Optical formed from merger of G.M. Smith Optical, Silbert Optical and Michaels, Bohling and Gibbs.

Zeiss produces improved scleral contact lens.

Continental introduces Kurova corrected curve single vision.

Wolverine Optical becomes Michigan division of White-Haines.

Peerless Optical opens in Columbus, OH.

Bradley Optical established in Los Angeles, succeeding Trojan.

Riggs Optical acquires Associated Optical of Los Angeles and all its branches.

Edwin Land announces first man-made polarizer.

Quintex bifocal released.

1933 AO celebrates 100th anniversary.

Shuron introduces Widesite A bifocal.

Homer White organizes Independent Optical Wholesalers Association.

NRA goes into effect.

B&L establishes 5 day/40 hour work week.

B&L introduces Greens refractor.

Ed Dietz opens Dietz Lab in Ft. Worth, Texas.

Mike Julian becomes BVI president.

1934 Quinton-Duffens repurchases Salinas office from Riggs Optical.

Barnett & Ramel buy Wahlgren-Carlson Optical in Omaha and Wahlgren Optical in Waterloo, IA.

Balester Optical opens in Wilkes-Barre.

Ira Webster opens Webster Lens Company.

1935 AO and B&L make Panoptik bifocal under license from Panoptik company.

AO acquires Spencer Optical which becomes the Scientific Instrument Division of AO.

Riggs Optical splits into two divisions, the Eastern based in Chicago and the Western in San Francisco.

Independent Optical Wholesalers Association consolidates with American Optical Wholesalers Association to become the Optical Wholesalers National Association.

NRA declared unconstitutional.

1936 American Optical signs contract for first polarized sun glasses.

Bausch & Lomb introduces Anti-Glare sunglasses.

Clair Lantz opens factory called Visionez.

1937 Bausch & Lomb changes Anti-Glare name to Ray-Ban.

Otto Kirscher establishes second Southwest Optical in Los Angeles.

Caldwell Optical and Wyandotte Optical established in Kansas City.

Ray-Ban sunglasses introduced to public.

1938 First Numont mounting patented by Uhlemann brothers.

Second Southern Optical Wholesalers Association established.

Reynolds Optical Department sold to AO.

B&L stock offered to public.

Ray McLain & Ed Dietz, Sr. open Dietz McLain.

1939 Continental Optical introduces Conoptex single vision torics, K Ultex and Flat Top bifocal.

Star Optical, Owl Lens Company and Olsmore Optical open in Kansas City.

Sutherlin Optical opens in Kansas City.

Association of Independent Wholesalers (AIOW) organized in Kansas City.

Michigan Wholesale Optical Distributors Association established.

California Optical wholesale sold to AO.

Famous Harlequin frame introduced.

Bauer Optical Export opens.

Arch Wakefield and wife open Wakefield Optical in Gastonia, N.C.

1940 Panoptik Trifocal patented.

95% of optical industry charged with monopoly and conspiracy to fix prices, using patented items. B&L and Zeiss charged with monopoly to split world between them on military optical goods. B&L pleads nolo contendere and is fined $40,000.

Central Optical Wholesalers Association established.

Kay Jewelers start laboratory that becomes Homer Optical.

1941 Pearl Harbor. U.S. enters war.

Government indicts leading manufacturers, their jobbers and OWNA for price fixing.

Defendants in optical trust suit to fix prices plead nolo contendere. Companies and individuals fined.

B&L and Soft-Lite indicted, charged with monopoly and conspiracy in supplying country with rose-colored glasses.

Ramel buys out Barnett. Barnett & Wright opens in Dallas.

Plastic artificial eyes announced.

Bell Optical opens in Dayton, Ohio.

1942 Heard Optical is established by Joe Heard in Long Beach, Calif.

1945 Jack Suddarth devises idea for generator sitting in a fox hole on Okinawa.

V-E day, May 8th. V-J Day, Aug. 14.

Gulf States Optical opens in New Orleans.

Harry Rack sets up Victory Opticians in Milwaukee.

Fred Soderberg opens Soderberg Optical in St. Paul, Minn.

Gerber Scientific incorporated.

1946 U.S. Justice Dept. Files suit against AO and Ophthalmologists for rebating.

1947 Celanese introduces cellulose acetate for frame material.

Shuron introduces first zyl/metal combination Browline frame.

Robert Graham starts Armorlite.

O.W. Coburn opens Wyoming Optical in Casper, Wyo.

1948 Bay State releases first molded frame *(Baylok)*.

Consent decree ends restrictive product licensing by AO and others.

Second consent decree eventually leads to B&L and AO leaving the retail business.

George Lee and Harold Thompson open Rite-Style Optical in Omaha.

Univis Lens suffers serious strike and moves plant to Puerto Rico and Florida.

Rockford Optical opens in Rockford, Illinois.

Eldon Siehl purchases Visionez.

Clair Lantz forms Lantz Lenses.

1949 Western Optical buys Wyoming Optical lab.

1950 Federal government bans use of nitrate for optical frames.

Sylvan Ray establishes Associated Optical in Dallas.

Coburn obtains rights to Fritzsche blocker.

1951 Midwest Optical Wholesalers Assn. *(MOWA)* formed in Kansas City.

Consent Decree signed eliminating all dispensing rebates.

1952 Guy Henry retires as OWNA secretary-manager, succeeded by Bill Tellefsen.

LOS develops ORMA 500 plexiglas lens in Europe.

Titmus Optical adds frames to their line.

Visionez name changed to Vision-Ease.

1953 B&L buys Soft-Lite.

Coburn Optical acquires Suddarth generator.

1954 Warner-Lambert buys American Optical.

La Lunette de Paris opens in New York City.

Optical Fair held in Chicago.

1955 Univis Lens buys Bay State Optical and enters frame business.

B&L receives Oscar for Cinemascope.

Continental Optical acquires Modern Optics.

Univis Lens and Vision-Ease briefly merge.

Irving Rips starts Younger Lens Company.

Coburn Optical introduces 501 cylinder machine.

1956 California Optical Laboratories Assn. *(COLA)* organized in San Luis Obispo bar.

LOS introduces ORMA 1000 CR-39 lens.

Coburn receives $140,000 machinery order from Dal-Tex Optical.

1957 Univis buys Bishop frame company.

1958 American Optical introduces first brand name frame called Schiaparelli.

Shuron Optical acquired by Textron.

1959 International Optical opened by Bill Benedict in Dallas.

Varilux I introduced in Europe by Essel.

1960 B&L name changed to Bausch & Lomb, Incorporated.

Scientific Optical Labs of Australia *(SOLA)* is formed.

Omnitech opens in Dudley, Mass.

1961 Fashion Eyewear Group of America *(FEGA)* formed to promote frame fashions.

Milwaukee Case filed against AO and B&L under Sherman Anti Trust Act.

1962 OWNA and AIOW join to form the Optical Wholesalers Association.

1963 Univis Lens acquires Zylite frame company.

Paramount and Northwest/ Northern labs merge.

Jack Suddarth made V.P. of Coburn.

Shuron acquires Continental Optical.

Dr. Otto Wichterle produces HEMA material for soft contact lenses.

1964 Federal law suit by Madison Optical requires AO and B&L to sell or close any lab branch not making profit, eventually leading to their closing lab branches.

1966 B&L sales exceed $100 million.

Milwaukee Case Consent Decree marks beginning of the end for AO and B&L lab systems.

B&L acquires rights to Czech soft contact lens material.

1967 Itek acquires Pennsylvania Optical

1968 Univis buys White Haines labs and sells combined company to Itek.

B&L advised by FDA that soft contacts require pre-market approval as medical device.

1969 B&L acquires Reese Optical's nine labs, giving them total of 163 branches.

LOR/Telgic joins SIL to form Silor.

Titmus Optical sold to Dal-Tex Optical.

Buckbee-Mears buys Vision-Ease.

1970 Itek buys Kelley & Hueber case company.

Itek acquires Balester Optical, TAT-Fairfield, Northwest-Northern and Merrit-Peninsula labs.

Gentex acquires Omnitech, launching them in optical products.

1971 FDA approves B&L Soft Contact Lens and releases lenses in U.S.

B&L acquires Bushnell Optical.

Essel and Silor merge to form Essilor International.

Coburn Optical enters lens business.

1972 B&L acquires two more labs, Peerless in Columbus, Ohio and Keller-Irwin, Johnston, Penn.

Omega Optical opened by Benedict.

Drop Ball testing mandated by FDA.

Varilux II lens introduced.

Silor casts first lens in US lens plant in Florida.

Titmus Optical acquired by Zeiss, West Germany.

Coburn Optical issues public stock offering.

1973 Schott Glass introduces 1.70 High-Lite glass.

1974 Marine Optical acquired by Barnes-Hind.

B&L acquires Standard Optical companies in South Africa.

B&L starts first consumer advertising of soft contact lenses.

Multi Optics Company established by Essilor.

First showing of LOH equipment in U.S.

1975 B&L discontinues manufacturing plastic lenses.

Rodenstock, USA opens in Danbury, Conn.

Sola USA opens in Sunnyvale, California.

Coburn Optical acquired by Revlon.

1976 OWA reorganizes and changes name to Optical Laboratories Assn.

Revlon buys Barnes-Hind.

B&L consolidates their U.S. labs *(from 139 to 127)*.

Signet Optical sold to Richard Ormsby and Robert Jepson.

American Optical introduces Ultravue progressive.

Sola begins producing lenses in U.S.

1977 B&L sells hard contact lens business in Mansfield to Dr. Platt.

B&L introduces Ray-Ban Ambermatic.

B&L advertises soft lenses on TV.

B&L labs reduced from 127 to 84.

1978 3M buys Armorlite.

Ted Izzi & Bob Kemp buy Marine Optical.

First OptiFair show held in N.Y. Hilton Hotel.

First OptiFair West held in Long Beach, Calif.

1979 Marine Optical ceases frame manufacturing.

B&L acquires Milton Roy toric soft lens production plant in Florida.

Otolaryngologists form their own organization.

Maurice Giss takes over as COLA Exec. Director.

Pilkington acquires Sola Optical.

1980 B&L discontinues lens manufacturing in Brazil and France.

Rodenstock acquires Felix Mendelson Company.

Omnitech name changed to Gentex.

1981 B&L announces plans to sell off worldwide ophthalmic products business.

AO releases photochromic plastic lens called Photolite.

Univis Lens purchased by Vision-Ease.

LOH establishes U.S. headquarters in Chicago.

1982 Coburn begins distributing Rodenstock R and Rodenstock lensometers.

1983 Signet buys Armorlite from 3M and merges.

B&L completes discontinuation of ophthalmic business.

B&L introduces cosmetic extended wear contacts in U.S.

B&L acquires Polymer Technology Corporation.

Boston Lens II material approved by FDA

B&L acquires Synemed.

1984 Optima established in U.S.

Sola produces first progressive lens.

1985 Bausch & Lomb Pharmaceuticals created.

1986 B&L closes glass plant.

Essilor opens lens plant in Puerto Rico.

1987 OLA launches OLA Awards of Excellence.

B&L sells microscope and diagnostic instrument businesses.

AO acquires United Kingdom Optical in the U.K

B&L introduces ReNu contact lenses.

First OLA Duty To Warn Kit released

Pilkington acquires Revlon's vision care business which includes Coburn Optical.

Sola takes over Coburn's glass lens operations.

Gerber Scientific sets up Gerber Optical division.

1988 B&L sells South Africa operations.

B&L announces Donna Karan sunglass line.

Rodenstock sets up U.S. Lens Division.

Sola international headquarters moved to California.

Multi Optics name changed to Varilux Corporation.

Gerber Optical introduces first multi-axis generator.

VICA takes over BVI.

1989 B&L sales exceed $1 billion.

Eagle Corporation buys Signet Armorlite from Jepson Corporation.

Essilor's Photocentron acquires AIT company.

1990 John Olsen, Michael Ferrara, David duFour and Don Everburg buy Marine Optical.

Bill and Donna Benedict open Benedict Optical in Dallas.

Essilor and PPG form joint venture called Transitions Optical and release Transitions lens.

1991 Rodenstock goes to direct selling of their frame line.

1992 Transitions Plus lenses introduced.

Pinnacle Group formed by OLA and frame manufacturers.

Varilux Corporation moves to Florida.

Coburn introduces IQ lens generator.

Coburn Optical sold to Jepson Corporation.

LOH moves to new facility in Milwaukee.

1993 Industree Ottiche Europee allies with Signet/Armorlite.

Vision Service Plan *(VSP)* starts importing frames *(Altair)*.

Pilkington sells Sola to AEA Investors.

1994 Benson Optical acquires Optical Radiation Corporation and the Omega Group.

Neolens acquires Sterling Optical.

Benson Optical sells retail branches to Optical Corp. of America.

Comfort progressive lens launched by Varilux.

Gerber Optical introduces thermoplastic blocking system.

THE BOOK THAT CHANGED AN INDUSTRY

Tom Lynch (Winchester Optical) was directly involved in Winchester's lab operations. He is credited with devising the "box measurement" system that has since become the industry standard. He got interested in the subject in 1950 when he noticed that using factory frame measurements for determining PD produced off-center lenses. There were no industry standards for measuring frames. Shuron's Ronsir frame is an example. One would expect a 48-20 frame to have a frame PD of 68mm. In fact, the Ronsir measured 48.6mm so the actual frame PD was 68.6mm. Spending months on the project, Lynch researched every commonly used frame and Winchester published the results in a book designed to guide anyone edging lenses on proper settings for the edger. Lynch's book was the first attempt to bring order out of chaos.

The response to his book was totally unexpected. Copies were sold all over the world and three editions were published. Shortly after the book appeared, however, the company had an upsetting experience. Roy Martin, then president of Winchester, was contacted by Shuron and threatened with a law suit for implying that Shuron's frame measurements were wrong. Shuron then made Martin an offer. If Lynch would come down to New York City to Shuron's next sales meeting and convince them their measurements were wrong, Shuron would pay his expenses and cancel the lawsuit. If he failed to convince them, he would pay his own trip expenses and Shuron would sue.

Lynch spent 10 minutes at that meeting and convinced them. They were so impressed, Jack Rohrbach, Shuron's vice president, took Lynch up to Harlem's Cotton Club for dinner and a Cab Calloway show. At that point, Shuron changed their frame markings. Shuron's decision led to other manufacturers doing the same thing and the Boxing System of frame measurements was unanimously adopted by all segments of the Ophthalmic industry on January 1, 1962 as a standard measuring system for all future frames designed in the United States.

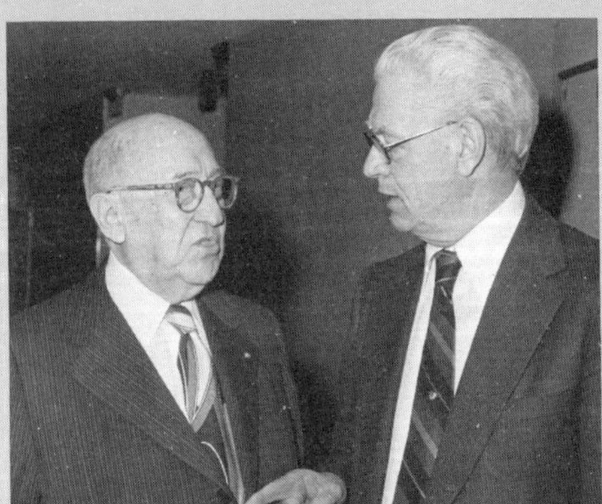

Tom Lynch, right, was president of the OWA when this photo was taken. Dr. Morris Fishbein, editor of the AMA Journal is at left.

Publication of the Lynch book produced another interesting result. George Bond had decided he wanted to start a service providing information and data on frames. He approached Tom Lynch asking if he'd like to participate but Lynch was too involved with Winchester to spare the time. As a result, Bond started the service he called FRAME-FAX without the help of Lynch. A short time later the FRAMES book published by Frames Data appeared, a positive acknowledgment that the type of information contained in Winchester's LENS & FRAME INFORMATION book was badly needed. Eventually, FRAME-FAX was absorbed by FRAMES and today FRAMES is the primary source of this information.

As an interesting sign of the times, the data appearing in FRAMES now includes 17,000 frames currently available in the U.S. More than 260 manufacturers and importers are represented. This frame data is now also available on disk for electronic use in computers. This important industry service all started that day in 1950 when Tom Lynch got tired of having lenses come out with incorrect P.D.'s.

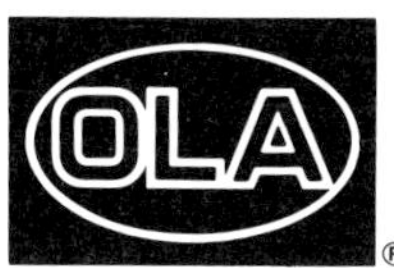

Presidents of the Optical Laboratories Association and Predecessors

These are the people who guided the organizations that merged into what has become today's Optical Laboratories Association. The original American Association of Wholesale Opticians (AAWO) was reorganized and changed its name to Optical Wholesalers National Association (OWNA) in December, 1935. Unfortunately, OWNA records are incomplete for the years 1936 to 1959 although we're told there were no meetings of the OWNA during the war years and probably no rotation of the officers.

American Association of Wholesale Opticians (AAWO)

1894	Dr. Julius King
1895	Dr. Julius King
1896	F. A. Hardy
1897	George Johnston
1898	D. V. Brown
1899	E. P. Wells
1900	F. H. Smith
1901	Walter G. King
1902	C. L. Merry
1903	A. G. Barber
1904	J. H. Hardin
1905	J. T. Brayton
1906	Leo Wormser
1907	A. Reed McIntire
1908	J. B. White
1909	Andrew V. Brown
1910	Andrew V. Brown
1911	R. C. Thompson
1912	R. C. Thompson
1913	A. Reed McIntire
1914	W. G. Wilkins
1915	Guy A. Henry
1916	Guy A. Henry
1917	Homer E. White
1918	Homer E. White
1919	Burnham W. King
1920	Burnham W. King
1921	V. R. Irvin
1922	D. D. Hubbell
1923	D. D. Hubbell
1924	Roy M. Wahlgren
1925	Roy M. Walgren
1926	S. D. Dempsey
1927	S. D. Dempsey
1928	A. Reed McIntire
1929	A. Reed McIntire
1930	Wm. B. Jones
1931	Wm. B. Jones
1932	Roy D. Martin
1933	Roy D. Martin
1934	Roy D. Martin
1935	Roy D. Martin
1936	William Dow

Optical Wholesalers National Association (OWNA)

1950-51	Roy Martin
1951-52	George P. Haas
1953-54	W.S. "Don" Gladstone
1955-56	William E. Driscoll
1957-58	George Nuthall
1958-59	Herman J. Muller
1959-60	Leon Totten
1960-61	Robert Bichel
1961-62	Richard L. Heilman

Association of Independent Optical Wholesalers (AIOW)

(Note: For a time there were two national Associations, AIOW and OWNA)

1940-43	Arthur G. Hager
1943-45	Leslie W. Myers
1945-47	Charles N. Fehr
1947-49	Norman A. MacLeod, Sr.
1949-50	J. Earl Lewis
1950-51	Phillip Dempsey
1951-52	Robert F. Duffens
1952-53	Dalton W. Bradley
1953-54	August R. Schrader
1954-55	Edward A. Dietz, Sr.
1955-56	Dean Cummins
1956-57	George W. Spratt
1957-58	Fred A. Soderberg
1958-59	J.A. Martin
1959-60	Clark Holmes
1960-61	Edward E. Ross
1961-62	Robert E. Duffens
1962-63	Harold V. Jones

Optical Wholesalers Association (OWA)

(This organization resulted from a merger of the AIOW and OWNA)

1963-64	Dan E. West, Jr.
1964-65	Albert L. Anderson
1965-66	Thomas P. Lynch
1966-67	Ted R. Uhlemann
1967-68	Tom Brown
1968-69	Thomas L. Neese, Jr.
1969-70	Roy A. Duffens
1970-71	George H. Grotelueschen
1971-72	Ellis S. Katz
1972-73	Gerald J. Dougher
1973-74	Edward A. Dietz, Jr.
1974-75	Ben E. Lynch
1975-76	Robert G. Hines

Optical Laboratories Association (OLA)

(The Association was reorganized with a name change)

1976-77	Robert A. Mueller
1977-78	Keith E. West
1978-79	Edward L. Sutherlin
1979-80	Phillip K. Eichelberger
1980-81	Robert T. Honsa
1981-82	James L. Hull
1982-83	Rolf Sulzberger
1983-84	Earnest F Swart
1984-85	Robert H. Dunn
1985-86	Richard J. Welch
1986-87	James R. LaLuzerne
1987-88	J. Keith Caudill
1988-89	Gary E. Duffens
1989-90	Bill A. West
1990-91	O.R. "Bud" Bargman
1991-92	J. Davis Lea
1992-93	Aloys E. Willenbring
1993-94	Thomas R. Styers, III
1994-95	Jack P. Dougherty

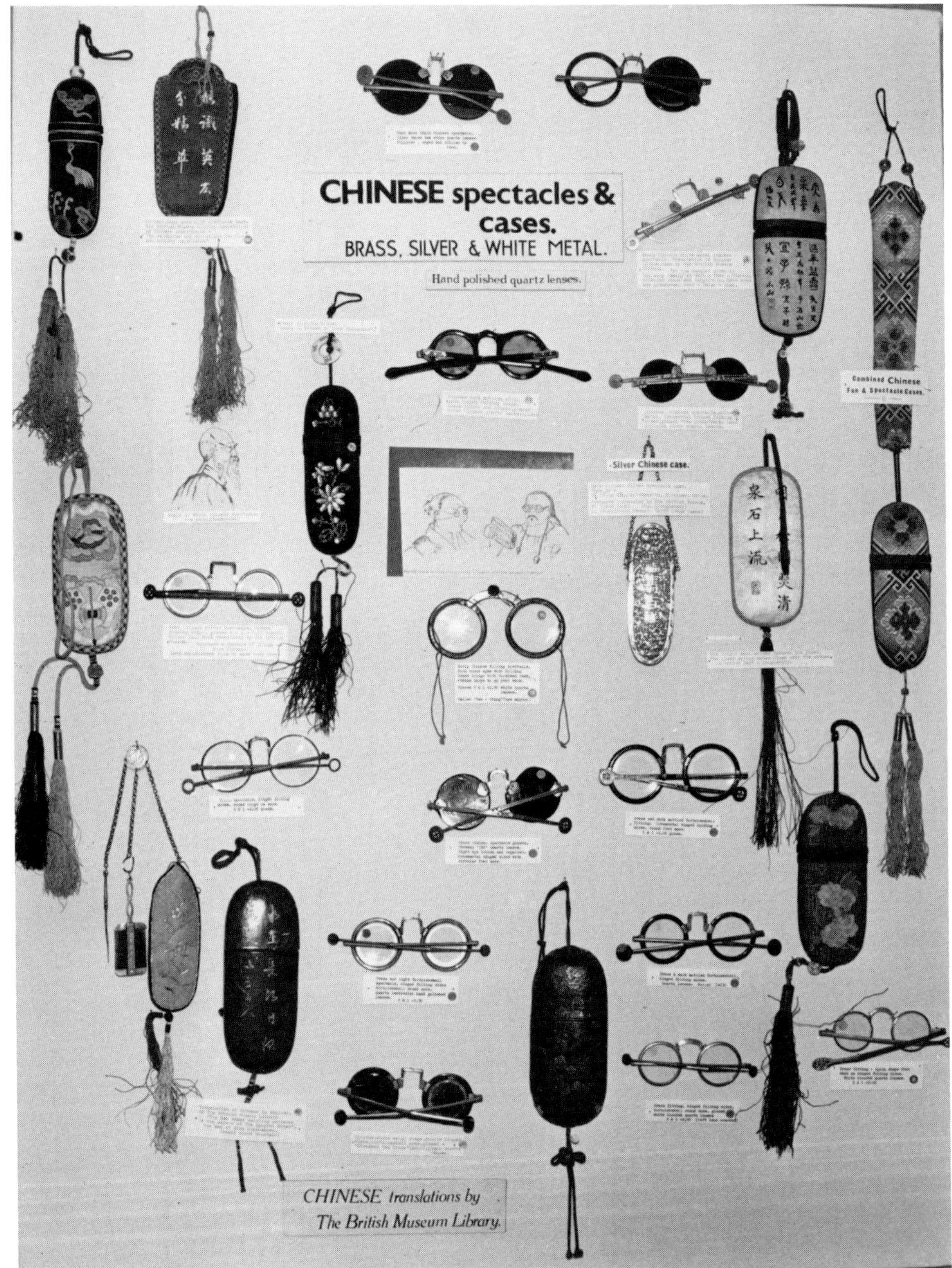

This remarkable assortment of Chinese spectacles and cases was collected by the British College of Optometrists and the photograph was made available by their Honorary Curator Hugh Orr. It was customary for dignitaries in China to often wear spectacles with no correction, sometimes with a tint, in a belief that the lenses had medicinal properties and lent the wearer an air of authority. The lenses in the pair at the top center are made of clear smoke "tea stone" quartz. The fourth spectacle down (rimless) in the center also has clear lenses made of streaky "Ink" quartz.

ILLUSTRATION - THE BRITISH COLLEGE OF OPTOMETRISTS

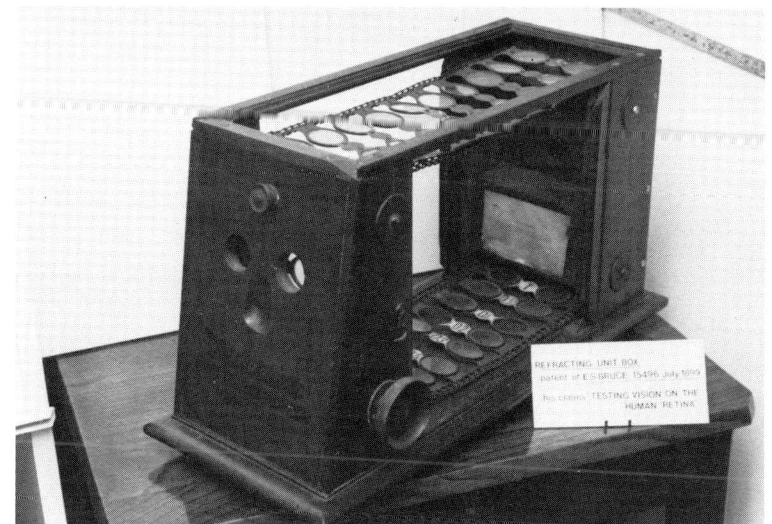

This fascinating "Refracting Unit Box" was one British optician's idea for a "self-refracting" machine, enabling the customer to determine their correction. It's an early mechanical version of today's "auto-refractors".

ILLUSTRATION – THE BRITISH COLLEGE OF OPTOMETRISTS

This early Chinese spectacle had wooden rims. While they don't show up in the photo, the rims have fine holes drilled through for the silk cords which held them in position on the nose. The brass bridge has a clever hook and eye fastener with a hinge which allows the glasses to be folded when not in use.

ILLUSTRATION – THE BRITISH COLLEGE OF OPTOMETRISTS

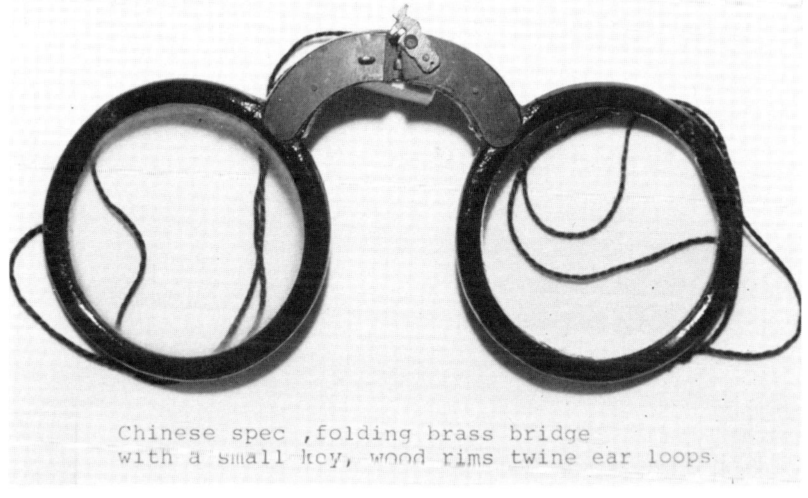

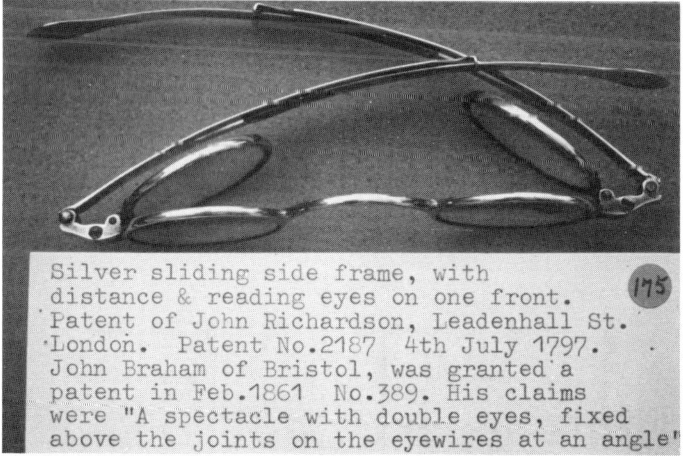

There was more than one way to approach the problem of providing near and distance vision. The design for this clever pair was patented in 1797. For reading, the wearer merely flipped the side lenses into position.

ILLUSTRATION – THE BRITISH COLLEGE OF OPTOMETRISTS

MISCELLANY

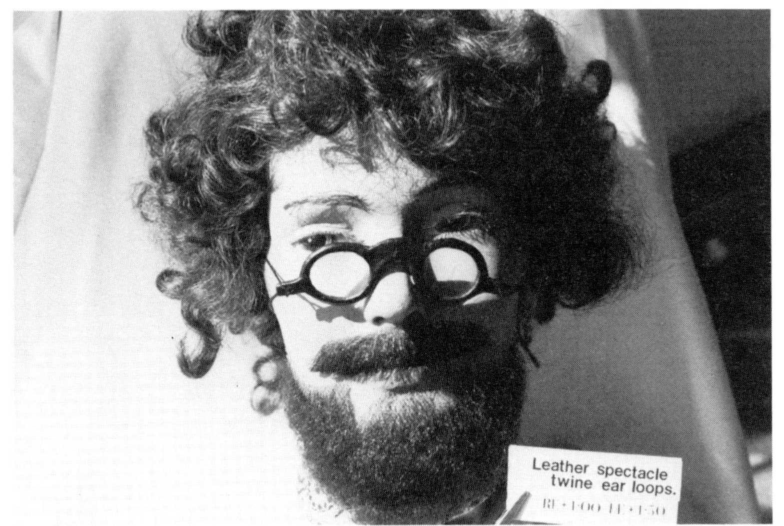

Displaying this ancient leather spectacle with cords on a model head provides a better idea of how such primitive spectacles appeared in use. It's unlikely they were worn for anything other than reading or close work. This pair has a +4.00 lens on the right and a +4.50 on the left, somewhat unusual since the majority of eyewear during that period had the same correction in each eye. These glasses are 300 years old.

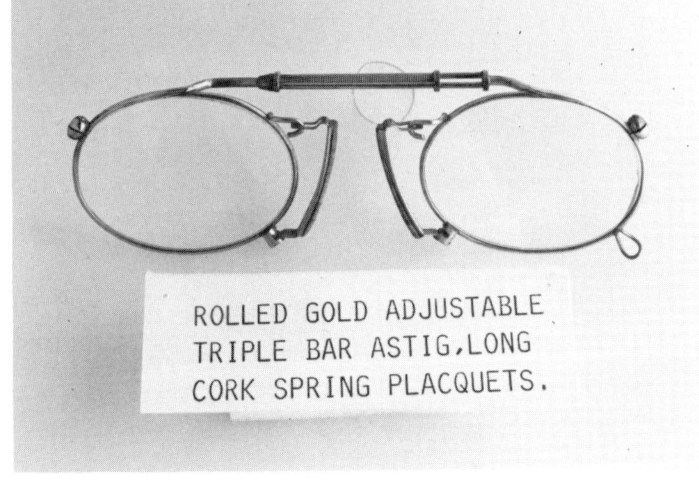

When cylinder lenses made it possible to correct astigmatism towards the end of the 19th century, it became obvious that traditional pince-nez frames would not keep the lenses and their cylinder axis properly aligned. This incredibly detailed pince-nez features a horizontal spring that grips the nose while precisely maintaining the lenses in position.

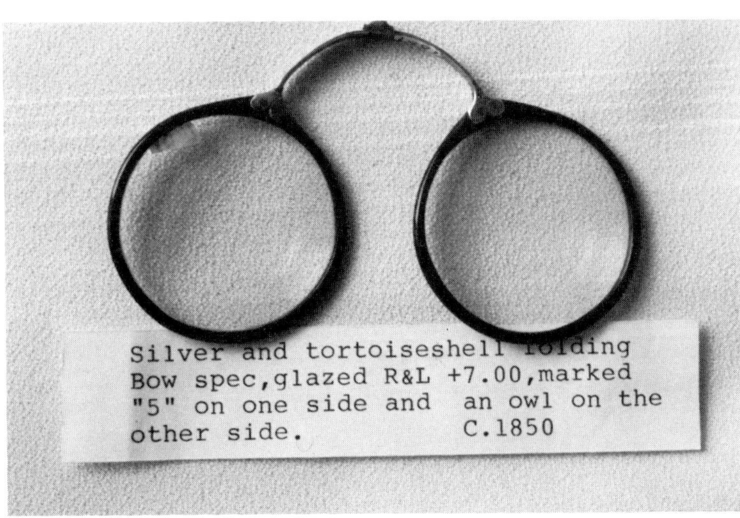

One can imagine the difficulty of holding glasses like these in position on the nose. Better opticians would identify their work and the optician who made this frame rather cleverly chose the owl as his "mark".

Index

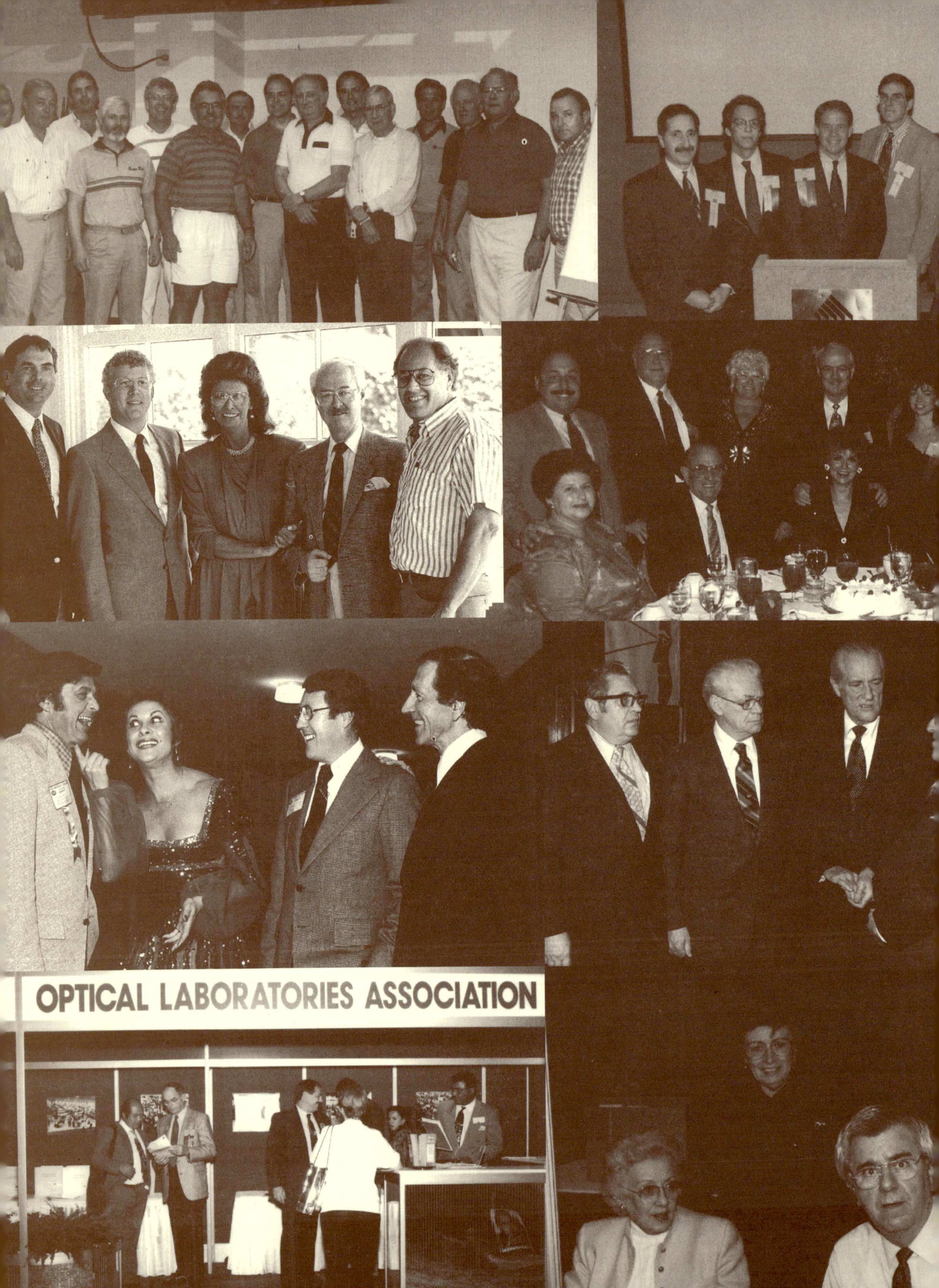
OPTICAL LABORATORIES ASSOCIATION